Endovascular and Open Vascular Reconstruction

Distilling a wide range of open vascular and endovascular reconstructive techniques into clear steps, this textbook provides insight and advice for vascular surgeons of all levels.

Written by experts from the world-leading Henry Ford Vascular and Endovascular Surgery team, each chapter includes a discussion of the indications for and planning of each procedure, detailed technical steps, and multiple-choice questions to improve comprehension of the subject matter. Unique "Tricks and Traps" boxes highlight important tips for successful procedures and common pitfalls to avoid. Whether studying for an exam or as a quick review of procedural steps prior to heading to the operating room, the stepwise approach and clear illustrations help readers perform vascular operations with a clear understanding of anatomical exposure, dissection, and angiographic imaging.

Vascular surgery trainees, junior and senior surgeons alike, will benefit from this practical advice when performing a wide range of vascular reconstructions. The collective expertise of the authors is invaluable to anyone looking to advance their understanding of the field.

Endovascular and Open Vascular Reconstruction

A Henry Ford Surgical Guide

Second Edition

Edited by
Alexander D. Shepard, Sachinder S. Hans,
Mitchell R. Weaver, and Timothy J. Nypaver

CRC Press
Taylor & Francis Group
Boca Raton London New York

CRC Press is an imprint of the
Taylor & Francis Group, an **informa** business

Second edition published 2025
by CRC Press
2385 NW Executive Center Drive, Suite 320, Boca Raton FL 33431

and by CRC Press
4 Park Square, Milton Park, Abingdon, Oxon, OX14 4RN

CRC Press is an imprint of Taylor & Francis Group, LLC

ISBN: 9781032589107 (hbk)
ISBN: 9781032433776 (pbk)
ISBN: 9781003452096 (ebk)

DOI: 10.1201/9781003452096

Typeset in Minion
by Deanta Global Publishing Services, Chennai, India

Dedication

This book is dedicated to the memory of Drs. Roger F. Smith and Joseph P. Elliott, who helped train some of us, inspired many of us with their hard work and dedication to Henry Ford, and together with Dr. Szilagyi, created the legacy of Henry Ford Vascular Surgery that forms the foundation of this text.

Contents

Editor biographies

Alexander D. Shepard is a Senior Staff Surgeon and past Division Head of Vascular Surgery at Henry Ford Hospital, Detroit, MI, where he holds the Betty Jane and Alfred J. Fisher Chair in Vascular Surgery. He is also a Professor of Surgery at the Wayne State University School of Medicine, Detroit, MI.

Sachinder S. Hans is the Medical Director Vascular and Endovascular Services, Henry Ford Macomb Hospital, Clinton Township, MI, and Clinical Assistant Professor of Surgery at the Wayne State University School of Medicine, Detroit, MI.

Mitchell R. Weaver is a Senior Staff Surgeon and the Clinical Director of the Noninvasive Vascular Laboratory in the Division of Vascular and Endovascular Surgery at Henry Ford Hospital, Detroit, MI. He is also a Clinical Assistant Professor of Surgery at the Wayne State University School of Medicine, Detroit, MI.

Timothy J. Nypaver is the Head of the Division of Vascular and Endovascular Surgery at Henry Ford Hospital, Detroit, MI, and the Director of the Vascular Surgery Service Line in the Heart and Vascular Institute of Henry Ford Health. He holds the Eve and D. Emerick Szilagyi Chair in Vascular Surgery and is an Assistant Professor of Surgery at the Wayne State University School of Medicine, Detroit, MI.

List of contributors

Ziad Al Adas, MD
Vanderbilt University Medical Center
Nashville, TN

Marwan Bahmad, MD
American University of Beirut
Beirut, Lebanon

Hisham Bassiouny, MD
Dar Al Fouad Hospital
Giza, Egypt

Tamer N. Boules, MD
Henry Ford West Bloomfield Hospital
West Bloomfield, MI

Joshua K. Burk, MD
Case Western Reserve University School of Medicine
University Hospitals
Cleveland, OH

Philip S. Chacko, DO
Henry Ford Macomb Hospital
Clinton Township, MI

Hassan Chamseddine, MD
Henry Ford Hospital
Detroit, MI

Jae S. Cho, MD
Case Western Reserve University School of Medicine
University Hospitals
Cleveland, OH

Daniel G. Clair, MD
Vanderbilt University Medical Center
Nashville, TN

Mark F. Conrad, MD, MMSc
St. Elizabeth's Medical Center
Boston University School of Medicine
Boston, MA

John L. Crawford, MD
Texas Health Vascular Surgical Specialists
Fort Worth, TX

Kaitlyn D. Dobesh, MD, JD
Henry Ford Hospital
Detroit, MI

Amr el Shafei, MbBch
Mansoura University
Mansoura, Egypt

Samia D. Ellias, MBBS
St. Elizabeth's Medical Center
Boston University School of Medicine
Boston, MA

Alison O. Flentje, MD
University of Maryland Medical Center
Baltimore, MD

Evan F. Guay, DO, PhD
McLaren Health
Grand Blanc, MI

Jacob W. Guerrant, DO
Henry Ford Jackson Hospital
Jackson, MI

Saurabh Gupta, MD
University of Maryland Medical Center
Baltimore, MD

Ali H. Hakim, MD
University of Nebraska Medical Center
Omaha, NE

Sachinder S. Hans, MD
Henry Ford Macomb Hospital
Clinton Township, MI

Mounir J. Haurani, MD, MPH
East Carolina Heart Institute at East Carolina University
Greenville, NC

Jamal Jawad Hoballah, MD, MBA
American University of Beirut
Beirut, Lebanon

Grant B. Hubbard, MD
Case Western Reserve University School of Medicine
University Hospitals
Cleveland, OH

Javaneh Jabbari, MD
University of Maryland Medical Center
Baltimore, MD

Miles Jackson, MD
Henry Ford Jackson Hospital
Jackson, MI

Layne G. Janda, MD
Vanderbilt University Medical Center
Nashville, TN

Loay S. Kabbani, MD, MHSA
Henry Ford Hospital
Detroit, MI

Stavros K. Kakkos, MD, MSc, PhD
University Hospital of Patras
Patras, Greece

Wasih Kamran, MD
Henry Ford Hospital
Detroit, MI

Joe Karam, MD, MBA
Minneapolis Heart Institute
Minneapolis, MN

Yasaman Kavousi, MD
Henry Ford Hospital
Detroit, MI

Nik Kolicaj, MD
Henry Ford Hospital
Detroit, MI

Alice Lee, DO
Henry Ford Hospital
Detroit, MI

Judith C. Lin, MD, MBA
Michigan State University Health Care Heart and Vascular Center
East Lansing, MI

Alexander K. Lu, DO
Henry Ford Macomb Hospital
Clinton Township, MI

M. Ashraf Mansour, MD, MBA
Corewell Health Medical Group, Vascular and Endovascular Surgery
Grand Rapids, MI

Kyle G. Miletic, MD
Henry Ford Hospital
Detroit, MI

Farah H.A. Mohammad, MD
Kaiser Permanente Medical Group
Fremont, CA

Robert G. Molnar, MD, MS
Michigan Vascular Center
Flint, MI

Mark D. Morasch, MD
George E. Whalen Veterans Affairs Medical Center
Salt Lake City, UT

Semeret T. Munie, MD
Marshall Health
Huntington WV

Abdul Kader Natour, MD
Mayo Medicine
Rochester, MN

Jake A. Nicholson, DO
Corewell Health
Grand Rapids, MI

Timothy J. Nypaver, MD
Henry Ford Hospital
Detroit, MI

Kevin T. Onofrey, MD
Henry Ford Hospital
Detroit, MI

Seyed S. Pairawan, MD
Henry Ford Hospital
Detroit, MI

Erin Pang, DO
Henry Ford Jackson Hospital
Jackson, MI

Chrysanthi P. Papageorgopoulou, MD, MSc, PhD
University Hospital of Patras
Patras, Greece

Woosup M. Park, MD
Case Western Reserve University School of Medicine
University Hospitals
Cleveland, OH

Andi N. Peshkepija, MD
Henry Ford Hospital
Detroit, MI

Iraklis I. Pipinos, MD, PhD
University of Nebraska Medical Center
Omaha, NE

Chinmayee Potti, MBBS
Ohio State Wexner Medical Center
Columbus, OH

Daniel J. Reddy, MD
Wayne State University School of Medicine (Ret.)
Detroit, MI

Kaitlyn M. Rountree, DO
Henry Ford Macomb Hospital
Clinton Township, MI

Ali Rteil, MD
Henry Ford Hospital
Detroit, MI

Hamzah Saleem, MD
Henry Ford Hospital
Detroit, MI

Guillermo P. Serra, MD
Henry Ford Macomb Hospital
Clinton Township, MI

Alexander D. Shepard, MD
Henry Ford Hospital
Detroit, MI

Victoria E. Simmons, MD
Michigan Vascular Center
Flint, MI

Jacqueline D. Stuber, MD
Henry Ford Hospital
Detroit, MI

Brian Sullivan, MD
Henry Ford Hospital
Detroit, MI

Yuqian Tian, MD
University of Nebraska Medical Center
Omaha, NE

Shahab A. Toursavadkohi, MD
University of Maryland Medical Center
Baltimore, MD

Michael P. Trpkowski, MD
Henry Ford Macomb Hospital
Clinton Township, MI

Mitchell R. Weaver, MD
Henry Ford Hospital
Detroit, MI

Charles A. West Jr, MD
Texas Health Vascular Surgical Specialists
Fort Worth, TX

Foreword

"There are no second chances in vascular surgery."

Allan D. Callow, MD
Professor of Surgery Emeritus,
Tufts University School of Medicine,
Past President, Society for Vascular Surgery

Dr. Callow used to regularly admonish the residents and fellows on the vascular service about the importance of performing the operation right the first time. As vascular surgeons, we are well aware of the consequences of imperfections. Technical failure often leads to thrombosis or bleeding, resulting in stroke, limb loss, or a return to the operating room. It is frequently difficult if not impossible to recover from such events and the patient pays the price. As vascular surgeons, one of our primary responsibilities is to avoid complications from technical failure. The performance of the operation from positioning to exposure and suturing, to wound closure requires meticulous attention to detail and must be done *right* the first time, which is why this textbook is so valuable.

The Vascular Surgery group at Henry Ford Hospital has a wealth of clinical experience and its members are highly regarded for their operative skills and technical expertise. The national reputation of this group allows them to write this authoritative textbook of vascular operations. Chapters cover the clinical scenario, indications, and contraindications in addition to operative techniques for commonly encountered vascular conditions. Detailed descriptions include technical tips and guidance that are usually only heard in the operating room and will be beneficial to the readers (and their patients). The text is nicely accompanied by clarifying illustrations.

The Henry Ford team has produced a compendium of knowledge, experience, and technique that is valuable for established surgeons as well as trainees. Doing it right and doing it right the first time will benefit both surgeon and patient alike as "there are no second chances in vascular surgery." This book is written to ensure that the operation is done right.

Jens Eldrup-Jorgensen, MD, DFSVS, FACS
Professor of Surgery, Tufts University School of Medicine
Medical Director, Society for Vascular Surgery, Patient Safety Organization, Vascular Quality Initiative

Preface to the 2nd edition

This is the second edition of this book. It was first published in 2018 as a "how-to" guide for vascular surgeons and was intended as a quick review of procedural steps prior to heading to the operating room or endovascular suite for a case. It is primarily a techniques text, explaining the steps of a procedure in the clearest terms from true experts in the field. Although the first edition proved very popular, particularly with vascular surgery trainees and early career surgeons, we have made several changes that we feel have improved the value of the book further. First among these is a boxed section for each chapter ("Tricks and Traps") highlighting important tips for a successful procedure as well as common pitfalls to avoid. A second addition is a multiple-choice question section for each chapter. This addition was at the request of many trainee readers who found the book useful when studying for certification. They felt such "practice" questions would help prepare them more thoroughly for their board exams.

A final change was the move to nearly all Henry Ford Health contributors, hence the change of subtitle from "A Practical Approach" to "A Henry Ford Surgical Guide." The reputation and strength of Henry Ford Vascular Surgery is indisputable. From the world's fifth abdominal aortic aneurysm repair by D. Emerick Szilagyi in 1952 to the creation of the first vascular registry in the 1960s, and the writing of multiple seminal papers that helped establish the foundations of our specialty, to our current position as the go-to vascular center in the region, the Division has been a leader from its beginnings. Dr. Szilagyi passed away in 2009, and since the publication of the first edition of this book, we have lost his two original partners, Dr. Roger F. Smith and Dr. Joseph P. Elliott—all were giants in the field. Together, these three helped birth our specialty and in the process pushed the name of Henry Ford to international prominence. Today, their impact lives on in the Division they formed, the vascular surgery training program they created, the legacy of innovation and quality they nurtured, and the tens of thousands of patients helped by successive generations of their trainees. The most valued product of this Division has been and always will be the quality vascular surgeons it has attracted and trained—residents, fellows, and staff alike—and it is to this group of surgeons we turned in putting together this second edition. Fifty of the 54 chapters have Henry Ford contributors, and it is the collective expertise of this group that ensures the quality of this book.

As we approach the publication of the second edition we need to recognize the contributions of several individuals. Chief among these is Sachinder Hans, the senior-most editor, who, as acknowledged in the Preface to the first edition, was really the driving force behind the creation of this book, believing that a techniques-focused text based on Henry Ford expertise would be a valuable addition to the literature. The popularity of the first edition taught us he was correct. He also pushed for a second edition, realizing that five years between editions was a very long interval in the fast-moving world of vascular surgery. Loay Kabbani was another voice of persistent support. Perhaps tired of referring trainees to past book chapters and papers by Henry Ford surgeons, he believed this text was the perfect response to a vascular fellow's queries: "How do you do this operation? What is the Henry Ford approach to …?" We also need to thank Miranda Bromage and Hudson Grieg of Taylor & Francis. Miranda recognized the value of the first edition and requested a second, while Hudson helped us through the difficult birthing process with patient guidance and support. Finally, we need to express our profound gratitude to the many vascular surgeons who selflessly gave their time and shared their expertise to help create this modern guide for *Endovascular and Open Vascular Reconstruction.*

For the editors,
Alexander D. Shepard, MD

1

Carotid angioplasty and stenting

ROBERT G. MOLNAR AND VICTORIA E. SIMMONS

INTRODUCTION

Carotid artery revascularization has evolved through several techniques since the mid-20th century, beginning in 1954 with the introduction of open carotid surgery by performing carotid endarterectomy (CEA). Carotid stenosis was first treated in an endovascular fashion by percutaneous balloon angioplasty in 1977, followed over a decade later by the placement of a balloon-expandable stent in 1989. Balloon-expandable stents were subsequently substituted with self-expanding stents, which have become the standard stent type used in endovascular carotid intervention. While several manufacturers have US Food and Drug Administration (FDA)-approved stent systems, this chapter concentrates on the techniques required to perform the procedure safely and effectively.

Several clinical trials have assessed the safety and efficacy of carotid artery stenting (CAS). The Carotid Revascularization Endarterectomy versus Stenting Trial (CREST) [1] is arguably the landmark trial that has influenced current practice regarding CEA and CAS. CREST enrolled symptomatic and asymptomatic standard risk patients. No statistical significance between the two groups existed in the primary composite end point of stroke, myocardial infarction (MI), or death from any cause during the periprocedural period, or ipsilateral stroke within four years of randomization. However, the periprocedural stroke rate was statistically more significant in the carotid stent group, and periprocedural MI was higher in the open carotid surgery group. Another notable trial is the Second Asymptomatic Carotid Surgery Trial (ACST-2) [2], which randomized asymptomatic standard risk patients to CEA or CAS. The 30-day risk of nondisabling stroke was significantly higher in the CAS group, and the rate of MI was higher in the CEA group, although the latter was not significant. The effects of the two procedures on disabling or fatal events were approximately equal up to five years of follow-up, suggesting that the protective effects of CAS and CEA are similar for at least the first few years after intervention.

While the Carotid Revascularization and Medical Management for Asymptomatic Carotid Stenosis Trial (CREST-2) will likely provide additional useful outcomes data, the determination for carotid stent placement has until very recently been driven by the Centers for Medicare and Medicaid Services (CMS) reimbursement criteria. Previously, CAS was only covered by Medicare in patients at high risk for CEA. According to the most recent reconsideration memorandum published in 2023 [3], CMS has expanded coverage of percutaneous transluminal angioplasty concurrent with stenting and use of an embolic protection device in standard risk patients to include:

- Patients with symptomatic carotid artery stenosis ≥50%.
- Patients with asymptomatic carotid artery stenosis ≥70%.

In addition, CMS approval will no longer be required by facilities to perform CAS. The decision to pursue open revascularization with CEA or CAS via a transfemoral approach or through transcarotid artery revascularization (TCAR) remains a shared decision-making process based on the individual patient. Of note, at this time, there are no verified shared decision-making tools available.

PROCEDURE PLANNING

When considering carotid stent placement, it may be helpful to evaluate the aortic arch with computed tomography angiography, magnetic resonance angiography, or an angiogram to assess arch anatomy and determine whether carotid cannulation can be performed safely and effectively from femoral artery access. The patient may be approached with an aortic arch and carotid arteriogram with the intent to treat, recognizing that unfavorable

DOI: 10.1201/9781003452096-1

arch anatomy, excessive calcification, or hostile carotid anatomy might lead to a diagnostic, rather than therapeutic, procedure. The presence of excessive calcification, tortuosity, or a severe type II or III aortic arch should be avoided and surgical endarterectomy or a transcarotid approach performed instead.

If planning for a transcarotid approach, there are several anatomic considerations that must be kept in mind. Duplex ultrasound and computed tomography angiography or magnetic resonance angiography can help to delineate patient anatomy and the morphology of carotid artery plaque. Instructions for use for placement of the ENROUTE® TCAR system (Silk Road Medical, Inc., Sunnyvale, CA, USA) include vessel diameter 4–9 mm at the target lesion, a common carotid artery diameter ≥6 mm, and ≥5 cm length from the clavicle to the carotid bifurcation. Additional considerations include depth of the common carotid artery, tortuosity of the internal carotid artery, plaque morphology, and degree of calcification in the common and internal carotid arteries. It is important to note that a meticulous approach to any carotid intervention is mandatory because the consequences of embolization or thrombosis are much more devastating than in other vascular beds treated by endovascular methods.

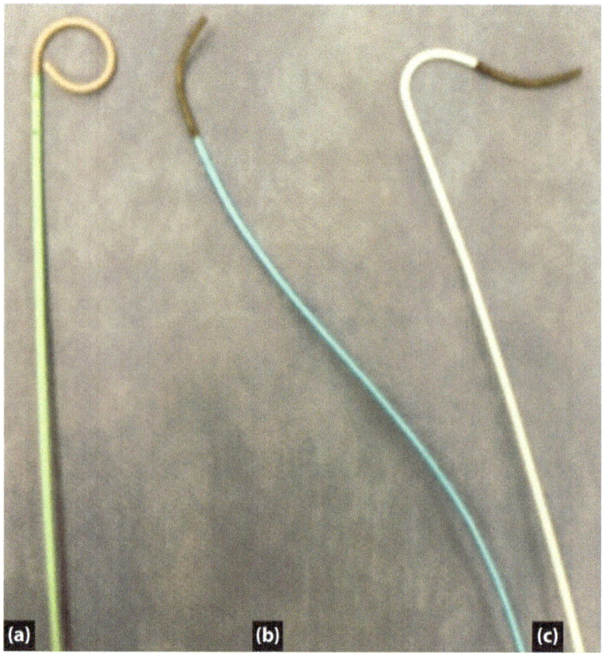

Figure 1.1 Basic diagnostic catheters: (a) Pigtail; (b) JB-1 or Berenstein; (c) Simmons 1.

PERIPROCEDURAL RECOMMENDATIONS

All patients should be counseled on expectations during the procedure and a detailed neurologic examination should be completed to document baseline neurologic status. Dual antiplatelet and lipid lowering therapy should be initiated if not contraindicated. If the procedure is to be done under sedation, the conduct of the procedure should be reviewed with the patient so they are comfortable with instructions on breathing and head positioning. It is often helpful to review the instructions that will be used during the procedure with the patient in the pre-procedure area to ensure they are familiar with what they will experience during the procedure. If the patient can anticipate these instructions and know that their breath hold will only be approximately eight seconds, image quality will be greatly enhanced.

PROCEDURES

Patients are placed in a standard supine position with arms tucked, and blood pressure (BP), electrocardiogram tracing, and pulse oximetry are monitored. Supplemental oxygen should be available and used routinely with conscious sedation. Whether planning for transfemoral or transcarotid access, both groins should be prepared to allow access to the optimal femoral vessels.

If planning for transfemoral carotid stenting, standard angiographic equipment is used, and strict attention to avoiding air embolization is critical. Once femoral access is obtained, the patient is fully anticoagulated, with goal activated clotting time (ACT) between 250 and 300 seconds. A pigtail catheter is inserted into the ascending aortic arch, and the image intensifier is rotated to visualize the aortic arch in its widest plane. Many textbooks recommend using a standard 30-degree left anterior oblique view; occasionally, the best angle may be up to 50 degrees. This becomes very important because some patients with an aortic arch that appears to be a steep type II at 30 degrees may be a type I or mild type II at a steeper angle (e.g., >30 degrees).

Once the anticoagulation level is confirmed by ACT, the contralateral carotid is cannulated with your catheter of choice (Figure 1.1). For a standard type I aortic arch and many mild type II aortic arches, a JB-1 or Berenstein catheter is usually an excellent selection. For a type II or severely angulated ascending aorta, we suggest a Simmons 1 or Vitek catheter. It is best to have a few catheters that are used routinely to develop familiarity with the "feel" for the catheter, including how it reacts with tortuosity, resistance, and operator manipulations.

The selective catheter should be advanced to the mid-common carotid artery (CCA); anterior-posterior (AP), lateral, and oblique images should be obtained, including intracerebral runs to assess for cross-filling between the cerebral hemispheres. Once the contralateral artery is assessed, the ipsilateral (treatment) side is selected. Again, baseline AP, lateral, and oblique images are obtained to quantify the degree of stenosis and vessel characteristics. Stent positioning and deployment can be assisted by visualizing bony landmarks in relation to the distal extent of the lesion or by an assistant marking the viewing monitor.

A stiff wire (e.g., Amplatz 1-cm floppy tip) is slowly advanced through the selective catheter, placing the wire tip in the distal CCA. The authors typically neither cross the bifurcation nor select the external carotid artery (ECA) to avoid traversing disease without distal protection. However, for extreme tortuosity or type II arches, selection of the ECA will help with safe sheath positioning. Maintaining fluoroscopic monitoring of the wire tip, the short femoral sheath is exchanged for a 90-cm sheath over the Amplatz wire. The sheath is slowly advanced into the CCA while monitoring the wire tip. Note that the sheath dilator may extend beyond the sheath tip by 4–6 cm. For this reason, the authors secure the dilator and slowly advance the sheath up to 2 cm proximal to a lesion in the CCA.

With the sheath in place, the wire and dilator are slowly removed, and the sheath is thoroughly debubbled. The sheath is connected to a power assisted injector, and the line is prepped and debubbled using the three-way stopcock. An additional magnified angiogram is obtained, centering the lesion on the viewing monitor to image from the proximal CCA to the distal internal carotid artery (ICA). Vessel reference measurements are made and include the diameter of the mid-to-distal ICA where filter placement would be anticipated. If the patient is not under general anesthesia, a pre-assessment neurologic check is made by having the patient squeeze a squeaky toy or follow motor commands with assessment by cath lab staff. Under fluoroscopic guidance, the distal protection device is advanced past the lesion and positioned in a straight segment of the distal ICA. Should there be significant tortuosity in the ICA, it may be safer to approach the lesion with retrograde flow protection using the Mo.Ma® Ultra (Medtronic, Minneapolis, MN, USA) device or with TCAR. With standard transfemoral approaches, after the filter is deployed, a small amount of contrast is delivered to ensure antegrade flow through the filter and to confirm lesion location. If stenosis is severe, pre-dilation should be considered to facilitate safe stent placement and stent delivery system removal. Angioplasty may cause bradycardia, and Atropine or Robinul should be readily available or given prophylactically. The CCA just proximal to the bifurcation determines the size of the stent used. Many operators select a 40-mm long stent in the majority of cases to fully cover the index lesion. The stent diameter should be a minimum of 1-mm wider than the CCA and may be a straight or tapered configuration. The stent is advanced over the wire and past the lesion, then slowly brought back to the diseased segment based on the bony landmarks or screen markings to remove any redundancy in the system and prevent the stent from "jumping" during deployment.

After the stent is deployed, another puff of contrast is administered to confirm antegrade flow and a neurologic test is performed. If the stent has a <30% residual stenosis, it is left as is. If the residual stenosis is >30%, angioplasty is performed based on the reference vessel diameter of the ICA. Two orthogonal views (including intracranial views) are obtained to ensure no additional intervention is required, the filter is recaptured, and another neurologic test is completed. The shuttle sheath is then withdrawn over a J-tipped wire and exchanged for a short sheath. There is no need to reselect the contralateral carotid artery for completion arteriogram. A closure device is used as needed.

TCAR utilizes a supraclavicular incision to gain access to the proximal CCA. Our approach is to use a Rummel tourniquet that is looped proximally on the CCA, and a purse-string suture is placed on the anterior arterial surface. The patient is anticoagulated with goal ACT between 250 and 300 seconds. The artery is accessed at the purse-string with a micro-access system, advancing the catheter only 2 cm into the CCA. An angiogram is taken, and the bifurcation is marked on the viewing screen. The TCAR sheath is placed over the 0.035" J-wire, taking care not to cross the bifurcation with the wire. The reverse flow system uses a femoral venous catheter (typically placed contralateral to the carotid artery being treated), which acts as the outflow from the sheath placed into the CCA. Between the two vascular accesses is a filter system and manifold that allows for confirming retrograde flow, as well as halting flow for arteriograms. The system initiates passive retrograde flow as soon as the conduit is connected between the sheath in the CCA and the sheath in the femoral vein.

Blood pressure should be maintained above 140 mmHg once the system is connected. Active retrograde flow is initiated by tightening the Rummel tourniquet. The 0.014" wire is advanced across the lesion. Typically, pre-dilation is performed to facilitate safe stent placement. The balloon should be sized according to the lumen at the area of disease. Diligent communication with the anesthesia team is critical, as the patient may become bradycardic or hypotensive with treatment at the carotid bulb, and Atropine, Robinul, or vasopressors may be required. The self-expanding stent is then placed, using the CCA diameter proximal to the bifurcation, to determine the size of the stent used. As with TFCAS, the stent is advanced slightly past the lesion and then slowly brought back to the target lesion. After the stent is deployed, the authors wait two minutes, allowing any debris to collect in the filter via the retrograde flow system. A completion angiogram is taken, with multiple orthogonal views. The stent may be post-dilated if there is residual stenosis >30%. The arteriotomy is closed using the previously placed purse-string suture, the neck incision is closed, and manual pressure is held on the femoral vein after the sheath is removed.

POSTPROCEDURAL CARE

Patients are admitted for 23-hour observation, which includes monitoring BP, evaluating the access site, and performing neurologic assessments. Any hypotension or hypertension should be appropriately treated and any change in the neurologic examination immediately assessed. Periprocedural strokes may occur due to late embolization through the stent struts or because of

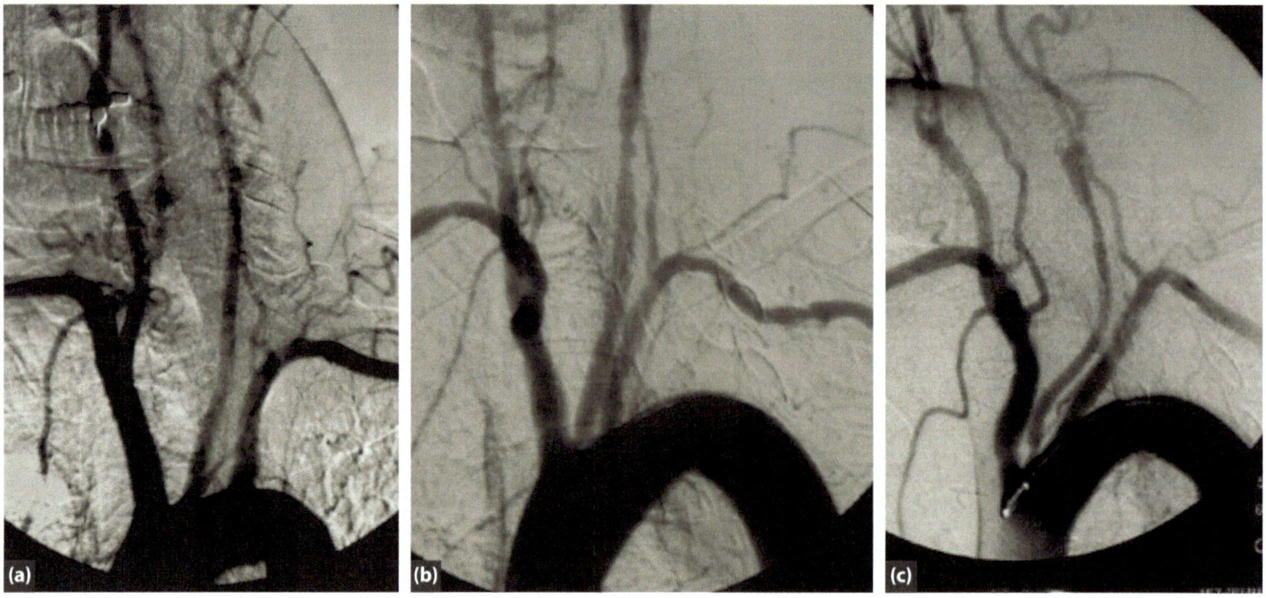

Figure 1.2 Proximal progressions of the origins of the great vessels for a (a) type I, (b) type II, (c) and type III aortic arch.

thrombus formation. Patients should be continued on dual antiplatelet medication as well as a cholesterol-lowering/stabilizing agent. Carotid duplex exams should be performed at one, six, and 18 months followed by yearly examinations to assess for restenosis.

CONTRAINDICATIONS AND PITFALLS TO AVOID

When performing transfemoral carotid artery stenting, aortic arch anatomy is an important detail that cannot be overlooked or its importance underestimated. Figure 1.2 provides angiographic depictions of three examples of aortic arch anatomy. Steep aortic arches in which the origins of the great vessels have shifted to a right/inferior orientation to the apex of the aortic arch make cannulation and safe placement of the stent delivery catheter difficult. Manipulation due to difficulty cannulating the great vessels can cause embolization from the aortic arch itself.

Concentric calcification or severe complexity of the lesion (Figure 1.3), thrombus/near-occlusion (Figure 1.4), and excessive tortuosity of the distal ICA (Figure 1.5) are all relative and, depending on severity, can be definitive contraindications to CAS.

CONCLUSIONS

CAS has been established as a safe and effective alternative to CEA. While transfemoral carotid intervention has become much less prevalent, it remains a valuable skill set for interventionalists. TCAR has rapidly gained popularity and appears to be a viable alternative to open carotid revascularization. The authors' analysis of carotid stent fractures highlights the question of stent durability long-term and points to a need to monitor longitudinal outcomes [4]. It remains important to critically assess carotid stent technology to finely focus on those characteristics that create a higher risk for patients undergoing CAS and to better define who is best suited for CAS versus CEA. While this clarity is being defined, it is of critical importance that interventionists who either perform or wish to perform carotid interventions have a meticulous approach to patient selection and procedural technique.

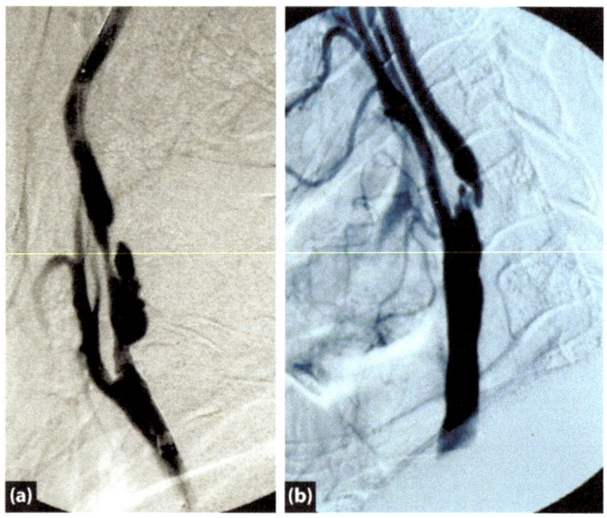

Figure 1.3 Complex lesions (a,b) prone to embolization with intervention.

TRICKS AND TRAPS

- While there are many brands and shapes available for selective catheterization of the great vessels, the proceduralist should identify a few catheters of choice

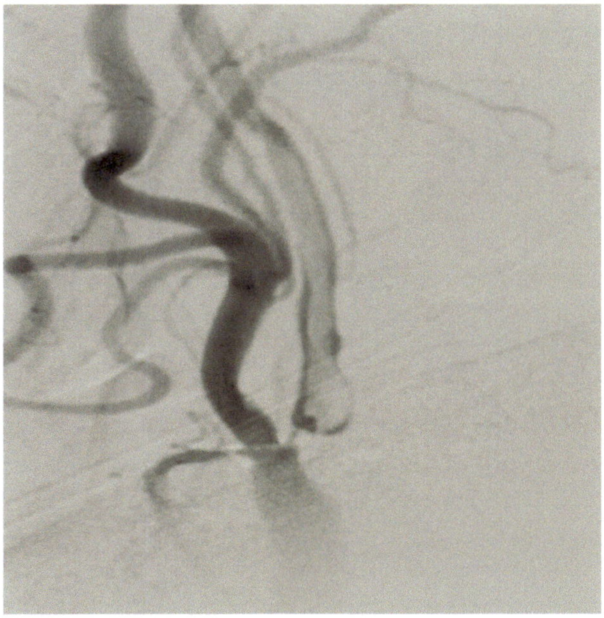

Figure 1.4 Thrombus present at severe carotid stenosis.

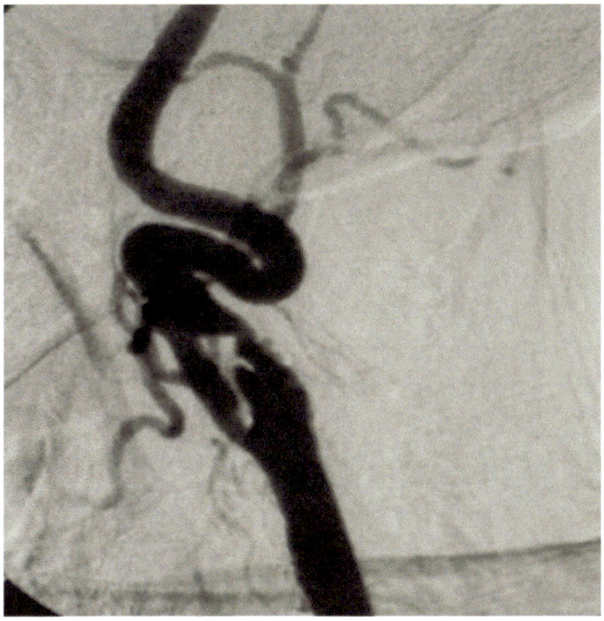

Figure 1.5 Excessive internal carotid artery tortuosity.

to allow for a reliable response during manipulation and avoid excessive "attempts" that increase the risk of embolization.

- Establishing sheath placement in the CCA is a critical component of TFCAS and carries a significant risk of embolization. It should be avoided in a type III arch and other methods of carotid revascularization should be considered in a type II arch.
- Crossing the lesion prior to systemic heparinization, or, in the case of TCAR, prior to initiation of active retrograde flow, should be avoided.
- The proceduralist must maintain communication with the anesthesia team, especially at critical portions of the case, and be prepared to treat the patient for hemodynamic changes associated with interventions at the carotid bulb.
- The decision to pursue open revascularization with CEA or CAS via a transfemoral or transcarotid approach should be individualized to the patient and results from a shared decision-making process.

QUESTIONS

1. Relevant contraindications for transfemoral carotid artery stenting include all of the following, except:
   a. Circumferential calcification
   b. A type I arch
   c. Thrombus
   d. Internal carotid artery tortuosity

   Answer: b

2. During transfemoral carotid stenting with filter protection, there is loss of antegrade flow, and the patient exhibits neurological changes. Bailout procedures include all of the following, except:
   a. Flushing the sheath
   b. Using an Export catheter
   c. Administering alteplase
   d. Aspirating the sheath

   Answer: a

3. Transcarotid artery revascularization (TCAR) might be a better approach to carotid stenting in which of the following circumstances?
   a. Disease in the common carotid artery 4 cm above the clavicle
   b. Patients with a type III aortic arch
   c. Patients with a contralateral recurrent laryngeal nerve injury
   d. Patients with bilateral common femoral venous thrombosis

   Answer: b

4. Which of the following regarding the procedure of carotid artery stenting is true?
   a. Patients should be on antiplatelet therapy, but anticoagulation is not needed
   b. TCAR should be performed with SBP <110
   c. Strokes will not occur if a distal protection filter is used
   d. A meticulous attention to detail is needed for those performing CAS

   Answer: d

REFERENCES

1. Brott TG, Hobson RW II, Howard G, et al. Stenting versus endarterectomy for treatment of carotid artery stenosis. *N Engl J Med.* 2010;363: 11–23.
2. Halliday A, Bulbulia R, Bonati LH, Chester J, Cradduck-Bamford A, Peto R, et al. Second asymptomatic carotid surgery trial. *Lancet.* 2021;398: 1065–1073.
3. Centers for Medicare & Medicaid Services. *Decision memo for Percutaneous Transluminal Angioplasty (PTA) of the carotid artery concurrent with stenting (CAG-00085R8).* Available from https://www.cms.gov/medicare-coverage-database/view/ncacal-decision-memo.aspx?proposed=N&NCAId=311 (accessed December 1, 2023).
4. Karani N, Corbitt K, Molnar R, Perla S. *RS03 – Carotid stent durability: The incidence of carotid stent fracture and the associated implications.* Paper presented at the SVS Vascular Annual Meeting, National Harbor, MD, June 14, 2023.

2

Trans-carotid artery revascularization

TIMOTHY J. NYPAVER

Trans-carotid artery revascularization (TCAR) is a hybrid method that obviates the need to manipulate both aortic arch disease and/or instrument carotid stenosis by utilizing a dynamic flow reversal system of cerebral protection. The hybrid designation, indicating both an open and endovascular procedure, is related to the need for a common carotid artery (CCA) exposure, and second, the endovascular means of placing a carotid stent. With TCAR, initial studies have demonstrated an extremely low stroke risk, between 1.0% and 1.7% and a combined stroke, death, and myocardial infarction rate of 1.3% to 3.5%. Long-term outcomes for TCAR are also favorable with outcomes similar to that of carotid endarterectomy (CEA) or trans-femoral carotid artery stenting (TF-CAS) in terms of patency and ipsilateral stroke-free survival. TCAR has the same limitations as TF-CAS in terms of severe calcific disease in which CEA may be more applicable. Thus, TCAR is a valuable procedure in the armamentarium of the treatment of appropriately selected patients with carotid artery disease.

INTRODUCTION

The management of atherosclerotic carotid artery occlusive disease has been one of the most studied of the vascular disease beds. While CEA remains a valuable tool and operation in the armory of carotid interventions, the addition of angioplasty and stenting procedures, introduced in 1977, has gained more acceptance as a technique for the management of carotid artery disease. There have been multiple studies comparing the outcomes and performance of CEA versus TF-CAS, examining both the asymptomatic and symptomatic cohorts of patients [1–4]. The major endpoint and outcome measures, inclusive of the risk of periprocedural neurologic events (transient ischemic attack [TIA] and stroke) as well as a long-term reduction in stroke risk, have consistently shown a better outcome with CEA than TF-CAS. The Carotid Revascularization Endarterectomy versus Stent Trial-2 (CREST-2) study is an ongoing longitudinal and international study attempting to define the optimal management of patients with asymptomatic carotid artery occlusive disease with patients randomized to either CEA or TF-CAS, with all patients receiving optimal medical management. As noted, earlier studies have indicated a higher risk of periprocedural stroke with TF-CAS when compared with CEA [1–5]. This higher periprocedural stroke risk may be due to the dislodgement of atherosclerotic debris due to the necessity of wire passage through the aortic arch, proximal carotid artery, and carotid bifurcation lesion before the establishment of any form of cerebral protection. No cerebral embolic protection is established until the wire has crossed the lesion and then the embolic protection device, also passed directly through the lesion, is deployed, prior to the balloon angioplasty or stent deployment. TCAR is a hybrid method that obviates the need to manipulate both aortic arch disease and/or instrument carotid stenosis by utilizing a dynamic flow reversal system of cerebral protection. The hybrid designation, indicating both an open technique and exposure combined with an endovascular procedure, is related to the need for a CCA exposure just above the clavicle, and second, the endovascular means of placing a carotid stent, with reversal of flow, and thus cerebral protection, established prior to any manipulation or instrumentation of the lesion. Thus, TCAR has the unique characteristic of establishing a highly reliable form of cerebral protection prior to wire crossing of the carotid lesion and has demonstrated results comparable to that of CEA, without the risk of cranial nerve injury. While initially restricted to high-risk patients, as defined by the Centers for Medicare and Medicaid Services (CMS), TCAR can now be utilized in the management of most patients with asymptomatic or symptomatic carotid artery stenosis, with the notable exception being those with anatomic contraindications for TCAR (see "Indications/contraindications for TCAR").

DOI: 10.1201/9781003452096-2

INDICATIONS/CONTRAINDICATIONS FOR TCAR

The indications for TCAR are essentially the same as CEA: atherosclerotic carotid artery bifurcation disease that may be either asymptomatic or symptomatic. Although approved for standard risk patients since 2022, in general, TCAR is favored over CEA in high-risk patients. Anatomic risk factors include recurrent stenosis, irradiated neck, or high plaque, while physiologic risk factors are largely cardiac in nature (e.g., advanced congestive heart failure, unstable angina, recent myocardial infarction). It is necessary to have a non-diseased CCA of adequate diameter (>6 mm) with 5 cm or greater of CCA length from the site of operative exposure to the bifurcation lesion. Thus, the relative anatomic contraindications for TCAR include the following: a previous intervention on the ipsilateral CCA, CCA disease at or near the anticipated exposure and entry site, less than 5 cm from the clavicle to the carotid artery bifurcation, a CCA diameter less than 6 mm, and severe ICA tortuosity and/or angulation. TCARs can be attempted in patients with a shorter clavicle to bifurcation length as well as a smaller CCA diameter (less than 6 mm), dependent upon the expertise and experience of the surgeon. In patients with severe calcific plaque, especially those with circumferential calcific disease, consideration should be given to CEA rather than risk an incompletely deployed stent performed via TCAR or TF-CAS. The role of a Shockwave balloon in or during the performance of TCAR is an invitingly intuitive option but one that should be considered experimental at this point until further data is available. Another contraindication to TCAR is the inability to take dual antiplatelet therapy.

Asymptomatic carotid artery disease

The current management of asymptomatic disease would appear to be in evolution. Presently, carotid artery disease with a greater than 70% stenosis should be considered for some type of carotid intervention unless the risk of the procedure is considered excessive (>3%) or if the patient longevity or life expectancy is less than three years such that the patient will not benefit from the stroke risk reduction. Unfortunately, in the realm of clinical practice, it is often difficult to reliably determine a patient's life expectancy. The role of isolated non-operative or non-procedural best medical therapy may show promise, especially if we can better define the risk factors or plaque characteristics associated with an increased risk of embolization or stroke emergence. Regardless, patients should be placed on optimal medical management with antiplatelets and aggressive means to reduce their lipid profile risk using statins or other novel lipid-lowering agents. Asymptomatic patients who have a reasonable life expectancy and perioperative risk should be considered for TCAR as long as the anatomic criteria are met. A further caveat to the decision-making process is the understanding of hospital and/or surgeons' outcomes with TCAR, such that more reliable decisions can be made based on benefits, risks, and outcomes.

Symptomatic carotid artery disease

As established in the North American Symptomatic Carotid Endarterectomy Trial (NASCET), the benefit of intervention in symptomatic carotid disease is much more established. In patients who are candidates anatomically for TCAR in whom a CEA may be a more extensive operation or have potential drawbacks, TCAR, with the appropriate anatomic criteria, should be strongly considered as the treatment of choice.

TECHNICAL CONSIDERATIONS

TCAR procedures can be performed under general anesthesia (GA) or regional anesthesia. The author prefers GA for TCAR as GA has not been associated with a higher myocardial infarction rate. The author does utilize electroencephalogram (EEG) monitoring, although it is recognized that EEG changes are infrequent, even with clamping of the CCA and establishment of active flow reversal. The patient is intubated, the head is rotated to the opposite side, and the shoulders are elevated to allow for maximal neck extension. This is critically important as this allows the maximum amount of distance between the CCA exposure site and the bifurcation. Ultrasound is utilized prior to prepping the patient to ascertain and mark out the course of the CCA, confirming not only the CCA diameter but also the absence of any significant disease. The author favors routine prophylactic administration of glycopyrrolate (dose 0.4 mg) intravenously immediately prior to initiating the procedure after GA is established. The TCAR procedure can be divided into three critical components (shown in the following sections).

Exposure

The author prefers a transverse incision, approximately 2.5 cm in length extending just over and between the heads of the sternocleidomastoid muscle (Figure 2.1). The dissection continues between the sternocleidomastoid heads, typically within an avascular plane, down to the carotid sheath. The vein is anterolateral, and the CCA is easily identified and dissected out for about 1.5–2 cm. The author utilizes an umbilical tape on the proximal CCA to allow for consistent traction when inserting the large bore 9F sheath. The patient is then anticoagulated with an ACT greater than or equal to 250 seconds. The author prefers the use of fish-hooks with silastic tubing to facilitate exposure yet they remain unobtrusive when placing the subsequent sheath. Concomitantly, access is gained in the left common femoral vein, and the specialized sheath is placed into the common femoral vein and secured.

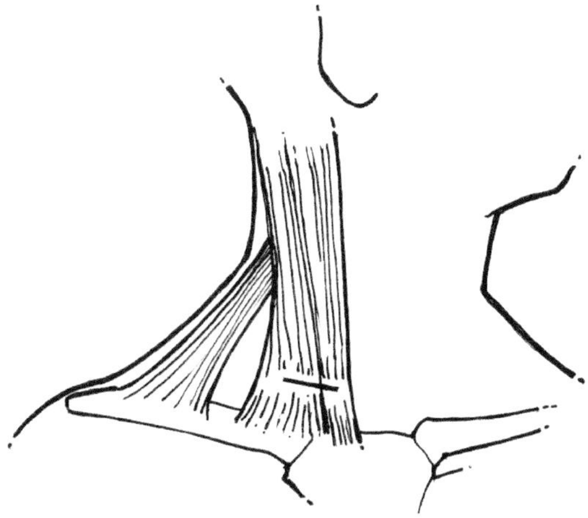

Figure 2.1 Location of the TCAR skin incision, one fingerbreadth above the clavicle, positioned between the heads of the sternocleidomastoid, approximately 2 cm in length.

Insertion of 9F specialized sheath and initiation of passive flow

Once the patient is confirmed to be normotensive, a U stitch with 5-0 proline is made on the anterior CCA at the anticipated puncture site. A microaccess kit, supplied by Silkroad Inc., is utilized, with a deliberate and careful anterior CCA puncture, bevel up with insertion of the supplied microaccess wire 3 cm beyond the CCA puncture. Without movement or change in position of the microwire, the micro sheath is then inserted approximately 3 cm into the CCA, the wire is withdrawn, and a preliminary angiogram is obtained in an orthogonal view from the bifurcation, allowing for easy identification of the location of internal carotid artery (ICA) disease, the location of the bifurcation, and the presence or absence of any proximal CCA disease. The decision is made at this point whether the next wire, the pre-supplied 0.035 stiff wire, will be inserted into and left short in the CCA, proximal to the patient's disease, or whether further efforts will be made to advance the micro sheath, over a wire, into the external carotid artery (ECA). This decision depends on the location of the disease and any CCA disease proximal to the bifurcation. If CCA disease is absent, and the disease is confined primarily to the ICA, the microaccess wire can be carefully manipulated only into the ECA, and the dilator and micro sheath are then advanced into the ECA. The stiff wire is then advanced into the ECA. With CCA bifurcation disease, the stiff wire is inserted up to 1 cm proximal to the disease. The micro sheath is then removed and the larger specialized sheath, designed by Silkroad Inc., is then inserted; this maneuver is facilitated by counter traction on the umbilical tape with the sheath inserted up to the designed cuff (Figure 2.2). The sheath is then quickly and efficiently secured to the patient's skin with two to three sutures of 3-0 silk. The dilator is

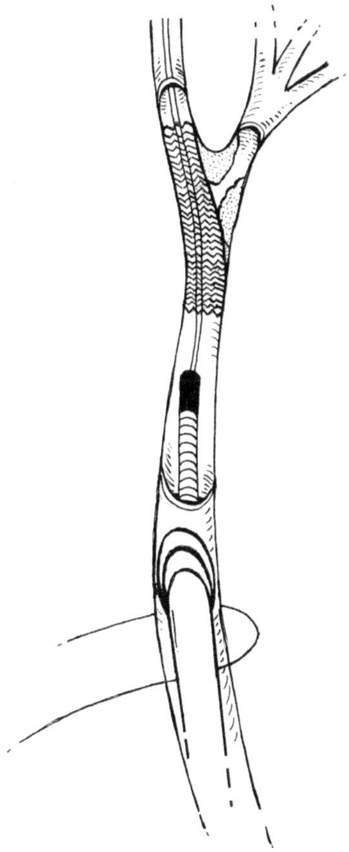

Figure 2.2 Schematic of the TCAR sheath inserted flush to the carotid artery with the sheath tip positioned proximal to the carotid disease (stent inserted).

removed, and the sheath is connected to the tubing with flow established through the filter and tubing apparatus after hooking it into the venous sheath (Figure 2.3). Passive flow in the circuit is then established, with the flow setting on high. The author confirms the appropriate location and positioning of the sheath tip by performing an angiogram in two separate orthogonal views.

Active flow and stent deployment

With the wire back-loaded on the selected balloon (typically, a 5 mm balloon is chosen but depends on the artery size), the balloon and its wire together are advanced into the sheath at the site of the CCA entry. The CCA is then clamped with an appropriate vascular clamp (the author utilizes a Gregory profunda femoral clamp) and active flow is initiated. In the appropriate view, an angiogram is performed through the sheath with the STOP button depressed during the angiogram to allow for visualization of the ICA in the neck and the intracerebral portion of the ICA. Now with active flow reversal, the wire is then advanced, crosses the lesion, and is positioned in the supraclinoid portion of the ICA. The balloon is advanced and the angioplasty is accomplished, following which the appropriately sized self-expanding nitinol stent is inserted

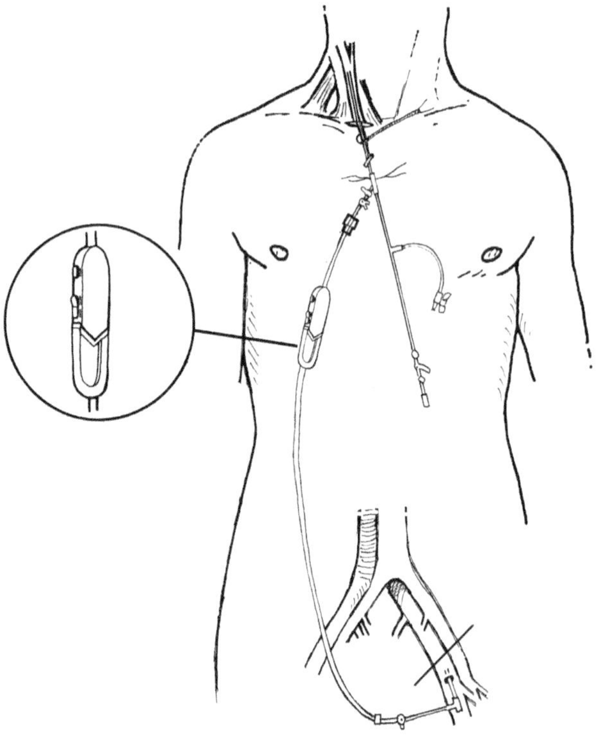

Figure 2.3 Overall TCAR setup illustrating the arterial sheath through the cervical incision, the flow reversal tubing apparatus, the flow controller (insert), and the venous sheath within the left femoral vein.

and deployed, covering all the disease, typically down into the CCA. Following stent deployment, flow reversal is allowed to run for two minutes. If the stent does not completely open, the stent can be ballooned, typically again with a 5 mm balloon. A completion angiogram is obtained in two separate views, and again it will be necessary to hit the STOP button on the device to allow the contrast to advance into the stent and just beyond prior to releasing the STOP button (Figure 2.4). Once the stent is determined to be technically sound, the wire is removed and then the proximal clamp is removed. The sheath is then removed by tying down the initial access suture. The heparin effect is reversed with protamine and the wound is closed. Following completion of the procedure, the filter can be checked for atherosclerotic debris (Figure 2.5).

There are various maneuvers the experienced surgeon should be familiar with when performing a TCAR. If cerebral ischemia is detected (as noted on EEG or with the patient awake), the patients' overall hemodynamics should initially be checked and optimized including a systolic blood pressure in the range of 140–160 mm Hg. If this is not immediately beneficial, the flow of the reversal system can be adjusted to the LOW setting. Intermittently adjusting the flow reversal from off to then back on may allow for the development of improved tolerance to the cerebral ischemia. Finally, the option exists for converting the stent procedure to a different method of cerebral embolic protection such as a distal embolic filter device and proceeding with standard stent deployment, or alternatively, in rare instances, the case can be converted to an open carotid endarterectomy.

RESULTS

It is worth noting that presently no randomized controlled trials exist regarding the comparison of TCAR to CEA or to TF-CAS. Despite this, initial studies, and subsequent registry studies, both state and national, have demonstrated an extremely low stroke risk, between 1.0% and 1.7%, and a stroke, death, and myocardial infarction rate of 1.3–3.5% [6,7]. TCAR appears to be worse when there is significant calcification defined as greater than 50% circumference of the lesion, implying that one should avoid TCAR (or stenting procedures in general) when significant calcification is present [8]. Circumferential calcifications may represent a contraindication to TCAR, and one should consider CEA in this circumstance. TCAR, or any stenting procedure inclusive of TF-CAS, may have worse peri-procedural outcomes in long carotid artery lesions (>25 mm in length), and consideration should be

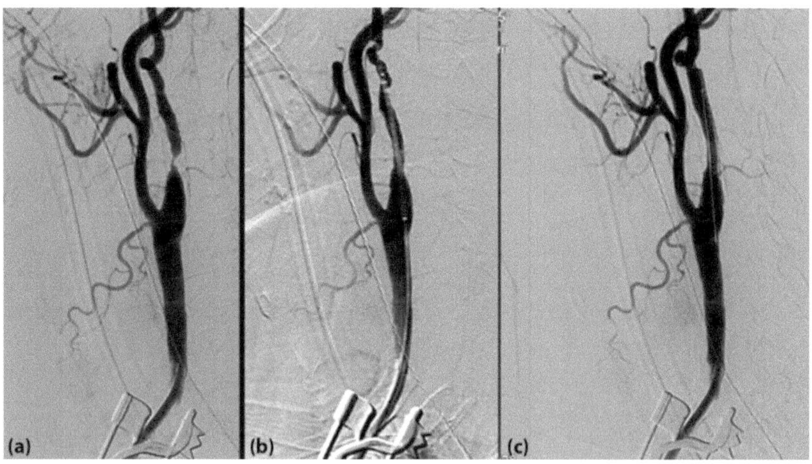

Figure 2.4 Angiogram series (all with active flow reversal) illustrating: (a) sheath insertion prior to lesion crossing; (b) angiogram with undeployed stent in place; and (c) completion study.

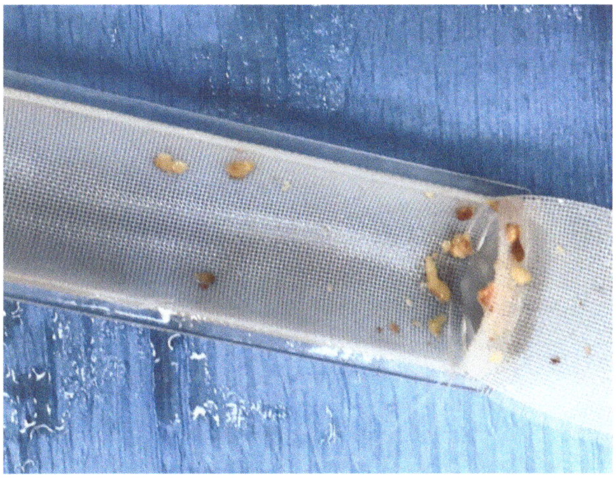

Figure 2.5 Finding of atherosclerotic debris within the filter (within the flow controller), indicative of effective flow reversal embolic protection, after TCAR completion.

given to CEA. TCAR has had comparable outcomes with CEA in octogenarians. Long-term outcomes for TCAR are also favorable with outcomes similar to that of CEA or TF-CAS in terms of patency and ipsilateral stroke-free survival [9].

COMPLICATIONS

The advantage of TCAR is the avoidance of manipulation of a diseased aortic arch and/or proximal CCA as well as the early establishment of a reliable method of cerebral protection. As with any revascularization procedure performed on the extra-cranial cervical carotid artery, there exists the risk of ipsilateral hemispheric stroke. In addition, there is the inherent risk of major adverse cardiac events inclusive of myocardial infarction or arrhythmia. Complications unique to TCAR include access site complications such as carotid artery dissection, antegrade or even retrograde, which may require conversion to open repair of the CCA access site. On follow-up, there exists a risk of recurrent stenosis within the stent, and a surveillance program with carotid duplex is warranted, especially over the first one to two years. It is imperative that prior to the procedure, the patient is maintained on dual antiplatelet therapy, typically aspirin and clopidogrel (Plavix), as well as an appropriate statin.

TCAR is unique in that the procedure hinges on uncomplicated carotid access and successful cannulation. Attention to the contraindications of TCAR allows for proper patient selection and successful TCAR performance. TCAR is ultimately a stent procedure and has the same limitations as TF-CAS in terms of calcific disease, circumferential calcification, and longer lesion length in which CEA may be more applicable. Thus, TCAR is a valuable procedure in the armamentarium in the treatment of patients with carotid artery occlusive disease in appropriately selected asymptomatic and symptomatic patients.

TRICKS AND TRAPS

1. TCAR is a hybrid procedure combining an open skill set with an endovascular means of carotid revascularization.
2. The success of TCAR directly hinges on successful common carotid artery cannulation without disturbance of the carotid lesion, providing cerebral protection by allowing dynamic flow reversal prior to any manipulation of the carotid disease.
3. Open exposure of the CCA is performed through a transverse 2 cm long incision at the base of the neck; appropriate countertraction on the CCA facilitates placement of the specialized 9F sheath.
4. Calcific disease, especially circumferential disease, long carotid lesions, and extremely tortuous/acutely angled ICAs are relative contraindications to TCAR, and consideration should be given to the performance of CEA.
5. Lesion crossing and angioplasty and stent deployment should always be performed with verified flow reversal.

QUESTIONS

1. Which of the following statements concerning the indications for TCAR is true?
   a. TCAR use is restricted to high-risk patients
   b. TCAR is indicated only if a carotid endarterectomy cannot be performed
   c. TCAR has a similar risk of periprocedural magnetic resonance imaging "hits" to that of carotid endarterectomy
   d. TCAR has better results with long carotid lesions

   Answer: c

2. Of the following, which is the most important critical step in the technical performance of TCAR?
   a. Placement of the appropriately sized venous sheath
   b. Placement of the 9F arterial sheath
   c. The total time of flow reversal
   d. The minimally disruptive dissection and exposure of a diseased common carotid artery

   Answer: b

3. Which of the following is a contraindication to the performance of a TCAR?
   a. Common carotid to internal carotid peak systolic velocity of greater than 2.0
   b. Aortic arch disease with a shaggy appearing aorta
   c. External carotid artery occlusion
   d. Access site to common carotid artery/internal carotid artery disease length of 3.5 cm in a common carotid artery with a diameter of 7 mm

   Answer: d

4. Which of the following statements concerning active flow reversal during TCAR is true?
   a. After cannulation of the common carotid artery and the femoral vein, flow reversal is established by turning up the controller to the HIGH setting
   b. Flow reversal is confirmed through a Doppler probe placed on the common carotid artery
   c. EEG changes occur frequently and can often be treated with blood pressure adjustment
   d. The time of flow reversal does not correlate directly with outcome measures

   Answer: d

REFERENCES

1. Rosenfield K, Matsumura JS, Chaturvedi S, Riles T, Ansel GM Metzger DC, et al. Randomized trial of stent versus surgery for asymptomatic carotid stenosis. *N Engl J Med.* 2016 Mar 17;37:1011–1020.
2. Mas JL, Chatellier G, Beyssen B, Branchereau A, Moulin T, Becquemin JP, et al. Endarterectomy versus stenting in patients with symptomatic severe carotid stenosis. *N Engl J Med.* 2006;19;355:1660–1671.
3. Halliday A, Bulbulia R, Bonati LH, Chester J, Cradduck-Bamford A, Peto R, Pan H, ACST-2 Collaborative Group. Second asymptomatic carotid surgery trial (ACST-2): A randomised comparison of carotid artery stenting versus carotid endarterectomy. *Lancet.* 2021 Sep 18;398:1065–1073.
4. Reiff T, Eckstein HH, Mansmann U, Jansen O, Fraedrich G, Mudra H, et al. Carotid endarterectomy or stenting or best medical treatment alone for moderate-to-severe asymptomatic carotid artery stenosis: 5-year results of a multicentre, randomised controlled trial. *Lancet Neurol.* 2022;21:877–888.
5. Mas JL, Chatellier G, Beyssen B, Branchereau A, Moulin T, Becquemin JP, et al. EVA-3S Investigators. Endarterectomy versus stenting in patients with symptomatic severe carotid stenosis. *N Engl J Med.* 2006;355:1660–1671.
6. Malas MB, Leal Lorenzo JI, Nejim B, Hanover TM, Mehta M, Kashyap V, Kwolek CJ, Cambria R. Analysis of the ROADSTER pivotal and extended-access cohorts shows excellent 1-year durability of transcarotid stenting with dynamic flow reversal. *J Vasc Surg.* 2019;69:1786–1796.
7. Malas MB, Dakour-Aridi H, Wang GJ, Kashyap VS, Motaganahalli RL, Eldrup-Jorgensen J, Cronenwett JL, Schermerhorn ML. Transcarotid artery revascularization versus transfemoral carotid artery stenting in the society for vascular surgery vascular quality initiative. *J Vasc Surg.* 2019;69:92–103.
8. Elsayed N, Yei KS, Naazie I, Goodney P, Clouse WD, Malas M. The impact of carotid lesion calcification on outcomes of carotid artery stenting. *J Vasc Surg.* 2022;75:921–929.
9. Malas MB, Elsayed N, Naazie I, Dakour-Aridi H, Yei KS, Schermerhorn ML. Propensity score-matched analysis of 1-year outcomes of transcarotid revascularization with dynamic flow reversal, carotid endarterectomy, and transfemoral carotid artery stenting. *J Vasc Surg.* 2022;75:213–222.

3

Open and endovascular treatment of aortic arch branches

MITCHELL R. WEAVER

INTRODUCTION

Symptomatic arterial occlusive disease of the branches of the aortic arch is not frequently encountered. When present, it is manifested by ischemia as the result of low flow or atheroembolism. Brachiocephalic artery (BCA) disease may present with upper extremity tissue loss or effort fatigue, or in the cerebral hemispheres with stroke, transient ischemic attack, or vertebrobasilar insufficiency. Patients with prior coronary artery bypass via an internal mammary artery may present with symptoms of coronary insufficiency. Atherosclerosis is the leading cause of BCA occlusive disease. However, other etiologies exist, including arteritis, congenital anomalies, and mechanical- or radiation-induced trauma. All may lead to symptoms and the need for intervention.

Advances in endovascular technology, along with its minimally invasive nature, have led to endovascular therapy becoming the first-line treatment for most proximal aortic arch lesions. A second option is extra-anatomic (cervical) revascularization, which is often ideal for isolated, single-vessel disease. In patients with multivessel disease, or in situations where complete arch debranching is indicated for aortic arch endografting, anatomic (transthoracic) revascularization may be the preferred or only option. Assessment of the patient's anatomy and physiologic status is used to determine the most appropriate therapeutic option.

PREOPERATIVE EVALUATION AND PLANNING

Non-invasive vascular laboratory studies are useful for screening for arterial occlusive disease and offering objective physiologic assessment. These studies include upper extremity segmental pressures that may reveal reduced distal extremity pressures or abnormal Doppler waveforms and carotid duplex imaging may document reduced flow velocities suggestive of proximal BCA occlusive disease. However, cross-sectional imaging with computed tomography angiography (CTA) (Figure 3.1) or magnetic resonance angiography are the studies of choice for confirming the diagnosis and planning of surgical intervention. It is important to image not only the aortic arch, but also the outflow, including the entire cervical and intracranial vasculature. This allows for the assessment for carotid bifurcation occlusive disease to be made to determine the need for concomitant carotid endarterectomy (CEA). Conventional catheter-based angiography may be of value in assessing aortic arch branch vessel

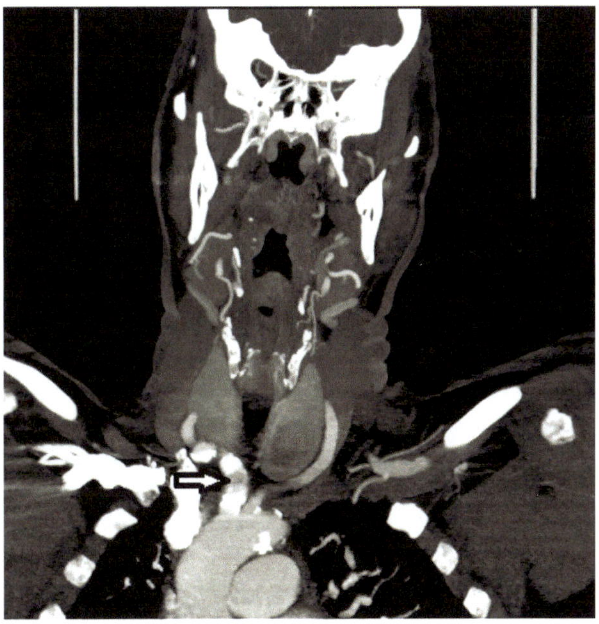

Figure 3.1 Reformatted computed tomography angiogram of the aortic arch with heavily calcified brachiocephalic artery (arrow).

DOI: 10.1201/9781003452096-3

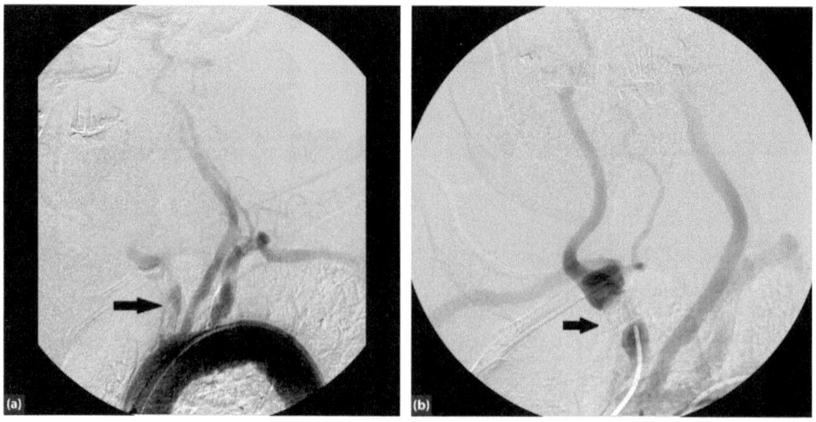

Figure 3.2 Nonselective aortic arch angiogram in a patient with right upper extremity effort fatigue and an ulcer on the little finger: (a) Severe calcified arterial occlusive disease is noted in the BCA (arrow); (b) selective angiogram of the BCA demonstrating severe stenosis of the BCA (arrow).

disease, especially when heavily calcified walls make it difficult to truly determine the degree of stenosis on cross-sectional imaging (Figure 3.2).

Important imaging considerations for surgical planning include the number of diseased arch vessels, stenosis versus complete occlusion, length of lesion, location of lesion (ostial versus non-ostial, relationship to branch vessels, i.e., vertebral artery), character of lesion (concentric versus eccentric), and degree of calcification. In general, endovascular procedures perform better in lesions that are shorter, non-ostial, concentric, lack heavy calcification, and are a stenosis as opposed to complete occlusion. Extra-anatomic bypass requires at least one widely patent supra-aortic branch to serve as an inflow source. Open arterial reconstructions require appropriate disease-free clamping sites, importantly for trans-thoracic direct arterial reconstruction, a site on the proximal ascending aorta and the distal targets for bypass, whether the distal BCA, the right subclavian artery (RSA), or either/both carotid arteries.

Given the nature of supra-aortic arch branch disease, appropriate preoperative cardiopulmonary assessment and optimization is required. This is important before trans-thoracic aortic arch reconstruction. The presence of any cardiac dysfunction, valvular heart disease, or coronary ischemia should be carefully ruled out. Non-invasive studies, such as echocardiography and myocardial perfusion scans, are useful in this evaluation. However, because these reconstructive procedures are performed via a median sternotomy, to ensure no other cardiac intervention is indicated, one should have a low threshold for obtaining catheter-based coronary angiography before proceeding with aortic arch surgery. Severe cardiopulmonary disease, a heavily calcified aortic arch, or prior sternotomy places patients at higher risk, makes the operation more difficult, and may occasionally preclude direct arch branch reconstruction.

ENDOVASCULAR THERAPY

Endovascular techniques, given their minimally invasive nature and satisfactory results, have become first-line therapy in appropriate candidates. Standard endovascular techniques are utilized in the treatment of supra-aortic trunk vessels. Important pre-procedural considerations include site of access, therapeutic intervention, and distal thromboembolic protection strategies.

Access options include an antegrade approach to the vessel via the femoral artery or the retrograde approach via the carotid, brachial, or radial arteries. The femoral approach has the advantages of familiarity with use for access, lack of need for surgical exposure, and lower access site complication rates compared with brachial artery access. Retrograde carotid, brachial, or radial approaches are beneficial when arch vessel origins are at unfavorable locations. Long sheaths are used to provide working support. The patient is anticoagulated with heparin prior to the manipulation of catheters within the aortic arch. Anatomy is defined with digital subtraction imaging and with injection of iodinated contrast via a flush catheter positioned in the ascending aorta. Typically, a left anterior oblique projection of the c-arm will splay out the aortic arch (Figure 3.2a). Additional digital subtraction angiography with the c-arm in the right anterior oblique projection with possible additional cranial or caudal angulation will better define the right brachiocephalic artery bifurcation. A long slightly angled catheter is the first choice for selecting the arch vessels (Figure 3.2b). Due to its location, the left subclavian is usually the easiest to access. If unsuccessful with the first catheter, specialized double-curved catheters are utilized.

Retrograde approaches via either the radial, brachial, or common carotid approach offer the advantage of a shorter distance to the lesion, which may allow for the greater response of catheters and wires to manipulation. A retrograde (hybrid) approach may also allow for

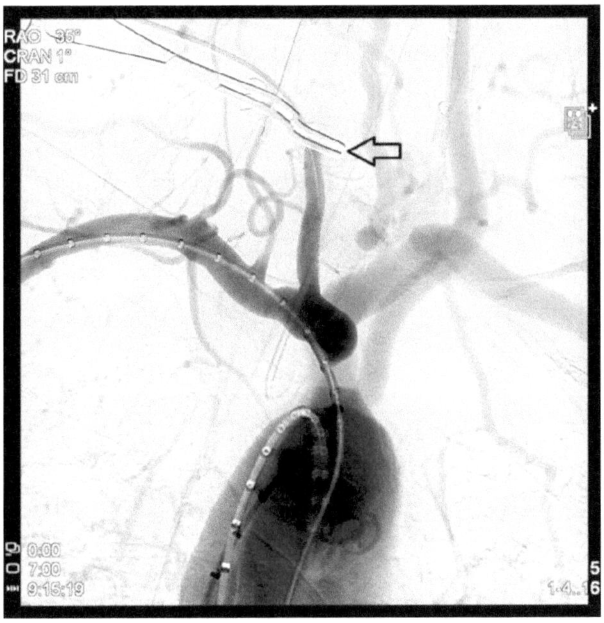

Figure 3.3 Digital subtraction angiogram demonstrating a retrograde (hybrid) approach with open exposure and distal clamping (arrow) of the common carotid artery with retrograde access as a precaution against atheroembolization.

distal clamping as a precaution against atheroembolization (Figure 3.3) and might be the only option when the angle of the vessel or degree of disease prevents the antegrade approach due to the inability to cannulate or gain enough purchase within the artery to advance therapeutic devices. The use of open exposure of the common carotid artery with retrograde access allows for clamping of the carotid artery distal to the access site during the intervention and "flushing" of the artery to remove any possible embolic debris prior to restoring flow after the intervention. This technique may be used in combination with carotid endarterectomy in the case of tandem lesions of the supra-aortic arch vessels and the carotid bifurcation [1,2]. When retrograde brachial artery access is used, we prefer open exposure because of the larger size sheaths that are required (6 French and larger) to limit access site complications. More recently, the radial artery has become a more frequently used access site with the availability of endovascular equipment specifically designed for radial access.

Once the lesion is crossed, therapeutic interventions include balloon angioplasty with provisional stenting for residual stenosis greater than 30% or flow limiting dissection, and primary stenting. Depending on the degree of stenosis, pre-dilation with a smaller balloon may be required in order to successfully and safely pass the stent. The use of through-and-through technique in which a wire is passed in a retrograde fashion and snared in the aorta from a femoral approach (or vice versa) can offer additional stability for passing and accurately deploying stents. Stent and final balloon sizing is based on preoperative cross-sectional imaging. If such imaging is not available, the diameter of the normal artery distal to the lesion on angiography is used as a guide for sizing. Primary stenting is more commonly performed, especially if heavy calcification is present or there is a complete occlusion. Both balloon-expandable as well as self-expanding stents may be deployed. Balloon-expandable stents are generally chosen for orificial lesions secondary to the precise deployment they allow. Generally, when treating orificial lesions, the stents are extended a few millimeters into the aorta. A "kissing" stent technique may be needed for treatment of the innominate artery bifurcation or if the origins of the innominate artery and left carotid arteries are adjacent. The current role of cover stents or lithotripsy balloons in the treatment of these lesions may have value but has not yet been defined. Postoperative care typically includes use of dual antiplatelet therapy of aspirin 81 mg and either clopidogrel or ticagrelor for six weeks.

Prevention of atheroembolism and stroke during these interventions is of great concern, but the role of available strategies to mitigate this has not been completely defined. Several series have demonstrated very low cerebrovascular event rates of 0–1.5% with the use of retrograde carotid access with distal clamping and flushing [3,4], even with the addition of carotid endarterectomy [2]. When transfemoral access is used, filter wires may be used for distal embolic protection of the carotid artery but its role is not completely defined as some authors report routine use of protective devices when treating common or innominate arteries, while others use them only in select cases, and still others report never using such devices [5–8]. The technical success rates for stenotic lesions are higher than those for occlusions. The procedure is associated with low morbidity and mortality with several studies reporting fewer than 3% combined 30-day stroke and death rates [3,4,5,8–11]. Primary patency is reported at 90–100% at one year [5,8–10] and greater than 70% after four years [9].

OPEN SURGICAL THERAPY

Extra-thoracic arterial reconstructions

Extra-thoracic arterial reconstructions for the treatment of supra-aortic branch pathology has played a substantial role due to the relative ease of exposure and elimination of the morbidity of a transthoracic exposure. All extra-thoracic reconstructions require at least one disease-free arch vessel to serve as the donor vessel. In the long term, as atherosclerosis is a progressive disease, the donor vessel is always at risk of stenosis itself, which may eventually lead to the decreased durability of extra-thoracic repairs. These operations include bypass between the carotid and subclavian arteries, transposition of the subclavian artery onto the carotid artery and vice versa, carotid-to-carotid artery bypass, and axillo-axillary bypass. Carotid-subclavian bypass/transposition is covered in Chapter 25.

Carotid-carotid artery bypass

This operation is performed under general anesthesia and the patient must be positioned, prepped, and draped in a manner that allows access to both sides of the neck. The common carotid arteries are exposed bilaterally in the standard manner. The tunnel connecting them will be in the retropharyngeal space. This tunnel is created by dissecting below the common carotid arteries over the vertebral bodies palpated behind the pharynx. The space behind the pharynx is entered and developed bilaterally using finger dissection. The shiny prevertebral fascia is visualized. Within this space, a short tunnel is created between the two common carotid arteries through which to pass the graft. The patient is systemically anticoagulated with heparin. With adequate anticoagulation, the donor common carotid artery is clamped and arteriotomy is made on the medial aspect of the donor common carotid artery. An end graft (usually 6–8 mm diameter) is sewn to the side of the donor carotid artery with 5-0 polypropylene suture. Next, the graft is taken through the tunnel and anastomosed to the recipient vessel in an end-to-end fashion. The arteries and graft are bled, before the final completion of anastomosis and restoration of flow. The arteries are interrogated with a Doppler probe and, if appropriate, signals are isonated; the heparin effect is reversed with protamine.

OUTCOMES

Ozsvath et. al [12] reported on 24 carotid-carotid artery bypasses with no perioperative mortality and one stroke. Three-year primary patency was 88% and secondary patency 92%, with a stroke-free survival at four years of 94%. In a review of carotid-carotid bypass procedures by Aziz et. al., [11] four studies were identified with a total of 67 patients. Perioperative mortality rate was 0–0.7% and stroke rate was 0–6.2%. Patency at five years reported in two studies was 70% and 94%.

Axillo-axillary bypass

Axillo-axillary bypass is an additional option that a vascular surgeon has for re-vascularizing the supra-aortic trunk vessels provided the contralateral axillo-subcalvian artery is widely patent. Advantages to this operation include both the safety and technical ease with which it can be performed compared with some of the other available surgical options. In situations of a hostile neck and or mediastinum, it may be a good option. Disadvantages include that the graft does produce a noticeable bulge across the sternum and its superficial position leads to concerns of skin erosion and infection.

The patient, under general anesthesia, is placed in a supine position with the arms along the side of the body with the elbows slightly flexed and the upper body elevated about 15 degrees. The operating table can then be tilted side to side depending on which side is being worked on so that the skin overlying the infra-clavicular fossa is in the horizontal plane. The incision is 1–2 cm below the clavicle overlying the deltopectoral groove starting just lateral to the sternal head of the clavicle and extending lateral about 7–8 cm toward the coracoid process. The incision is ended laterally slightly more inferiorly (2 cm below clavicle), roughly paralleling the muscles of the pectoralis major muscle. The fascia of the pectoralis major muscle is incised and the muscle fibers split. The clavipectoral fascia is incised. If necessary, the pectoralis minor muscle fibers, which are at the lateral limits of the dissection, may be divided to improve exposure. Arterial branches of the thoracoacromial trunk and accompanying veins may be encountered and require ligation and division. The axillary vein is mobilized and retracted to expose the axillary artery.

The axillary artery is exposed for 3–4 cm and encircled with vessel loops. After completing this dissection bilaterally, a subcutaneous tunnel is then created superficial to the sternum at the level of the first interspace. This can often be accomplished with finger dissection alone. Once the tunnel is completed, the patient is systemically anticoagulated and anastomosis is performed. Prosthetic grafts of 7–8 mm diameter are typically chosen for conduit. The grafts are usually cut at a 30- to 45-degree angle for their anastomosis to the artery. Once the artery is controlled with atraumatic vascular clamps, an appropriate length longitudinal arteriotomy is created removing a small ellipse of the artery, which is usually on the anteromedial aspect of the artery. The donor side anastomosis is performed first in a running fashion, usually with running 5-0 or 6-0 polypropylene suture. Once the anastomosis is completed, the proximal and distal arteries are vented and the graft is arterialized. After ensuring the anastomosis is hemostatic, the graft is taken through the previously created tunnel, taking care not to twist or kink it. After creation of an arteriotomy in the recipient artery in like fashion to the donor artery, the graft is cut in a beveled fashion so as not to be redundant or under tension. The outflow anastomosis is then completed in like fashion. Just before completion of the anastomosis, the artery and graft are vented, then the anastomosis is completed and flow is restored. Distal flow in the upper extremities is accessed by pulse exam and continuous wave Doppler evaluation. Once the flow is noted to be satisfactory, the heparin effect is reversed with protamine, hemostasis within the wounds is ensured, and the extremities are closed.

OUTCOMES

Overall, this operation can be performed with minimal morbidity and mortality. Perioperative mortality and stroke are reported at 0.5% (0–3%) and 1.1% (0–10%), respectively, with patency of up to 90% at five years [11].

Transthoracic arterial reconstructions

PREPARATION

Procedures are performed under general anesthesia (GA). Appropriate preoperative antibiotics are administered within one hour before incision. Preoperative discussion with the anesthesiology team regarding arterial line placement and venous access is important. Considerations include which arteries are diseased, which arteries are going to be clamped, and the plans for any concomitant procedures (i.e., CEA). The authors generally avoid electroencephalography monitoring unless carotid bifurcation clamping is planned. The patient is placed in a supine position with a posterior shoulder roll to extend the neck and elevate the sternal notch after GA is induced. The midline is marked with a pen before prepping and draping. A chlorhexidine-based solution is used for prepping the skin. The field should be large enough to incorporate the neck should an extension of the skin incision be needed to expose the proximal carotid arteries (Figure 3.4). The field should also include both groins in case emergency access to the femoral vessels is needed for cardiopulmonary bypass.

EXPOSURE

Median sternotomy is performed by incising the skin from the sternal notch to the xiphoid process with a No. 10 blade scalpel. Electrocautery is then used to divide the subcutaneous tissues until the sternum is reached. The interclavicular ligament is then split and the midline of the sternum is marked from the sternal notch to the xiphoid process. After having the anesthesiologist suspend ventilation, a standard pneumatic saw is used to divide the sternum in the midline. The saw can be used from cranial-to-caudal or caudal-to-cranial depending on surgeon preference. After controlling any periosteal bleeding points, a sternal retractor is placed on the mid-to-lower aspect of the sternal edges.

A ministernotomy or upper hemisternotomy is another slightly less invasive option that can provide adequate exposure of the aortic arch and great vessels. This exposure is performed by limiting the incision to just below the angle of Louis (sternal angle). The sternotomy is performed from the sternal notch to the level of the third intercostal space. The saw is then turned at a right angle to "T-off" the sternotomy into the right or left intercostal space. Care must be taken not to injure the underlying internal mammary artery.

After placing a sternal retractor, the pericardium is divided in the midline and three heavy silk stay sutures are placed on both edges of the pericardium to elevate the mediastinal structures and create a pericardial well. The thymic fat that typically covers the aortic arch and proximal arch vessels is either divided in the middle or excised until the left brachiocephalic vein (BCV) is identified. This vein is dissected circumferentially and encircled with a vessel loop that is used to retract the vein superiorly or inferiorly to provide exposure of the underlying structures (Figure 3.5). The ascending aorta may be dissected free from the main pulmonary trunk laterally and the right pulmonary artery inferiorly to provide additional mobility and excellent proximal control.

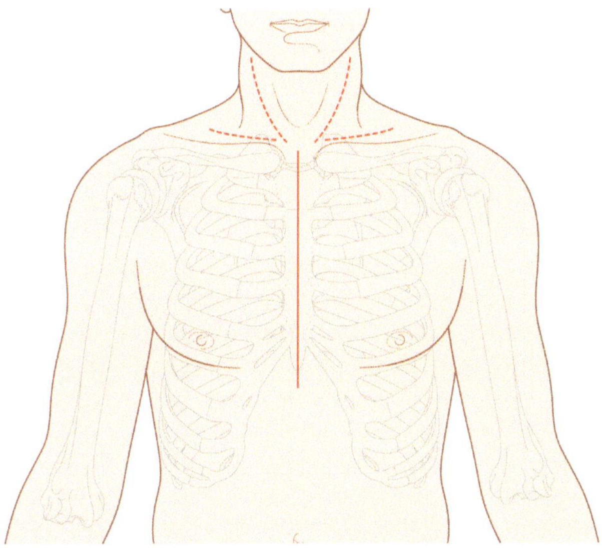

Figure 3.4 Incision for median sternotomy (solid line) and optional cervical extensions (dotted lines).

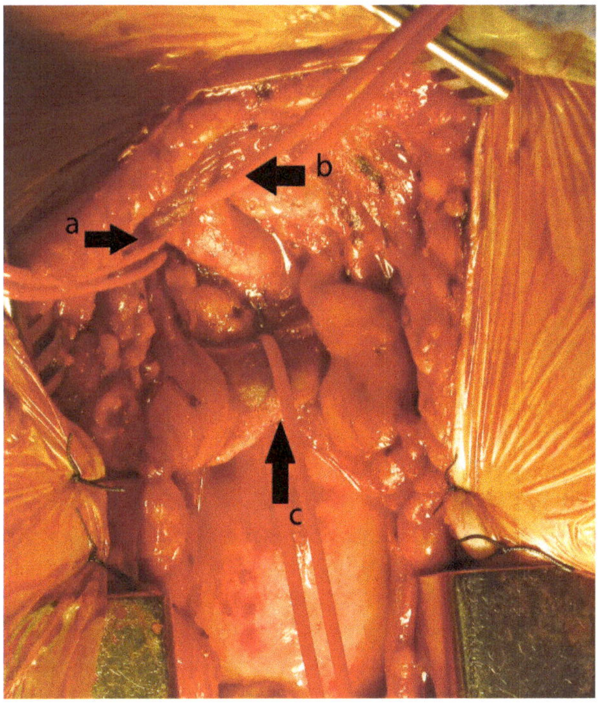

Figure 3.5 Intraoperative photograph demonstrating exposure of the brachiocephalic artery. Proximal right subclavian artery (a arrow); proximal right common carotid artery (b arrow); left brachiocephalic vein (c arrow). Both arteries and the vein have been circled with vessel loops.

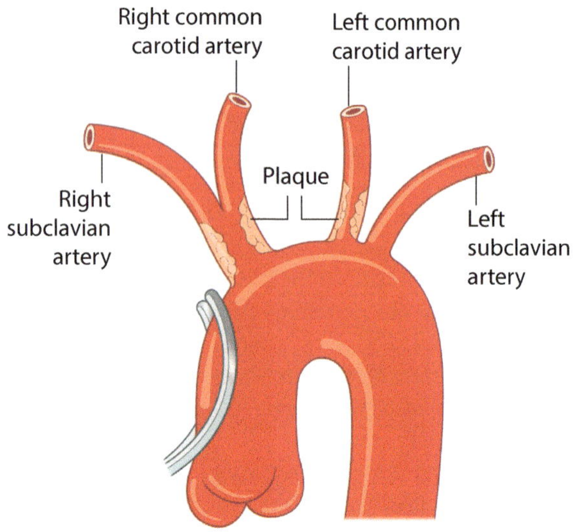

Figure 3.6 Placement of a side-biting aortic clamp on the ascending aorta in preparation for the performance of proximal anastomosis.

The arch is then further exposed by dividing the pericardial reflection. The BCA, the left carotid artery (LCA), and as needed, the left subclavian artery (LSA) are then dissected and encircled with vessel loops. In the case of BCA reconstruction, the BCA is dissected distally until a soft spot is identified to clamp or, more commonly, the proximal most right common carotid artery (CCA) and RSA are exposed and controlled. When controlling the RSA, care should be exercised to avoid injury to the vagus and recurrent laryngeal nerves. While BCA endarterectomy can occasionally be performed on a very focal mid-BCA stenosis, most brachiocephalic lesions are best served with a bypass originating from the ascending aorta.

After completing dissection, heparin is given intravenously to achieve an activated clotting time of 200–250 seconds. An appropriately sized graft is then brought to the field (typically 8–12 mm). After lowering the mean blood pressure (BP) to <70 mmHg, a deep and strong side-biting clamp is then applied to the ascending aorta slightly lateral and to the right (Figure 3.6). The authors prefer a LEMOLE-STRONG aortic clamp (Becton, Dickinson and Company, Franklin Lakes, NJ, USA) for this (Figure 3.7). The graft is beveled appropriately to lay comfortably on the anterolateral (right) side of the ascending aorta. An aortotomy is performed with a No. 11 blade scalpel and extended with Potts scissors; if the aorta is dilated, the authors frequently remove a small ellipse of aortic wall. Proximal anastomosis is performed with 4-0 polypropylene running suture. After assuring hemostasis, attention is directed distally to the BCA.

While it is sometimes possible to clamp a disease-free segment of the distal BCA, in most situations it is necessary to clamp the RSA and CCA separately. Clamp application on calcified vessels should be avoided because of the risk of embolization. After clamping these arteries, the proximal BCA needs to be ligated and a segment resected to provide more room. A stapler works nicely for this purpose if the vessel is not calcified. Otherwise, it needs to be clamped and oversewn in two layers with 4-0 polypropylene suture. A distal cuff of BCA is prepared for anastomosis; limited plaque at the BCA bifurcation can be endarterectomized. The graft is tunneled distally, usually under the BCV to avoid compression; it is pressurized and cut to length to reach the distal anastomosis site. This anastomosis is usually performed under slight tension because of the tendency for the field to collapse after removal of the sternal retractor predisposing to graft redundancy. If there is any doubt, the sternal retractor should be temporarily loosened before graft transection. The distal anastomosis is then performed with a 5-0 polypropylene running suture (Figure 3.8). When the disease extends beyond the BCA bifurcation, the authors prefer to perform the distal anastomosis to the right CCA after sewing a sidearm on for RSA bypass. While a tempting option, bifurcated aortic grafts should be avoided because of their increased bulk, which can lead to compression following the removal of the sternal retractor.

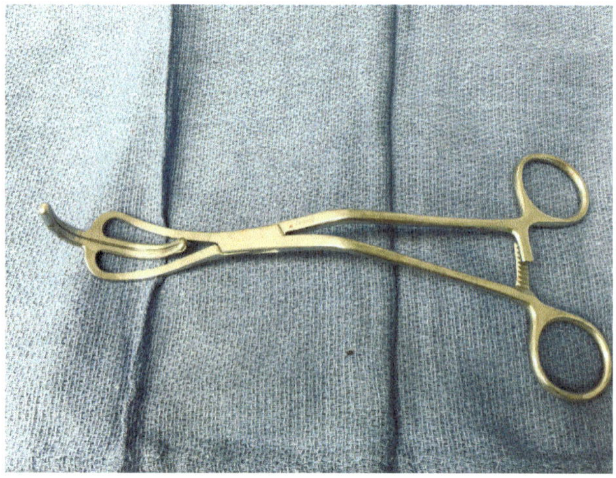

Figure 3.7 LEMOLE-STRONG aortic clamp (Becton, Dickinson and Company, Franklin Lakes, NJ, USA) used for partial (side-biting) clamping of the ascending aorta.

The same technique can be applied to bypass the LCA or LSA when they are involved. A side branch graft can be anastomosed to the larger main graft, ideally after performing the aortic anastomosis and checking the lay of the graft (Figure 3.9). Branded grafts are commercially available that are designed for bypassing more than one arch vessel. Bypass to the LCA should be performed only after BCA flow has been restored. Again, the proximal vessel can be stapled or oversewn. Depending on the anatomy of the LSA, specifically how laterally and posteriorly it is positioned, adequate exposure for performing arterial reconstruction via a median sternotomy may not be possible. If revascularization of this vessel is required, an extra-anatomic reconstruction (i.e., carotid-subclavian bypass or carotid-subclavian transposition) may be considered after revascularization of the LCA.

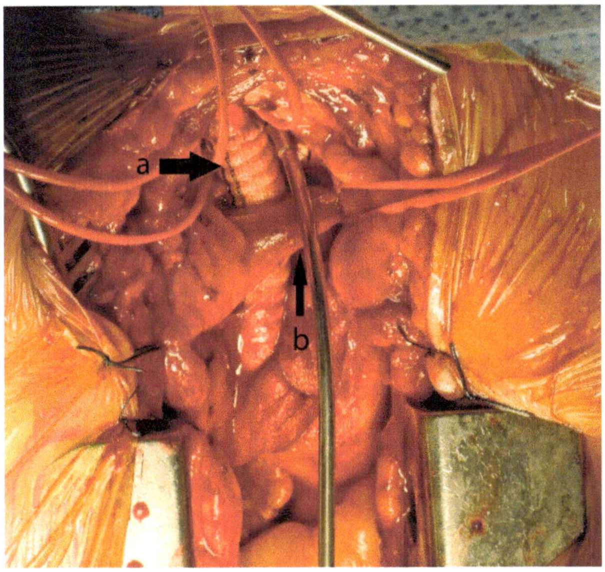

Figure 3.8 Intraoperative photograph demonstrating aorta-to-BCA bypass. End-to-end anastomosis to BCA (a arrow); bypass graft passes beneath the left brachiocephalic vein (b arrow).

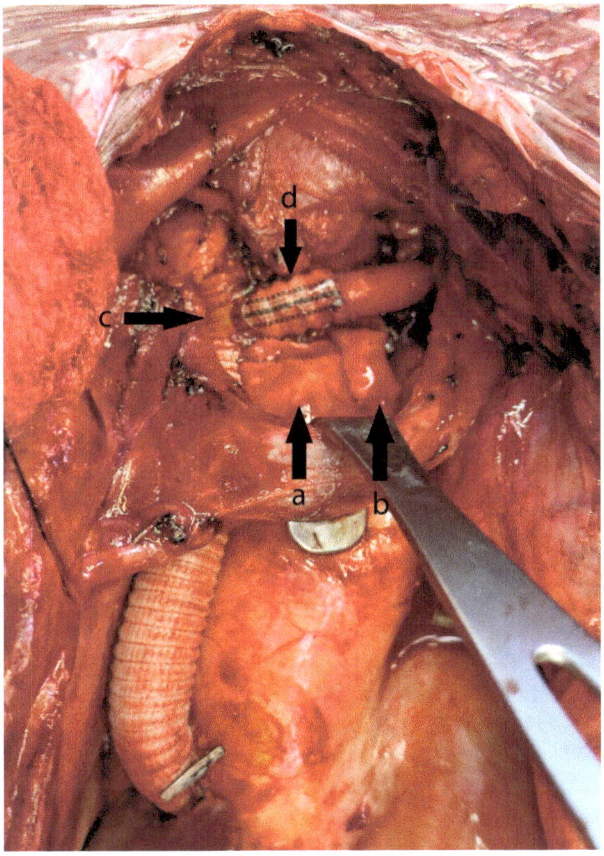

Figure 3.9 Intraoperative photograph demonstrating ligated (stapled) BCA (a arrow); ligated (stapled) left carotid artery (b arrow); ascending aorta-to-BCA bypass (c arrow), with side branch bypass to the left common carotid artery (d arrow).

CLOSURE

Having completed the bypass, heparin is reversed with protamine sulfate and hemostasis is ensured with cautery and hemostatic agents as needed. Typically, one large-bore (36-Fr) drainage tube is used to drain the mediastinum. It is exteriorized inferiorly and sutured to the skin. The sternum is closed with interrupted sternal wires. Soft tissues and skin are then closed with absorbable suture in a layered fashion.

OUTCOMES

Outcomes are generally very satisfactory when performed for BCA occlusive disease. Early complications typically involve cardiopulmonary events or stroke. Mortality rates range from 2.7% to 8%. Stroke rates from 2.7% to 8% and myocardial infarction rates from 1.5% to 3% have been reported. Survival rates at five and ten years are 77.5–87% and 51.9–81%, respectively. Graft patency at five and ten years is reported from 94% to 98% and 88% to 96%, respectively [13–15].

TRICKS AND TRAPS

- Careful study of high-quality cross-sectional computed tomography angiography (CTA) imaging to choose and plan for arterial reconstruction.
- Avoid excess manipulation of catheters within the arch that may increase the risk of embolic stroke.
- Avoid unnecessary flushing of catheters and sheaths into the aortic arch and cerebrovascular system, and always back-bleed catheters and sheaths prior to flushing.
- Through-and-through wire control via two access sites allows for greater stability in performing endovascular intervention.
- When operating simultaneously on both carotid arteries, identify and treat the vagus nerve with the greatest care as a bilateral recurrent nerve injury and vocal cord paralysis will lead to a tracheostomy.
- Significant postoperative chyle leaks should prompt an early return to the OR for wound exploration.
- Prefabricated bifurcated grafts can be bulky and make the closure of a sternotomy difficult without distorting grafts and are usually avoided.

QUESTIONS

1. The most commonly injured nerve during carotid-carotid bypass is:
   a. Phrenic nerve
   b. Hypoglossal nerve
   c. Vagus nerve
   d. Long thoracic nerve

   Answer: c

2. A "bovine" arch refers to:
   a. A single origin of the left and right common carotid arteries
   b. The left common carotid arising from the innominate artery with single origin
   c. A single origin of the right and left carotid arteries and left subclavian artery
   d. An accurate reflection of a cow's arch anatomy

   Answer: b

3. A 35-year-old woman presents with symptoms of dizziness and has effort ischemia of both upper extremities. A CT scan shows stenosis of the proximal left subclavian artery and left common carotid artery and complete occlusion of the proximal innominate artery. Her erythrocyte sedimentation rate (ESR) is 3 mm/hr. What is the most appropriate treatment of this condition?
   a. Anticoagulation with warfarin
   b. Percutaneous transluminal angioplasty and stenting of the innominate, left carotid, and left subclavian artery
   c. Stenting of the innominate artery with right to left carotid and left carotid to left subclavian bypass
   d. Ascending aorta to the innominate, left carotid, and left subclavian artery bypass
   e. Carotid-carotid bypass

   Answer: d

4) Anatomic findings that affect both procedural and long-term outcomes when using endovascular techniques to treat arch vessel occlusive disease include:
   a. Complete occlusion versus stenosis
   b. Length of lesion
   c. Calcification
   d. All of the above
   e. None of the above

   Answer: d

REFERENCES

1. Takach TJ, Reul GJ, Cooley DA, et al. Brachiocephalic reconstruction I: Operative and long-term results for complex disease. *J Vasc Surg.* 2005;42:47–54.
2. Sfyroeras GS, Karathanos C, Antoniou GA, Saleptsis V, Giannoukas AD. A meta-analysis of combined endarterectomy and proximal balloon angioplasty for tandem disease of the arch vessels and carotid bifurcation. *J Vasc Surg.* 2011;54(2):534–40.
3. Queral LA, Criado FJ. The treatment of focal aortic arch branch lesions with Palmaz stents. *J Vasc Surg.* 1996;23(2):368–375.
4. Payne DA, Hayes PD, Bolia A, Fishwick G, Bell PRF, Naylor AR. Cerebral protection during open retrograde angioplasty/stenting of common carotid and innominate artery stenoses. *Br J Surg.* 2006;93(2):187–190. doi:10.1002/bjs.5232.
5. Ben Ahmed S, Benezit M, Hazart J, Brouat A, Daniel G, Rosset E. Outcomes of the endovascular treatment for the supra-aortic trunks occlusive disease: A 14-year monocentric experience. *Ann Vasc Surg.* 2016;33:55–66.
6. Soga Y, Tomoi Y, Fujihara M, Okazaki S, Yamauchi Y, Shintani Y, Suzuki K, SCALLOP Investigators. Perioperative and long-term outcomes of endovascular treatment for subclavian artery disease from a large multicenter registry. *J Endovasc Ther.* 2015 Aug;22(4):626–633.
7. Payne DA, Hayes PD, Bolia A, Fishwick G, Bell PRF, Naylor AR. Cerebral protection during open retrograde angioplasty/stenting of common carotid and innominate artery stenoses. *Br J Surg.* 2006;93(2):187–190. doi:10.1002/bjs.5232.
8. AbuRahma AF, Robinson PA, Jennings TG. Carotid-subclavian bypass grafting with polytetrafluoroethylene grafts for symptomatic subclavian artery stenosis or occlusion: A 20-year experience. *J Vasc Surg.* 2000;32(3):411–419.
9. Sullivan TM, Gray BH, Bacharach JM, Perl J II, Childs MB, Modzelewski L, et al. Angioplasty and primary stenting of the subclavian, innominate, and common carotid arteries in 83 patients. *J Vasc Surg.* 1998;28(6):1059–1065.
10. Clouse WD, Ergul EA, Cambria RP, Brewster DC, Kwolek CJ, LaMuraglia GM, et al. Retrograde stenting of proximal lesions with carotid endarterectomy increases risk. *J Vasc Surg.* 2016;63(6):1517–1523.
11. Aiello F, Morrissey NJ. Open and endovascular management of subclavian and innominate arterial pathology. *Semin Vasc Surg.* 2011 Mar;24(1):31–35.
12. AbuRahma AF, Robinson PA, Khan, et al. Brachiocephalic revascularization: A comparison between carotid-subclavian artery bypass and axilloaxillary artery bypass. *Surgery.* 1992;112:84.
13. Aziz F, Gravett MH, Comerota AJ. Endovascular and open surgical treatment of brachiocephalic arteries. *Ann Vasc Surg.* 2011 Jan 31.
14. Kieffer E, Sabatier J, Koskas F, et al. Atherosclerotic innominate artery occlusive disease: Early and long-term results of surgical reconstruction. *J Vasc Surg.* 1995;21:326–336.
15. Berguer R, Morasch MD, Kline RA. Transthoracic repair of innominate and common carotid artery disease: Immediate and long-term outcome for 100 consecutive surgical reconstructions. *J Vasc Surg.* 1998;27:34–41.

4

Endovascular intervention for mesenteric and renal artery occlusive disease

TIMOTHY J. NYPAVER AND JACQUELINE D. STUBER

INTRODUCTION

The management approach to mesenteric arterial occlusive disease and renal artery occlusive disease differs significantly. However, for both mesenteric and renal artery occlusive disease, endovascular revascularization has emerged as a first-line therapy of choice with open revascularizations reserved for specific problems or conditions. In addition, the techniques for intervention are very similar. Both mesenteric and renal artery occlusive disease presentations are divided into chronic disease states, with slow often insidiously developing patient complaints, and acute arterial occlusion, or acute ischemia, in which interventions and revascularizations are considered emergent if an optimal outcome is to be achieved. The practicing vascular surgeon needs to attain a level of familiarity, skill, and confidence in the approach to and with endovascular management of these high-stakes complex disease conditions.

INDICATIONS FOR INTERVENTION

Chronic mesenteric ischemia

Chronic mesenteric ischemia (CMI) is defined as inadequate perfusion of the gastrointestinal tract, resulting in ischemic symptoms or "intestinal angina" of at least three months' duration [1]. The most common etiology is atherosclerotic disease with infrequent cases attributed to fibromuscular dysplasia, chronic dissection, vasculitis, or external compression. Presenting symptoms classically include post-prandial abdominal pain and diarrhea resulting in food aversion and weight loss. Diagnosis requires symptomatology with evidence of hemodynamically significant stenosis (>70%) in at least two of the three major visceral arteries inclusive of the celiac axis (CA), superior mesenteric artery (SMA), or inferior mesenteric artery (IMA). Occasionally, significant isolated involvement of the SMA, the primary gatekeeper vessel to intestinal perfusion, can produce symptoms of CMI. The redundant collateral networks among these arteries will often allow for single-vessel disease to remain asymptomatic unless collateral networks have been disrupted by prior abdominal surgery. Duplex ultrasonography is the screening modality of choice with computed tomography angiography (CTA) required after a positive study to confirm and delineate the anatomic pattern of the disease, as well as plan for operative or endovascular intervention (Figure 4.1). Magnetic resonance angiography (MRA) may be useful in patients who are intolerant of iodinated contrast but provides limited visualization of the distal mesenteric vessels. Once the diagnosis is confirmed, revascularization should not be significantly delayed. The goals of treatment include relief of symptoms, recovery of weight loss, prevention of intestinal necrosis, and improvement in survivability and quality of life. Treatment of asymptomatic disease is typically deferred as a low percentage of these patients (less than 10%) become symptomatic while short-term mortality is high, secondary to comorbid conditions [2]. An exception may be considered in patients with high-grade, simultaneous CA and SMA disease as a series demonstrated that patients who became symptomatic were exclusively those with multi-vessel disease [2].

Current guidelines from the Society for Vascular Surgery (SVS) recommend endovascular intervention as the initial treatment modality of choice due to comparable technical success to open revascularization but with benefits of lower perioperative complications, shorter hospital length of stay, and lower hospital costs with comparable short- and long-term mortality [3]. Open repair may be considered at the index operation based upon anatomic factors that impact endovascular success, including poor access vessels, long-segment occlusions, tandem lesions, small mesenteric vessel diameter,

DOI: 10.1201/9781003452096-4

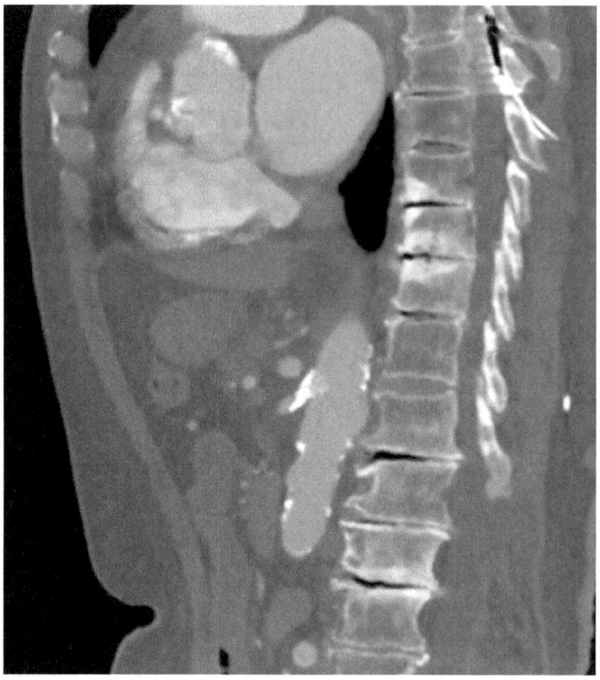

Figure 4.1 Sagittal computerized tomography arteriography (CTA) demonstrating significant orifical superior mesenteric artery calcific disease.

circumferential calcification, and major aortic occlusive disease in proximity to the visceral vessels. Lastly, select young (age <60) patients may benefit from open repair as the primary patency of endovascular interventions tends to be lower with more frequent reinterventions and symptom recurrence [4]. The SMA should be the primary target for revascularization [5]. Revascularization of both the CA and the SMA (multi-vessel treatment) has been found to be protective against symptom recurrence and the need for reintervention [6]. The authors, therefore, perform synchronous treatment of chronic CA and SMA disease if technically feasible. For recurrent symptomatic mesenteric artery stenosis or occlusion, the authors will attempt an endovascular reintervention, if possible, consistent with SVS guidelines [3].

Acute mesenteric ischemia

Acute mesenteric ischemia (AMI) is defined as the abrupt development of intestinal hypoperfusion with resulting intestinal ischemia presenting as severe abdominal pain that may progress to peritonitis. The most common etiologies are thromboembolism of cardiac or aortic origin and in-situ thrombosis of mesenteric atherosclerotic occlusive disease. A timely intervention is essential to prevent the development of intestinal ischemia and sepsis. Treatment is conducted in a multidisciplinary setting as evaluation of intestinal viability is required by either diagnostic laparoscopy, exploratory laparotomy, or serial abdominal exams. Revascularization is completed with an endovascular, open, or hybrid retrograde open mesenteric stenting (ROMS) procedure. In the setting of a classic embolic occlusion, the authors will often proceed with an open embolectomy as this allows for the timely restoration of perfusion and control of distal branch vessels for the prevention of embolization. In the setting of a thrombotic occlusion of pre-existing mesenteric occlusive disease, endovascular intervention is recommended due to lower rates of bowel resection and mortality when compared with open revascularization [1].

Chronic renal artery occlusive disease

Atherosclerotic disease remains the most common cause of renal artery occlusive disease and typically occurs at the origin of the renal arteries. While previously a more common practice, endovascular revascularization of the renal arteries in the setting of atherosclerotic occlusive disease has fallen out of favor due to a lack of benefit identified in randomized clinical trials. The Cardiovascular Outcomes in Renal Atherosclerotic Lesion (CORAL) and the Angioplasty and Stenting for Renal Artery Lesions (ASTRAL) trials demonstrated no benefit of endovascular intervention over medical therapy alone in improving cardiac outcomes, preventing ischemic nephropathy, or improving mortality [7, 8]. However, these trials had several important limitations, including non-standardized inclusion criteria, variable methods for determining degree of renal artery stenosis, and exclusion of high-risk patients most likely to benefit from treatment. Therefore, endovascular revascularization of the renal arteries is still offered in highly selected patients likely to benefit from revascularization. This patient population includes those with high-grade stenoses (>70%) of the bilateral renal arteries or a single functioning kidney associated with at least one of the following: a) refractory hypertension despite compliance with three classes of antihypertensives; b) hypertension associated with flash pulmonary edema or recurrent congestive heart failure exacerbation; c) hypertension intolerant to initiation of ACE inhibitor or ARB therapy (>30% decrease in eGFR after initiation); d) acutely elevated blood pressure associated with a simultaneous deterioration in renal function; and e) renal artery stenosis in a transplanted kidney [9]. Due to lower perioperative complications and shorter length of stay, endovascular therapy is preferred over open surgical revascularization.

The second most common etiology of chronic renal artery occlusive disease is fibromuscular dysplasia (FMD). Unlike in atherosclerotic occlusive disease, FMD lesions occur more frequently in the mid or distal renal artery than at the vessel origin. In further contrast, these lesions respond well to percutaneous transluminal angioplasty (PTA) alone with stenting reserved for the treatment of complications (dissection, pseudoaneurysm, or perforation) or for the primary treatment of aneurysm or select dissections. Intervention with PTA is indicated for hemodynamically significant stenoses associated with medically refractory hypertension, accelerated or malignant hypertension, or deteriorating renal function.

Overall, isolated endovascular interventions for renal artery occlusive disease have been decreasing. However, a renal endovascular skill set remains essential to the vascular surgeon with the evolution of advanced endovascular techniques for the treatment of complex abdominal and thoracoabdominal aortic aneurysms including the Zenith® Fenestrated platform (Cook Medical Inc., Bloomington, IN, USA), the TAMBE platform (Gore Medical, Newark, DE, USA), parallel grafting, or physician modified endografts. In each of these procedures, cannulation and stenting of the renal arteries (covered stents) are instrumental to maintaining kidney perfusion and achieving successful exclusion of the aneurysm.

Acute occlusion of the renal arteries

With the advent of advanced endograft techniques for the treatment of abdominal and thoracoabdominal aortic aneurysms, immediate or long-term complications following fenestrated and/or branched endovascular aneurysm repair (F/BEVAR) are becoming a more frequent cause of acute renal artery occlusion. Additional etiologies include thromboembolism, in-situ thrombosis, iatrogenic injury, or trauma. Controversy exists regarding the timeframe after which renal salvage is unlikely. A recent multi-institutional retrospective study of renal artery occlusions following F/BEVAR demonstrated successful recovery of renal function in 64% of patients with occluded bilateral renal arteries or a single renal artery of a solitary functioning kidney after a median time to revascularization of 27.5 hours [10]. This study challenges previous teaching that renal recovery is unlikely after greater than six hours of occlusion. For thromboembolic disease, an attempt at endovascular revascularization would be appropriate if it is within six hours from the onset of symptoms. If greater than six hours, with renal recovery less likely, the decision to proceed with an attempt at renal revascularization must consider the overall risk to the patient balanced with the risk of renal function loss (solitary kidney versus a functioning contralateral kidney).

TECHNIQUES FOR INTERVENTION

Endovascular approach to treatment of mesenteric arteries

Access to the abdominal aorta is obtained by either the femoral artery or the left brachial artery. With the advent of shapeable guiding catheters, the author now favors percutaneous femoral access. Upper extremity access may be necessary in the presence of aortoiliac occlusive disease, prior endovascular aneurysm repair (EVAR), hostile or difficult femoral access, a calcified angulated pararenal aorta, or the steep trajectory of the SMA in relationship to the aorta. For upper extremity access, percutaneous access is used when the brachial artery is greater than 5 mm in diameter with open exposure reserved for smaller diameter vessels. In the setting of a small left brachial artery, the axillary artery may be selected. For femoral access, the artery is accessed first with a micropuncture technique following which a standard 5F sheath is placed. It is important to review the CTA to define the optimal view orthogonal to the takeoff of the involved vessel. An aortogram in this projection should identify the SMA and the underlying disease, or, if there is an occlusion, typically one can visualize a short stump representing the vessel orifice. Failure to identify the exact location of the visceral vessel will result in frustration and failed attempts at vessel cannulation. The patient is fully heparinized to maintain an ACT greater than 250. While a number of different catheters—renal double curved (RDC) (Merit Medical OEM, Salt Lake City, UT, USA), Van Shie 2 and 3 (Cook Medical Inc.), and Cobra 2 (Merit Medical OEM)—have been utilized in directing the wire through the orifice and into the SMA or celiac artery, a 7F steerable sheath (Tour Guide™, Medtronic Inc., Santa Clara CA, USA) is preferably utilized due to its simplicity and allowance for multiple different shapes and angles. Alternately, if a tour guide sheath is not available, a standard 7F Destination sheath is utilized (45 cm) and the orifice is crossed with one of the catheters above (Figure 4.2). The authors favor a "no-touch" technique, if possible, without engagement of the sheath or catheter directly into the arterial disease. Rather, one forms the shape of the steerable sheath to the appropriate anticipated angle and direction that will allow gentle probing of the disease with the crossing wire. If difficulty in sheath manipulation is encountered (due to tortuosity or adherence to the access vessel), one can upsize the sheath to a 10F sheath and reinsert the steerable guide catheter. Wires that facilitate crossing of the atherosclerotic disease include the soft Glidewire, the stiff Glidewire, and the Glide Advantage® (Terumo Medical Corp., Somerset, NJ, USA). Occasionally, when there is a very tight stenosis, a smaller diameter wire such as the 0.018 V-18 wire (Boston Scientific, Marlborough, MA), the 0.014 Command ES wire (Abbott, Lake County, IL, USA), or the 0.014 Spartacore wire (Abbott) may be necessary.

The lesion is traversed, and a crossing catheter is placed to obtain a distal angiogram for confirmation of true intraluminal position. The wire is then exchanged for a stiffer wire for stent delivery, such as a Rosen wire (Cook Medical Inc.). With significant occlusive disease, the authors do pre-dilatation with a 4–6 mm balloon to allow for subsequent passage of the stent or stent graft. For orifical disease, the authors prefer to use a balloon-expandable covered stent. For more distal lesions, balloon-expandable bare metal stents may be used to preserve the perfusion of branch vessels. Stents are typically sized 1:1 with target vessel diameter from preoperative CTA or intravascular ultrasound (IVUS) (Philips Healthcare,

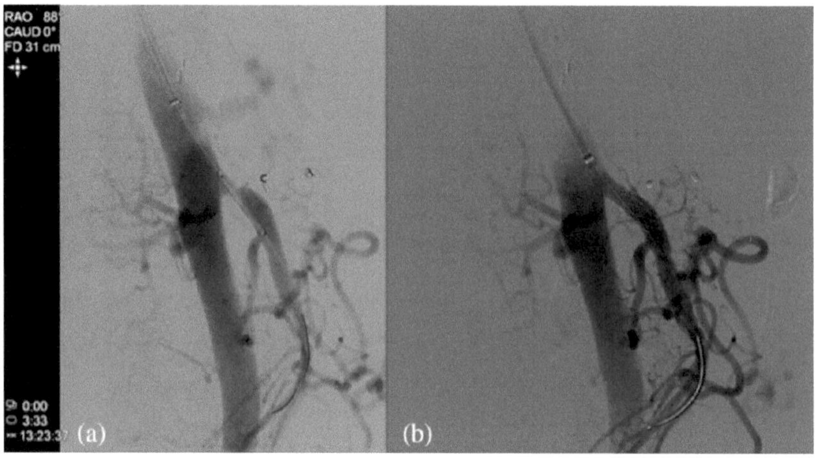

Figure 4.2 Angiogram series showing appropriate orthogonal view with (a) the pre-angioplasty/stent stenosis, and (b), the completion study after stent deployment.

Andover, MA, USA). Stent length is selected based on lesion length. A selective angiogram of the target vessel is completed from the steerable sheath to mark the location of early branches and ensure inadvertent coverage is avoided. Primary PTA alone should be avoided due to the high risk of recurrence. Stents should be deployed with approximately 5 mm of overlap into the abdominal aorta as orifical mesenteric disease is often an extension of aortic atherosclerotic disease. A completion angiogram is then obtained to ensure satisfactory stent expansion and avoidance of distal embolization or dissection. Residual stenosis over 30% should be treated by additional angioplasty. In general, shorter-length stents or stent grafts are utilized in the CA, sized to avoid branch vessel coverage. The CA typically extends 1.5–2.0 cm prior to branching into the left gastric, common hepatic, and splenic arteries. The completion study should show no residual stenosis, good flow through the stent (or stent graft) and the outflow target vessel, and reflux into the aorta to ensure that the stent extends into the aortic lumen beyond the aortic disease. While not routinely used by the author, IVUS may be useful for stent sizing, identification of early branch vessel takeoffs, and detection of postoperative complications such as dissection or inadequate stent expansion. Postoperatively, patients are typically started on dual antiplatelet therapy (DAPT) or a single antiplatelet agent with anticoagulation if not already initiated. The choice of regimen depends on patient comorbidities and etiology of mesenteric ischemia (e.g., embolic versus atherosclerotic). Evidence supporting a specific duration of DAPT is not established, but guidelines suggest a duration of three to 12 months [1].

BRACHIAL ACCESS

When using the brachial or axillary artery for access, the authors prefer to use a 6.5F steerable sheath "bareback." Whether one performs a cutdown or performs the procedure percutaneously is dependent on the size of the artery (the senior author uses 5 mm as the cutoff), the size and thickness of the arm, and the ability to hold pressure against the humerus afterward. For the most part, due to the relatively small size of the vessel, closure devices are avoided. Importantly, with the brachial approach, one needs to traverse the origin of the subclavian and direct the wire and subsequent sheath into the descending aorta. The Rim catheter (Merit Medical OEM), Omni flush catheter (Angiodynamics, Latham, NY, USA), the vertebral catheter (Merit Medical OEM), and the Shepard hook catheter (Merit Medical OEM) have all been utilized to allow the wire to be positioned distally within the descending and distal aorta. A prior CTA study showing the proximal subclavian and the aortic arch is ideal but not always necessary. As noted earlier, the preoperative CTA is used to determine an appropriate image intensifier parallax for the visualization of the target vessel origin. Using a steerable sheath, the origin of the vessel is targeted and one of the previously noted wires is utilized to engage the disease and then be manipulated through the stenosis with the crossing of the lesion (Figure 4.3). The remaining interventional procedure continues as noted earlier with the exception that longer wires and catheter lengths (balloons, balloon-expandable stents, balloon-expandable stent grafts) are necessary to reach and treat the lesion.

SUPERIOR MESENTERIC ARTERY AND CELIAC ARTERY OCCLUSIONS

In chronic total occlusions or high-grade stenoses, cannulation of the target vessel can prove difficult and remains challenging, even in the most experienced hands. In this setting, a review of the patient's preoperative imaging is essential to identify optimal image intensifier parallax for arterial visualization. Obtaining angiography in multiple projections may be necessary to select an optimal view. Magnification may aid in the detection of small channels within high-grade stenoses that may be selected to cross a lesion. The wire selection is greatly expanded including those developed as crossing wires. With wire advancement

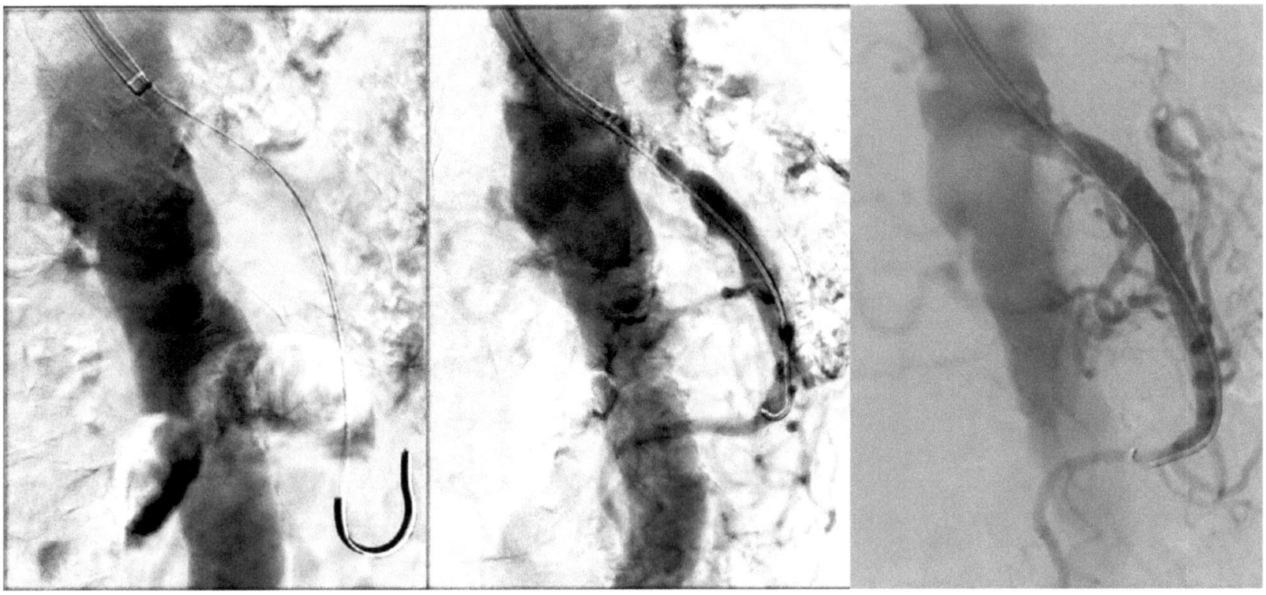

Figure 4.3 Angiogram series showing severe calcific near-occlusion of the SMA, successfully crossed via an upper extremity approach with pre-angioplasty and stent-graft placement extending appropriately into the aortic lumen.

and "purchase" into the area of the occlusion, the use of crossing catheters (Navicross®, Terumo Medical Corp.; Quick-Cross, Philips Healthcare) become instrumental in providing support. Occasionally, a coaxial system with a steerable sheath and an internal shaped catheter are used to gain wire traction on the involved or occluded vessel. A Torque™ device (Terumo Medical Corp.) or angled catheter may assist in navigating the wire through or across a lesion. If aortic angulation precludes cannulation, an alternative access site may be selected. Like all endovascular interventions on occlusions, it is critically important to control the reentry location and ensure that reentry has been accomplished. This prevents one from advancing the wire distally within a false plane. The vessel length from the aortic lumen to the area of reentry will all need to be treated to enable unrestricted flow in the artery distal to the stent.

INFERIOR MESENTERIC ARTERY INTERVENTIONS

The benefit of complete CA and SMA revascularization, whenever possible, had been established in open revascularization as well as in series of endovascular revascularizations. For the most part, the IMA, if diseased, is not intervened upon. However, when *direct* revascularization of the SMA territory cannot be achieved, there may be a role for indirect revascularization by stenting the IMA. Most series of isolated IMA interventions are restricted to case studies. Despite the small numbers, there is good long-term patency in this highly selected patient group when other options were prohibitive [11]. In high-risk patients, with additional comorbid conditions, inclusive of frailty and nutritional depletion, prioritization of IMA stenting over an open procedure for SMA revascularization may be preferable, either as a temporary or long-term solution.

ACUTE MESENTERIC ISCHEMIA

AMI occurs in the setting of acute mesenteric artery occlusion usually related to an embolus, most often cardioembolic in etiology, or acute visceral arterial thrombosis, related to underlying SMA occlusive disease. As such, the removal of the embolism or thrombus is required. The procedure is typically performed in the emergent setting and demands a multidisciplinary approach for the assessment of bowel viability and determining the need for bowel resection. The endovascular setup, access, and approach to the patient are similar to the CMI patient with the notable exception that the surgeon needs to be prepared for both brachial or femoral access, as well as the potential need for diagnostic laparoscopy, exploratory laparotomy, or open SMA exposure. The femoral or brachial approach can be used, but again, the femoral approach is favored. Access to the involved vessel is carried out as previously noted. Once the vessel occlusion has been crossed and distal vessel cannulation confirmed, the next step is endovascular thrombectomy/thrombolysis. Several percutaneous thrombectomy devices are on the market and may be utilized. Most commonly, a suction thrombectomy system is used (e.g., Angioget™, Boston Scientific; JETI™, Abbott; Lightning Bolt™, Penumbra, Alameda, CA, USA). In this setting, to avoid distal embolization, we have utilized distal embolic protection wires (SpiderFx™, Medtronic Inc.) that are retrievable. Residual stenosis following the thrombectomy is common, and whether from residual, adherent thrombus, or atherosclerotic disease, it should be treated by angioplasty

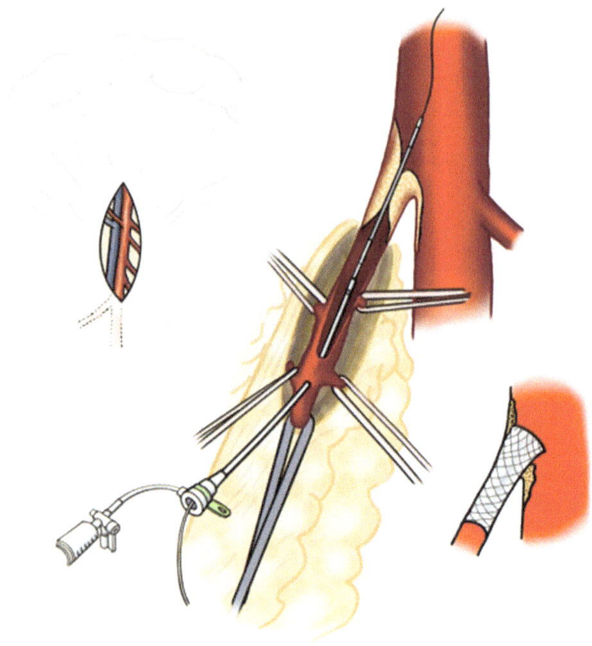

Figure 4.4 Schematic representing retrograde open mesenteric revascularization showing the dissection and exposure of the superior mesenteric artery at the base of the colonic mesentery (left insert) and completion stent-graft deployment (right insert).

and, if orifical, placement of a stent. Recoil, persistent stenosis, or any dissection are indications for stent or stent-graft placement. Completion angiographic images with visualization of the entirety of the vessel and distal vascular bed is mandatory and cannot be over-emphasized. In instances in which all thrombus or embolus cannot be removed, and there is still significant impedance to flow, the surgeon will have to convert to an open procedure to extract the residual thrombus via standard balloon catheter thrombectomy. If the mesenteric vessel cannot be crossed successfully, the authors proceed with open SMA exposure with the intent of performing a ROMS procedure.

RETROGRADE OPEN MESENTERIC STENTING

As noted, if percutaneous techniques are unsuccessful, one proceeds with transabdominal open SMA exposure with the intent of performing a ROMS procedure. Open access of the SMA is performed via an infra-mesocolic approach with exposure of the SMA. The SMA and its corresponding vein can be palpated at the base of the mesentery with the vein lateral to the artery. One can trace the middle colic artery backward down to the SMA, and the SMA is exposed just distal to the middle colic for approximately 4 cm in length. A micropuncture kit is used to access the artery and a short 5 or 6F sheath is placed 1–2 cm into the artery. Angiography is used to identify the occlusive lesion, which may be removed by suction thrombectomy or Fogarty embolectomy. Typically, the wire (Soft Glidewire, Stiff Glidewire, Glidewire Advantage®; Terumo Medical Corp.) can be manipulated through the occlusive lesion in the proximal SMA with reentry into the paravisceral abdominal aorta. Via a retrograde approach, there is direct pushability of the wire and crossing is more likely to be successful. After upsizing the sheath, stenting of the residual atherosclerotic disease and aortic or orifical disease can also be completed, most often with a covered stent graft, sized 1:1 with the artery diameter (Figure 4.4). After obtaining a completion angiogram, the sheath is removed and the arteriotomy is closed, primarily with Proline sutures or by patch angioplasty. This hybrid technique allows for the visualization of the immediate effect of bowel revascularization and a determination of bowel viability.

Endovascular approach to the treatment of renal arteries

Access for renovascular intervention may be via the femoral artery or brachial artery. With the exception of aortoiliac occlusion or hostile femoral artery disease (calcific occlusive disease, aneurysms, open groins, or recent femoral incisions), brachial access is rarely required in primary interventions. As in mesenteric disease, the authors proceed with an initial aortogram to define the location and extent of disease within each renal artery, performed through a 5F flush catheter. Anteroposterior (AP) projections are often satisfactory, but anteriorly or posteriorly displaced renal arteries may require more lateral oblique views. Any preoperative studies (CTA or MRA) as well as intraprocedural angiography are used to delineate the origin and direction of the target renal artery. When intervening upon renal artery occlusive disease, even if bilateral disease is present, the senior author would intervene on only one side at a time. Once the disease is confirmed, the patient is anticoagulated, and the sheath is upsized to a 6F or 7F sheath with insertion of a 6F or 7F guiding catheter (RDC or an appropriately shaped guide) up to the area of the renal artery disease. Again, a "no-touch" technique is employed as much as possible to avoid plowing of the atherosclerotic disease and resultant dissection. The author typically initially utilizes a 0.014 platform, such as the Spartacore wire (Abbott), for crossing of the lesion, and many times, the entire intervention can be carried out on the 0.014 platform. The author finds that for cannulation, it is rarely necessary to upsize to a larger but potentially more traumatic 0.035 wire. Alternately, one can insert a steerable 6.5F sheath bareback that will allow for the appropriate directionality, which can greatly facilitate cannulation. If there is significant angulation, one would then place a crossing catheter and replace the wire with a stiffer 0.035 wire such as the Rosen wire (Cook Medical Inc.) (Figure 4.5). It is imperative in renal artery interventions that one carefully monitors the location of the wire tip, inclusive of the initial cannulation,

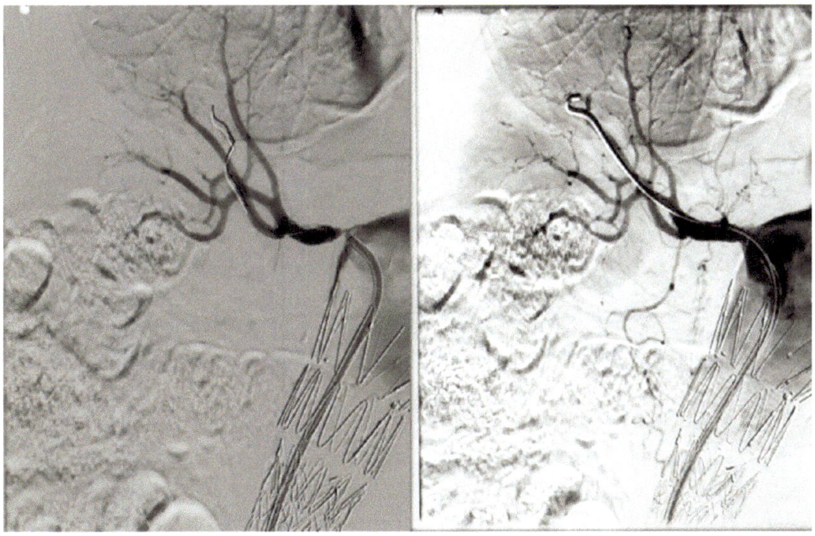

Figure 4.5 Angiogram series showing high-grade right artery stenosis in a patient with a prior endograft who presented with flash pulmonary edema (left renal artery chronically occluded); the right renal artery successfully treated with angioplasty and stenting.

the process of upsizing to a stiffer wire, or subsequent exchanges or interventions. The wire must remain in place within a secondary or tertiary branch, avoiding the loss of renal artery access or risking perforation of smaller branches or even the renal parenchyma. As one frequently intervenes in significantly severe atherosclerotic disease, the author does favor pre-dilatation to ensure non-traumatic passage of the balloon-expandable stent; this also allows for a better size selection of the following stent. When performed on a 0.014 platform, the lesions can be treated with a balloon-expandable stent on a monorail platform, allowing for a smaller-sized sheath and guide catheter. There is no difference in outcomes between balloon-expandable bare metal stents and covered stents. Primary angioplasty alone is not recommended, with the exception of fibromuscular dysplasia, as recurrence rates are high. Angiography or IVUS is utilized to mark early branches and ensure coverage is avoided. Stents should be deployed with 5 mm of overlap into the abdominal aorta as orifical disease is often an extension of aortic atherosclerotic disease. A completion angiogram is obtained to verify stent expansion and detect any complications. As in the endovascular treatment of the mesenteric vessels, IVUS may be useful in renal artery revascularization for stent sizing, identification of early branch vessel takeoffs, or detection of postoperative complications such as dissection or inadequate stent expansion. Patients should be observed for blood pressure lability postoperatively with appropriate adjustments made to their home antihypertensive regimen.

TROUBLESHOOTING

Due to angulation of the target vessel and aorta, passing the stent across a lesion may prove difficult and cause the wire to bow into the aorta. This can be avoided by using a stiffer wire or by advancing the wire further into the target vessel. Pre-dilation of the lesion with a small diameter balloon and swallowing the balloon with the steerable sheath can be used to then un-sheath the balloon-expandable stent when the stent will not easily cross the stenosis.

CONSIDERATIONS IN INADVERTENT COVERAGE OF THE RENAL ARTERIES DURING EVAR

Techniques for the treatment of inadvertent coverage of the renal arteries depend on when the coverage is identified. If identified during the index procedure, techniques exist to mobilize the endograft caudally. Some endografts have options to re-constrain and redeploy the endograft in a more caudal location. If such options are not available, a wire may be snared from the contralateral femoral artery and withdrawn to create a "flossing," "through-and-through" access. A long crossing catheter is placed over the wire to prevent shearing of the endograft. Both ends are pulled caudally to displace the endograft. However, this technique should be employed with utmost caution as injury to the aorta or crushing of the iliac limbs may occur. Alternatively, the affected renal artery may be cannulated and covered or bare metal stents deployed across the origin to maintain patency. In this setting, it is imperative to extend the stents approximately at least 5 mm into the aorta and to flare the proximal stent to allow for the sealing and prevention of stent migration. Brachial access is often required in these cases to cannulate the renal arteries on the outside of the aortic endograft.

COMPLICATIONS

Complications following mesenteric or renal artery interventions are most frequently related to access site issues including hematoma (<4–5%), pseudoaneurysm (<1%), dissection (<1%), and vessel thrombosis (<1%). Brachial access hematomas are particularly worrisome due to the risk of median nerve compression, which requires emergent hematoma evacuation. Additional target vessel complications include perforation, dissection, or embolization. In the setting of target vessel dissection, a self-expanding stent may be deployed to prevent propagation. Perforation may be treated with stent-graft placement or coil embolization of the branch vessels, recognizing that renal artery branches are end vessels. Atheroembolization may result from uncontrolled wire and sheath manipulation in a diseased aorta or during the crossing of lesions. This may lead to bowel ischemia, renal compromise, or lower extremity ischemia depending on the affected vessel. The use of embolic protection devices has been described, but insufficient evidence exists to support routine use. The creation of a dissection plane and stent deployment into a target vessel false lumen can create a serious complication, especially if left undetected. As such, it is crucial to confirm the true intraluminal position with catheter angiography or IVUS after crossing all lesions. False lumen stenting can be salvaged by gaining true lumen position and stenting past the malpositioned stent. However, this can prove extremely difficult, and aborting endovascular techniques for open revascularization may be necessary. Long-term complications include in-stent stenosis, stent occlusion, or stent migration.

POSTOPERATIVE RESULTS AND SURVEILLANCE

Endovascular techniques are utilized with high rates of technical success in the revascularization of the mesenteric and renal arteries, with most studies reporting technical success exceeding 95% [12]. These results are reproducible in the setting of acute mesenteric ischemia with endovascular success rates of 90% [13]. Less data is available on endovascular salvage of occluded renal arteries following EVAR or B/FEVAR. Thirty-day mortality following endovascular treatment of CMI is near 2% with significantly higher mortality rates of 20% in the setting of AMI [6, 13, 14]. Technical success and in-hospital mortality following ROMS are comparable to percutaneous endovascular treatment of AMI [15]. Lifelong surveillance after mesenteric stenting begins with a one-month clinic visit and mesenteric duplex ultrasound. Follow-up may then be increased to every six months for two years and then annually. Any stenosis should be followed up with CTA. Follow-up should be sooner if recurrent symptoms develop. Reintervention is warranted in the setting of recurrent symptoms with imaging demonstrating recurrent stenosis or occlusion. If re-stenosis or occlusion occurs in the absence of symptoms, we would recommend shared decision-making between patient and provider to decide upon intervention, the clinician assessing the overall risk of recurrent symptoms developing. The author prefers to manage re-stenosis or occlusion aggressively with an endovascular first approach to prevent recurrent symptoms, provided the patient has a reasonable life expectancy. Similar follow-up is initiated after renal artery interventions. Antiplatelet therapy and lipid-lowering agents should be continued lifelong. It is recommended that DAPT is initiated for the initial first three to 12 months following mesenteric and renal revascularization, although the long-term benefits of DAPT over single antiplatelet therapy are unproven [1].

In summary, endovascular revascularization is the treatment of choice on mesenteric or renal occlusive disease (whether acute or chronic) once the patient meets the criteria for intervention. The benefit established by a less invasive means of renal or mesenteric revascularization more than offsets the reduction in patency, especially as most recurrent disease can also be managed endovascularly.

TRICKS AND TRAPS

1. Endovascular revascularization for CMI is the preferred revascularization method with less morbidity and hospital stays and costs, yet comparable long-term mortality when compared to open revascularization procedures.
2. For successful CMI endovascular revascularization, the vascular surgeon needs to be familiar and comfortable with both femoral and upper extremity access.
3. For CMI visceral vessel occlusion, special techniques are required with successful wire reintervention into the distal patent lumen, thus ensuring a successful endovascular intervention.
4. For AMI, an emergent multidisciplinary approach is mandated, and thrombectomy/thrombolysis devices and techniques are necessary to achieve a successful patient outcome.
5. For AMI, retrograde open mesenteric revascularization is a life-saving option (when other first-line efforts fail or are unable to be performed) that all vascular specialists need to be familiar with.
6. Renal artery interventions for both chronic real artery occlusive disease and acute renal artery occlusion, although uncommonly performed, are deemed complex with special attention paid to wire selection and positioning, mandating a high-level endovascular skill set, avoiding renal artery dissection, occlusion, or perforation.

QUESTIONS

1. Endovascular techniques are recommended over open surgical revascularization in chronic mesenteric ischemia due to:

a. Lower rates of symptom recurrence
b. Lower perioperative complications
c. Improved long-term survival
d. Lower rates of re-stenosis requiring intervention

Answer: b

2. When treating orificial mesenteric artery disease, which of the following stents is recommended?
   a. Balloon-expandable covered stent
   b. Self-expanding covered stent
   c. Angioplasty alone
   d. Self-expanding bare metal stent

   Answer: a

3. Which of the following is an accepted indication for renal artery stenting?
   a. Bilateral renal artery stenosis (>70%) in a patient with concurrent SMA stenosis (>70%)
   b. Unilateral renal artery stenosis in a single functioning kidney associated with hypertension controlled on a maximum dose of a beta-blocker and calcium channel blocker
   c. Bilateral renal artery stenosis (>70%) in a patient associated with an episode of flash pulmonary edema
   d. Bilateral renal artery stenosis (>70%) in a patient less than 50 years of age

   Answer: c

4. Guidelines recommend follow-up after mesenteric stenting according to which schedule in the absence of recurrent symptoms?
   a. Clinic visit and CT angiography at one-month post-op; every six months until two years post-op; and then annually
   b. Clinic visit and mesenteric duplex ultrasound at one-month post-op; every six months until two years post-op; and then annually
   c. Clinic visit and mesenteric duplex annually
   d. Clinic visit and CT angiography at one-month post-op and then annually

   Answer: b

REFERENCES

1. Bjorck, M., et al., Editor's choice - management of the diseases of mesenteric arteries and veins: Clinical practice guidelines of the European society of vascular surgery (ESVS). *Eur J Vasc Endovasc Surg*, 2017. 53(4): p. 460–510.
2. Thomas, J.H., et al., The clinical course of asymptomatic mesenteric arterial stenosis. *J Vasc Surg*, 1998. 27(5): p. 840–4.
3. Huber, T.S., et al., Chronic mesenteric ischemia: Clinical practice guidelines from the society for vascular surgery. *J Vasc Surg*, 2021. 73(1S): p. 87S–115S.
4. Hogendoorn, W., et al., A comparison of open and endovascular revascularization for chronic mesenteric ischemia in a clinical decision model. *J Vasc Surg*, 2014. 60(3): p. 715–25 e2.
5. Malgor, R.D., et al., Results of single- and two-vessel mesenteric artery stents for chronic mesenteric ischemia. *Ann Vasc Surg*, 2010. 24(8): p. 1094–101.
6. Peck, M.A., et al., Intermediate-term outcomes of endovascular treatment for symptomatic chronic mesenteric ischemia. *J Vasc Surg*, 2010. 51(1): p. 140–7 e1-2.
7. Cooper, C.J., et al., Stenting and medical therapy for atherosclerotic renal-artery stenosis. *N Engl J Med*, 2014. 370(1): p. 13–22.
8. Investigators, A., et al., Revascularization versus medical therapy for renal-artery stenosis. *N Engl J Med*, 2009. 361(20): p. 1953–62.
9. Sarafidis, P.A., et al., Atherosclerotic renovascular disease: a clinical practice document by the European Renal Best Practice (ERBP) board of the European Renal Association (ERA) and the Working Group Hypertension and the Kidney of the European Society of Hypertension (ESH). *Nephrol Dial Transplant*, 2023. 38(12): p. 2835–50.
10. Konstantinou, N., et al., Revascularization of occluded renal artery stent grafts after complex endovascular aortic repair and its impact on renal function. *J Vasc Surg*, 2021. 73(5): p. 1566–72.
11. Schneider, D.B., et al., Isolated inferior mesenteric artery revascularization for chronic visceral ischemia. *J Vasc Surg*, 1999. 30(1): p. 51–8.
12. Nana, P., et al., A systematic review of endovascular repair outcomes in atherosclerotic chronic mesenteric ischaemia. *Eur J Vasc Endovasc Surg*, 2023. 66(5): p. 632–43.
13. Li, W., et al., Treatment outcomes in patients with acute thromboembolic occlusion of the superior mesenteric artery. *J Cardiothorac Surg*, 2024. 19(1): p. 235.
14. Alahdab, F., et al., A systematic review and meta-analysis of endovascular versus open surgical revascularization for chronic mesenteric ischemia. *J Vasc Surg*, 2018. 67(5): p. 1598–605.
15. Habib, S.G., et al., A decade's experience with retrograde open mesenteric stenting for acute mesenteric ischemia. *J Vasc Surg*, 2024. 80(3): p. 831–7.

5

Endovascular management of aortoiliac occlusive disease

SACHINDER S. HANS

INTRODUCTION

Aortoiliac occlusive disease (AIOD) is a chronic atherosclerotic arterial occlusive disease that typically involves the aortic bifurcation and iliac arteries but can gradually progress both proximally up the aorta and distally down to and into the femoral arteries. Clinical presentation depends on the extent of the involved segments and can vary from intermittent claudication of the hip (buttock-gluteal region), thigh, or calf to ischemic rest pain and/or tissue loss (chronic limb-threatening ischemia [CLTI]) in the foot secondary to multilevel occlusive disease. Vascular interventions are typically indicated for patients presenting with severe claudication, CLTI (Rutherford class 3–6), or distal embolization resulting in blue toe syndrome. As a result of advances in imaging, stent technology, and intravascular lithotripsy (IVL; Shockwave Medical, Santa Clara, CA, USA) over the past decade, endovascular management of AIOD has demonstrated high rates of successful revascularization and limb salvage with low morbidity. Direct surgical reconstruction with an aortofemoral bypass graft provides superior primary patency but at the cost of increased morbidity and mortality [1–4].

Clinical examination of the patient should include complete pulse examination and noninvasive arterial testing (segmental pressure testing including waveforms and toe pressures). A diminished femoral pulse with bruit, decreased thigh segmental pressure with diminished amplitude, and a monophasic common femoral artery Doppler waveform are all suggestive of AIOD. In a small number of patients, a normal pulse exam and normal ABI can be obtained in the presence of hemodynamically significant AIOD. In these patients, exercise testing on a treadmill with resting and post-exercise ABI can help diagnose the presence of a significant stenosis. However, other causes of claudication (i.e., neurogenic due to lumbar stenosis or herniated disc) should be ruled out in patients with normal exercise testing. Computed tomographic angiography (CTA) is extremely useful in procedural planning because of its ability to define the arterial anatomy, severity of disease, and degree of calcification in three-dimensional views. Magnetic resonance angiography (MRA) has a limited role except in patients with a history of anaphylaxis to iodinated contrast agents as it frequently overestimates the degree of stenosis and cannot determine the morphology of occlusive lesions (e.g., associated calcification). Diagnosis of concomitant aortic, common femoral, and profunda femoris disease helps in determining the feasibility of endovascular versus open revascularization and if a percutaneous versus hybrid approach is necessary. In addition, for percutaneous endoluminal interventions, the most appropriate type of access (ipsilateral femoral, contralateral femoral, or brachial access) can be selected.

The hemodynamic significance of questionable lesions can be determined at the time of angiography by measuring intraarterial pressures using a "pullback" method. Significant concomitant common femoral disease and in particular orifical profunda stenosis usually requires a hybrid approach with groin cutdown for exposure/endarterectomy of the femoral artery [2].

TECHNIQUES FOR INTERVENTION

Arterial access is usually obtained via ipsilateral retrograde or a contralateral common femoral artery (CFA) approach depending on the extent of disease, tortuosity of the aortoiliac arteries, and severity of calcification. If a femoral approach appears to be unsatisfactory, left brachial access (either percutaneous or by cutdown) is also a good option. For aortoiliac lesions, ipsilateral retrograde transfemoral access is typically obtained using ultrasound guidance and a micropuncture needle, microwire,

DOI: 10.1201/9781003452096-5

and microsheath (Angiodynamics, Marlborough, MA, USA). Following the passage of a microsheath over the microwire, a short 0.035" J-wire is advanced and a short 5F sheath is inserted. This sheath is upsized depending on the type of intervention planned and the need for bare metal or covered stenting. Full-dose anticoagulation should be obtained prior to intervention and should be continuously monitored with an activated clotting time (ACT) machine. We usually administer 100 units/kg of heparin prior to crossing a significant stenosis and maintain an ACT > 250 sec for the duration of the procedure. For lesions in the contralateral iliac, a longer sheath (45 cm long 6F Pinnacle; Terumo Medical, Tokyo, Japan) can be placed after confirmatory angiography. A contralateral up-and-over technique should be used in patients with mid to distal common iliac artery (CIA) lesions or for external iliac artery (EIA) stenosis or occlusion. For lesions involving the most proximal segment of the CIA, an ipsilateral retrograde femoral approach or a left brachial approach should be considered. In patients with tortuous iliac anatomy or a steeply angled bifurcation (frequently encountered in patients with prior aortic endografts or aortoiliac/femoral bifurcation grafts), it is virtually impossible to use the contralateral femoral approach to pass a catheter "up and over" the aortic bifurcation.

In these uncommon situations, trans-brachial access is a more useful alternative if ipsilateral retrograde femoral access is not possible or successful. Left brachial artery access is far preferable to right brachial artery access as there is a potentially higher risk of cerebral embolization from crossing the aortic arch from the right side. Trans-brachial access using brachial artery cutdown is preferable if larger than a 6F sheath is necessary. The incidence of brachial artery complications is greater in women due to their smaller diameter brachial arteries. Careful manipulation of the wire and catheter in the distal aortic arch should be performed when using trans-brachial access to reduce the risk of embolic complications. We prefer to use an Omniflush (5F) catheter (Angiodynamics Inc, Latham, NY, USA) with its tip pointing toward the left shoulder in LAO projection in order to advance a stiff angled glide wire into the descending thoracic aorta and subsequently into the abdominal aorta followed by the Omniflush catheter over the wire.

Crossing an iliac stenosis/occlusion is often helped using a torque device on the guide wire and a support catheter (Kumpe catheter). In general, flush occlusions are more difficult to cross than those with a short stump at the origin of the common iliac artery. Most occlusions can be crossed without resorting to a special re-entry catheter. Special considerations in patients with heavily calcified, eccentric, near occlusive lesions in the iliac arteries are necessary. Retrograde femoral access in this type of lesion may result in inadvertent entry of the wire into a subintimal plane with further attempts to enter the true lumen being unsuccessful. Contralateral femoral access with up-and-over placement of a long 6 Fr sheath (45cm) with attempted passage of a regular (soft) glide wire with an appropriate support catheter (we prefer a 4 Fr glide catheter) is often successful. A stiff glide wire may result in prolapse of the sheath and catheters cephalad with an inability to advance the wire toward the groin. Using a torque device with rapid clockwise spinning of the 0.035" floppy glide wire tip like a drill with catheter support can be successful in most cases.

Puncture of the brachial artery should be performed in its distal portion in the antecubital fossa under ultrasound guidance. The artery is relatively superficial, and after sheath removal, it can be compressed against the humerus to obtain hemostasis. The use of radial artery access is expanding, and data supports its use for iliac artery interventions. Left radial access is preferred. Longer sheaths and catheters (110–125 cm) are required before initiating an intervention; one should have the availability of catheters with 6 Fr compatibility.

In 10–15% of cases, plaque morphology (severely fibrotic and calcified lesions) may necessitate a subintimal approach and use of crossing catheters. While there are a variety of such catheters available, we prefer the Pioneer Plus re-entry device with intravascular ultrasound (IVUS) guided clarity (Philips Inc-Volcano). This catheter consists of a monorail double-lumen catheter, integrated with an IVUS array (Volcano, San Diego, CA, USA) and equipped with a curved needle allowing for passage of a 0.014" non-hydrophilic guidewire back into the lumen [5]. Once the 0.035" guidewire penetrates the subintimal place, it is exchanged for a 0.014" guidewire and the Pioneer catheter is advanced. With the catheter in place, the IVUS system is activated to detect the position of the true lumen and the quality of the blood flow through a color-flow mode (chromoflow) feature. Using this modality, the operator can choose the best area to cross back into the lumen from the subintimal space. By turning the handlebar at the bottom of the catheter to push the needle out (7 mm below the IVUS array), the intimal layer is perforated, allowing the passage of the re-entry guidewire into the true lumen. The length of the needle can be modified through the handlebar of the catheter with a range varying from 1 to 7 mm. Occasionally, the needle may not be able to penetrate heavily calcified plaque.

The Outback catheter (Cordis Corp., Bridgewater, NJ, USA) is an older monorail single lumen crossing catheter with a curved needle at its top for penetrating the intima. It is more commonly used for re-entry into the distal superficial femoral and popliteal artery than for iliac artery occlusions [5].

STENT SELECTION

Preoperative assessment of the diameter of a stenotic or occluded segment can be obtained by CTA measurements. If a preoperative imaging study is inadequate or not available, pretreatment measurement of the vessel

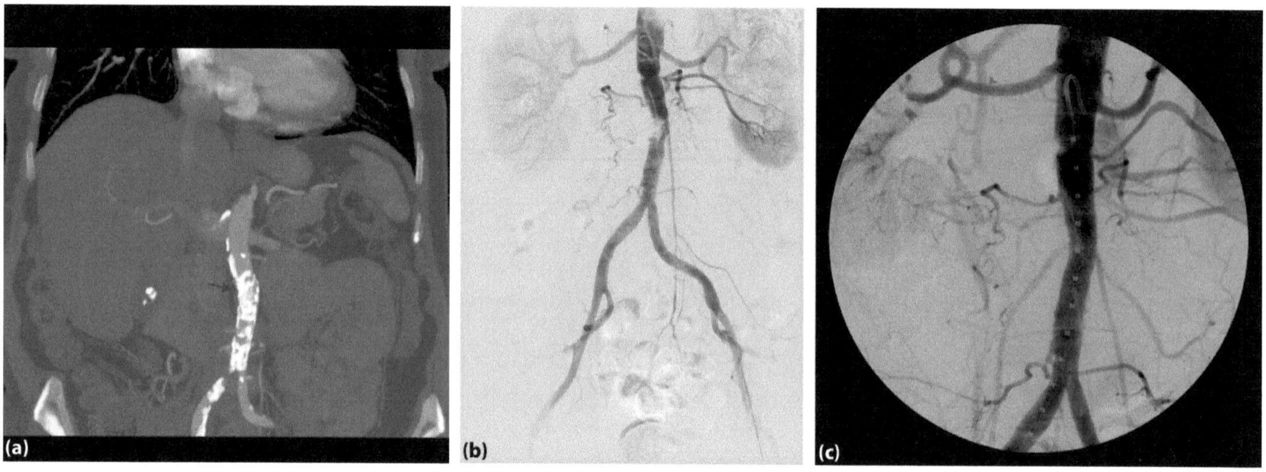

Figure 5.1 (a) CTA arteriogram showing a calcified, eccentric, severe (80%), and focal infrarenal aortic stenosis; (b) aortogram confirming the presence of this infrarenal aortic stenosis; (c) post-deployment of a balloon-expandable covered stent.

diameter and length can be performed simply with a marker catheter or more accurately from arteriographic images using the integrated computer system in the intervention suite. For heavily calcified lesions, we prefer using an intravascular lithotripsy (IVL) catheter (Shockwave Medical) that is passed across a calcified lesion on a 0.014" wire and activated after expanding the integrated balloon to a pressure of 4 atmospheres. The length of the balloon or stent used for iliac lesions should only cover the diseased segment without causing intimal damage in the relative normal artery proximally and distally. Slow balloon insufflation with a gradual increase in the size of the balloon is helpful if the lesion is eccentric and heavily calcified. In general, oversized stents (5–10%) are used except in severely calcified lesions where there is an increased risk of arterial rupture. Stent types include bare metal stents and covered stents in both self-expanding and balloon-expandable varieties. In proximal CIA lesions, covered balloon-expandable stents are preferable (VBX WL Gore Newark, DE, USA or iCAST Medimack, NH, USA) [6]. A careful measurement of the required stent length should be obtained to avoid inadvertent coverage of the internal iliac artery. Balloon-expandable stents allow for precise stent placement and provide strong hoop strength and excellent radiolucency on fluoroscopy. The disadvantage of balloon-expandable stents is that there is a small risk of deformity of the stent in the presence of heavy arterial wall calcification. Self-expanding stents are often preferable in EIA lesions or even in CIA lesions if there is significant tortuosity, but the precision of stent placement is not as good as with balloon-expandable stents.

AORTIC AND AORTIC BIFURCATION AND ILIAC ARTERY LESIONS

For isolated localized infrarenal aortic high-grade stenosis/occlusion, covered balloon-expandable stents are preferable (Figure 5.1). In patients with distal aortic stenosis/occlusion extending into the proximal CIAs, "kissing" stents, i.e., with simultaneous balloon insufflation or stent deployment, are typically used. Even in the presence of a unilateral lesion, treatment of one side can result in plaque shifting with contralateral CIA luminal compression, plaque embolization, or dissection. In the presence of distal aortic disease just proximal to the bifurcation, stents can be deployed from just above the aortic plaque down into the CIAs in a "kissing" stent manner (Figure 5.2). In patients with total CIA occlusions, retrograde ipsilateral or contralateral access may result in the passage of the wire into a subintimal plane. Despite the availability of crossing catheters, true lumen re-entry into the proximal CIA may be unsuccessful. In this situation, arm access via the left brachial artery should be considered (Figure 5.3).

COVERED ENDOVASCULAR RECONSTRUCTION OF AORTIC BIFURCATION

The randomized covered versus balloon expandable stent trial (COBEST) has reported encouraging results highlighting the benefits of covered stents in both the distal aorta and the iliac arteries [7]. This trial showed the superiority of covered stents for TASC II C and D lesions as compared with bare metal stents. In addition, such lesions are complex and may be difficult to cross with the potential of flow limiting dissection, perforation, and distal embolization, the risks of which can be minimized by the deployment of a covered stent [7].

Most reported studies comparing aortobifemoral graft with iliac stenting are non-randomized case series with results showing equivalent limb salvage rates and secondary patencies. Primary patency is superior with aortobifemoral grafting but at the cost of significant morbidity, some mortality, increased length of stay, and longer return to work. Moreover, the comparison is only

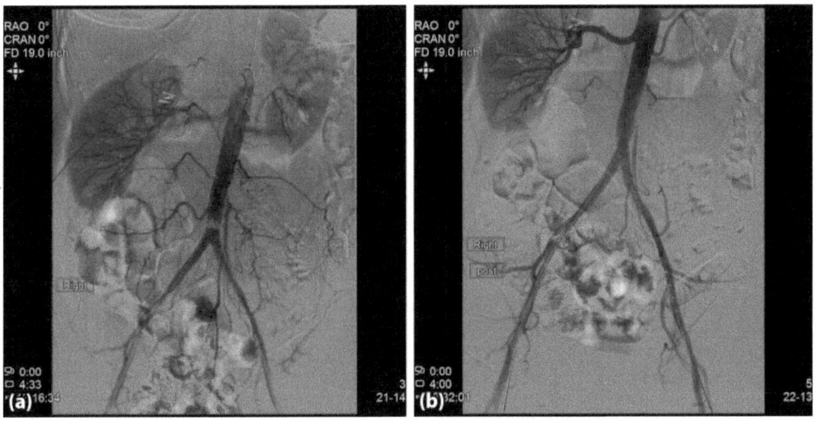

Figure 5.2 (a) Severe focal aortic stenosis just proximal to aortic bifurcation; (b) following treatment with bilateral "kissing," balloon-expandable covered stents.

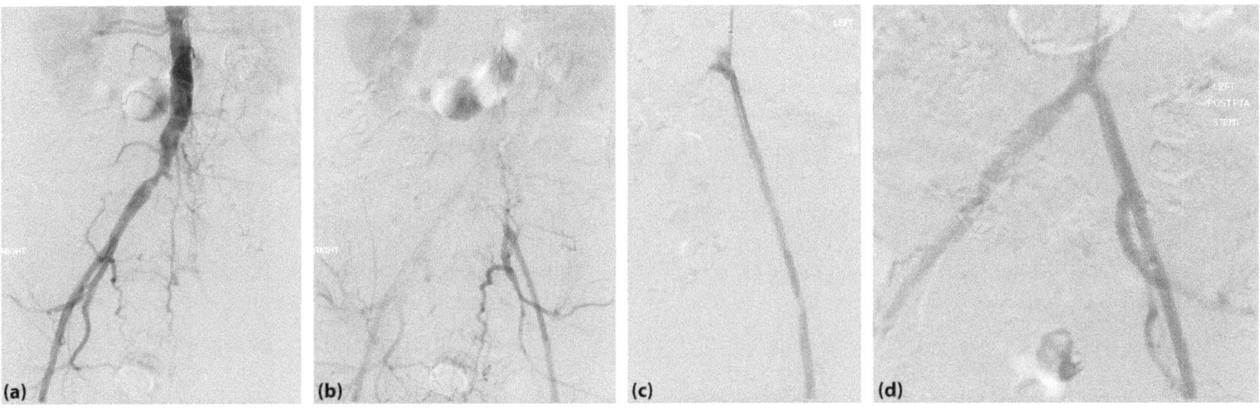

Figure 5.3 (a) TASC-B lesion with occlusion of the left common iliac artery and reconstitution of left common iliac artery bifurcation; (b) continued; (c) crossing of the lesion with 0.035" exchange wire using left brachial access and deployment of a left common iliac stent; (d) continued.

valid if the lesions can be crossed—in a small number of cases, an endovascular intervention may not be technically feasible. The author prefers open arterial reconstruction in younger, good risk patients with TASC C and D lesions, patients with a hypoplastic aorta, and cases of infrarenal aortic occlusion. In the last group, crossing a total occlusion can be extremely challenging, and even if successful, the risk of complications is higher. An endovascular approach is clearly more suited for patients with advanced age and multiple medical comorbidities. The author prefers an endovascular approach to extra-anatomic grafting (i.e., femoral-femoral or axillo-femoral bypass) in such patients.

MAJOR COMPLICATIONS

Iliac artery perforation/rupture is the most serious complication of iliac stenting and needs immediate diagnosis by contrast injection followed by balloon insufflation (tamponade) and placement of a covered stent. Delay in diagnosis/treatment can result in significant morbidity and even mortality due to severe bleeding. Arterial access-related complications include arterial dissection, pseudoaneurysm, arteriovenous fistula, and retroperitoneal hematoma in patients with an arterial access puncture close to or above the inguinal ligament, usually cephalad to the origins of the inferior superficial epigastric and lateral circumflex iliac arteries. These two branches are a landmark for the EIA-CFA junction. Ultrasound guided arterial access has been shown to reduce access-related complications and should be used universally.

Stent-related complications include stent dislodgement, migration, misplacement, and embolization, often due to undersizing. Stent fracture, and rarely, infection and nickel allergy have been reported. In stent re-stenosis from intimal hyperplasia, progression of atherosclerotic disease and thrombosis in the stent are more commonly recognized problems in follow-up. Though closure devices (femoral access) are increasingly used, particularly for larger caliber punctures, it should be noted that manual compression is a satisfactory method of obtaining hemostasis. Complete reversal of heparin and adequate blood pressure control are recommended prior to manual compression. Several studies have found there is no overall benefit in clinical outcomes using vascular closure devices compared with manual compression; however, there is a significant reduction in time to hemostasis and time to ambulation with the use of these devices. Closure device placement is often contraindicated in the presence of heavy femoral artery calcification. Post-procedure, the patient is given a loading dose of clopidogrel (300 mg) if not already on it, followed by 75 mg daily for one month along with long-term use of aspirin 81 mg daily. Post-intervention follow-up includes a complete pulse exam immediately after the intervention and a noninvasive arterial study of the lower extremities at one-month and three-month intervals for one year followed by yearly noninvasive and clinical assessment. Statins should be started prior to the intervention and continued indefinitely post-intervention.

TRICKS AND TRAPS

1. High-quality CTA imaging for preprocedural planning is very helpful.
2. The access site (ipsilateral femoral, contralateral femoral, or left brachial) should be selected on the basis of the location of the lesion to be treated, the extent of calcification, and the presence of concomitant common femoral and profunda disease. Access should be obtained under ultrasound guidance.
3. In the presence of common femoral/profunda disease, a hybrid procedure consisting of cutdown and femoral endarterectomy with simultaneous iliac intervention (stenting) should be performed.
4. Brachial artery cutdown is preferred over percutaneous puncture for brachial access if a 6F or larger sheath is required; this step reduces access site complications, particularly in women with small size arteries.
5. Bilateral "kissing" stents are often used for proximal CIA lesions even if the disease is unilateral to prevent complications (i.e., contralateral luminal compression).
6. In general, balloon-expandable stents are preferred for CIA lesions and self-expanding stents for EIA lesions.
7. Covered balloon-expandable stents are preferable for infrarenal aortic pathology and proximal CIA lesions in the presence of heavy calcification.
8. A sudden drop in blood pressure with concomitant tachycardia or any complaints of abdominal discomfort, nausea, or diaphoresis mandates an on-table arteriography to rule out rupture/perforation of the iliac artery, which is treated with immediate balloon insufflation and deployment of a covered stent.

QUESTIONS

1. A 68-year-old woman with severe right hip claudication has a right common iliac artery occlusion (4 cm in length) and a 70% stenosis at the origin of her left common iliac artery. She has a known left subclavian artery occlusion. Attempted interventions from ipsilateral femoral access and contralateral femoral access were unsuccessful. The next best option is:
   a. Aortobifemoral graft
   b. Stenting of the left common iliac artery and cross-over femoral-femoral graft
   c. Right brachial access for right common iliac artery intervention and retrograde access of the left iliac lesion from the left common femoral artery for placement of bilateral "kissing" stents
   d. Right axillary access for percutaneous common iliac artery intervention

   Answer: c

2. A 72-year-old woman has bilateral hip and thigh claudication on walking 50 yards. Ankle brachial index on the right is 0.64 and on the left is 0.66. CTA shows focal calcified 90% stenosis of the infrarenal abdominal aorta just above the origin of a small diameter inferior mesenteric artery. The best management option is:
   a. Aortic endarterectomy
   b. Self-expanding bare metal stent
   c. Balloon-expandable bare metal stent
   d. Balloon-expandable covered stent

   Answer: d

3. The reported complications of iliac stenting are:
   a. Iliac artery rupture
   b. Maldeployment of the stent
   c. Distal embolization
   d. All of the above

   Answer: d

4. The following statement best reflects the results of iliac stenting as compared with aortobifemoral grafting for TASC C and D lesions:
   a. Iliac stenting has superior primary patency and equal secondary patency
   b. Iliac stenting has inferior primary patency but equal secondary patency
   c. Iliac stenting has both superior primary and secondary patency
   d. Aortobifemoral grafting has superior primary patency and a superior secondary patency

   Answer: b

REFERENCES

1. Hans S.S., DeSantis D., Siddiqui R., Khoury M. Results of endovascular therapy and aortobifemoral grafting for trans-Atlantic inter-society type C and D aortoiliac occlusive disease. *Surgery* 2008; 144: 583–589.

2. Kashyap V.S., Parkop M.L., Bena J.F. et al. The management of severe aortoiliac occlusive disease: Endovascular therapy rivals open reconstruction. *J. Vasc. Surg.* 2008; 48: 1451–1457.
3. Sachwani G.R., Hans S.S., Khoury M.D. et al. Results of iliac stenting and aortobifemoral grafting for iliac artery occlusion. *J. Vasc. Surg.* 2013; 577: 1030–1037.
4. Premratne S., Newman J., Hobbs S. et al. Meta-analysis of direct surgical versus endovascular revascularization for aortoiliac occlusive disease. *J. Vasc. Surg.* 2020; 72: 726–737.
5. Pescatori L.C., Tacher V., Kobeiter H. The use of re-entry devices in aortoiliac occlusive disease. *Front Cardiovasc Med.* 2020; 7: 144. PMID:33062643.
6. Mwipatyi B.P., Ourel K., Anwari T. et al. A systematic review of covered balloon expandable stent for treating aortoiliac occlusive disease. *J. Vasc. Surg.* 2020; 72(4): 1473–1486.
7. Mwipatyi B.P., Sharma S., Daneshmand A. et al. Durability of the balloon expandable covered stents versus bare-metal stents in the covered versus balloon expandable stent trial (COBEST) for the treatment of aortoiliac occlusive disease. *J. Vasc. Surg.* 2016; 64: 83–94.

6

Percutaneous intervention for femoropopliteal artery occlusive disease

TIMOTHY J. NYPAVER

INTRODUCTION

The femoropopliteal segment is the most common location of lower extremity peripheral arterial occlusive disease. Atherosclerotic lesions within the superficial femoral artery (SFA) tend to be long and diffuse, making interventions more challenging, both in their approach and durability. Furthermore, the SFA and popliteal arteries are high resistance and low flow in character and subject to mechanical stresses from joint flexion, variables that adversely affect the long-term patency of any endovascular intervention. The decision to intervene is based on three major factors: (1) symptoms; (2) the natural history of the disease process; and (3) whether the patient will experience a meaningful benefit from a technically successful procedure. Most important is the distinction between claudication, which is non-limb-threatening, from critical limb-threatening ischemia (CLTI), which is associated with major limb loss. Multiple anatomical classification systems can guide the decision-making process for the type of intervention, the most common of which is the TransAtlantic Inter-Society Consensus (TASC) II classification. General recommendations from the TASC Working Group include endovascular treatment for type A and B lesions, open surgical treatment for type D lesions, and either endovascular or open options for type C lesions [1]. The choice of the best first option for patients with lower extremity peripheral arterial disease, especially those with CLTI, continues to be debated. Recent randomized studies have attempted to delineate the best option for CLTI patients. The Best Endovascular versus Best Surgical Therapy in Patients with CLTI (BEST-CLI) trial was an international multicenter randomized superiority trial where CLTI patients were randomized to either open bypass or endovascular intervention conducted over an approximately six-year period. The study consisted of two separate cohorts dependent on the availability and use of the single segment greater saphenous vein (SSGSV) as the bypass conduit versus the need for an alternate conduit for patients randomized to open revascularization [2]. The findings of the study were as follows: for CLTI patients who had an adequate SSGSV and were considered suitable candidates for either endovascular revascularization or open revascularization, there was an associated 32% lower risk of major adverse limb events or death in the open bypass group compared with an endovascular-first approach (median follow-up: 2.7 years; 42.6 vs 57.4%, respectively; hazard ratio: 0.68; 95% confidence interval: 0.59–0.79; $p<0.001$). The BEST-CLI study concluded that for those CLTI patients with an adequate SSGSV for surgical revascularization, surgical intervention was favored due to a lower incidence of a major adverse limb event (MALE) or death. MALE was defined as above-ankle amputation of the index limb or a major index-limb reintervention (new bypass, interposition graft revision, thrombectomy or thrombolysis). Among the CLTI patients who lacked an adequate SSGSV vein conduit, the outcomes in the two groups were similar [2]. In contrast, in the United Kingdom Bypass versus Angioplasty for Severe Ischemia of the Leg Trial (BASIL-2), a surgical revascularization strategy was associated with a 35% increase in relative risk of amputation or death compared with endovascular intervention [3]. The difference in these studies in terms of patient enrollment, and both operative and endovascular outcomes, are being subjected to increasing scrutiny to define and expand upon their respective findings. In practice, the vascular surgeon must consider a variety of factors to make the most appropriate treatment recommendation, which includes the patient's surgical risk, symptom severity, wound depth and extent, ambulatory ability, living status, and the durability of the planned intervention [4,5].

DOI: 10.1201/9781003452096-6

INDICATION FOR INTERVENTION: CLAUDICATION

Claudication is defined as major muscle group pain with ambulation that occurs at a level below that of the atherosclerotic disease. For lesions within the SFA and popliteal artery, this typically occurs in the calf. The natural history of claudication secondary to SFA and popliteal artery occlusive disease is relatively benign with <5% patients progressing to CLTI [1, 4–7]. Confirmation of the disease with the measurement of an ankle-brachial pressure index (ABPI) and risk factor modification are the mandatory initial steps in patient management. Intervention is recommended if the claudication symptoms are severe, progressive, and not well managed with a 45–90-day trial of medical therapy. Many patients improve their ambulation distance with cessation of tobacco use, a supervised exercise program, lipid-lowering agents, antiplatelet agents, and selective use of cilostazol, and may never require intervention [6,7]. For those with persistent lifestyle-limiting or disabling claudication, evaluation with computed tomography angiography (CTA) is indicated to define the anatomic disease pattern and suitability for endovascular intervention. As lesion length is the major factor affecting long-term patency, it is accurate to imply that the shorter the lesion (i.e., the lower the TASC classification), the more likely the patient is to experience a beneficial and durable intervention.

INDICATION FOR INTERVENTION: CLTI

CLTI is defined as a chronic limb-threatening peripheral arterial disease with either ischemic rest pain or tissue loss with non-healing ulcers or gangrene. This is often associated with an ankle pressure of <40 mmHg or toe pressure of <30 mmHg for rest pain or an ankle pressure of <60 mmHg in patients with tissue loss. The WIfI (Wound, Ischemia, and foot Infection) classification scheme, adopted by the Society for Vascular Surgery, is a validated scoring system correlating with the overall risk of major amputation [8,9]. The natural history of CLTI, compared with claudication, is considerably worse with >25% of patients progressing to major limb amputation within one year of diagnosis. Of those patients initially presenting with CLTI, 10–40% will require primary amputation because of major tissue loss, infection, non-reconstructible occlusive disease, non-ambulatory status, or high risk of revascularization failure [10,11]. Revascularization is recommended in functional patients whenever possible. Notably, within the BEST-CLI study, there was significant and meaningful improvement in health-related quality of life within the three-month post-procedural period, irrespective of whether an endovascular or open revascularization was performed [2].

An endovascular-first approach has been adopted by many centers specializing in limb salvage. Several studies have now directly compared open and endovascular options. The BEST-CLI study, noted earlier, demonstrated the benefit and superiority of an adequate SSGSV [2]. The BASIL-2 found survival benefit for those patients undergoing endovascular revascularization compared with open bypass [3]. Both procedures are viewed as complementary; there exists patients who will do better with endovascular revascularization and those who will do better with open bypass.

TECHNIQUES FOR INTERVENTION

Endovascular approach and set-up

Once an endovascular approach has been deemed warranted, the set-up in terms of access, imaging, wire crossing, and intervention is critically important to achieve optimal patient outcomes. A hybrid operating endovascular suite provides the optimal resolution and field of view to accomplish these complex percutaneous interventions. Groin access is used in most cases; however, the following arteries have also been used: brachial; radial; popliteal; posterior tibial; anterior tibial, and even the peroneal artery. Alternate sites are chosen depending on disease location, any previous aortic operation, and the success of prior attempts. Except in rare cases, the patient is positioned supine; the left arm is tucked, padded, and supported (unless brachial access is used), and the right arm is left out for IV access and monitoring. Common femoral access options include a retrograde puncture contralateral to the SFA disease versus anterograde ipsilateral to the side of the disease. A retrograde approach is preferred unless there is a contraindication, such as a prior aortofemoral bypass graft or endovascular aneurysm repair, in which the graft bifurcation angle may be too steep to successfully pass a sheath to the contralateral side. The presence of significant contralateral common femoral artery (CFA) disease would also represent a relative contraindication to the retrograde approach. Preprocedural maneuvers to limit access site complications include control of hypertension (HTN) and the review of any previous diagnostic angiograms or CTAs. Details about the access artery including its length, concomitant atherosclerotic disease, and the presence of any previously inserted stents are easily noted.

Vascular access/diagnostic angiography

While topographic and fluoroscopic anatomy can assist femoral artery access, the anatomic relation of the groin crease to the CFA is unreliable. Thus, the authors use adjunctive ultrasound (US) guidance in all cases. US not only guides identification of the CFA and its bifurcation but also demonstrates arterial calcification and the external iliac-CFA junction. The adjacent common femoral vein is evident by its compressibility. A review of the anatomic relationship of the CFA to the vein, nerve, and adjacent structures is warranted (Figures 6.1 and 6.2). If US is

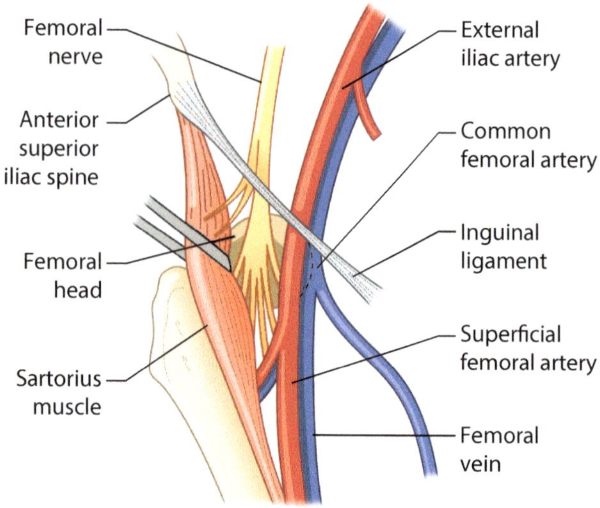

Figure 6.1 Anatomy of the femoral artery and its relationship with the femoral vein and nerve and the underlying femoral head.

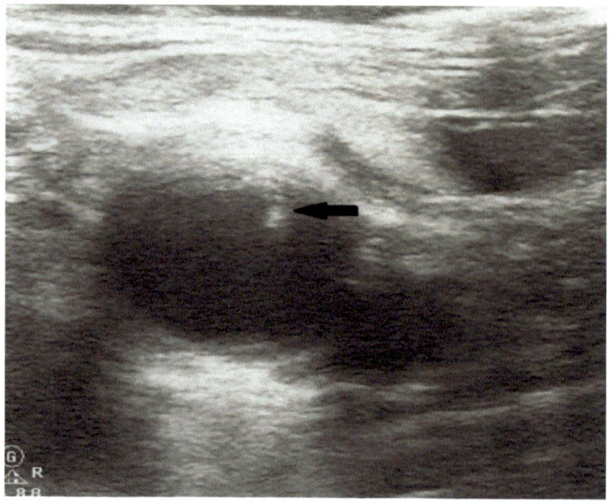

Figure 6.3 Access ultrasound demonstrating the tip of the needle in the lumen of the femoral artery (arrow).

not available, fluoroscopic imaging identifies the probable location of the CFA. In >80% of patients, the CFA overlies the medial one-third of the femoral head.

From a procedural standpoint, the US probe and gel are placed in a sterile sleeve. A micropuncture access needle is inserted at 45 degrees directly over the CFA, and in most cases, can be visualized in the CFA lumen (Figure 6.3). With blood return, the wire is inserted and the microaccess sheath is placed. Arterial flow is confirmed, a J wire is advanced, and the microaccess sheath is exchanged for a 5-Fr sheath. If no prior imaging is available, a full diagnostic aortogram with runoff is performed. With recent imaging available, the plan is for immediate access to the symptomatic limb through a retrograde approach from the contralateral extremity and an "up-and-over" technique. The authors favor the Omni™ flush catheter for wire passage to the contralateral extremity; however, many catheters can serve this purpose (e.g., Rösch inferior mesenteric; Cobra 1, 2, 3; pigtail, Contra-2) (Figure 6.4). A stiff 260 cm, 0.035-inch guidewire (Glidewire®; Terumo Medical Corporation, Somerset, NJ, USA) is used for passage to the contralateral extremity. If there is known proximal SFA disease, the Glidewire is passed into the profunda femoris artery. If the SFA is free of disease, the Glidewire is positioned into the proximal or mid-SFA. The 5F sheath is removed while maintaining wire position and a 45-cm, 6F Destination® guiding sheath (Terumo Medical Corporation) is advanced over the bifurcation into the CFA. Occasionally, and especially in patients with iliac artery calcification, it may be difficult to obtain contralateral access, and the authors have used other

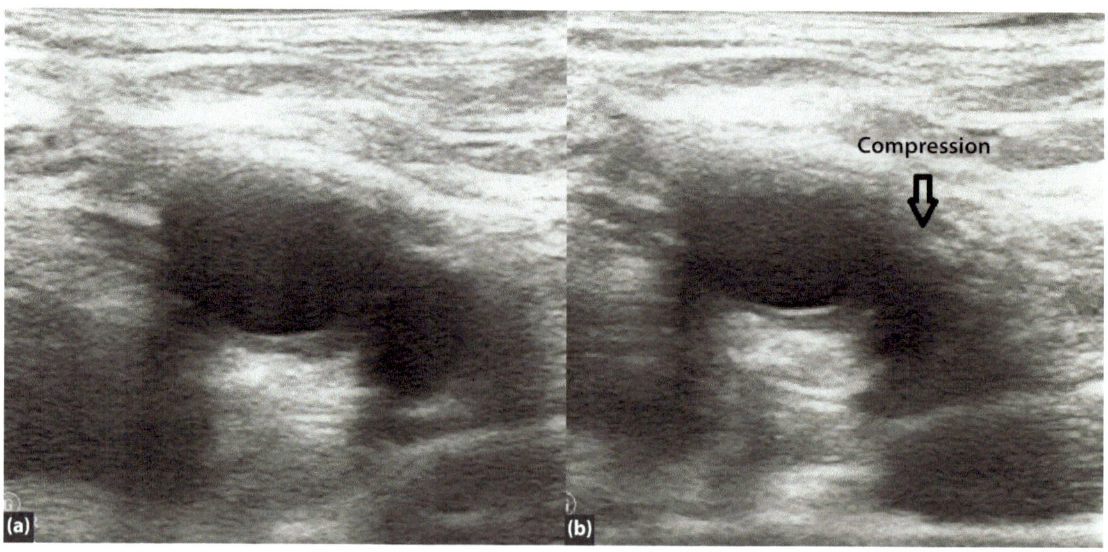

Figure 6.2 Access ultrasound demonstrating the compression of the femoral vein: (a) the non-compressed image; (b) the image showing femoral vein compression.

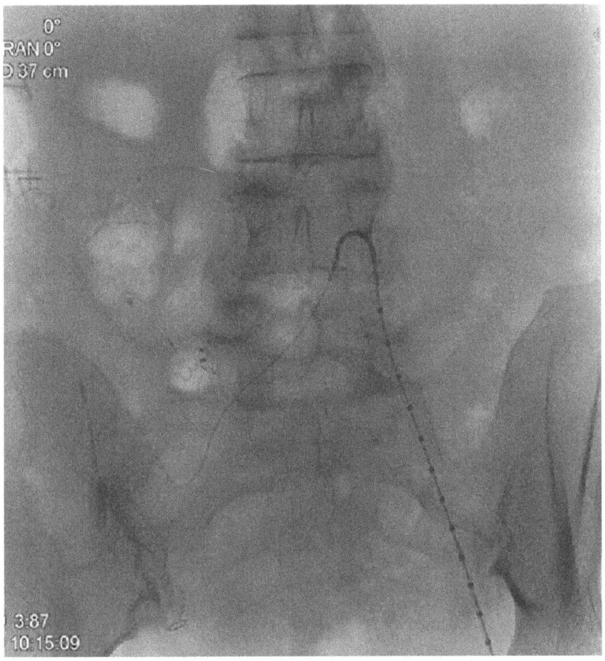

Figure 6.4 Fluoroscopy image of a patient where a flush catheter and advancing guidewire up and over the aortic bifurcation were used.

guidewires of increasing stiffness (Amplatz Super Stiff™; Boston Scientific Corporation, Marlborough, MA, USA) to facilitate placement. An additional technique for crossing a difficult aortic bifurcation is with an angioplasty balloon in the contralateral iliac artery. The balloon is inflated to maintain the position of the stiff guidewire and enhances the ability to track the sheath over the aortic bifurcation. The balloon is slowly deflated while simultaneously advancing the sheath over the balloon catheter. Once access to the contralateral side is achieved, IV heparin is administered (70 U/kg) and a confirmatory lower extremity angiogram is obtained. To reduce contrast volume, carbon dioxide (CO_2) angiography may be utilized. This is performed via a closed circuit with a slow injection of 30 cc of CO_2; it is prudent to wait two minutes between injections so that the extra CO_2 equilibrates.

Crossing the lesion

The success of the procedure is directly tied to the ability of the interventionalist to cross the lesion. The author uses a stiff Glidewire or a Glide Advantage wire (Terumo Interventional Systems) with an angled tip supported by a 135-cm support catheter (Quick-Cross®; Spectranetics Corporation, Colorado Springs, CO, USA) for the initial attempt. If the SFA or popliteal disease has been determined to be a stenosis, the success of crossing these lesions approaches 100%. The Glidewire (either the stiff Glidewire or the Glidewire Advantage) and catheter are advanced together with the Glidewire out 2–3 cm. One looks for deflection of the Glidewire tip and feels for any resistance in advancing the guidewire/catheter combination. The Glidewire is advanced outward in areas of the disease to "test" or feel the stenosis to maintain the wire intraluminally. Once the lesion is crossed, wire resistance dissipates, and one advances the support catheter over the Glidewire, a distal angiogram is performed to confirm the intraluminal position. The author then passes a stiff 0.014-inch wire through the support catheter, allowing for subsequent passage of any balloons, devices, and stents for the intervention being performed. When the artery is occluded, the author initially attempts to remain "intraluminal" with a similar approach. If this is unsuccessful, after a relatively short period of time, one proceeds with crossing the lesion in the subintimal plane—this is accomplished by allowing a loop to form and then advancing the loop past the disease to a predetermined area where the artery reconstitutes and is relatively disease-free (Figure 6.5). With the passage of the catheter, the guidewire is straightened out and one attempts to regain access intraluminally. This often occurs spontaneously or with the assistance of an angled catheter. It is important not to allow the subintimal dissection to continue beyond the designated arterial re-entry point so as not to destroy a potential target artery for bypass. When unsuccessful, the author has used re-entry devices, such as the Outback® LTD® Re-Entry (Cordis Corporation, Baar, Switzerland) with very good success in regaining entry into the lumen (Figure 6.6). This is performed by passing the device to the area of re-entry, orienting it to the lumen, and then thrusting the needle forward with the goal of positioning the needle tip intraluminally (Figure 6.7). Retrograde access from a distal reconstituted vessel beyond the lesion with a bidirectional crossing of the lesion is gaining in popularity and often greatly facilitates the successful crossing of the lesion. Retrograde pedal access is safe and technically feasible and is increasingly being used primarily rather than as a bailout approach. Using ultrasound guidance, access is gained into the pedal vessel, either the dorsalis pedis or common plantar artery. Alternatively, the anterior or posterior tibial artery, at or above the ankle level, can be accessed. This is done preferably using a pedal access kit (Micropuncture Pedal Introducer Access Kit, Cook Medical, Bloomington, IN, USA) or a standard micropuncture kit. It is preferable to avoid sheath insertion to limit the access injury to the small outflow artery. If deemed necessary, a 4F specialized sheath can be inserted. Using a 0.014-inch or 0.018-inch wire, the lesion within the SFA or popliteal is crossed from below, and the wire is then snared through the contralateral access (or ipsilateral antegrade access) positioned in the CFA or SFA. The procedure then ensues through the standard endovascular maneuvers. At the end of the procedure, hemostasis at the pedal access site is achieved via manual pressure.

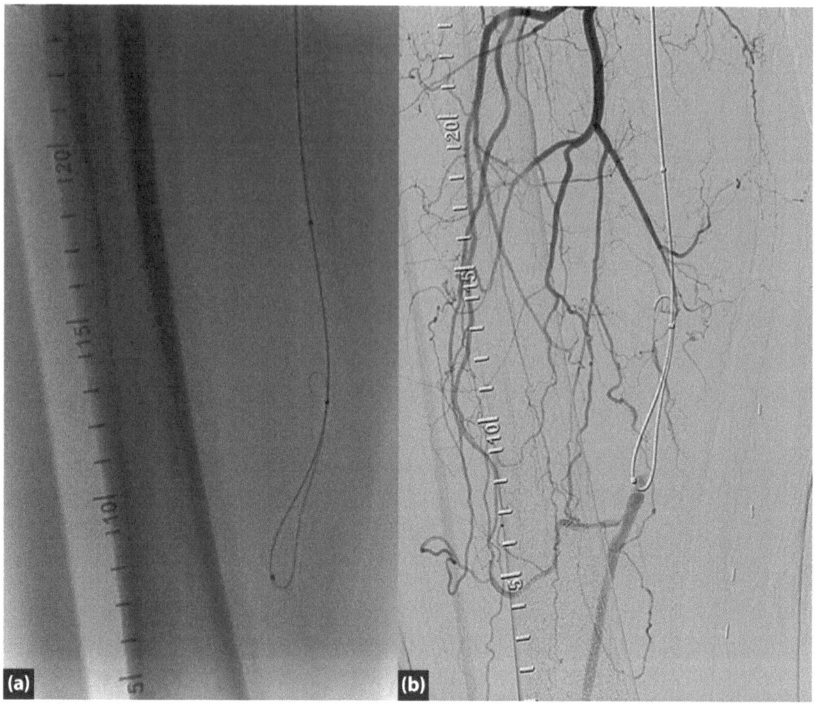

Figure 6.5 The success of the procedure is directly linked to crossing the lesion: (a) fluoroscopy image showing loop created with the stiff GlidewireR (Terumo Medical Corporation, Somerset, NJ, USA) to allow subintimal passage and advancement; (b) subtraction image showing the location of the loop in relationship to the reconstituted popliteal artery.

Endovascular management of femoropopliteal stenosis

When the lesion is relatively short (<10 cm in length), the author presently favors drug-coated balloons (DCBs) (Lutonix®, BARD Peripheral Vascular, Inc., Tempe, AZ, USA; IN.PACT Admiral, Medtronic, Minneapolis, MN, USA) for the intervention. Pre-dilation of the lesion is performed with a similarly sized balloon to that of the DCB, selected based on the diameter of the artery. The DCB is then used to treat the lesion. If a good technical result is obtained, no further intervention is required. If the lesion intervention results in a significant dissection or residual stenosis (>30%), a self-expanding stent is placed, sizing the stent 1–2 mm greater than the diameter of the artery. Longer lesions are treated similarly; however, as the likelihood of requiring placement of a self-expanding nitinol stent increases, the author would be less likely to use DCBs. One avoids stents in the popliteal artery if possible, preferring to use a scoring percutaneous transluminal angioplasty (PTA) balloon catheter (AngioSculpt® PTA Scoring Balloon, Spectranetics Corporation). Pre-angioplasty vessel prep, particularly with atherectomy devices (DiamondBack 360° Peripheral Orbital Atherectomy System; Cardiovascular Systems Inc., St. Paul, MN, USA), has gained in popularity despite minimal evidence supporting its use. The intention is to debulk the lesion allowing for improved fluoroscopic angioplasty results, which would hopefully translate into improved patency. Additionally, there does not appear to be any difference in the type of atherectomy device utilized. When deemed necessary by the extent and bulkiness of the underlying disease, the author has favored the Diamondback 360 orbital atherectomy system, the Rotarex Rotational excisional atherectomy system (BD Interventions Inc., Franklin Lakes, NJ, USA), or occasionally the HawkOne Directional Atherectomy System (Medtronic Medical Inc., Minneapolis, MN, USA). The latter device is particularly useful in eccentric plaque or plaque at or near a bifurcation. Distal embolization is a real and potentially under-recognized complication of atherectomy devices that has persisted despite the use of distal embolic protection filters.

Endovascular management of femoropopliteal occlusion

The management of occlusion, once the lesion is crossed, does not vary significantly from what has been discussed previously. The lesion is dilated with an appropriately sized balloon and re-evaluated angiographically. Once the post-angioplasty angiogram is obtained, the authors selectively stent the areas of significant residual disease or dissection. The author tries to reserve DCBs for patients with relatively short occlusions or for those lesions through which the wire was thought to pass intraluminally. Alternately, for occluded lesions that are successfully crossed, the author has used debulking devices, such

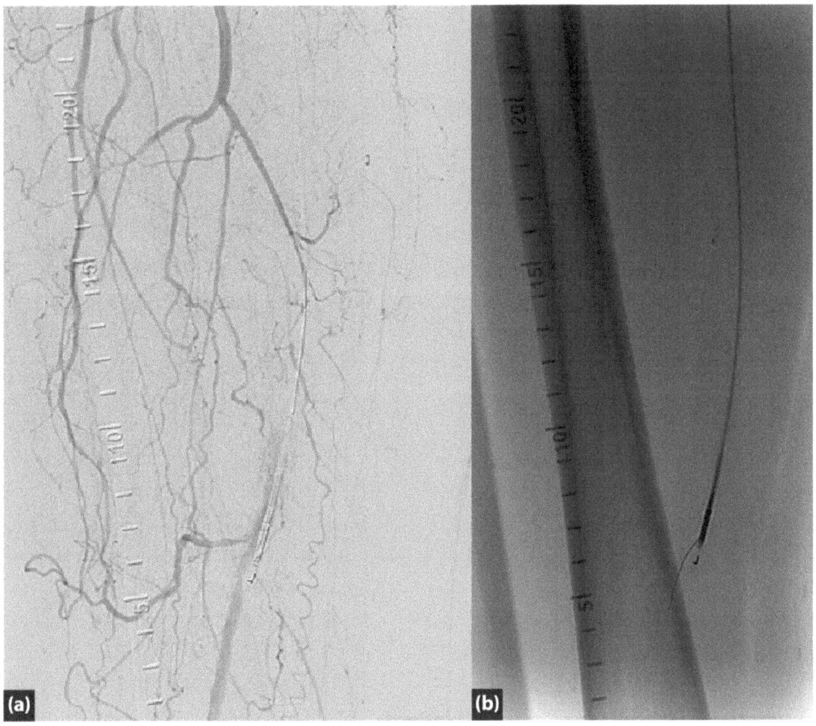

Figure 6.6 Using re-entry devices to regain entry back into the lumen: (a) subtraction image showing the appropriate orientation of the re-entry catheter in relationship to the artery in preparation for re-entry; (b) fluoroscopy image showing successful advancement of the tip of the 0.014-inch wire into the lumen.

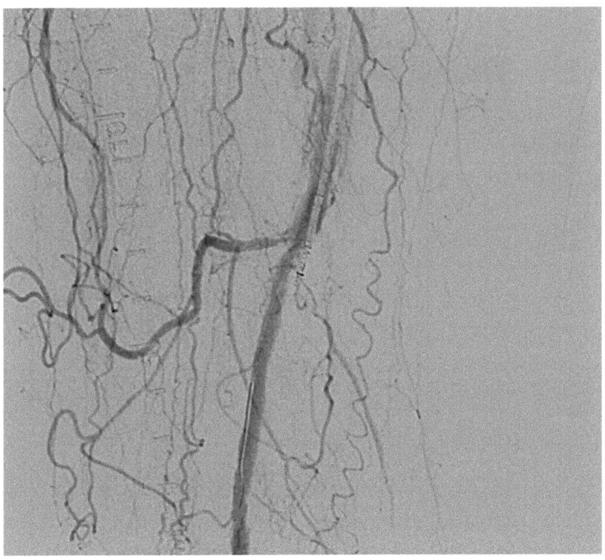

Figure 6.7 Subtraction image showing the 0.014-inch guidewire passed further down into the lumen with confirmation of intraluminal position.

as the orbital atherectomy device (DiamondBack 360° Peripheral Orbital Atherectomy System; Cardiovascular Systems Inc.). The theoretical advantage would be to debulk the lesion following which a DCB is used to try to reduce the likelihood of stent insertion and potentially improve patency. The author has reserved the use of these debulking devices for lesions that show a high degree of eccentric calcification. Deposition of calcium into the arterial wall has a negative impact on the technical and procedural success of femoropopliteal interventions. This is especially true in those lesions characterized by focal irregular and eccentric calcified atherosclerotic plaque. Calcified lesions decrease the ability to manipulate and advance devices because of the inherent drag that builds up, preventing and limiting advancement and successful positioning. Sequential balloon dilation to allow for the passage of larger devices may be necessary. Additionally, in highly calcified lesions, the author has liberalized use of Shockwave balloon angioplasty, or intravascular lithotripsy (Shockwave Medical Inc., Santa Clara, CA), which utilizes sonic pressure waves to soften the calcified plaque, rendering it more amenable to angioplasty to allow luminal restoration. In addition, while the author has used intravascular ultrasound (IVUS) very selectively, there may be benefit to a more routine-use adoption of IVUS to peripheral interventions in terms of appropriate sizing, determination of lesion length, and post-procedural completion studies.

COMPLICATIONS

Complications can be divided into access site complications (ASCs) and procedural complications (involving the artery being treated). Risk factors for ASCs include the following: older age; female sex; smaller body mass index; use of antiplatelets and anticoagulants; uncontrolled HTN; arterial calcification; larger sheath size; therapeutic procedures; and a history of previous catheterization.

Common ASCs include hematoma and acute bleeding with an incidence rate of 1.2–8.9%. Multiple unsuccessful access attempts, puncturing of back wall, and inadequate manual pressure can result in a hematoma and a pseudoaneurysm. Closure devices, inclusive of those that are suture based, plug based or external clip/star based, allow for shorter recover and earlier ambulation, but have not consistently reduced ASCs. The author has used closure devices whenever a 7F sheath or larger is utilized; for a 6F sheath, the closure devises are used frequently, although selectively. For 5F sheaths, manual pressure is typically used and has proven to be satisfactory if performed correctly. Other rare complications include dissection (0.4%), arteriovenous fistula (0.6%), and thrombosis (0.1%). Nerve injury is rare in femoral access (0.2%) but well documented in transbrachial access with an incidence of 0.4–12.7%. Overall, with the selective use of appropriate closure devices, reversal of anticoagulation (IV protamine sulfate is routinely administered), and enactment of a post-procedural sheath removal policy, including timing and technique of manual compression, the author has reduced the risk of all ASCs to <2%. Procedural complications include stent maldeployment, embolization of friable plaque or thrombus, and arterial wall dissection or perforation. Perforation is relatively rare and typically does not lead to significant bleeding. It can be managed with the inflation of a balloon matching the size of the artery, providing internal compression. Rarely, a stent graft will have to be deployed. Embolization occurs more frequently with atherectomy devices, although it can occur with any endovascular intervention; a careful and complete post-revascularization angiogram concentrating on the distal and foot vasculature will ensure the absence of distal embolization. If an embolus is present and is occlusive of any major arterial outflow, an endovascular salvage procedure can usually restore patency via a thrombectomy catheter or device.

POST-OPERATIVE RESULTS AND SURVEILLANCE

In general, for stenotic lesions, technical success is at or near 100%. For occlusions, the authors have found that with the noted approach, technical success is nearly 95%. Endovascular procedures have decreased patency rates compared with open surgery bypass; however, the benefits of a less invasive and morbid procedure often outweigh this reduction in patency. For SFA interventions, patency results have been as poor as 50% at 1–2 years and as high as 75% at three years [4,12]. Of course, endovascular interventions, especially for those lesions in the femoropopliteal segment, are continually evolving with newer devices and approaches influencing long-term durability. Post-procedurally, the author has followed any endovascular intervention as is performed with a bypass patient: performance of an ABPI and arterial imaging every four months for the first year; every six months for the second year; and annually thereafter [13]. While the technical success of femoropopliteal interventions is expected to be high, one must employ sound judgment in the decision and justification to intervene, thereby optimizing patient outcomes both in terms of symptom relief and limb salvage.

TRICKS AND TRAPS

1. Superficial femoral and popliteal artery endovascular interventions should be based on symptomatology, reserved for those claudicants who have failed a trial of medical therapy or those patients with CLTI.
2. When performing an endovascular procedure, it is important to consider future or subsequent possible interventions so as to not jeopardize additional or alternate attempts at limb salvage.
3. Some methods used have proven benefits, i.e., drug-coated balloons, whereas other interventional methods (atherectomy, lesion debulking, IVUS) have theoretical yet potentially promising benefits; the vascular interventionist should be prepared to employ these techniques as deemed necessary to optimize treatment outcomes.
4. Intravascular complications, including but not limited to rupture, dissection, and embolization, can typically also be managed endovascularly at the time of complication recognition.
5. In general, one starts with a 0.035-inch wire but once the lesion is crossed, it is beneficial to convert to a 0.014-inch or 0.018-inch platform to facilitate balloon or device selection.

QUESTIONS

1. A 68-year-old male prior smoker presents to you for the first time with right calf 1.5 block claudication; his femoral pulse is present and the popliteal pulse is absent. His ankle-brachial index is 0.55. The most appropriate next step in the patient's management would consists of:
    a. Performance of a CTA to evaluate the patient's anatomic disease and rule out other causes of SFA occlusion
    b. Medical therapy consisting of tobacco cessation, lipid-lowering agents, antiplatelet therapy, and an exercise program
    c. An angiogram with an intervention into his SFA occlusion
    d. Vein mapping and if the single segment greater saphenous vein is found, proceed with bypass
    e. Medical therapy consisting of vasodilators

    Answer: b

2. During an endovascular procedure on an occluded superficial femoral artery, a wire loop traverses the course of the occlusion but one is unable to have the wire directed into the patent proximal popliteal artery beyond the lesion. The next most appropriate step would be:
   a. Arterial cutdown at the popliteal artery above the knee
   b. Stent the artery down to the area of patent popliteal artery
   c. Ultrasound the tip of the wire percutaneously to ascertain how close you are to gaining entry into the patent popliteal artery
   d. Perform a retrograde puncture and get the wires to meet
   e. Use a re-entry device, i.e., the Outback

   Answer: e

3. The findings of the BEST-CLI study can be best summarized by which of the following statements regarding treatment of CLTI patients:
   a. Alternate bypass was superior to endovascular intervention
   b. In patients with single segment greater saphenous vein, bypass was associated with fewer major adverse limb events
   c. In patients with single segment greater saphenous vein, bypass was associated with higher mortality
   d. In patients with single segment great saphenous vein, bypass was associated with improved quality of life
   e. In patients without a single segment greater saphenous vein, endovascular therapy was associated with less death and fewer major adverse limb events

   Answer: b

4. Regarding access site complications, which of the following is associated with a higher risk of access site complications:
   a. Right femoral access
   b. Femoral artery measuring 6 mm in diameter
   c. Use of closure devices
   d. Female gender
   e. Anterior wall puncture

   Answer: d

REFERENCES

1. Norgren L, Hiatt WR, Dormandy JA, et al. Inter-society consensus for the management of peripheral arterial disease (TASC II). *J Vasc Surg.* 2007;45(Suppl S):S5–S67.
2. Farber A, Menard MT, Conte MS, Kaufman JA, Powell RJ, Choudhry NK, et al. BEST-CLI investigators: Surgery or endovascular therapy for chronic limb-threatening ischemia. *N Engl J Med.* 2022 Dec 22;387(25):2305–2316.
3. Bradbury AW, Moakes CA, Popplewell M, Meecham L, Bate GR, Kelly L, et al. BASIL-2 Investigators: A vein bypass first versus a best endovascular treatment first revascularization strategy for patients with chronic limb threatening ischemia who required an infra-popliteal, with or without an additional more proximal infra-inguinal revascularization procedure to restore limb perfusion (BASIL-2): An open-label, randomized, multicenter, phase 3 trial. *Lancet.* 2023 May 27;401(10390):1798–1809.
4. Conte MS, Bradbury AW, Kolh P, White JV, Dick F, Fitridge R, et al. Global vascular guidelines on the management of chronic limb-threatening ischemia. *J Vasc Surg.* 2019 Jun;69(6S):3S–125S.e40. (Comprehensive update review and guidelines in the management of chronic limb-threatening ischemia).
5. Conte MS, Pomposelli FB, Clair DG, et al. Society for vascular surgery practice guidelines for atherosclerotic occlusive disease of the lower extremities: Management of asymptomatic disease and claudication. *J Vasc Surg.* 2015;61(Suppl 3):2S–41S.
6. Greenhalgh RM, Belch JJ, Brown LC, et al. The adjuvant benefit of angioplasty in patients with mild to moderate intermittent claudication (MIMIC) managed by supervised exercise, smoking cessation advice and best medical therapy: Results from two randomised trials for stenotic femoropopliteal and aortoiliac arterial disease. *Eur J Vasc Endovasc Surg.* 2008;36:680–688.
7. Kannel WB, Skinner JJ Jr., Schwartz MJ, et al. Intermittent claudication: Incidence in the Framingham study. *Circulation.* 1970;41:875–883.
8. Stoner MC, Calligaro KD, Chaer RA, et al. Reporting standards of the society for vascular surgery for endovascular treatment of chronic lower extremity peripheral artery disease. *J Vasc Surg.* 2016;64:e1–e21.
9. Mills JL Sr, Conte MS, Armstrong DG, et al. The society for vascular surgery lower extremity threatened limb classification system: Risk stratification based on wound, ischemia, and foot infection (WIfI). *J Vasc Surg.* 2014;59:220–234.e1–2.
10. Bradbury AW, Ada DJ, Bell J, et al. Bypass versus angioplasty in severe ischaemia of the leg (BASIL) trial: Analysis of amputation free and overall survival by treatment received. *J Vasc Surg* 2010;51(Suppl 5): 18S–31S.

11. Abou-Zamzam AM Jr, Gomes NR, Molkara A, et al. A prospective analysis of critical limb ischemia: Factors leading to major primary amputation versus revascularization. *Ann Vasc Surg*, 2007;21:458–463.
12. Landry GJ. Functional outcome of critical limb ischemia. *J Vasc Surg*. 2007;45(Suppl A):A141–A148.
13. Draxler MS, Al-Adas Z, Abbas D, et al. Outcome benefit of arterial duplex stent imaging after superficial femoral artery stent implantation. *J Vasc Surg*. 2021;73:179–188.
14. AbuRahma AF, Robinson PA, Boland JP, et al. Complications of arteriography in a recent series of 707 cases: Factors affecting outcome. *Ann Vasc Surg*. 1993;7:122–129.

7

Percutaneous intervention for infrapopliteal arterial occlusive disease

LAYNE G. JANDA, ZIAD AL ADAS, AND DANIEL G. CLAIR

INTRODUCTION

Historically, the treatment for infrapopliteal disease in the setting of critical limb-threatening ischemia (CLTI) has been managed with open surgical bypass in appropriate patients with adequate autologous conduit in order to achieve in-line flow to the foot. With an aging population combined with an increase in advanced comorbid conditions (e.g., diabetes mellitus, coronary artery disease, end-stage renal disease), these patients are at a significantly higher risk of morbidity and mortality when undergoing an open procedure. This has prompted a shift from a "bypass first approach" to a tailored approach utilizing definitive treatment with endovascular therapy (EVT) in appropriate high-risk patients using diverse strategies to achieve a successful intervention. Early studies have shown suboptimal results with endovascular treatment of infrapopliteal lesions [1], however, advancements in endovascular technology, increasingly skilled interventionalists, coupled with a better understanding of target lesion anatomy, and patient and device selection have led to improved outcomes with enhanced rates of technical and procedural success making endoluminal strategies an attractive option for limb salvage [2]. This chapter discusses standard endovascular techniques for intervention in the infrapopliteal segment.

PATIENT SELECTION

Patient selection plays an important role in the decision-making process for endovascular strategies. Factors such as age, functional status, disease severity, patient frailty, and associated comorbid conditions are important when considering candidates for intervention. Generally, younger patients with good functional status, fewer comorbid conditions, and adequate autologous conduit are better suited for open bypass surgery. EVT, on the other hand, is more strongly considered in patients with comorbid conditions, absent autologous conduit, and shorter life expectancy. The treatment indication, claudication versus CLTI, should also augment the decision-making process. Patients suffering from claudication should receive optimal medical therapy, risk factor modification, and supervised exercise therapy prior to proceeding with any intervention. On the other hand, patients with CLTI, especially tissue loss, require reconstruction of in-line flow to the foot for maximum wound healing potential. For those patients who ultimately undergo treatment, inflow lesions in the aortoiliac and femoro-popliteal arterial segments should be addressed initially, especially in patients with rest pain. If they continue to be symptomatic, consideration for infrapopliteal revascularization via EVT is reasonable.

ACCESS APPROACHES AND CROSSING INFRAPOPLITEAL LESIONS

Treatment of the infrapopliteal segment includes the tibioperonal trunk, tibial vessels, the anterior tibial, posterior tibial, and peroneal arteries, as well as the pedal vessels and pedal arch. Arteries in this segment can have variable degrees of atherosclerosis, from focal high-grade stenosis to long-segment chronic total occlusion with variable amounts of calcium burden. Prior to intervention, it is important to understand the arterial anatomy. Axial imaging can be helpful to evaluate more proximal disease in the aortoiliac or femoral segment that may warrant treatment, preclude access, or be difficult to navigate; it can also help quantify the extent of calcific burden.

Antegrade common femoral access

To address infrapopliteal disease, it is advisable to prep both groins as well as the foot and lower leg in the event

DOI: 10.1201/9781003452096-7

an alternative approach is necessary. Ideally, EVT is performed through ipsilateral antegrade access in the common femoral artery (CFA), with access gained over the femoral head under ultrasound guidance using a 21G micropuncture needle. The proximal CFA should be accessed to allow for working room to navigate to the superficial femoral artery (SFA). Alternatively, if the proximal SFA is disease free and of adequate caliber on preoperative imaging, the proximal SFA can be accessed in an antegrade fashion. Although this can be challenging in obese patients, this technique allows very distal disease at the level of the ankle or foot to be accessible for treatment, in addition to better control and pushability of the wire and catheter, and shorter device and sheath lengths.

Once the CFA has been accessed, a guidewire is navigated anteromedially to cannulate the SFA, and the access sheath positioned in this vessel. Positioning the imaging system in the ipsilateral lateral anterior oblique position will better expose the femoral bifurcation, allowing easier advancement of the wire from the common femoral artery into the SFA. Once the wire is in the SFA, the access sheath (usually 5F) is advanced over the wire, and diagnostic angiography is performed. The guidewire is navigated down to the popliteal artery and a longer guide sheath can be positioned in the popliteal artery to provide additional support for distal intervention. The patient is systemically heparinized with 50–100 IU/kg maintaining an ACT of >250 seconds. Digital subtraction angiography is performed to delineate the tibial vessels and the runoff into the foot to determine target lesion anatomy.

Initial attempts to cannulate and cross tibial stenosis may be made with a 0.035-inch hydrophilic wire (e.g., Glidewire; Terumo Medical, Somerset, NJ, USA) and a crossing catheter of the operators' choice, Quick-Cross (Spectranetics, Colorado Springs, CO, USA) or Navicross (Terumo Medical) for support. There are advantages to using a braided catheter in performing this procedure as they improve torque control and allow better pushability. Smaller platform wires such as 0.018-inch or 0.014-inch hydrophilic, floppy tipped wires are often preferable to cross stenotic lesions, but hard or calcified plaque can cause these wires to coil, making crossing unsuccessful. The Command 0.018 wire (Abbott Vascular, Santa Clara, CA, USA) with its floppy tip is adept at crossing tibial stenoses. The V18 wire (Boston Scientific, Natick, MA, USA) is often useful in crossing tibial stenoses and provides excellent weight for advancing balloon catheters through challenging stenoses. While initial attempts to cross occlusions can be made with these hydrophilic tipped wires, increasingly weighted tip wires (3–40g) can be helpful in crossing complex lesions with heavy calcification and/or a tough fibrous cap. Utilizing a crossing catheter in conjunction with these weighted tip wires allows further escalation of the strength of the wire tip, and the catheter should be advanced across the occlusion so distal angiography can be performed to confirm presence in the vessel beyond the area of occlusion. This assures interventions are performed in connection to the patent distal segment of the artery.

Retrograde common femoral access

Retrograde common femoral access via the contralateral limb may also be considered. Traditionally, this has been the access of choice for treating supra- and infrainguinal disease and allows for treatment of proximal tibial disease. This approach may be necessary if there is disease in the proximal SFA that will require treatment at the same time. Additionally, it can be helpful in treating concomitant iliac or femoropopliteal disease. However, it can limit your ability to treat distal tibial or pedal lesions due to the lengths of guidewires, catheters, and devices required. Moreover, the tortuosity of the aortic bifurcation can also be a limitation, compromising control of the catheter and wire and "pushabilty" of devices. This "up-and-over technique" can be achieved using a stiff Glidewire (Terumo Medical) and a hooked catheter that sits at the aortic bifurcation. Once the guidewire is navigated through the iliac and femoral popliteal segment as mentioned earlier, a ring-reinforced sheath of appropriate length is advanced as far distally as feasible to attempt to cross infrapopliteal target lesions as described previously.

Retrograde tibiopedal access

Retrograde tibial or pedal access is an additional option to cross infrapopliteal lesions as antegrade vessel recanalization may be unsuccessful in up to 15–20% of patients [3]. Retrograde pedal access is safe and technically feasible and is increasingly being used primarily rather than as a bailout approach in select patients. Using ultrasound guidance, access is gained into the pedal vessel, either the dorsalis pedis or common plantar artery. Alternatively, the anterior or posterior tibial artery, at or above the level of the ankle, can be accessed. This is done preferably using a pedal access kit (Micropuncture Pedal Introducer Access Kit, Cook Medical, Bloomington, IN, USA) or a standard micropuncture kit. If needed, a 4 French sheath can be inserted, but it is advisable to work sheathless to prevent damage to the distal access vessel. Using a 0.014-inch or 0.018-inch wire, the lesion is crossed from below, and the wire is then snared from the proximal femoral access and exteriorized so that therapy may be delivered in an antegrade fashion. At the end of the procedure, hemostasis at the pedal access site is achieved via manual pressure.

TREATMENT

Angioplasty

Once a stenosis or an occlusion has been crossed with the wire followed by the catheter, angiography is performed to confirm true lumen position and patent distal runoff.

Balloon angioplasty with an appropriately sized balloon is then performed. There are a variety of balloons for treatment including plain angioplasty balloons, cutting balloons, lithoplasty balloons, and drug-coated balloons (DCB). While DCBs have proven efficacy in the femoropopliteal segment compared with plain balloon angioplasty (POBA), the results in the infrapopliteal vessels have not been as promising, and trials have shown inconsistent results [4,5]. thus DCBs are not currently FDA approved for use in the infrapopliteal segment.

Stenting

Stenting for infrapopliteal atherosclerotic occlusive lesions has been described, either primarily in an effort to prevent the elastic recoil of tibial vessels after angioplasty or as a bailout technique for flow-limiting dissections after balloon angioplasty. Bare metal self-expanding stents and balloon-expandable stents, in addition to drug eluting stents, have been utilized. However, trials and meta-analysis have failed to show a significant short- or long-term patency benefit for primary stenting of infrapopliteal lesions [6,7]. With this being noted, the use of coronary drug eluting stents in the setting of significant recoil or dissection is useful and should be considered in these settings.

Shock wave lithotripsy

Balloon lithoplasty using Shockwave Intravascular System (Shockwave Medical, Fremont, CA, USA) utilizes balloons that transmit pulsatile sonic pressure waves that interact with intimal and medial calcium resulting in fracture of the calcified plaque allowing intraluminal expansion. The use of this technology is most effective in heavily calcified tibial lesions. Shockwave balloon diameters start at 2.5 mm and early pilot studies have shown promising results for calcified stenotic tibial vessels [8].

Atherectomy

Atherectomy is performed to treat CLTI and acts to remove endoluminal plaque and increase luminal diameter. Several types of devices exist including directional, orbital, rotational, and laser atherectomy and these devices work by cutting, coring, or shaving lesions to reduce the plaque burden. This comes at the risk of distal embolization which may ultimately result in limb loss, therefore, appropriate patient selection is imperative, and consideration of a distal embolic protection device should be considered, particularly with directional atherectomy. Data on the long-term benefit of infrapopliteal atherectomy is limited, therefore, more research is necessary before appropriate recommendations may be made.

Deep venous arterialization

Deep venous arterialization (DVA) is considered a "last resort" and reserved for patients with tissue loss who do not have any named arterial outflow in the foot, frequently referred to as "desert foot," and thus are not candidates for standard endovascular arterial recanalization or surgical bypass. Patients being considered for DVA should be reasonable candidates for limb salvage, from both a tissue loss and global health standpoint. Patients with extensive soft tissue and bone infection with an unsalvageable foot as well as those who are bed-bound and non-ambulatory are not good candidates for DVA. From a vascular standpoint, patients considered for DVA should have the following: adequate inflow in the femoropopliteal arterial segment; a patent tibial artery proximally, ideally the posterior tibial

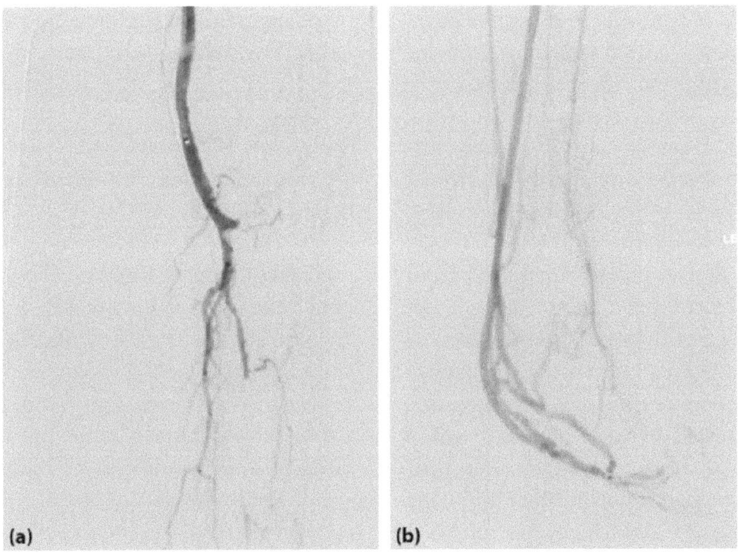

Figure 7.1 (a) Left lower extremity with occluded anterior tibial at the origin and occluded posterior tibial and peroneal arteries a few centimeters after their origins in a patient who underwent DVA; (b) completion angiogram after deep venous arterialization of the left lower extremity.

artery (PTA) (Figure 7.1a); a patent lateral plantar vein in the foot; and no arterial reconstruction option. DVA has been shown to be safe and effective in the PROMISE I and II trials using the LimFLow system [9,10].

To briefly describe the procedure using off-the-shelf devices, the patient is placed supine on the operating room table and the bilateral groins and affected leg are circumferentially prepped and draped. Venous access is established by accessing the lateral plantar vein at the distal third of the food under ultrasound guidance. The latter can be tedious and can be facilitated by the inflation of a tourniquet at the lower leg to dilate the venous system. A 5 French Glidesheath Slender (Terumo Medical) is placed for access in the lateral plantar vein and an 0.018 wire is advanced through the PTV to the level of the patent PTA, which is exchanged for a 4 mm Gooseneck snare that is positioned at the vein at the planned cross-over point. Antegrade arterial access is established and a sheath is positioned in the ipsilateral popliteal artery. The proximal PTA is selected using an angled wire and catheter. A re-entry catheter is used to create the arteriovenous connection between the proximal PTA and distal PTV, snaring the wire in the vein with the previously positioned venous snare. The wire is then externalized to create through-and-through wire access. After establishing through-and-though wire access, the arteriovenous fistula (AVF) is dilated with a 3.0 mm angioplasty balloon to allow devices to be delivered to the venous system. The venous valves are then lysed with a valvulotome introduced from the venous sheath in the foot. Following this, the vein is dilated with a 5 mm angioplasty balloon to ensure the venous stent graft will expand as needed in the calf and proximal foot vein. Following stenting of the venous system, the cross-over point is then stented with a 5 mm self-expanding covered stent. This crossing stent can be transitioned into the arterial system with a balloon-expandable coronary stent to ensure adequate inflow into the venous arterialization. Stents will extend from the PTA through the AVF cross-over point, all the way down to the PTV, and into the common plantar vein at the level of the calcaneus. The valves in the foot beyond the stent are lysed using a cutting balloon or valvulotome, again introduced through the venous sheath positioned on the plantar surface of the foot. Ideally, completion will involve obtaining wire access around the pedal venous arch and dilation of the arch to ensure an adequate extent of the venous filling out near the metatarsal heads. A completion angiogram (Figure 7.1b) is performed to evaluate forward flow to the foot via the venous system to determine if any further valves need to be lysed, or any stealing venous branches need to be embolized, which can also be accomplished in subsequent sessions. It is critical to maintain antegrade arterial flow to the foot as the venous arterialization takes six to ten weeks to establish an oxygen delivery pathway to the foot. In this period, the pre-existing arterial system is the only source of oxygenated blood to the foot.

Pedal loop revascularization

The pedal loop technique is primarily used in order to provide in-line flow for CLTI and tissue loss by restoring flow through the pedal arch. This technique requires antegrade puncture in the ipsilateral common femoral artery and the placement of a long 6F sheath to the popliteal artery. Using a 0.014 in platform with preferred wire and microcatheter, the pedal arch is navigated from either the direction of the ATA or the PTA while crossing over through the perforating plantar artery to complete the loop connecting the lateral plantar artery with the dorsalis pedis artery. Obtaining quality images of the foot and understanding the anatomy is paramount to facilitating the passage of the wire successfully. If the antegrade approach fails, a retrograde attempt can be made, ideally ensuring to stay transluminal with crossing. The arteries here are prone to spasm so using vasodilators may be necessary. Once across the pedal loop, balloon angioplasty of the pedal vessels is the primary treatment and is performed using 2–2.5 mm angioplasty balloons with inflation times of three minutes.

CONCLUSIONS

Endovascular treatment for infrapopliteal arterial lesions is feasible and effective, as supported by a growing body of evidence. While long-term data is less complete, this approach provides an attractive treatment option for older patients and poor surgical candidates with limited open revascularization options. The continued advancement of endovascular technologies, combined with increased operator experience, is likely to expand the use of endovascular treatment of infrapopliteal disease and provide promise for improved outcomes. To conclude, the treatment of patients with infrapopliteal disease requires an individualized multidisciplinary approach, including optimal medical therapy, wound care, revascularization, and continued surveillance.

CASE

A 69-year-old female with a history of insulin dependent diabetes mellitus now with non-healing wounds with underlying osteomyelitis along the right lateral plantar foot (Figure 7.2a). Her ankle brachial index was non-compressible, but her toe brachial index was 0.12.

A right lower extremity angiogram via left percutaneous femoral access showed widely patent inflow and superficial femoral and profunda femoris. There was a moderate stenosis in the P1 popliteal and occluded P2 and P3 popliteal, in addition to a diseased tibioperoneal trunk (TPT) with reconstitution of the anterior tibial (AT) and peroneal arteries at their origin and posterior tibial artery (PTA) at the mid-leg (Figure 7.2b). A 6 French × 90 cm sheath was advanced from the left femoral to the level of the P1 popliteal. The P2-P3 popliteal and TPT occlusions

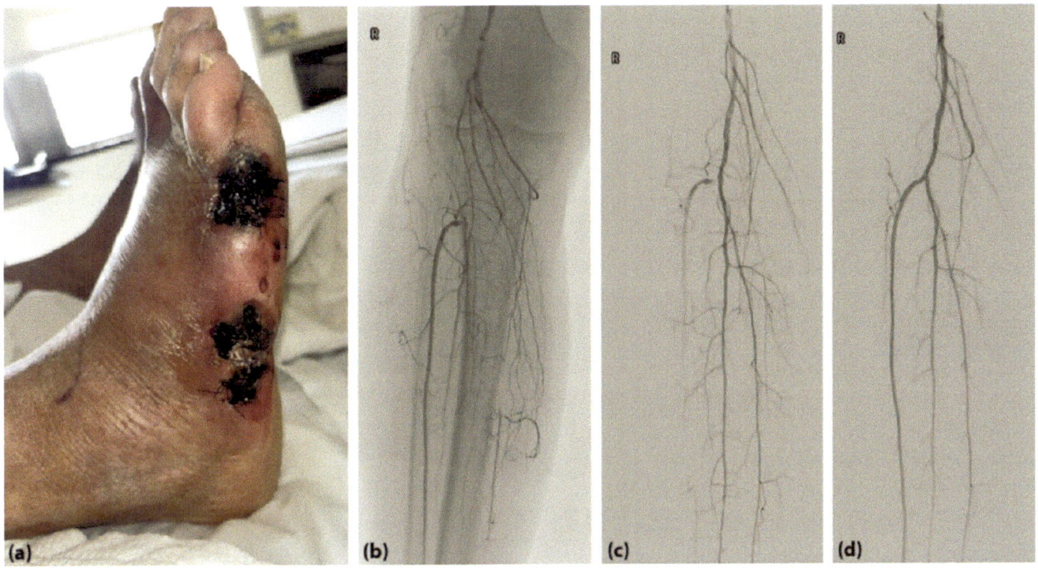

Figure 7.2 (a) Right foot with tissue loss and underlying osteomyelitis; (b) pre-treatment angiogram; (c) recanalization of the P3 popliteal, TPT, PT, and peroneal with high-grade stenosis at the AT origin; (d) completion angiogram with three-vessel runoff.

were traversed using a stiff Glidewire and a 0.035 straight Navicross. After confirming the intraluminal position, a V18 Guidewire was advanced and parked in the distal peroneal artery. The TPT and P2/P3 popliteal artery were dilated with a 4 mm balloon followed by a 4 mm drug-coated balloon. Using a Command 0.014 wire (Abbott Cardiovascular, Santa Clara, CA, USA) and an angled 0.014 TrailBlazer catheter (Medtronic, Minneapolis, MN, USA), the PT was cannulated; after confirming intraluminal position in the mid-leg, it was dilated using a 2.5 mm plain balloon. This resulted in an excellent filling of the PT and peroneal with delayed filling of the AT secondary to a high-grade stenosis at the AT origin (Figure 7.2c). Using the same wire/catheter system, the AT was selected and the origin was treated using a 3 mm plain balloon. The sheath was pulled and the P1 popliteal artery was treated with a 5 mm plain balloon followed by a 5 mm drug-coated balloon (Figure 7.2d). There was a dissection in the distal TPT that was treated successfully with prolonged inflation of a 3.5 mm balloon.

TRICKS AND TRAPS

- Patient selection, lesion characteristics, vessel anatomy, and patient overall health are important factors to consider when identifying patients suitable for endovascular therapy.
- Percutaneous femoral arterial access, whether antegrade or retrograde, should always be performed under ultrasound guidance.
- Consider avoiding aggressive endovascular interventions in patients with single-vessel runoff to the foot.
- Retrograde pedal access is preferably performed sheathless and simply with a catheter to minimize tibial artery complications such as dissection or thrombosis. Hemostasis may be achieved with manual pressure after procedure completion.
- Avoid retrograde pedal access in patients with a single-vessel runoff, especially if the vessel is a potential distal target for a surgical bypass.
- After crossing a subtotal occlusion or chronic total occlusion, angiography is important to ensure intraluminal position and patent distal runoff before performing angioplasty.
- When crossing lesions in the tibial or pedal distributions, it is preferable to remain transluminal rather than subintimal as re-entry is more challenging in these smaller vessels, and perforation can be more common with non-transluminal passage.
- Maintain a therapeutic ACT of greater than 250 seconds throughout the intervention to avoid vessel thrombosis.
- Judicious use of vasodilators may help prevent spasm and a low-flow state potentially leading to thrombosis.
- Close surveillance following intervention is important to maintain patency and optimize limb salvage, as restenosis rates in this arterial bed are not insignificant.

QUESTIONS

1. What strategy can help minimize the risk of distal embolization?
   a. Minimal use of anticoagulation
   b. Performing aggressive vessel dilation
   c. Using larger contrast volumes
   d. The use of distal protection devices

Answer: d

2. Which adjunctive therapy has been consistently shown to improve long-term patency rates in infrapopliteal endovascular intervention?
   a. Atherectomy
   b. Primary stenting
   c. Drug-coated balloon angioplasty
   d. No specific adjunctive therapy has consistently shown to improve long-term patency with infrapopliteal endovascular interventions

   Answer: d

3. Antegrade access is useful and beneficial in all of the following *except:*
   a. Treatment of a TP trunk stenosis
   b. Allows for ease of access in large, obese patients
   c. Allows for better wire and catheter control and "pushability" when crossing a lesion
   d. Allows for treatment of distal tibial and pedal disease due to the length of catheters while avoiding a tortuous aortic or iliac bifurcation

   Answer: b

4. Deep venous arterialization is considered for
   a. Bed-bound patients
   b. Patients who have an SFA occlusion with reconstitution of their above knee popliteal
   c. Patients who have a patent inflow and femoropopliteal segment with no named outflow to the foot
   d. Patients with iliac occlusive disease

   Answer: c

REFERENCES

1. Ihnat DM, Mills JL. Current assessment of endovascular therapy for infrainguinal arterial occlusive disease in patients with diabetes. *Journal of Vascular Surgery* [Internet]. 2010 Sep 1;52(3, Supplement):92S95S. [cited 2020 Mar 27]. Available from: https://www.sciencedirect.com/science/article/pii/S0741521410013352
2. Treiman GS, Treiman RL, Ichikawa L, Van Allan R. Should percutaneous transluminal angioplasty be recommended for treatment of infrageniculate popliteal artery or tibioperoneal trunk stenosis? *Journal of Vascular Surgery.* 1995 Oct;22(4):457–65.
3. Montero-Baker M, Schmidt A, Bräunlich S, Ulrich M, Thieme M, Biamino G, et al. Retrograde approach for complex popliteal and tibioperoneal occlusions. *Journal of Endovascular Therapy.* 2008 Oct;15(5):594–604.
4. Cassese S, Gjin Ndrepepa, Liïstro F, Fanelli F, Kufner S, Ott I, et al. Drug-coated balloons for revascularization of infrapopliteal arteries. *JACC: Cardiovascular Interventions.* 2016 May 1;9(10):1072–80.
5. Liistro F, Porto I, Angioli P, Grotti S, Ricci L, Ducci K, et al. Drug-eluting balloon in peripheral intervention for below the knee angioplasty evaluation (DEBATE-BTK). *Circulation.* 2013 Aug 6;128(6):615–21.
6. Schulte KL, Pilger E, Schellong S, Tan KT, Baumann F, Langhoff R, et al. Primary self-EXPANDing Nitinol stenting vs balloon angioplasty with optional bailout stenting for the treatment of infrapopliteal artery disease in patients with severe intermittent claudication or critical limb ischemia (EXPAND Study). *Journal of Endovascular Therapy.* 2015 Aug 5;22(5):690–7.
7. Hsu C C-T, Nga G, Singh D, Rophael JA, Anthony CA, van Driel ML. Angioplasty versus stenting for infrapopliteal arterial lesions in chronic limb-threatening ischaemia. *The Cochrane Library.* 2018 Dec 8;2018(12).
8. Brodmann M, Holden A, Zeller T. Safety and feasibility of intravascular lithotripsy for treatment of below-the-knee arterial stenoses. *Journal of Endovascular Therapy.* 2018 Jun 18;25(4):499–503.
9. Shishehbor MH, Powell RJ, Montero-Baker MF, Dua A, Martínez-Trabal JL, Bunte MC, et al. Transcatheter arterialization of deep veins in chronic limb-threatening ischemia. *New England Journal of Medicine.* 2023 Mar 30;388(13):1171–80.
10. Clair DG, Mustapha JA, Shishehbor MH, Schneider PA, Henao S, Bernardo NN, Deaton DH. PROMISE I: Early feasibility study of the LimFlow System for percutaneous deep vein arterialization in no-option chronic limb-threatening ischemia: 12-month results. *J Vasc Surg.* 2021 Nov;74(5):1626–35.

8

Endovascular repair of non-ruptured infrarenal abdominal aortic and iliac artery aneurysms

TAMER N. BOULES

INTRODUCTION/PATIENT SELECTION

Endovascular AAA repair (EVAR) has emerged as the primary treatment for anatomically appropriate patients with infrarenal aortoiliac aneurysms. Based on the results of landmark randomized trials, the indications for abdominal aortic aneurysm (AAA) repair include expansion to diameters greater than 5.5 cm in men, 5.0 cm in women, or by 0.5 cm over six months. Repair of iliac artery aneurysms (IAA) is indicated for a diameter greater than 3.5–4 cm [1, 2].

Decisions to intervene are individualized based on a risk/benefit analysis that includes the consideration of patient comorbidities, life expectancy, and expected operative mortality. Randomized trials comparing EVAR to open AAA repair demonstrated improved perioperative mortality and morbidity, with its advantages waning at 8–12 years following intervention, albeit with early generation devices [3, 4].

ANATOMIC CONSIDERATIONS

Anatomic candidacy for EVAR with or without iliac involvement includes assessment of proximal and distal seal zone diameter, length, and quality, neck angulation, iliac tortuosity and calcific disease, and femoral access vessel patency, diameter, and disease. This is based on CT angiography (CTA) with 3D reconstructions and centerline measurements (Figure 8.1). Although there are various fixation (suprarenal vs infrarenal) and sealing (radial force vs polymer-ring) methods available on commercially available stent grafts that may alter the anatomic requirements detailed in their instructions-for-use (IFU, Figure 8.2), the majority require at least 10–15 mm of non-conical aortic neck (between 16 and 32 mm diameter) free of significant calcium and thrombus, with less than 60° aortic neck angulation, and 2 cm of distal common iliac artery (between 8 and 25 mm in diameter) (Table 8.1).

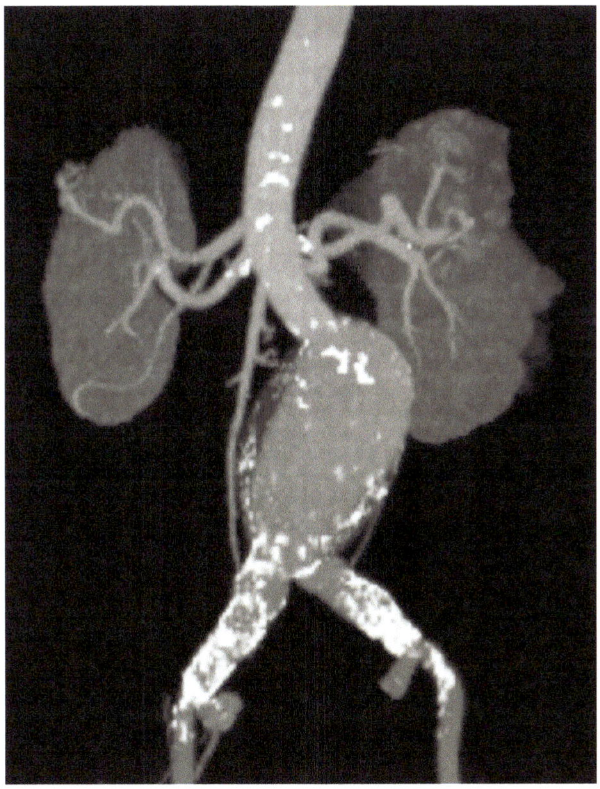

Figure 8.1 Reformatted CTA demonstrating a clear anatomic candidate for EVAR.

DOI: 10.1201/9781003452096-8

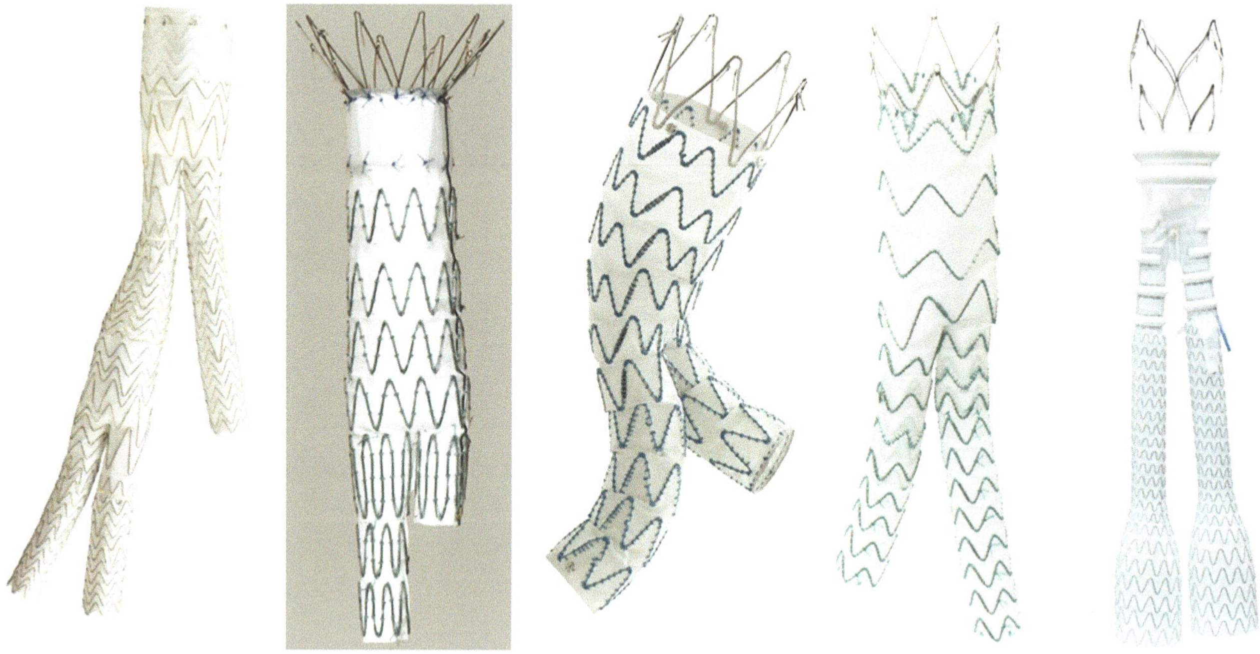

Figure 8.2 Commercially available stent grafts: (a) Gore Excluder; (b) Cook Zenith Flex; (c) Medtronic Endurant II/IIs; (d) Terumo Treo; (e) Endologix Alto.

Table 8.1 Characteristics of commercially available AAA stent grafts

Device	Graft/stent material	Treatable aortic neck diameter (mm)	Minimum aortic neck length (mm)	Treatable iliac artery diameter (mm)	Proximal aortic neck angulation (degrees)	OD delivery sheath (main body—contralateral limb, French)	Fixation
Gore Excluder	ePTFE/ nitinol	19–32	15	8–25	<60	16–18/12–15	Infrarenal
Cook Zenith Flex	Polyester/ stainless steel	18–32	15	7.5–20	<60	18–22/14–16	Suprarenal
Medtronic Endurant II/IIs	Polyester/ nitinol	19–32	10	8–25	<60	18–20/14–16	Suprarenal
Terumo Treo	Polyester/ nitinol	17–32	15	8–20	<60	18–19/12–14	Suprarenal and infrarenal
Endologix Alto	ePTFE/ nitinol	16–30	7	8–25	<60	14–15/12–15	Suprarenal

ePTFE, expanded polytetrafluoroethylene.

Device selection is dependent on knowledge of the unique advantages of each system in situations of suboptimal neck length or severe angulation, and small diameter or tortuous iliac arteries. General principles of successful durable repair include coverage of the iliac arteries to their bifurcations when iliac aneurysmal disease is absent for greatest axial support, and adherence to IFU when possible for proximal neck seal. In the modern era, it is preferable to consider more proximal branched or fenestrated devices to seal in normal aorta than to accept short-term results with a tenuous seal in a compromised short or diseased infrarenal neck.

SURGICAL TECHNIQUE

Access to a hybrid endovascular environment, preferably with fixed imaging, is critical to maximizing EVAR success. Although general endotracheal anesthesia may have advantages for controlling respiratory motion during device deployment, EVAR can be performed under regional or local anesthesia for patients with advanced cardiopulmonary disease or ruptured aneurysms.

Percutaneous access has become increasingly utilized despite the need for larger sheath access with the development of closure devices, most commonly using suture mediated methods and a "pre-close" technique to deploy sutures prior to large sheath (8.5 to 24F) arterial dilation under ultrasound guidance. This technique affords patients more rapid recovery, lower length of stay, and reduced risks of wound complications including infections and seromas [5].

Relative contraindications to percutaneous access include small iliofemoral arterial diameter, heavy anterior calcification, and the presence of femoral occlusive disease precluding sheath delivery. In these cases, open exposure is an acceptable alternative and allows for necessary adjunctive procedures such as femoral endarterectomy reducing the risk of ischemic complications.

Iliac occlusive disease also poses a challenge during EVAR but can be mitigated with preemptive external iliac angioplasty and covered stenting, now with the option of arterial lithotripsy in severely calcified stenotic arteries [6]. Although some devices can be delivered through iliac arteries as small as 5 mm, a surgically created iliac prosthetic conduit with anastomosis to the distal common iliac artery via a retroperitoneal approach is also an option.

Once bilateral femoral access has been achieved, aortography with a marker pigtail placed at the level of the renal arteries is performed to confirm distances to the iliac bifurcation and select a main-body ipsilateral limb length for anticipated two-piece cases. However, this is not routinely performed in cases where bilateral iliac limbs are extended from a shorter main body. Stiff 0.035 in Lunderquist or Amplatz wires are delivered to the proximal thoracic aorta bilaterally, maximizing support for the delivery of device components, and in some cases, larger sheaths. This also allows for the "preview" of wire and sheath trajectories at the bifurcation that will aid in the planning of contralateral gate positioning and cannulation after main body deployment.

With magnified pararenal aortography, using cranial and oblique gantry angulation, the main device is deployed below the lowest renal artery (Figure 8.3). Most EVAR systems allow for stepwise deployment where repeat angiography and gantry position optimization (accounting for parallax) can be performed prior to committing to final main-body stent deployment. This allows for the maximization of seal zone overlap by precise positioning of the stent graft often partially or nearly completely deployed, but still mobile to allow for cephalad/caudal or rotary positional "fine-tuning." One common strategy to take account for "stored energy" as the device is pushed cephalad into position (which may result in unanticipated renal encroachment once released) is to release this energy with partial deployment of the stent in a more proximal position just above the target renal origin and pull it down caudally to its final desired position. If inadvertent renal ostial encroachment or coverage has occurred, the surgeon must be prepared for renal stenting (frequently from a brachial approach). Main body deployment continues until the contralateral gate is exposed and available for cannulation using contralateral femoral access.

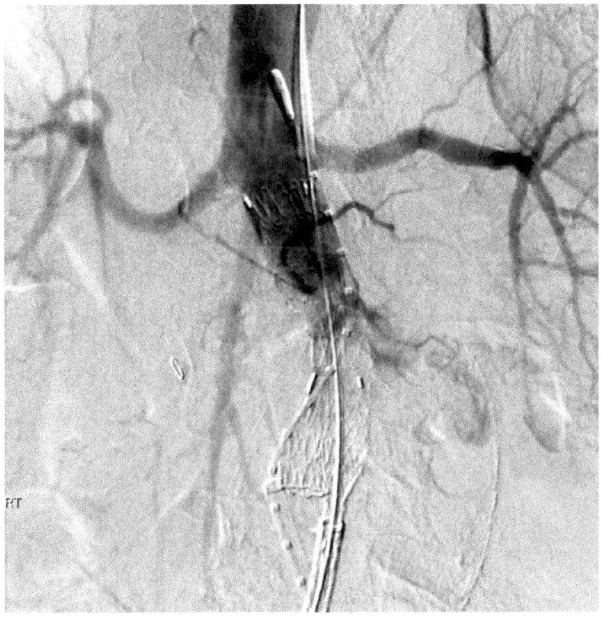

Figure 8.3 Angiogram demonstrating the position of the main body of the stent graft after deployment below the lowest renal artery.

Contralateral gate cannulation can be accomplished with a simple angled catheter such as the Berenstein and a steerable 0.035 in Glidewire (Figure 8.4). Once the gate is cannulated, a "spin test" is performed in which a formed pigtail is spun after positioning in the main body of the stent graft, confirming it is intraluminal prior to limb delivery. Alternatively, this is confirmed with the inflation of a molding balloon within the main body, allowing its visualized deformation over the flow divider as the gantry is rotated.

When encountering challenges in cannulation, a systematic approach is necessary:

1. Changing gantry position while "live" imaging allows for the anterior/posterior redirection of catheters and wires.
2. Alternative catheters, including the C2 and Van Schie 5, with secondary angles that allow wires to reach the opposite sides of the aneurysm sacs, may also assist

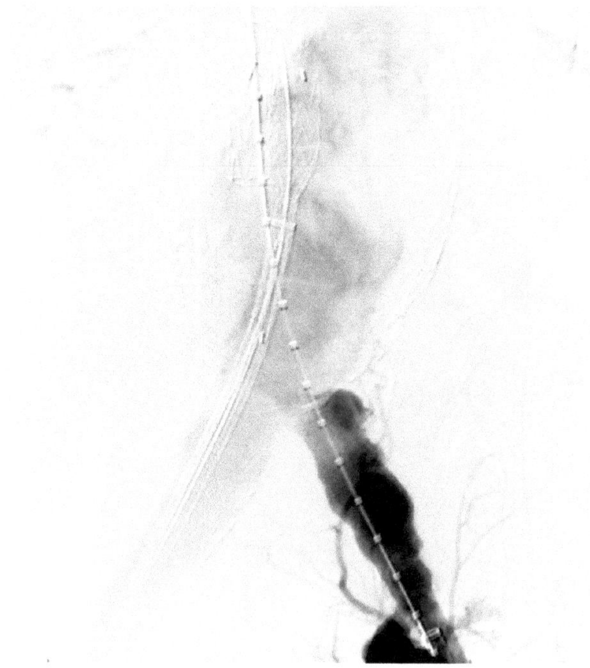

Figure 8.4 Retrograde angiogram with marker pigtail in place performed after successful cannulation of contralateral gate noting distance to the hypogastric artery and intended iliac limb seal zone.

in difficult retrograde cannulation such as in larger AAAs with little space occupying mural thrombus.

3. Especially useful is the mating of a 25 cm 8F angled sheath or guiding catheter (MPA or Hockey-Stick) with the 5F Berenstein catheter to allow for the controlled roticulation of the angles in series with each other.
4. EVAR systems such as the Gore Excluder allow for cannulation of the gate prior to commitment to permanent fixation at the infrarenal level, leaving the option of rotating the main body to a gate position that is more favorable.
5. "Up-and-over" antegrade delivery of a wire through the gate can be performed to allow for snaring of the wire from the contralateral femoral approach either within the AAA sac or the contralateral iliac artery.
6. If the gate is compressed or incompletely deployed (as may be encountered with a small distal aorta), delivery of an antegrade sheath through the gate from a brachial/radial approach should be considered, with snaring of the wire once the zone of compression is traversed.
7. Finally, rarely needed, is conversion to the aorto-uni-iliac configuration with coverage of the contralateral gate and plugging of the contralateral iliac artery with femoral-femoral bypass.

Once cannulation has been confirmed, a stiff wire is once again positioned, and a marker catheter is used to select the appropriate length of contralateral limb based on the necessary overlap with the gate and distance to the hypogastric origin viewed in opposite-oblique and caudal gantry angulation. This is repeated for the ipsilateral limb in three-piece modular systems.

A non-compliant molding balloon is then used at the aortic neck, zones of overlap within each limb, and distal iliac seal zones, avoiding inflation outside the proximal and distal extents of the stent graft to avoid native arterial dissection or rupture. Some prefer the use of simultaneous "kissing" non-compliant balloons in the limbs as they traverse a small distal aorta or bifurcation where asymmetric or incomplete expansion of a limb can predispose to limb thrombosis. Although rarely needed with modern well-supported stent graft limbs, reinforcement of these zones with balloon expandable stents is an option. Similarly, self-expanding stents can be used to support limbs in zones of iliac tortuosity or angulation when limb kinking is encountered.

Prior to sheath removal and vessel closure, a completion angiogram is performed to assess patency of the renal arteries and hypogastric arteries, symmetric brisk flow in the iliac limbs without kinks, and all seal zones for early appearing type I or III endoleaks, differentiating them from late-appearing type II endoleak (Figure 8.5). Oblique or lateral imaging can be helpful to differentiate a subtle slow filling type IA endoleak from lumbar arteries adjacent to the neck contributing to a type II endoleak (Table 8.2).

Most patients can be discharged on the first postoperative day after EVAR. Postoperative non-contrast, arterial, and delayed phase CTA is obtained within 30 days and at

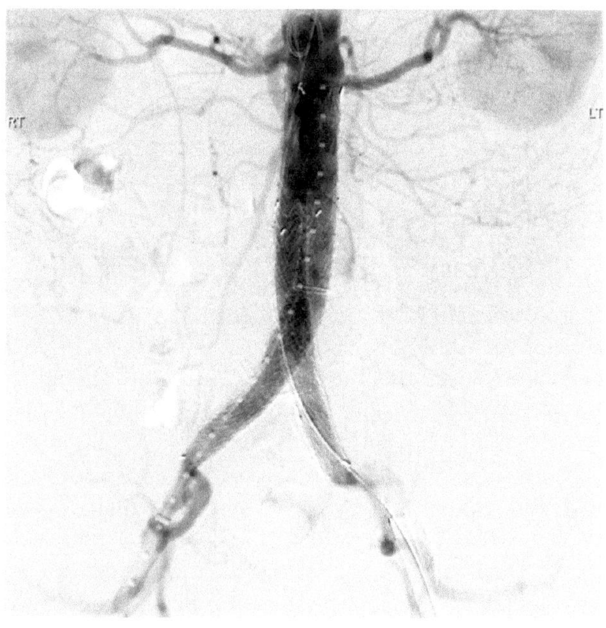

Figure 8.5 Completion aortogram demonstrating patency of the graft and native anatomy without obvious endoleak.

Table 8.2 Types of endoleak

Type of endoleak	Definition
Type I	Incomplete seal at proximal (type IA) or distal (type IIB) grafts
Type II	Retrograde branch flow (lumbar or inferior mesenteric arteries)
Type III	Defect in graft, separation, or inadequate overlap of graft components
Type IV	Porosity of graft fabric
Type V	Sac expansion without clear evidence of endoleak

one year prior to conversion to Duplex-based yearly surveillance (in the absence of sac expansion and type I/III endoleaks). Triple-phase protocol is necessary for monitoring stent graft patency and sac size/volume, detection of early and late filling endoleak, and differentiation of contrast within the sac from calcified thrombus. Once duplex-based surveillance is established, CTA is reserved for sac expansion to assess for endoleak requiring intervention. CTA should also be considered every five years to assess proximal or distal seal zone degeneration and to detect not uncommon adjacent metachronous aortoiliac aneurysmal disease.

MANAGEMENT OF ENDOLEAKS DURING EVAR

Although type II endoleaks are managed conservatively, type I(a/b) or III endoleaks are treated with molding balloon angioplasty if poor vessel apposition is thought to be the cause, and if unsuccessful, extension of coverage proximally or distally with cuffs or other stent grafts, respectively. In the case of type I(b) endoleaks, coil embolization or plug occlusion of the hypogastric artery with extension into the external iliac artery is an option if an adequate seal cannot be achieved with coverage to the iliac bifurcation.

Other adjuncts to managing type I(a) proximal endoleaks include use of Palmaz stents or endoanchors to facilitate apposition or fixation of graft material to the aortic wall when further proximal extension with cuffs is not possible. This is less likely to be successful if the neck is heavily calcified or contains circumferential thrombus, emphasizing the importance of preoperative planning for success. Alternatively, in the modern era, the use of renal covered stents (delivered through a brachial approach) as "snorkels" with even more proximal cuff placement or intentional partial encroachment is an option. Staged extension with fenestrated devices to achieve a proximal seal at the visceral level can be considered if no other durable endovascular options exist.

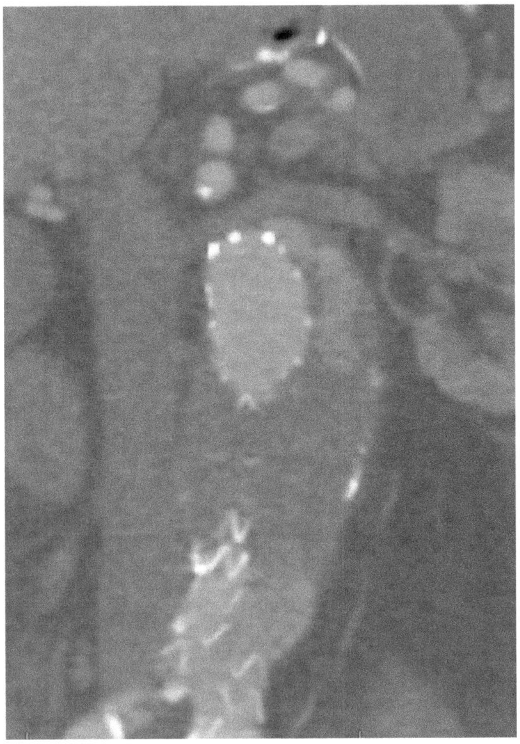

Figure 8.6 CTA with coronal reconstructions demonstrating a type IA endoleak.

MANAGEMENT OF LATE ENDOLEAKS

Late type I(a) endoleaks typically reflect neck degeneration with or without caudal migration of the main body of the stent graft (Figure 8.6). Some believe that the risks of caudal migration can also be reduced by the use of suprarenal fixation, coverage of the iliac arteries to their bifurcations, or by the use of stent grafts where the components are interlocking (such as the Terumo Treo device), but strong evidence for this is lacking. If the previously described options are not successful in managing late type I(a) endoleaks, coil or glue embolization of the endoleak cavity has been used with variable success. More frequently, proximal extension with fenestrated or branched endografts to seal in normal aorta is used at centers with expertise in thoracoabdominal stent grafting. Elective open conversion is a final option but is rarely necessary if the anatomic IFU requirements noted for each stent graft have been adhered to.

Late type II endoleaks are managed conservatively if they persist unless sac expansion is noted on serial imaging studies. However, it is critical to exclude occult type I/III endoleaks at the time of angiography as the true cause of sac expansion, even if not seen on CTA. The association of larger and multiple sac branch vessels with late sac expansion from a type II endoleak has led some to consider pre-emptive lumbar or inferior mesenteric artery embolization for larger branches, prior to EVAR, but strong evidence for this remains sparse. If intervention

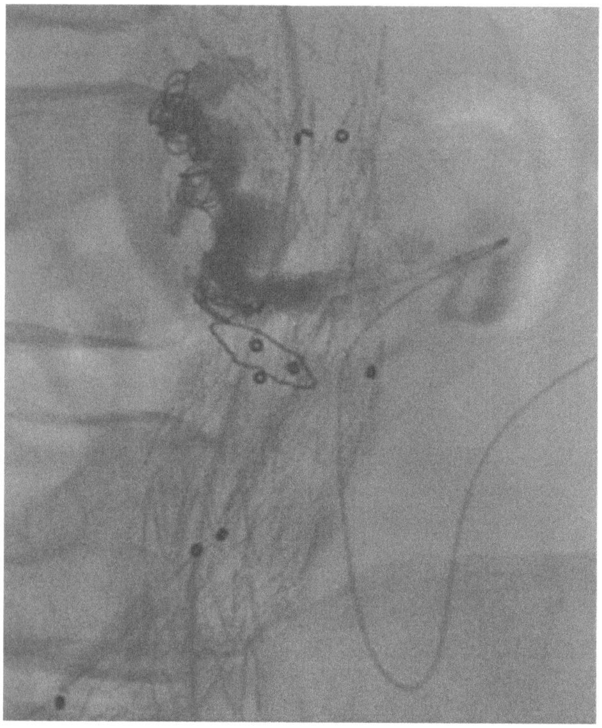

Figure 8.7 Coil embolization of the inferior mesenteric artery through the superior mesenteric and marginal arteries.

for a type II endoleak is indicated, the most common targets for treatment include coil embolization via trans-femoral iliolumbar (via hypogastric artery) or inferior mesenteric artery approach (via superior mesenteric artery and marginal artery; Figure 8.7), or CT-guided trans-lumbar direct aortic sac access and branch occlusion. Ideally, both inflow and outflow vessel occlusion are necessary for successful resolution of the endoleak, but this can be challenging and may require staged sessions. Other less common strategies, depending on the location of the endoleak, include accessing the sac through a venous trans-caval approach or by entering the sac through a catheter supported channel created between the stent graft limb and its iliac artery. Even sac access directly through a stent graft limb with perpendicular needle puncture, wire access, and catheter placement has been described with relining of the limb after endoleak intervention is completed. Finally, transabdominal lumbar/inferior mesenteric arterial ligation via a laparoscopic approach can be performed.

A late type IV endoleak relates to graft porosity and is listed for historical reasons, as modern grafts are less porous and not susceptible to this. A type V endoleak (endotension) reflects sac expansion in the absence of a CTA or angiographically detectable endoleak and frequently results in an open conversion for definitive treatment.

The management of other late complications of EVAR including limb thrombosis, graft migration, and infection is beyond the scope of this chapter but must be considered in the long-term surveillance after EVAR. In addition to intervention for endoleak, these complications contribute to the 10–20% risk of secondary intervention.

ENDOVASCULAR REPAIR OF ILIAC ANEURYSMS

Common Iliac artery aneurysms

In the setting of coexisting AAA, although "bell-bottom" limbs or larger cuffs can seal in iliac arteries already aneurysmal up to 25 mm or larger in diameter, this approach may be best reserved for the patient with limited life expectancy, with no other option for the maintenance of ipsilateral hypogastric patency with contralateral hypogastric occlusion, or with ruptured AAA under urgent/emergent conditions when expeditious sealing is the primary goal.

In those where the indication for intervention is the common iliac artery aneurysm (CIAA), younger patients who would have higher long-term risk of a type I(b) endoleak with further iliac aneurysmal degeneration, and those whose iliac artery is not amenable to bell-bottom limbs, several options exist:

1. Coil embolization or plugging of the ipsilateral internal iliac artery (IIA) origin with extension of the iliac stent limb to the external iliac artery (EIA) remains commonplace. Preservation of the contralateral IIA and avoiding extension of the coil/plug distal to the ipsilateral IIA bifurcation is critical to reducing risks of pelvic ischemia and buttock claudication.
2. Using the Gore Iliac Branch Endoprosthesis (IBE), even CIAAs that extend to the iliac bifurcation can be treated successfully, with distal seal achieved in the preserved normal IIA and EIA using bifurcated components. This approach is rapidly gaining favor over sacrifice of the IIA, even with a patent contralateral IIA, as there is mounting evidence of heightened morbidity from unilateral IIA sacrifice [7] (Figure 8.8).
3. Although most CIAAs are treated as extensions of aortic aneurysmal disease, if the CIAA is isolated with an adequate proximal CIA seal zone, it can be treated with simple stent graft exclusion rather than with a modular bifurcated aortoiliac device.

Internal iliac artery aneurysms

Internal iliac artery aneurysms (IIAAs) with or without CIA involvement require embolization/plugging of each outflow branch with stent graft coverage of the origin of the IIA. Rarely, when bilateral sizable IIAs require treatment, use of an IBE with extension to a dominant relatively normal anterior or posterior pelvic branch can be performed with sacrifice of the other branches to preserve some pelvic perfusion and reduce the risks of pelvic

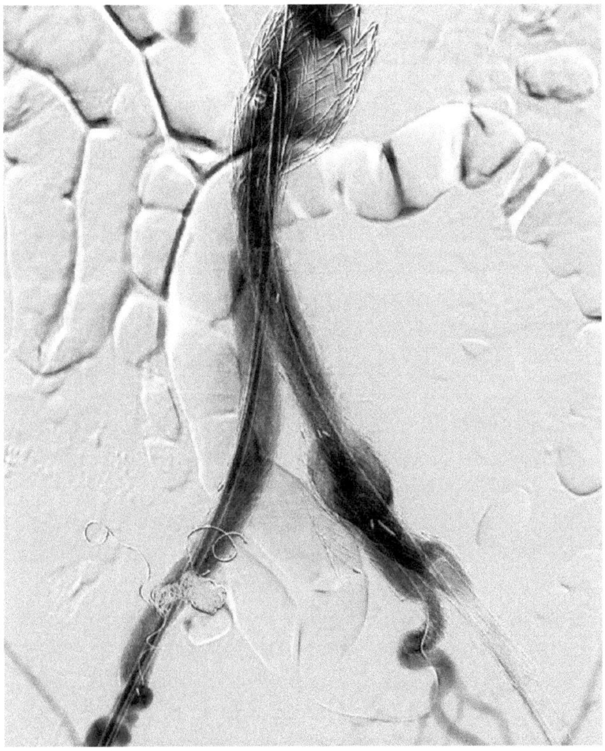

Figure 8.8 Completion angiogram demonstrating successful deployment of left-sided IBE as well as right IIA coiling with extension of the limb to the right EIA in a patient with bilateral CIAA.

ischemia. When this is not possible, staged bilateral sacrifice, with reliance on deep femoral artery and IMA collaterals (when the infrarenal aorta does not require treatment) becomes necessary.

In both CIAAs and IIAAs, when IBE is not an option and preservation of the hypogastric artery is necessary, a distal EIA to IIA bypass can be performed with ligation of the internal iliac origin ("relocating" the iliac bifurcation) prior to stent graft repair with extension into the EIA now available just proximal to the bypass origin. This hybrid option can be performed simultaneous to or staged with the endovascular portion.

TRICKS AND TRAPS

- Adhering to IFU-based anatomic guidelines is a high predictor of procedural success and long-term durability of repair.
- If adequate normal seal zones proximally and distally are not available, consider alternatives such as fenestrated or iliac bifurcated devices if possible.
- Percutaneous access should be considered in all patients when anatomically possible to reduce morbidity of open femoral exposure.
- Be prepared for renal stenting from a brachial approach, if necessary, when renal ostial encroachment or coverage is encountered.
- When encountering challenges in gate cannulation, a systematic algorithmic approach to alternative technical strategies is necessary.
- In the absence of sac expansion, type II endoleaks can be managed conservatively, while all type I and III leaks should be treated with secondary intervention regardless of changes in sac size.
- Every effort should be made to preserve at least one IIA when planning endovascular treatment of iliac aneurysms using either iliac bifurcated devices or open IIA revascularization as part of hybrid approaches.

QUESTIONS

1. Which of the following is considered a contraindication to percutaneous femoral access to EVAR?
   a. Common femoral artery with eccentric coral-reef circumferential calcific occlusive disease
   b. External iliac artery stenosis
   c. Morbid obesity
   d. Access sheath greater than 18 French
   e. Prior closure of femoral artery with another closure device

Answer: a

Percutaneous closure in EVAR is contraindicated in the setting of severe CFA disease, especially in the setting of thick circumferential calcific involvement or coral-reef bulky intraluminal disease that is unavoidable. In these cases, open exposure with associated endarterectomy or other reconstruction may reduce ischemic complication. The other listed choices are not contraindications, although the presence of significant obesity or scar can make percutaneous closure technically difficult. Sheath access up to 24 French has been closed successfully, especially if the vessel is relatively disease free.

2. Which of the following anatomical characteristics is considered unfavorable for EVAR using commercially available infrarenal grafts?
   a. Infrarenal neck length of 15 mm
   b. Infrarenal neck diameter 30 mm
   c. Proximal neck angulation of 80 degrees
   d. Presence of bilateral common iliac aneurysms
   e. External iliac artery diameter 6 mm

Answer: c

Severe angulation greater than 60 degrees is considered unfavorable for EVAR with most commercially available stent grafts. All other anatomic characteristics in the other options are not considered universally unfavorable. Certain devices may be more favorable than others, especially with shorter neck length (<15 mm) or smaller iliofemoral diameters.

3. Which of the following is the least commonly used strategy for challenges in gate cannulation?
   a. Conversion to the aorto-uni-iliac configuration with femoral-femoral bypass
   b. Alternative complex catheter or guide catheter shapes to direct a wire through the gate
   c. Snare capture of wire with up-and-over or brachial access
   d. Rotating partially deployed main body to change gate position
   e. Changing gantry position with "live" imaging to reveal anterior/posterior gate position

   Answer: a

   Unplanned conversion to the aorto-uni-iliac configuration with femoral-femoral bypass is very rarely needed when challenges in gate cannulation are encountered. Simple changes in gantry position, use of alternative shape catheters, and less frequently, snare-assisted techniques are all more common initial options.

4. Which of the following patient anatomies is associated with the highest risk of pelvic ischemia or buttock claudication with endovascular repair?
   a. AAA with bilateral common iliac artery aneurysm
   b. Bilateral internal iliac aneurysms extending to bifurcations bilaterally
   c. AAA with common iliac with ipsilateral internal iliac aneurysm and no contralateral iliac aneurysm
   d. AAA with common iliac aneurysm with contralateral internal iliac artery occluded
   e. AAA with bilateral internal iliac artery stenosis

   Answer: b

   Bilateral internal iliac aneurysms requiring treatment have the highest risk of long-term buttock claudication or pelvic ischemia, given the need to sacrifice both internal iliac arteries and their branches. This scenario frequently occurs in the setting of associated inferior mesenteric artery occlusion, leaving the pelvis reliant on only deep femoral or lumbar collaterals. All of the other listed scenarios have lower risk due to the need for only unilateral internal iliac treatment (frequently requiring only origin plugging rather than branch coiling) or are more likely to be candidates for iliac bifurcated endovascular (IBE) devices.

REFERENCES

1. Chaikof, E.L., Dalman, R.L., Eskandari, M.K., Jackson, B.M., Lee, W.A., Mansour, M.A., Mastracci, T.M., Mell, M., Murad, M.H., Nguyen, L.L. and Oderich, G.S., 2018. The society for vascular surgery practice guidelines on the care of patients with an abdominal aortic aneurysm. *Journal of Vascular Surgery*, *67*(1), pp. 2–77.
2. Charisis, N., Bouris, V., Rakic, A., Landau, D. and Labropoulos, N., 2021. A systematic review on endovascular repair of isolated common iliac artery aneurysms and suggestions regarding diameter thresholds for intervention. *Journal of Vascular Surgery*, *74*(5), pp. 1752–1762.
3. Patel, R., Sweeting, M.J., Powell, J.T. and Greenhalgh, R.M., 2016. Endovascular versus open repair of abdominal aortic aneurysm in 15-years' follow-up of the UK endovascular aneurysm repair trial 1 (EVAR trial 1): a randomised controlled trial. *The Lancet*, *388*(10058), pp. 2366–2374.
4. van Schaik, T.G., Yeung, K.K., Verhagen, H.J., de Bruin, J.L., van Sambeek, M.R., Balm, R., Zeebregts, C.J., van Herwaarden, J.A., Blankensteijn, J.D., Grobbee, D.E. and Blankensteijn, J.D., 2017. Long-term survival and secondary procedures after open or endovascular repair of abdominal aortic aneurysms. *Journal of Vascular Surgery*, *66*(5), pp. 1379–1389.
5. Agrusa, C.J., Meltzer, A.J., Schneider, D.B. and Connolly, P.H., 2017. Safety and effectiveness of a "percutaneous-first" approach to endovascular aortic aneurysm repair. *Annals of Vascular Surgery*, *43*, pp. 79–84.
6. Price, L.Z., Safir, S.R., Faries, P.L., McKinsey, J.F., Tang, G.H. and Tadros, R.O., 2021. Shockwave lithotripsy facilitates large-bore vascular access through calcified arteries. *Journal of Vascular Surgery Cases, Innovations and Techniques*, *7*(1), pp. 164–170.
7. Kouvelos, G.N., Katsargyris, A., Antoniou, G.A., Oikonomou, K. and Verhoeven, E.L.G., 2016. Outcome after interruption or preservation of internal iliac artery flow during endovascular repair of abdominal aorto-iliac aneurysms. *European Journal of Vascular and Endovascular Surgery*, *52*(5), pp. 621–634.

9

Endovascular repair of ruptured abdominal aortic aneurysms

M. ASHRAF MANSOUR AND JAKE A. NICHOLSON

INTRODUCTION

The National Vital Statistics in the United States show that abdominal aortic aneurysms (AAA) are the direct or indirect cause of death in over 17,000 individuals annually [1]. Screening programs, using abdominal ultrasound, in Europe and the USA have been useful in the detection of patients with aortic aneurysms [2,3]. The SAAAVE Act authorized payment for a screening abdominal ultrasound in males qualifying for Medicare, however, it has not had a significant impact on the rate of elective repair or AAA rupture in the USA [4]. It is clear that the outcomes of elective repair, whether open or endovascular, will always be more favorable than waiting for the AAA to rupture [5].

Endovascular aneurysm repair (EVAR) was first described by Volodos in 1986 [6], then modified by Parodi in 1991 [7]. Several graft prototypes were tested in the 1990s in Europe and Australia. In the USA, the FDA approved the first two grafts, AneuRx (Medtronic, Minneapolis, MN, USA) and Ancure (Guidant, Indianapolis, IN, USA) in September 1999. Since then, many other devices have received approval and are being used in patients routinely. Currently in the USA, the three most commonly used devices are the Gore *Excluder* (W. L. Gore, Flagstaff, AZ, USA), the Cook *Zenith* (Cook Medical, Bloomington, IN, USA), and the Medtronic *Endurant* II (Medtronic, Minneapolis, MN, USA). Several randomized trials comparing elective EVAR to open repair have shown improved outcomes, especially in frail patients [8,9]. On the other hand, randomized trials of ruptured AAA comparing EVAR to open repair failed to demonstrate a significant advantage [10–12]. However, many of the trials were flawed and thus their results should be interpreted with caution.

Recent data from the US Medicare population indicate that the rate of ruptured AAA in the last few years has been cut in half [13], arguably due to improved screening and detection programs. The same database depicts a significant shift from open repair to EVAR over time. EVAR is now the preferred method of treatment in elective patients [14]. Although randomized trials have been conducted to evaluate EVAR versus open repair for ruptured AAA, the results have been mixed [15–17]. We, along with many investigators, however, are firmly convinced that an endovascular first approach for ruptured AAA is best [18]. A recent population study has shown that patients undergoing EVAR for ruptured AAA have a lower hazard all-cause mortality and major adverse cardiovascular events when compared with patients having open repair [19]. The purpose of this chapter is to describe the preoperative planning and intraoperative technique of EVAR for ruptured AAA.

PREOPERATIVE PLANNING

In order to achieve good outcomes, a multidisciplinary and coordinated approach affords the best chance for the patient [20–22]. As in many complex surgical cases, the assignment of roles and rehearsing the steps help with good preparation for the event. A true multidisciplinary approach should involve emergency and operating room personnel. The vascular surgeon and anesthesiologist should be informed as early as possible. Open lines of communication between team members are essential to be able to execute plans and secure a good outcome.

Clinical presentation

Although the triad of abdominal or back pain, pulsatile mass, and shock are pathognomonic of ruptured AAA, the vast majority of stable patients will receive a bedside ultrasound and a CT scan to confirm the diagnosis (Figures 9.1 and 9.2). In order to obtain accurate

DOI: 10.1201/9781003452096-9

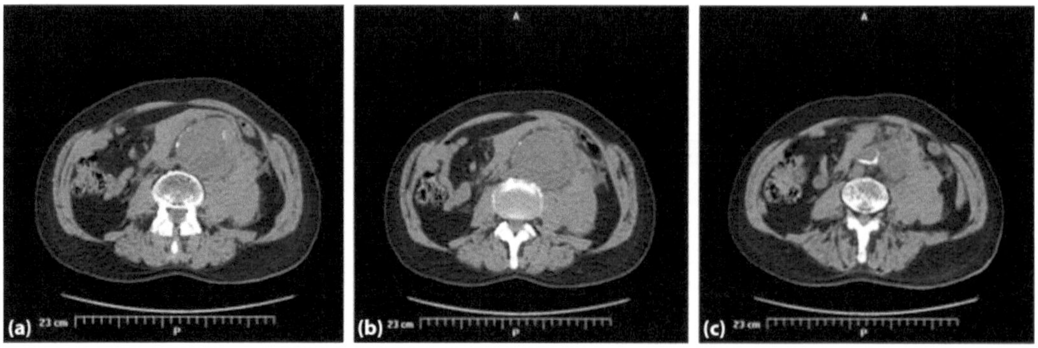

Figure 9.1 Abdominal computed tomographic images without intravenous contrast showing a 7 cm abdominal aortic aneurysm with a left retroperitoneal rupture going from proximal (a) to distal (c).

measurements for graft selection, a thin cut (2–3 mm) spiral CT angiogram is ideal. With compromised renal function, there may be a reluctance to administer intravenous contrast, and in some hypotensive unstable patients, it may be more prudent to proceed directly to the operating room without imaging (see Algorithm 9.1). It is still possible to get measurements of the aortic neck diameter from a non-contrast abdominal CT scan and confirm on initial aortogram (Figure 9.3).

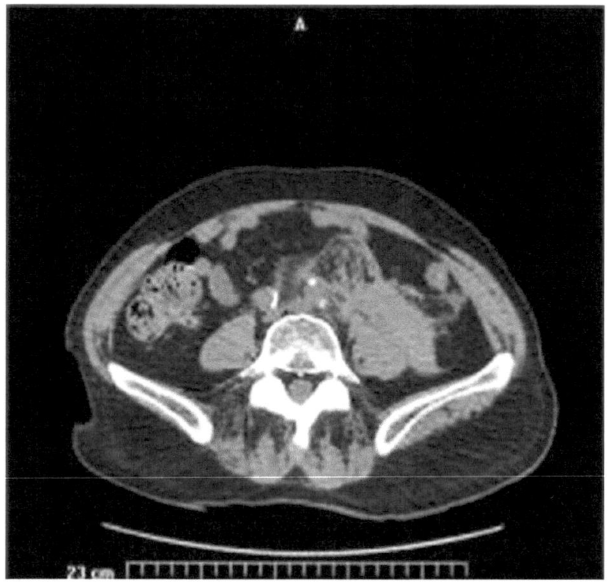

Figure 9.2 Pelvic CT, without IV contrast, showing common iliacs with calcifications, and suitable for EVAR.

Algorithm 9.1:

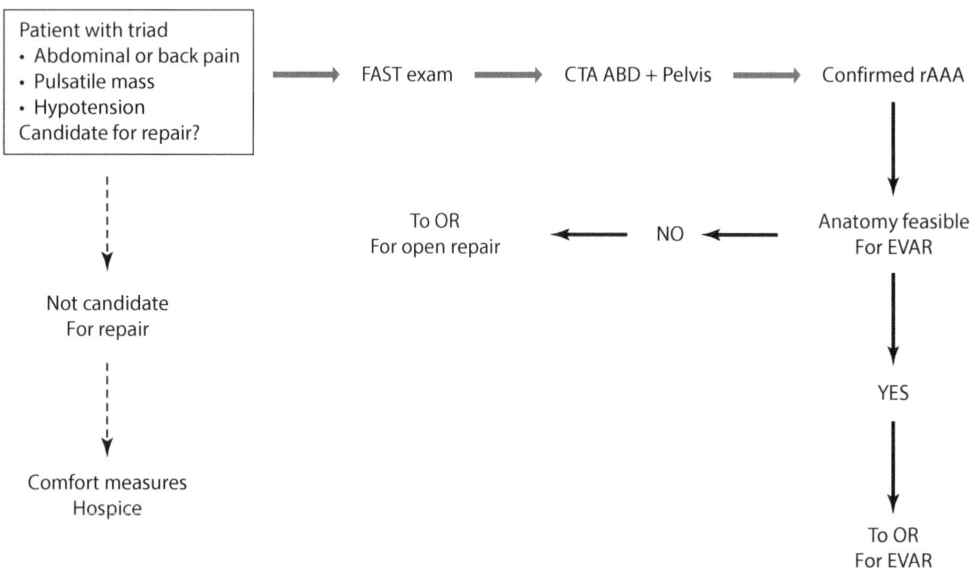

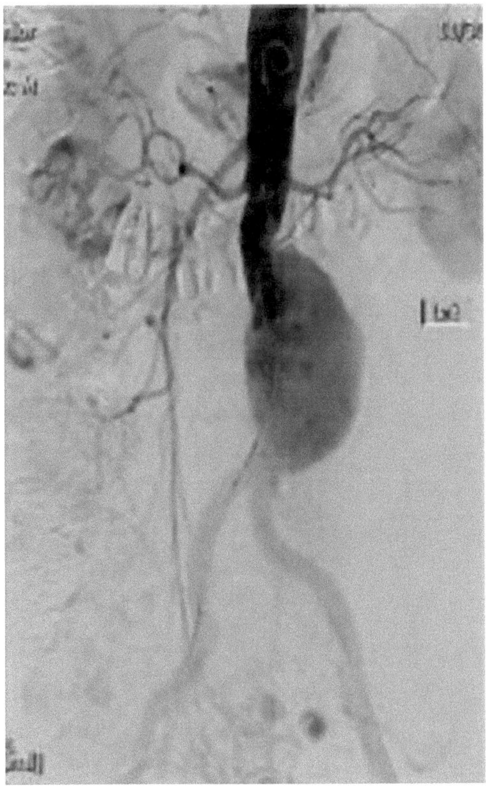

Figure 9.3 Initial intraoperative angiogram, showing a slightly angulated neck, and suitable for EVAR.

Graft selection

Many surgeons have a favorite aortic endograft they are comfortable using. It is important to select the graft the surgeon is most familiar with and certainly not one they have never seen or used. In our hospital, we stock two types of endografts on the shelf and our choice of graft largely depends on the following features: proximal neck diameter and length, diameter of the external iliacs, and general tortuosity of the aortic neck and iliacs.

A hybrid endovascular surgical suite is ideal to treat patients with ruptured AAA. Even if the patient is not suitable for EVAR, a percutaneous placement of an intra-aortic occlusion balloon may be life-saving and certainly less morbid than an emergency thoracotomy or open supraceliac cross-clamp [23].

Procedure

The primary objective of the "team" is to get the patient to the endovascular suite as soon as possible. Everyone should be working purposefully and expeditiously. Any undue delay is not in the patient's best interest. In the pre-operative period, permissive hypotension is a good option to help maintain any temporary seal following the rupture. Keeping the room and the patient warm is important to avoid the worsening of a coagulopathy [24]. The patient may be given mild sedation to relieve stress and anxiety, such as a small dose of Versed and fentanyl.

But most importantly, avoiding anesthesia induction and muscle paralysis, until the patient is prepared and the surgeon is gowned and ready to access the groin, are crucial to avoiding a sudden drop in blood pressure. Many experienced surgeons prefer to have the patient awake to maintain sympathetic tone just to avoid this potential problem.

Preparation

Skin preparation from the chest to thighs (nipples to knees) as with any open AAA repair is essential. Adherence to best practice to avoid skin infection, including the use of clippers for hair removal in the groin and a chlorhexidine-based solution to cleanse the skin, should be emphasized. A foley catheter and radial arterial line are ideal but could be omitted in certain cases. Placing a central line is not necessary and should never be the cause of delaying the start of the case. Many experienced anesthesiologists will use intraoperative TEE monitoring to guide fluid resuscitation.

Emergent EVAR

The first step, after the patient is prepared and draped, is to perform a percutaneous ultrasound guided puncture of the femoral artery. Unless the femoral arteries are severely diseased and calcified, we typically use the "preclose" technique, deploying two Proglide sutures at 10 and 2 o'clock for later closure. If the surgeon is uncomfortable with this technique, an open femoral cutdown can be performed. Once the femoral artery is accessed with a micropuncture kit, an 8Fr sheath is placed, the first diagnostic angiogram can be performed using a pigtail catheter (Figure 9.3). In the event the patient is hypotensive or more unstable, a supraceliac aortic occlusion balloon can be placed [23]. In cases where intra-aortic balloon occlusion is performed, it is important to keep track of how long it is inflated to avoid sequelae of prolonged organ ischemia. In addition, it is preferable to use a longer sheath, either 55 or 90 cm long, to support the balloon and avoid its distal migration.

After the diagnostic angiogram, the surgeon now has a firm idea of what type of graft to use and if, indeed, EVAR is the best option (Figure 9.3). At this point, we typically give a heparin dose. In most cases, a full heparin dose is not necessary and we usually opt for a moderate dose of 50–70 units/kg. It is possible to proceed without additional anticoagulation if the patient is already coagulopathic.

Insertion of the main body of the graft is usually from the right side, however, in some cases, the surgeon may opt to use the left side to avoid calcification or narrowing of the right iliac artery, or to address an aortic neck angulation. Whether to keep the graft's short limb anatomical or cross the legs depends on the angle of the aorto-iliac bifurcation (Figure 9.4). In general, angles of 90° or greater favor crossing the graft legs. This simple

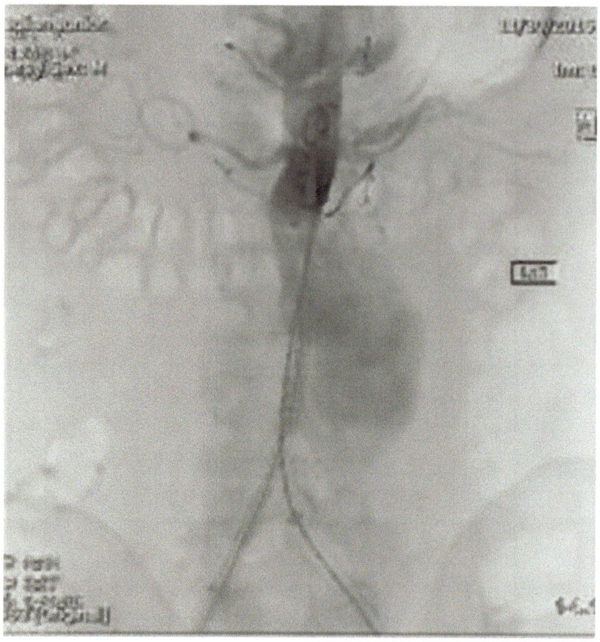

Figure 9.4 Angiogram with device in place, accessory renals are now seen. Also note that the wires cross at the iliac bifurcation, which favors crossing the limbs of the graft (see Figure 9.7).

maneuver can save a lot of time in trying to cannulate the short leg of the graft, especially when time is a factor. There are many techniques that have been described to help speed up the process of short gate cannulation. We typically use a Kumpe catheter and an angled glide wire, and less frequently use other preformed catheters, such as a Sos or Van Schie (Cook Medical) for more difficult cannulations. Once the short gate is cannulated, the distance from the gate to the hypogastric is measured, and an appropriate graft overlap is factored in, the proper length of limb is then selected and inserted (Figure 9.5). The ipsilateral side is then addressed. With the Excluder C-3 (W. L. Gore), most of the time no additional pieces are necessary.

With the Zenith (Cook Medical), the ipsilateral limb is selected based on the length from the graft to the hypogastric and the diameter of the distal landing zone. It is generally a good policy to try to line the aorta and the iliacs from the renals to the hypogastrics, especially if the exact location of the rupture or leak is not known. This will save a lot of time after graft deployment and a persistent contrast blush is observed. If one iliac is aneurysmal, coverage of the hypogastric can be done by landing in the external iliac. In an unstable patient, coiling is not advised (Figure 9.6).

Once the endograft is deployed, balloon inflation at the proximal end, graft to graft, and distal junctions, a completion angiogram is performed (Figure 9.7). If no type I or type III endoleaks are observed, it is time to complete the procedure. If percutaneous access was used, and the preclose technique employed, these sutures are carefully

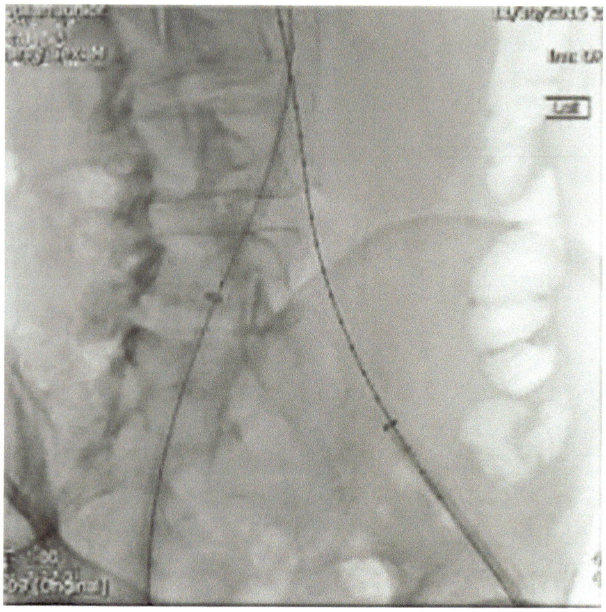

Figure 9.5 The device has been deployed and a pigtail catheter with centimeter markers to measure the distance between the short leg of graft and the left hypogastric, in an oblique view.

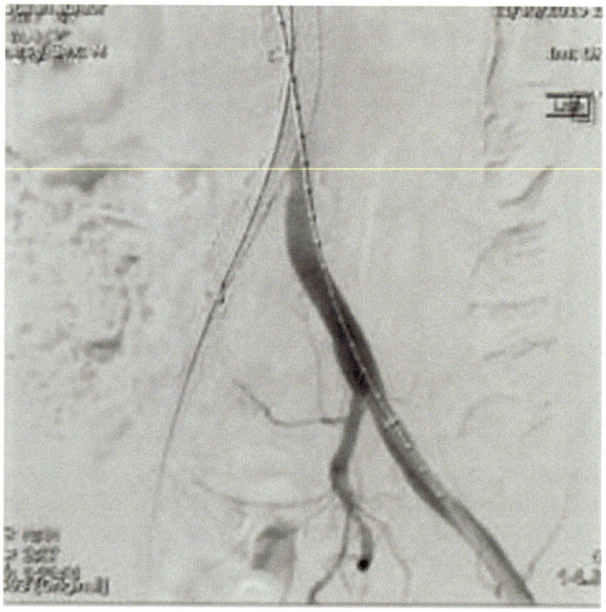

Figure 9.6 Angiogram showing distance from the gate to the hypogastric to select the correct limb length.

tied, and gentle manual compression for five minutes is done. It is reasonable to reverse the heparin effect with some protamine at this point, especially if there is evidence of unusual oozing.

If an open cutdown was done, the femoral artery is repaired with 5.0 or 6.0 Prolene and the wound is closed in layers. After closure, it is important to examine the legs and feet and palpate pedal pulses or check for Doppler signals. The abdomen is also examined. If the abdomen

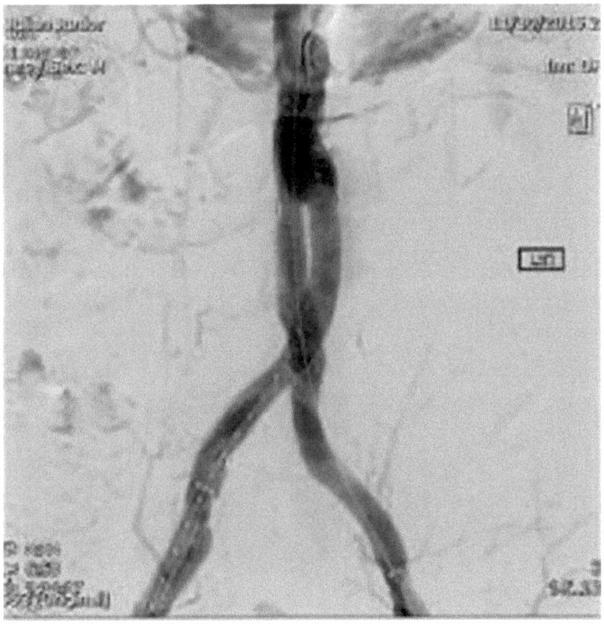

Figure 9.7 Completion angiogram: note the legs are crossed.

is tense, bladder pressure can be measured. If the anesthesiologist reports the need for high ventilator pressures, and the abdomen is tense, careful consideration should be given for releasing the abdominal compartment [25]. In our experience, this is necessary in only about 10–15% of cases with ruptured AAA.

Complications

Access site. With percutaneous access and the preclose technique, careful selection of the puncture site to avoid anterior calcification is important. Despite proper technique, preclose can fail in up to 5–8% of cases and an open femoral cutdown has to be performed. Other complications at the access site include inadvertently raising a flap causing ischemia, or distal embolization. Occasionally, with the preclose technique, the sutures break and open femoral artery repair is needed. If the femoral artery is badly diseased, it is sometimes necessary to perform an endarterectomy and patch closure.

Myocardial infarction. Patients with severe coronary artery disease do not tolerate hypotension and hemodynamic instability. ECG changes or arrhythmias intra- or postoperatively should prompt a cardiology consultation.

Contrast induced nephropathy. Contrast induced nephropathy (CIN) is a known complication after EVAR. Using proper technique and avoiding excessive contrast volume are essential.

Maintaining a normal blood pressure postoperatively and crystalloid hydration can lessen the incidence of CIN.

Distal embolization. Atheroembolization occurs when the aortic graft snowplows through unstable aortic plaque or thrombus or there is excessive graft manipulation and torsion in the AAA. These maneuvers should be avoided if possible.

Abdominal compartment syndrome. If the ruptured AAA has caused excessive retroperitoneal bleeding, a large hematoma may lead to an abdominal compartment syndrome. Release of the abdominal compartment and placement of an abdominal vacuum dressing is our preference. It is often feasible to close the abdomen in 36–48 hours when the hematoma is resorbed.

Graft limb occlusion. Acute graft limb occlusion can occur in cases of a severely diseased iliac artery or a tortuous one. If the endograft is not fully expanded in a narrow iliac artery, this could lead to limb thrombosis. On the other hand, in very tortuous iliac arteries, the rigid graft may end up distorting the iliac artery and causing a functional occlusion. The latter problem can sometimes be averted by performing the completion angiogram without the stiff wire in place.

CONCLUSION

To ensure the ideal outcomes for patients with ruptured AAA, a multidisciplinary and coordinated approach needs to be adopted. While many randomized trials comparing EVAR for ruptured AAA to traditional open repair have failed to show a conclusive benefit for EVAR, most experts agree that an "EVAR first" stance is best [26,27]. It is recognized that there will be patients with difficult anatomy or hostile necks who are not good candidates for EVAR. However, if EVAR is feasible in a ruptured AAA, patients will be afforded the best chance of surviving this catastrophe. Complication rates after emergent EVAR may be slightly higher than elective cases, but overall survival is improved over open repair.

TRICKS AND TRAPS

- In patients undergoing endovascular repair of ruptured AAA, induction and muscular paralysis with anesthesia should be postponed until the patient is prepped and the surgeon is ready to gain groin access to avoid sudden hypotension as sympathetic tone is lost with induction.
- Supraceliac balloon occlusion should be performed in hemodynamically unstable patients. A longer sheath (55.0 cm long) should be used to avoid distal migration of the balloon.
- Diagnostic arteriogram should be performed using a marker pigtail or Omniflush catheter to aid in the selection of the type of endograft to be used, and in most cases, endovascular repair is often the most appropriate choice.
- Abdominal compartment syndrome may occur in patients with excessive retroperitoneal bleeding or

those with a large retroperitoneal hematoma. Release of the abdominal compartment and vacuum-assisted closure using a non-adherent sponge would be performed.

- In patients with ruptured AAA, the anatomical situation favors endovascular repair; the patient has a better chance of survival as compared with open repair.

QUESTIONS

1. A 74-year-old male with a known AAA presents to the ER with a sudden onset of back pain and hypotension. After careful fluid resuscitation, blood pressure reaches 100 mmHg systolic. The patient should now undergo
   a. Immediate thin section CTA of the abdomen and pelvis
   b. Abdominal aortogram
   c. Emergency open repair without further delay
   d. MRA abdomen

   Answer: a

2. While being taken to a CT scan, the patient becomes hemodynamically unstable with BP dropping to 60 mmHg systolic and is pale, diaphoretic, and difficult to arouse. What is the next best course of action?
   a. Continue with CTA imaging
   b. Take the patient to hybrid OR immediately; use left brachial access and balloon occlusion of the suprarenal artery
   c. Using femoral access to obtain immediate supraceliac balloon occlusion of the aorta
   d. Immediate open repair

   Answer: c

3. In the recovery room, the patient requires 100% FIO_2 to maintain a saturation of 90, peak airway pressure of 40 cm water. The patient is oliguric and has normal coagulation, BP is 100 mmHg systolic with sinus tachycardia (118/min). The next course of action is
   a. Start ECMO
   b. Increase PEEP
   c. Ionotropic support
   d. Measure intraabdominal pressure using a Foley catheter in the bladder

   Answer: d

4. Intraabdominal pressure is 24 mmHg and PEEP is increased to 15 cm/water. The patient is administered neuromuscular blockade, albumin, and furosemide. However, the patient remains oliguric with a further increase in abdominal girth; you should now consider:
   a. Decompressive laparotomy with closure of linea alba only
   b. Decompressive laparotomy with leaving open the abdomen and vacuum-assisted temporary closure using AbThera™ open dressing
   c. Open decompression using a retroperitoneal approach and evacuation of periaortic hematoma
   d. Fiberoptic sigmoidostomy

   Answer: b

REFERENCES

1. www.CDC.gov
2. Kim LG et al. How cost effective is screening for abdominal aortic aneurysms? *J Med Screen* 14:46–52; 2007
3. Thompson SG et al. Screening for abdominal aortic aneurysm: 10 year mortality and cost effectiveness results from the randomized multicenter aneurysm screening study. *BMJ* 338:b2307; 2009
4. Shreibati JB et al. Impact of the screening abdominal aortic aneurysm very efficiently (SAAAVE) act on abdominal ultrasonography use among Medicare beneficiaries. *Arch Int Med* 172:1456–1462; 2012
5. Soden PA et al. Outcomes for symptomatic abdominal aortic aneurysms in the American college of surgeons national surgical quality improvement program. *J Vasc Surg* 64:297; 2016
6. Volodos NL et al. A self-fixing synthetic blood vessel endoprosthesis. *Vestn Khir Il Grek* 137:123; 1986
7. Parodi JC et al. Transfemoral intraluminal graft implantation for abdominal aortic aneurysms. *Ann Vasc Surg* 5;491–499; 1991
8. Endovascular aneurysm repair versus open repair in patients with abdominal aortic aneurysms (EVAR trial 1): randomized cotrolled trial. *Lancet* 365:2179–2186; 2005
9. Endovascular aneurysm repair and outcome in patients unfit for open repair of abdominal aortic aneurysm (EVAR trial 2): randomized controlled trial. *Lancet* 365:2187–2192; 2005
10. Endovascular strategy or open repair for ruptured abdominal aortic aneurysm: one-year outcomes from the IMPROVE randomized trial. *Eur Heart J* 36:2061–2069; 2015
11. Powell JT et al. Endovascular or open repair strategy for ruptured abdominal aortic aneurysm: 30-day outcomes from IMPROVE randomized trial. *BMJ* 348:f7661; 2014
12. Reimerink JJ et al. Endovascular repair versus open repair of ruptured abdominal aortic aneurysms: a multicenter randomized controlled trial. *Ann Surg* 258:248–256; 2013

13. Schermerhorn ML et al. Changes in abdominal aortic aneurysm rupture and short-term mortality, 1995–2008: a retrospective observational study. *Ann Surg* 256:651–658; 2012
14. Chang DC et al. Survival after endovascular vs. open aortic aneurysm repairs. *JAMA Surg* 150:1160–1166; 2015
15. Egorova N et al. National outcomes for the treatment of ruptured abdominal aortic aneurysm: comparison of open versus endovascular repairs. *J Vasc Surg* 48:1092–1100; 2008
16. Veith FJ et al. Collected world and single center experience with endovascular treatment of ruptured abdominal aortic aneurysms. *Ann Surg* 250:818–824; 2009
17. Sweeting MJ et al. Individual patient meta-analysis of three randomized trials comparing endovascular versus open repair for ruptured abdominal aortic aneurysm. *Br J Surg* 102:1229–1239; 2015
18. McPhee J et al. Endovascular treatment of ruptured abdominal aortic aneurysms in the United States (2001–2006): a significant survival benefit over open repair is independently associated with increase institutional volume. *J Vasc Surg* 49:817–826; 2009
19. Salata K et al. Population-based long-term outcomes of open versus endovascular repair of ruptured abdominal aortic aneurysms. *J Vasc Surg* 71(6):1867–1878; 2020
20. Mehta M et al. Establishing a protocol for endovascular treatment of ruptured abdominal aortic aneurysms: outcomes of a prospective analysis. *J Vasc Surg* 44:1–8; 2006
21. Starnes BW et al. Management of ruptured abdominal aortic aneurysm in the endovascular era. *J Vasc Surg* 51:9–17; 2010
22. Mehta M et al. Ruptured abdominal aortic aneurysm: endovascular program development and results. *Semin Vasc Surg* 23:206–214; 2010
23. Malina M, Holst J. Balloon control for ruptured AAAs: when and when not to use? *J Cardiovasc Surg* 55:161–167; 2014
24. Quiroga E et al. Hypothermia is associated with increased mortality in patients undergoing repair of ruptured abdominal aortic aneurysm. *J Endovasc Ther* 17:434–438; 2010
25. Ersryd S et al. Abdominal compartment syndrome after surgery for abdominal aortic aneurysm: a nationwide population based study. *Eur J Vasc Endovasc Surg* 58:671; 2019
26. Holst J et al. Early and intermediate outcome of emergency endovascular aneurysm repair of ruptured infrarenal aortic aneurysm: a single-centre experience of 90 consecutive patients. *Eur J Vasc Endovasc Surg* 37:413–419; 2009
27. Kapma MR et al. Cost-effectiveness and cost-utility of endovascular versus open repair of ruptured abdominal aortic aneurysm in the Amsterdam Acute Aneurysm Trial. *Br J Surg* 101:208–215; 2014

10

Popliteal artery aneurysm

KEVIN T. ONOFREY, HASSAN CHAMSEDDINE, AND ALI RTEIL

INTRODUCTION

Aneurysms are defined as vessel enlargement greater than 1.5 times the diameter of the normal adjacent artery segments. As the normal diameter of the popliteal artery ranges from 5 to 11 mm, any popliteal artery greater than 1.5 cm is considered aneurysmal. Popliteal artery aneurysms (PAA) less than 20 mm in diameter are expected to have growth rates between 0.3 and 1.5 mm annually. Those greater than 20 mm in diameter have significant variability in growth rates.

PAA have a 20:1 male to female ratio with approximately 50% of individuals having bilateral PAA and 40% having a concurrent abdominal aortic aneurysm. The mean age at presentation is 65 years with an incidence of 7/100,000 in males and 1/100,000 in females. PAA often have asymptomatic presentations and are found incidentally on imaging or on physical examination manifesting as a prominent pulse. Symptomatic presentations are often dire and include acute limb threatening ischemia secondary to thrombosis, distal embolization, or a combination of both. Limb swelling and pain from vein or nerve compression are additional manifestations, as well as symptoms of chronic ischemia associated with chronic thromboembolism, making it indistinguishable from atherosclerotic arterial occlusive disease. While rare, the first presenting symptom of PAA can be rupture. Major amputation rates exceed 15–20% following acute presentations.

While most surgeons use 2 cm as a threshold for consideration for elective repair, it is important to consider the presence of mural thrombus, the status of runoff vessels, the ambulatory status, as well as patients' underlying comorbid conditions in the decision-making process when treating PAA. The most recent Society for Vascular Surgery clinical practice guidelines published in January of 2022 suggest that PAA less than 20 mm with identifiable thrombus, with compromised distal runoff vessels, or those with severe angulation >45 degrees, could be considered for earlier repair [1]. Conversely, patients with higher surgical risk could be deferred until the aneurysm grows to over 30 mm, especially in the absence of thrombus.

Traditional repair of PAA has consisted of open surgical bypass, preferably using autologous saphenous vein with excision or exclusion of the aneurysm (open popliteal artery repair; OPAR). Advances in endovascular technology have, however, opened up opportunities for endovascular popliteal aneurysm repair (EPAR) in appropriate patients.

Pre-operative evaluation

Duplex ultrasound, computed tomography angiography (CTA), magnetic resonance angiography (MRA), and catheter-based digital subtraction angiography are all modalities used for both diagnosing and guiding management of PAA (Figure 10.1). Duplex ultrasound is the least invasive, cheapest, and most useful in both identification and surveillance of asymptomatic PAA that have not yet met size criteria for repair. Patients with PAA should also undergo baseline ankle-brachial indices (ABI) with digital photoplethysmography to objectively document limb perfusion status. Regardless of repair modality, there are several considerations, including anatomy and the degree of atherosclerotic disease within the proximal inflow and the outflow vessels, which have implications on the success of repair. While there are no endografts approved for the treatment of PAA, EPAR using the GORE VIABAHN endoprosthesis, a covered stent composed of polytetrafluoroethylene (PTFE) with a nitinol exoskeleton, has been used successfully. Important considerations for EPAR include normal proximal and distal landing zones at least 2 cm in length, diameter discrepancy between the proximal and distal landing zones of less than 1 mm, vessel tortuosity less than 45°, aneurysm diameter less than 5 cm, and ideally at least a two vessel runoff to the ipsilateral foot. Additional relative contraindications to EPAR

DOI: 10.1201/9781003452096-10

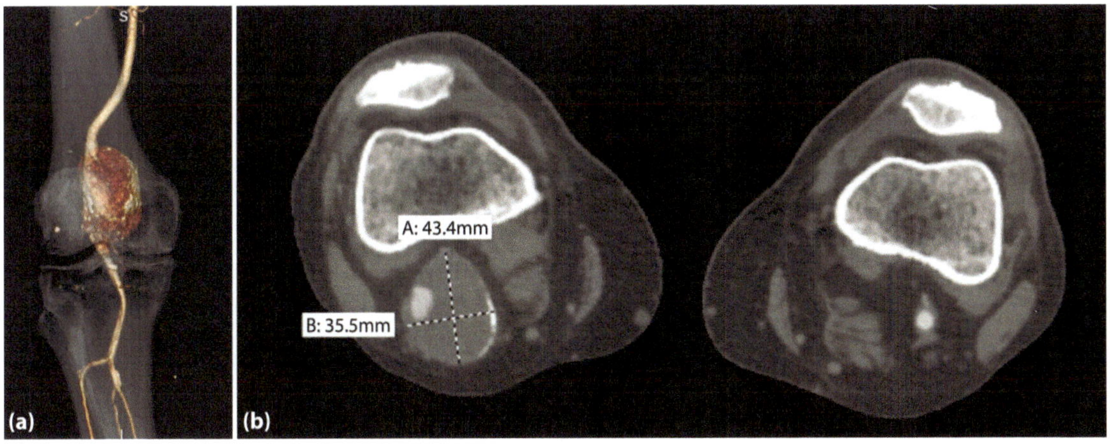

Figure 10.1 (a) Three-dimensional reconstruction of popliteal artery aneurysm and (b) cross-sectional CTA showing 4.3 cm popliteal artery aneurysm.

include occupations or hobbies that require prolonged bending at the knee, which may predispose the stent graft to thrombosis.

MANAGEMENT

Open surgical treatment: Medial approach

Open surgical treatment of PAA can be performed via either a medial or posterior approach. The medial approach is most commonly utilized and is particularly useful in aneurysmal disease that extends beyond the popliteal fossa requiring a more distal bypass target or a more proximal inflow site. It also allows for the easy exposure of the greater saphenous vein (GSV) as a bypass conduit. A notable disadvantage with this approach is that it is usually performed with proximal and distal arterial ligation without decompression, thus posing a risk of continued aneurysm mass effect in addition to geniculate perfusion of the aneurysm sac with growth, persistence of symptoms, and possibly rupture. As such, many vascular surgeons are proponents of concomitant decompression and suture ligation of side branches.

In this technique, the patient is placed supine with the involved leg externally rotated. Proximally, a medial above-the-knee incision is fashioned longitudinally between the sartorius and the vastus medialis muscles. The popliteal artery can be located posterior to the femur. Care should be taken to preserve the saphenous nerve, which exits alongside the popliteal artery from the adductor hiatus, with special attention given to the popliteal vein that lies posteromedial to the artery. A non-aneurysmal segment of the popliteal/superficial femoral artery (SFA) is then circumferentially controlled with silicon vessel loops. When the aneurysmal process involves the entire SFA, it is sometimes necessary to originate a graft in the groin.

Distally, a medial incision 1 cm posterior to the tibia is made to obtain access to the deep posterior compartment. The gastrocnemius is retracted further posteriorly and blunt dissection is used to isolate the below knee popliteal artery. For more distal exposure of the below knee popliteal artery, the insertion of the upper portion of the soleus muscle may be divided. Special care should be taken in handling the popliteal vein, which will again be encountered along with the tibial nerve; both should be retracted posteriorly.

After controlling the proximal and distal non-aneurysmal segments of the popliteal artery, a tunnel traversing the medial and lateral heads of the gastrocnemius muscle is created. In the presence of large PAA, this step can be quite challenging. The patient is then heparinized with 80–100 units of heparin per kilogram of body weight with a goal activated clotting time (ACT) of more than 250 seconds. A bypass graft is then performed from the normal segment of the popliteal artery proximal to the PAA to a normal segment of the popliteal artery distal to the PAA. Both end-to-end and end-to-side anastomoses are acceptable depending on the size discrepancy between the artery and GSV. The procedure is then concluded by ligating the proximal and distal popliteal arteries, preferably as close to the aneurysm sac as possible, to promote aneurysm thrombosis and decrease the probability of continued expansion.

Open surgical treatment: Posterior approach

In patients with PAA confined to the popliteal fossa, a posterior approach may be considered (Figure 10.2). In this approach, the patient is positioned prone after harvesting an adequate length of GSV from the contralateral groin to perform an interposition graft. An S-shaped incision is made starting superomedial to expose the proximal popliteal artery, extended transversely across

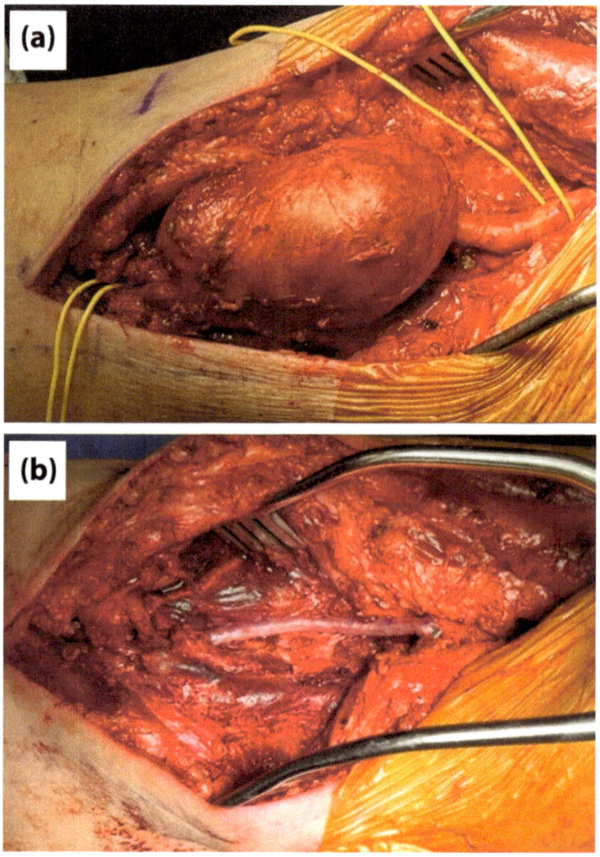

Figure 10.2 (a) Open posterior approach to popliteal artery aneurysm repaired with (b) interposition greater saphenous vein harvested from the ankle after completely excising the aneurysm sac. Proximal popliteal artery (encircled with yellow vessel loop) is to the right and distal popliteal artery (also encircled with a yellow vessel loop) is to the left.

the popliteal crease, before being carried vertically below the knee. Using this approach, the popliteal vein is encountered superficial to the artery and is best retracted medially to expose the artery. Proximally, the popliteal artery is exposed by separating the semimembranosus and semitendinosus muscles from the long head of the biceps femoris. Care must be taken to avoid injury to the tibial and peroneal nerves that may be encountered traversing laterally. A large branch of the tibial nerve to the lateral head of the gastrocnemius is frequently encountered coursing over the artery and usually requires sacrifice to achieve adequate exposure. Distally, the two heads of the gastrocnemius muscle serve as a landmark to identify the distal popliteal artery. Exposure of the tibioperoneal trunk beyond the origin of the anterior tibial artery can be achieved with the division of the upper portion of the soleus muscle but is much more difficult from this approach. After proximal and distal control is achieved, the patient is heparinized to a goal ACT of 250 seconds. The aneurysmal sac is opened and intraluminal thrombus is removed and any backbleeding branches oversewn. Alternatively, the entire aneurysm sac can be excised, but this increases the risk of injury to the vein and nerve. An interposition GSV graft reconstruction is usually performed with end-to-end anastomoses. In rare situations, GSV can be harvested from the ankle if of adequate caliber by inverting and slightly elevating the foot. The short saphenous vein can also be used if large enough.

Comparable primary patency rates have been reported between the medial and posterior approaches. The choice of conduit, however, is of increased significance. While a prosthetic conduit may be utilized, especially when using the posterior approach and when a short segment interposition is needed, saphenous vein conduit is always preferred because of its superior primary and secondary patency rates [2, 3, 4].

Endovascular repair

Endovascular repair of PAA, first described in 1994, utilizes fundamentals similar to endovascular aortic aneurysm repair, namely, the utilization of a covered stent with adequate healthy proximal and distal landing zones to achieve an appropriate seal. As such, the first contraindication to EPAR is the lack of adequate landing zones. Additionally, at least two good outflow vessels and a size discrepancy less than 1 mm between the inflow and outflow vessels is required for endovascular repair to be considered [5].

EPAR is usually performed with ipsilateral antegrade or contralateral retrograde groin access. The PAA is traversed using a straight tip catheter and the borders of the aneurysm are marked using radio-opaque needles. The overall length of the aneurysm and inflow/outflow vessel diameter dictates stent choice. The recommended proximal and distal landing zone length is 2 cm or more. In cases where more than one stent is required to traverse the lesion, a minimum of 3 cm of overlap is recommended. However, care should be taken to avoid overlap at major hinge points of the native popliteal artery. This is followed by balloon dilatation to ensure adequate stent opposition to the arterial wall with complete sac exclusion, which is confirmed on completion angiography (Figure 10.3).

Post-operatively, dual antiplatelet therapy is recommended with aspirin 81 mg and Plavix 75 mg for one year, and aspirin monotherapy thereafter. Additionally, duplex ultrasonography is performed at the first outpatient follow-up visit, at six months, and then annually along with ABIs.

Complications of endovascular PAA repair include stenosis, occlusion, stent fracture, and stent migration. Stenosis often occurs secondary to intimal hyperplasia at the borders of the stent graft, with occlusion being the most feared ensuing complication. Stent graft thrombosis can also be caused by prolonged bending at the knee, poor runoff secondary to prior embolization, and atherosclerotic disease. Type II endoleak can also complicate endovascular repair with back bleeding from popliteal

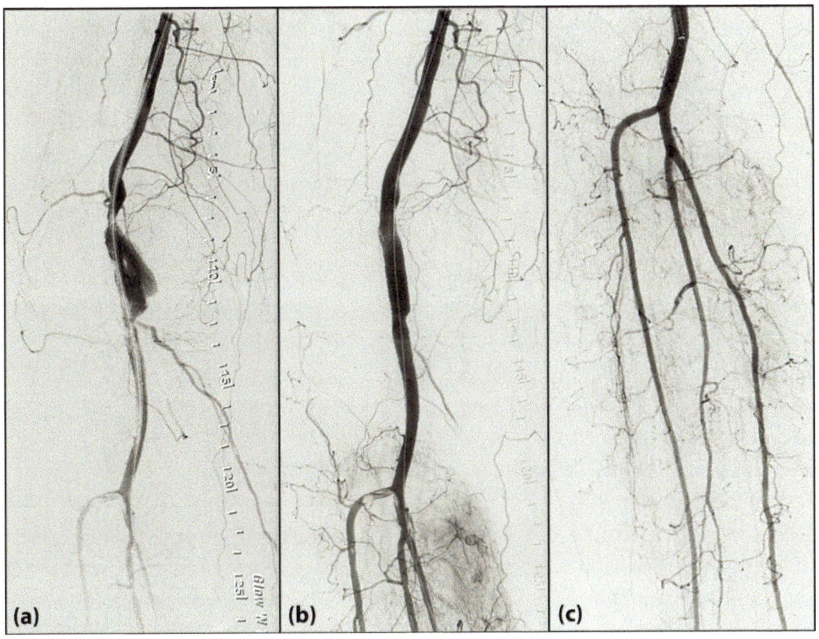

Figure 10.3 Angiography showing (a) popliteal artery aneurysm with thrombus in the anterior tibial artery; (b) complete aneurysm sac exclusion after deployment of an endovascular stent graft; and (c) completion angiography after clearance of thrombus from the anterior tibial artery.

side branches as discussed previously in the open repair section.

URGENT CONSIDERATIONS

The most common emergent presentation of PAA is acute limb ischemia secondary to thrombosis of the aneurysm. In such cases, the degree of arterial occlusion is often severe enough that no distal runoff is visualized on angiography. In this setting, a timely intervention is required to salvage the limb, with amputation rates as high as 15–20%. Principles of management in patients presenting with acute thromboembolism secondary to PAA include immediate initiation of anticoagulation followed by operative intervention. Care should be taken in the assessment of reperfusion and consequent compartment syndrome.

Intraoperatively, if the aneurysm is completely occluded and a distal patent target vessel is identified, a bypass should be attempted. In the absence of a patent tibial artery, exposure of the popliteal trifurcation is advised with gentle Fogarty balloon catheter thromboembolectomy of the affected distal vessels in an attempt to establish an appropriate distal target. At case conclusion and post-operatively, the surgeon should have a high index of suspicion for compartment syndrome and a four-compartment fasciotomy may be required.

Additionally, peri-operative thrombolysis can also be considered. When no good outflow vessel is identifiable preoperatively, and the limb is not immediately threatened, catheter-directed thrombolysis can be attempted to restore patency to a potential distal bypass target. Unfortunately, in this situation, the distal outflow may be so chronically damaged by repetitive prior embolism of aneurysm mural thrombus that limb salvage is not possible. Intraoperative thrombolysis has also been utilized with an intent to clear residual aneurysm-related thrombus, but this is usually of limited utility in our experience.

Rupture is a rare presentation of PAA, and hemorrhage is self-limiting given the anatomic restriction of the popliteal fossa. Limb loss, however, remains a real and common outcome in this patient population.

TRICKS AND TRAPS

- Repair of PAA is indicated in all symptomatic patients and in asymptomatic patients when the diameter exceeds 2 cm in appropriate risk patients.
- In high-risk patients with no thrombus, repair can be deferred until a diameter of 3 cm is reached.
- Open PAA repair is the gold standard, and options include a medial approach with vein bypass and PAA exclusion, or a posterior approach with vein interposition and aneurysmorrhaphy or aneurysmectomy.
- When performing an open repair using the posterior approach, the greater saphenous vein should be harvested prior to positioning the patient prone.
- Endovascular repair of PAA requires 2 cm of similar diameter (within 1 mm) healthy artery above and below the aneurysm and a minimum of a two vessel runoff.
- When performing endovascular repair of PAA, oversize the stent graft by 10–15% compared with the normal artery diameter.

- In acute presentations with a thrombosed PAA and no discernible tibial artery outflow, we recommend catheter-directed thrombolysis in an attempt to re-establish an outflow target.
- In acute presentations with Rutherford 2b ischemia and no runoff vessels, we recommend operative therapy with attempted thrombectomy to establish a target vessel for bypass repair.

QUESTIONS

1. An 86-year-old patient presents with a symptomatic 2.8 cm popliteal artery aneurysm. He has a past medical history of coronary artery bypass without remnant saphenous vein to utilize. What is the optimal management strategy moving forward?
   a. Surveillance with duplex ultrasound every year
   b. Operative repair of the popliteal artery aneurysm
   c. Peri-operative evaluation of the abdominal aorta and contralateral popliteal artery
   d. B and C

   Answer: d

2. A 55-year-old patient presents with a 1.7 cm popliteal artery aneurysm. He is asymptomatic and his aneurysm was noted incidentally on a lower extremity venous duplex. What is the most next appropriate step in management?
   a. Urgent open repair
   b. Urgent endovascular repair
   c. Evaluation of the contralateral limb and abdominal aorta followed by operative repair
   d. Evaluation of the contralateral limb and abdominal aorta followed by serial duplex observation at 6–12 months intervals

   Answer: d

3. A 48-year-old presents for follow-up after an endovascular repair of a 3 cm popliteal aneurysm. What are the principles of medical therapy in this patient?
   a. Lifelong dual antiplatelet therapy
   b. Aspirin 100 mg and Plavix 75 mg for one year only
   c. Aspirin 100 mg and Plavix 75 mg for one year, followed by lifelong aspirin monotherapy
   d. No need for medical therapy if the patient receives duplex ultrasonography at the first outpatient visit

   Answer: c

4. A 50-year-old patient is being evaluated for a 1.8 cm popliteal artery aneurysm. On duplex ultrasonography, there is intraluminal thrombus with abrupt occlusion of the anterior tibial artery distally, and diminished ankle-brachial indices. What is the recommended management strategy?
   a. Follow-up with surveillance imaging
   b. Follow-up with surveillance imaging and dual antiplatelet therapy
   c. Evaluate the patient for operative repair
   d. Perform an exercise ankle-brachial index test

   Answer: c

REFERENCES

1. Farber A, Angle N, Avgerinos E, et al. The society for vascular surgery clinical practice guidelines on popliteal artery aneurysms. *J Vasc Surg*. 2022;75(1S):109S–120S. doi:10.1016/j.jvs.2021.04.040
2. Beseth BD, Moore WS. The posterior approach for repair of popliteal artery aneurysms. *J Vasc Surg*. 2006;43:940–944. discussion 4–5.
3. Ravn H, Wanhainen A, Björck M, et al. Surgical technique and long-term results after popliteal artery aneurysm repair: Results from 717 legs. *J Vasc Surg*. 2007;46:236–243.
4. Huang Y, Gloviczki P, Noel AA, et al. Early complications and long-term outcome after open surgical treatment of popliteal artery aneurysms: Is exclusion with saphenous vein bypass still the gold standard?. *J Vasc Surg*. 2007;45:706–715.
5. Shah NG, Rokosh RS, Garg K, et al. Endovascular treatment of popliteal artery aneurysms has comparable long-term outcomes to open repair with shorter lengths of stay. *J Vasc Surg*. 2021;74(5):1565–1572.e1. doi:10.1016/j.jvs.2021.04.046

11

Complex endovascular repair of pararenal and thoracoabdominal aneurysms utilizing physician-modified endografts

SAURABH GUPTA, ANDI N. PESHKEPIJA, AND SHAHAB A. TOURSAVADKOHI

INTRODUCTION

Open aortic aneurysm repair remains the gold standard repair for pararenal and thoracoabdominal aneurysms. However, national trends demonstrate a significant decline in open surgical volume with endovascular repair becoming the dominant method [1]. Endovascular repairs have shown a significant decrease in morbidity and mortality in infra-renal aortic aneurysms, a decrease in operative time, intraoperative blood loss, and hospital length of stay [2]. However, for patients with hostile infra-renal aortic necks, a significant portion of these aneurysms are treated outside of the device instructions for use (IFU). In patients with higher physiological risks, this departure from guidelines becomes even larger. Resulting in a poor repair with a higher incidence of a type 1A endoleak and lower five- and ten-year survival [3].

When compared with infra-renal endovascular repair, endovascular management of pararenal and thoracoabdominal aneurysms remains coveted. The utilization of fenestrated and branched devices adds a significant level of complexity to the operation and access to *off-the-shelf* or custom-made devices (CMD) is limited to a select number of centers. Planning and technical mistakes can result in significant morbidity and mortality. Currently, the only Food and Drug Administration (FDA) approved fenestrated device is for the treatment of juxtarenal and short-necked infra-renal aneurysms, the Zenith Fenestrated AAA Endovascular Graft (ZFEN; William A. Cook Australia, Brisbane, Australia). The ZFEN device has physical and design constraints with a 4 mm infra-renal neck indication, maximum seal zone only up to the celiac trunk along, and four-to-six-week manufacturing time, essentially placing restrictions on its utility for more anatomically complex aneurysms and urgent, emergent situations.

In the United States, multiple industry- and physician-sponsored trials are studying the feasibility and durability of endograft implantation in the supra-renal aorta. These trials are occurring at select centers throughout the United States with a large portion of the population left without access to custom patient-specific devices. Physicians who seek to treat these aneurysms endovascularly may choose to perform physician-modified endografts (PMEG), an alternative to CMD devices left to the surgeon's discretion. Endografts are considered significant-risk devices and therefore modification should be performed under a physician-sponsored investigational device exemption (IDE) from the FDA. Unfortunately, this process is lengthy and requires significant investment from the sponsoring institution.

In the previous edition of this textbook, this chapter discussed industry-supplied CMD devices. At that time, and unfortunately still now, most vascular surgeons did not have access to these devices, therefore, we have shifted the focus of the chapter to a practical approach discussing the methods to modify the grafts on your own to treat complex aortic aneurysms. We will also describe adjunctive techniques to facilitate these operations. Techniques such as in-situ fenestration and parallel grafts are noteworthy, however, with the utilization of PMEG, we believe these should be reserved for unique situations. In this current environment, as we await FDA-approved devices for the management of complex aortic aneurysms, PMEG will help bridge the gap in available technology for the management of high-risk patients unfit for open surgical repair.

CASE EXAMPLE

A 57-year-old woman who suffered a Stanford type A dissection in 2016. This was followed with immediate

DOI: 10.1201/9781003452096-11

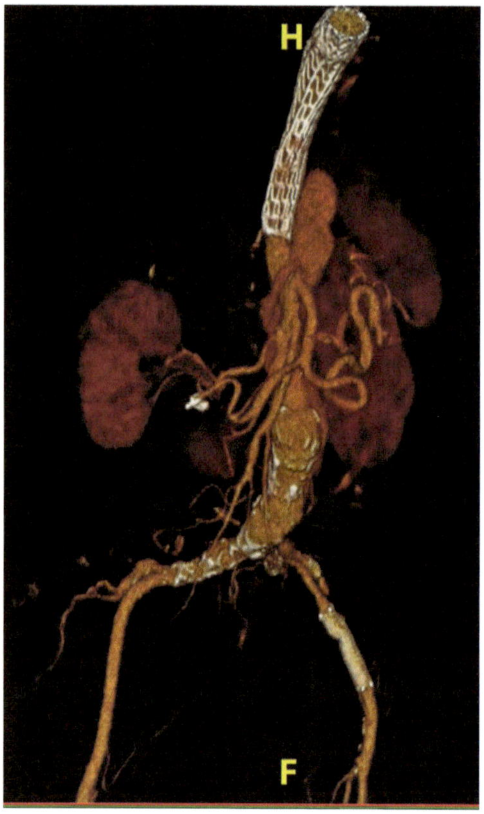

Figure 11.1 Dissection thoracoabdominal aneurysm with TEVAR extension to the level of the celiac artery. Aneurysm involving false lumen; aortic diameter at this level now measuring 6 cm.

hemiarch replacement and valve suspension. Over the subsequent years, her residual arch and thoracic aorta degenerated requiring a redo sternotomy with total arch replacement with a frozen elephant trunk repair. On follow-up, it was noted that she had progressive enlargement of the descending thoracic aorta from retrograde flow into the false lumen—now measuring approximately 6 cm at the level of the diaphragm. She was offered a staged total endovascular repair of her extent two dissection thoracoabdominal aneurysm. Stage one of her repair consisted of descending thoracic aortic endograft extension to the level of the celiac artery (Figure 11.1).

PREOPERATIVE PLANNING AND DEVICE SELECTION

Meticulous preoperative planning is mandatory to successfully perform PMEG repair. A careful review of a thin-cut, high-quality computed tomography angiography (CTA) of the chest abdomen, and pelvis post-processed on a centerline reconstruction software is paramount [4]. This will outline the anatomy and help determine the required specifications for aortic endografts and bridging stents for aneurysm exclusion and visceral vessel incorporation. Challenging iliac and femoral access can hinder the passage of large bore devices and may require adjunctive procedures.[5]

When planning a PMEG repair, the proximal landing zone of the graft must be within a disease-free portion of parallel aorta for at least 2 cm or within an existing endograft or surgical graft. With this mantra in mind, the incorporation of all four visceral vessels is usually required for the treatment of supra-renal aneurysms with the proximal sealing stent within the supra-celiac aorta. Extension of the proximal edge of the endograft fabric at least 2 cm above the celiac fenestration into the supra-celiac aorta allows for future proximal extension if the supra-celiac aorta is to degenerate resulting in a type 1A endoleak. This extension cephalad can be executed safely to the level below the next set of intercostal arteries, balancing the risk of spinal cord ischemia and maximizing seal.

On the contrary, if one plans an "easier" case where all four vessels are not incorporated (authors are against this strategy), there is an increased risk of a type 1A endoleak if further aortic degeneration is to occur. This will result in a very challenging repair as there will not be a suitable landing/overlap zone within the fenestrated graft for proximal extension as the fenestrations/scallops will be within the first few millimeters of the PMEG [6]. This would require an open conversion or an additional PMEG incorporating the previous fenestrated endograft and branches.

If ilio-femoral access allows, our preference is to modify the Zenith TX2® thoracic stent graft (Cook Medical Inc., Bloomington, IN, USA) typically measuring around 150 mm in length with a diameter approximately 10–20% oversized to that of proximal healthy aorta. As most visceral vessels are within a 50 cm segment, this allows a good proximal seal and a suitable infra-renal overlap for the infra-renal device. If there is significant narrowing of the iliac arteries, then a low-profile graft such as the Zenith Alpha™ (Cook Medical Inc.), Terumo Relay®Pro or Terumo TREO® graft (Terumo Aortic/Bolton Medical Inc., Sunrise, FL, USA) can be considered for modification. Each manufacturer has a device catalog with specific endograft dimensions such as lengths, diameters, tapers, and delivery sheath diameters.

Straightened geometric centerline reconstruction will then allow the planning of the location of fenestrations/branches for the target vessels. Usually, the automatic geometric centerline generated by the program will suffice, however, in a tortuous visceral aorta, the surgeon will need to adjust the centerline to mimic that of a stiff wire and predicted graft behavior. Distances to each target vessel are calculated from the intended proximal fabric edge of the graft along with their respective clock positions/arch lengths. If the endograft diameter is larger than the aorta, the arch length is based on the diameter of the aorta. However, if the aorta is larger than the endograft, the arch length is corrected for the endograft diameter. In the latter case, if there is a large gap between the endograft and target vessel ostium (greater than 5 mm gap), it is suggested to utilize a mini-cuff or a branch to prevent branch instability [7].

During operative planning, one of the critical considerations will be how to handle stenotic, tortuous, or dissected target vessels. In such situations, there are specific strategies to address each condition. Severe stenosis typically requires pre-cannulation with stenting, often using the iCast covered stent system (Getinge, Gothenburg, Sweden). When dealing with dissections, the approach involves stenting the true lumen open by identifying the reentry point of the false lumen and using a self-expandable covered stent such as the Gore® Viabahn® (W.L. Gore & Associates, Flagstaff, AZ, USA). In cases of tortuous branches, the recommended course of action is stenting with a self-expandable bare metal stent to prevent kinks distal to the bridging balloon expandable stent graft.

The infra-renal implant is then planned like a typical case with attention to the lengths from the lowest renal artery to the hypogastric arteries noted for potential iliac branch device implantation. An aortoiliac stent graft without supra-renal fixation is ideal such as the Gore® Excluder® AAA Endoprosthesis (W. L. Gore & Associates) to prevent disruption of bridging stents. This graft is slightly oversized to ensure proper seal within the PMEG graft (Figures 11.2–11.4).

SPECIAL SCENARIOS

In patients with dissection thoracoabdominal aneurysms, as shown in the case example, the goal of this operation is to seal the false lumen and treat the aneurysm. This may require adjective procedures such as endovascular thermal septostomy to increase the size of the true lumen, cannulate target vessels arising from the false lumen, and create a distal landing zone [8,9]. The decision to perform a septostomy requires thoughtful evaluation of the aorta and consideration of true lumen diameter, existing endograft diameters, existing landing zones, and the presence of thrombus within the false lumen. If the true lumen is large enough and there is a contraindication to septostomy, vessels arising off the false lumen can be individually cannulated by controlled septal penetration without the need for a full septostomy. Retrograde flow into the false lumen at the iliac level may require iliac branch endoprosthesis and extension of stent grafts into the external and/or internal iliac arteries.

Utilizing a physician-modified endograft to repair an aorta that has degenerated after a previous endovascular infra-renal repair also requires special considerations. The existing implants should be noted and the endoleak present should be clearly defined. The presence of supra-renal fixation, rigid iliac stents, and endoskeleton stent structure can complicate a planned PMEG repair. Isolated proximal degeneration with a type 1A endoleak can be

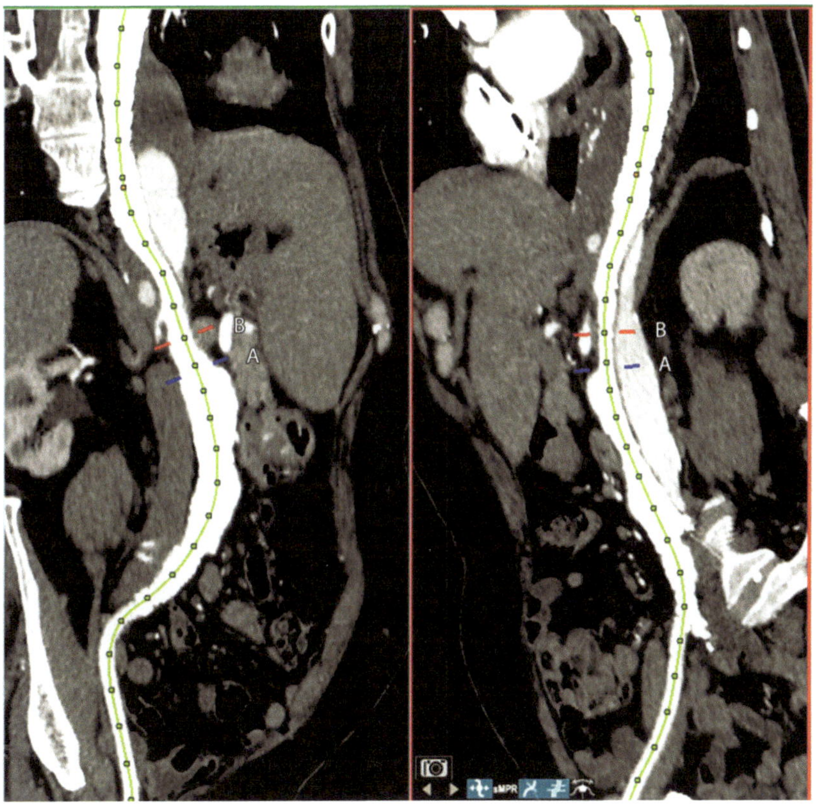

Figure 11.2 The geometric centerline is adjusted by the physician to ensure the path is through the true lumen of the aorta.

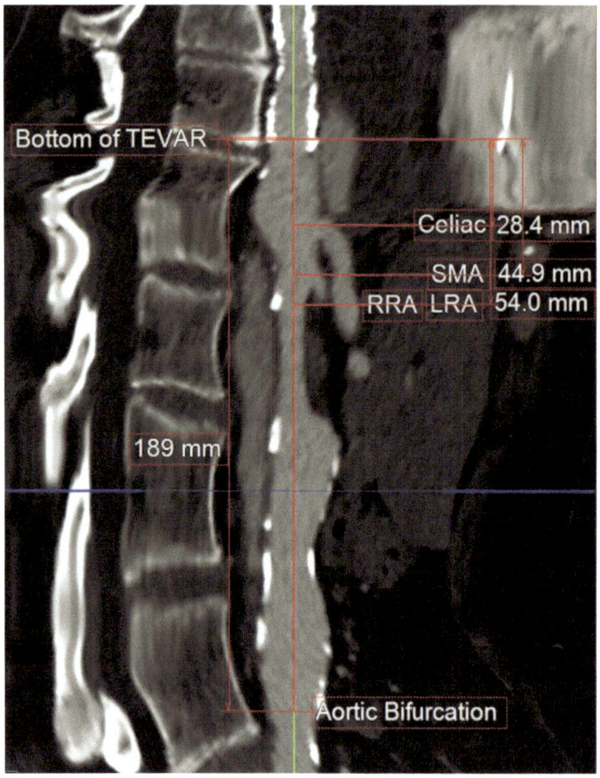

Figure 11.3 Straightened centerline reconstruction allowing calculation of visceral vessel fenestrations.

potentially treated with a physician-modified aortic cuff or a thoracic stent graft landed into the existing endograft main body. However, it is our preference to utilize a bifurcate graft to mitigate the risk of a type 3 endoleak between the aortic components. To implant a bifurcated graft safely, the distance from the lowest renal artery to the existing endograft flow divider will determine the need for inverted limbs or visceral artery branches to prevent difficulty with visceral/renal artery incorporation. The Zenith Flex ® AAA Endovascular Bifurcated Main Body Graft (Cook Medical Inc.) has the shortest contralateral gate measuring 22 mm, which makes it ideal for implantation within an existing endograft. It can also be modified to invert the contralateral gate; however, this is rarely required. It is important to consider the orientation of the existing endograft gate and iliac limb configuration to plan the clock position of the bifurcated physician-modified graft for easy cannulation.

PHYSICIAN-MODIFIED ENDOGRAFT CONSTRUCTION

Until custom industry-manufactured devices are disseminated, most surgeons must prepare the grafts themselves. Once a device has been selected for the visceral aorta, utilizing preoperative measurements, one must modify the graft in the operating room. Most devices currently available on the market can be modified utilizing the same sequence of steps. Sterile deployment, marking of fenestrations, meticulous construction of the fenestrations, orientation markers, diameter reduction, and re-sheathing.

We will describe the modification steps for the Zenith TX2® thoracic stent graft (Cook Medical Inc.).

1. The graft is opened sterile, preserving the inner sterile sleeve. A portion of the clear plastic is cut and set aside for creating a stencil.

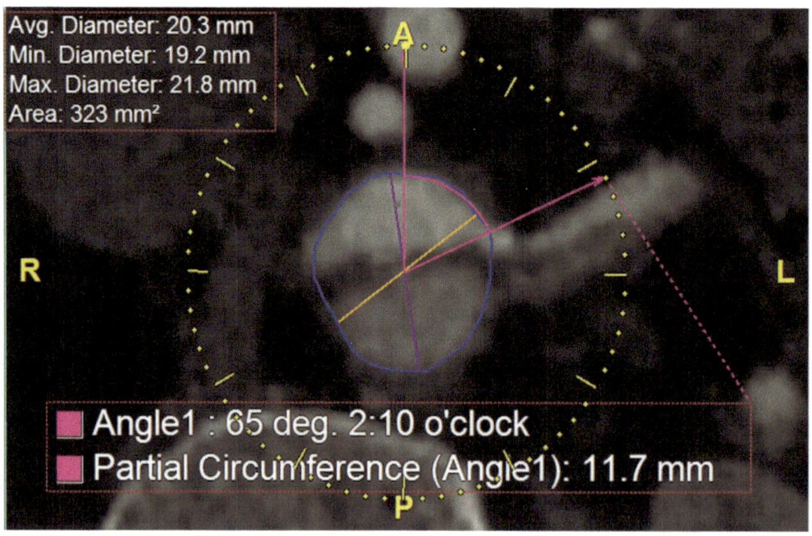

Figure 11.4 Arch length measurement for the left renal artery that is involved by the dissection and supplied by both true and false lumen. Axial view of the aorta demonstrating significant narrowing of the true lumen.

2. The preloaded peel-away sheath is advanced past the valve of the delivery sheath and the light gray delivery catheter is pulled retrograde, removing the endograft from the delivery sheath.

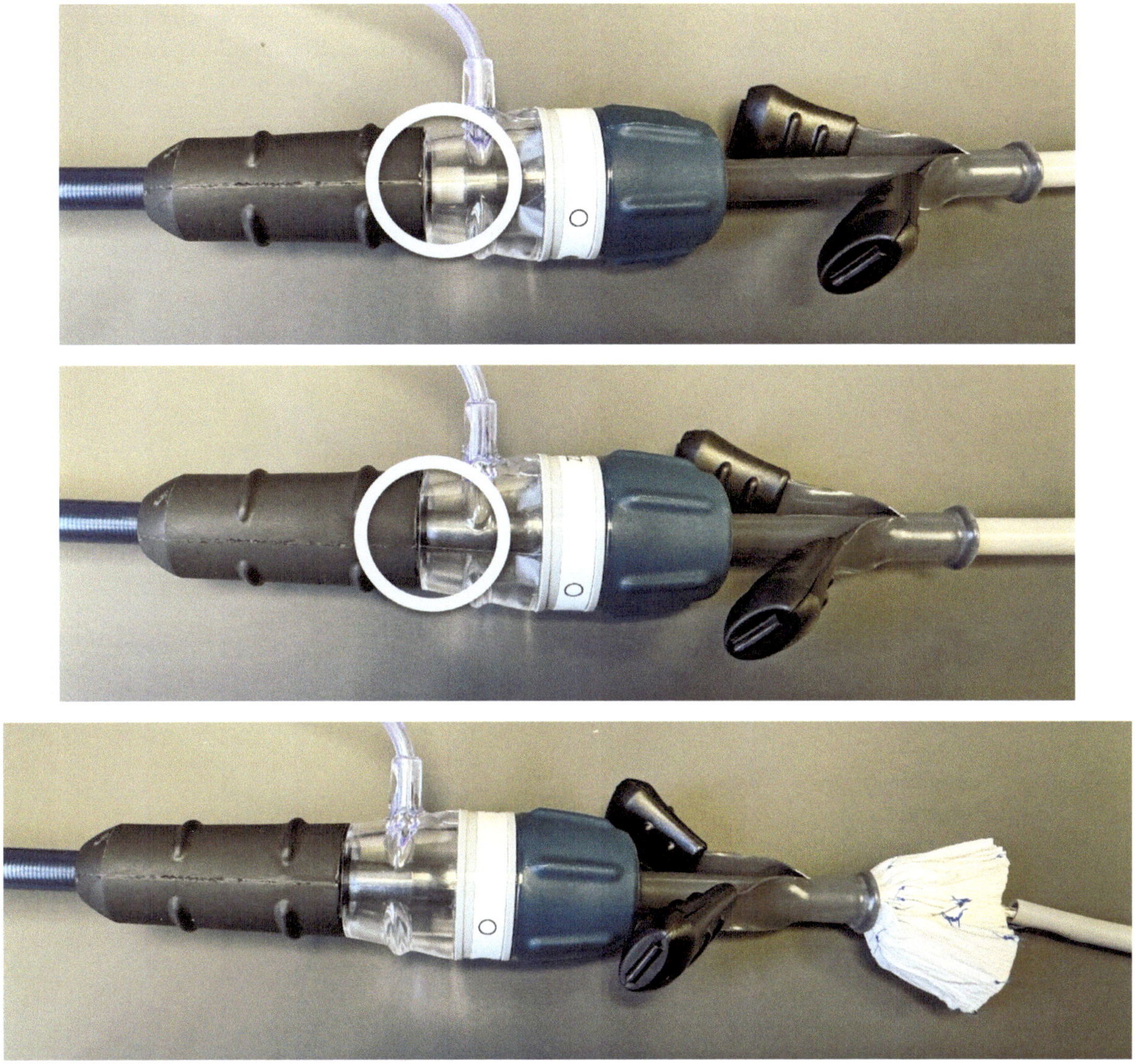

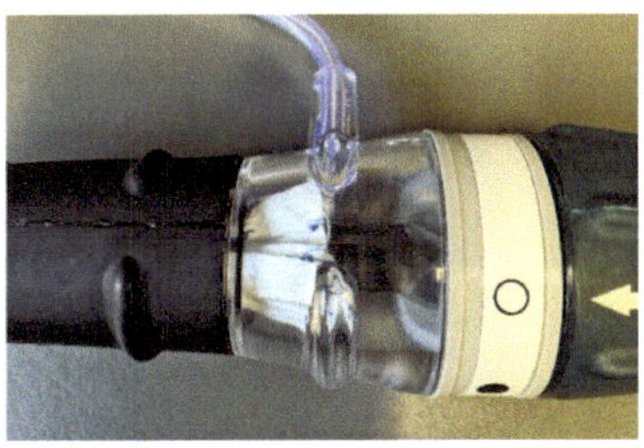

Peel-away not advanced past the valve, therefore when gray delivery catheter was retracted, the graft deployed into valve

3. A clear stencil is created, utilizing distance from the top of the fabric edge and arch length measurements for the target vessels. The top edge of the plastic is aligned with the top edge of the endograft fabric and adjustments are performed, allowing optimal positioning of the fenestrations to avoid stent struts.

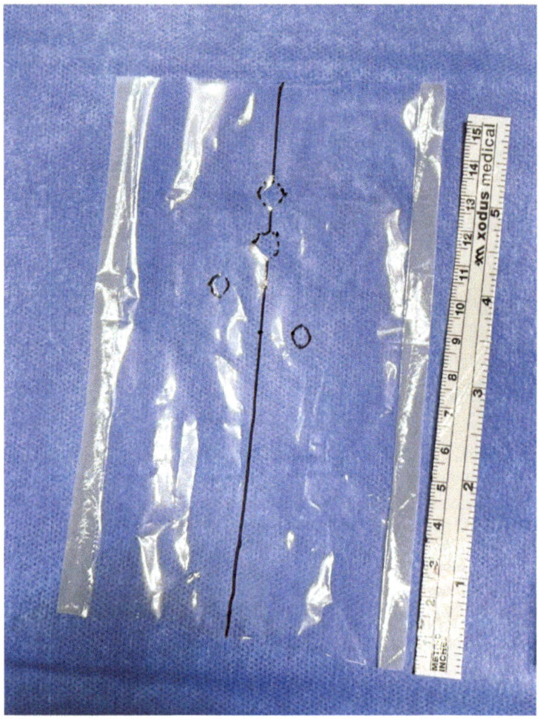

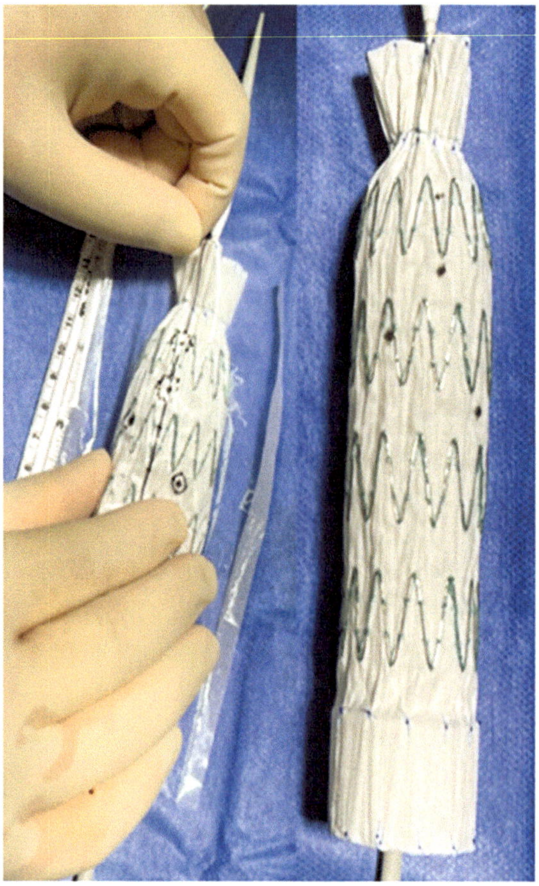

4. Fenestrations are then meticulously created in the graft material utilizing ophthalmologic cautery sized for the intended target vessel diameter.
5. Fenestrations are reinforced with a nitinol-based wire that is sewn circumferentially utilizing 5-0 multifilament braided polyester suture.
6. Utilizing the gold markers off a marking catheter or residual wire, orientation markers are applied to the 12 o'clock position along the first stent row and typically the 3 o'clock or 9 o'clock positions between the celiac and superior mesenteric artery fenestration. This helps ensure the correct rotation of the graft within the patient and maintains an anterior-posterior orientation.

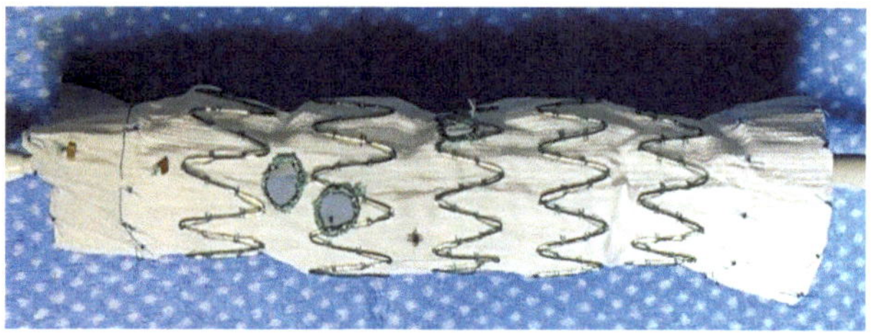

7. Diameter reduction can be performed in two ways, the easiest being to utilize a 4-0 chromic suture and either to perform a circumferential reduction or posterior reduction (A). Techniques for re-routing the trigger wire in the Cook grafts have been described and create a system that is nearly identical to that of a custom-manufactured fenestrated device (B) [10].

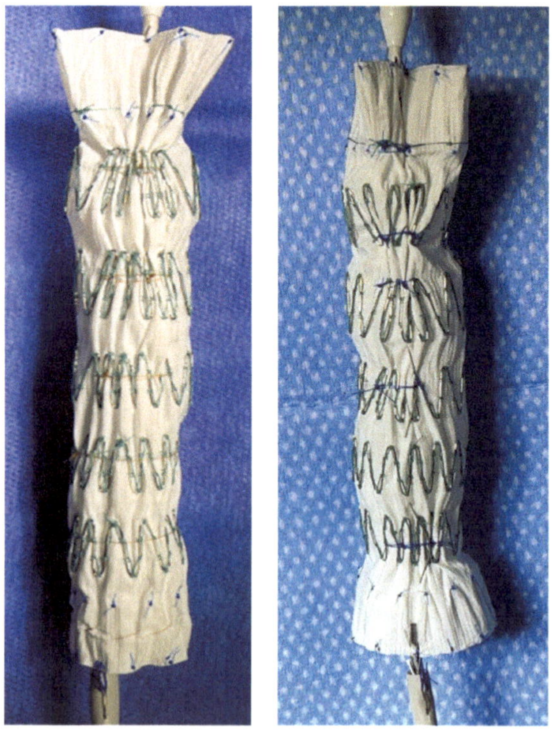

8. The graft is then replaced into the original delivery sheath by inserting it into the peel-away sheath that was advanced past the valve while removing the graft.

9. 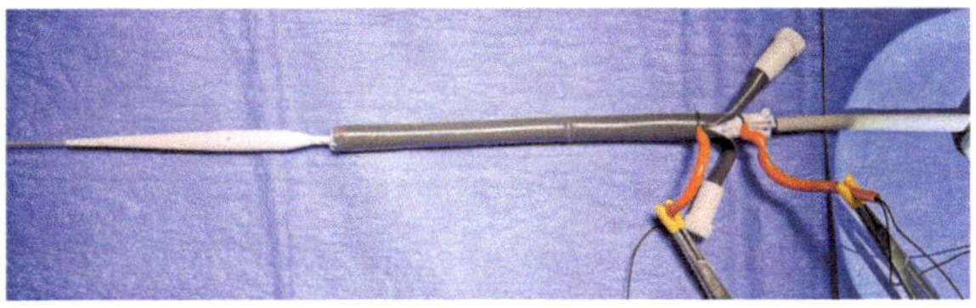

It is helpful to have the orientation of the graft before replacing it into the sheath, for example, with the knobs of the trigger wires on the Zenith (Cook Medical Inc.) platform. Replacing the graft is a tedious process and can be performed with the assistance of Rummel tourniquets, peel-away sheaths, silk sutures, or umbilical tape. It is critical to ensure that the graft is not being twisted/candy-wrapped and that the stent structure is not being damaged.

Removal and replacement of the Zenith TX2® thoracic stent graft and Zenith Flex ® AAA Endovascular Bifurcated Main Body Graft (Cook Medical Inc.) from the delivery sheath is performed with ease as these grafts come with a preloaded peel-away sheath allowing retrograde removal of the graft. This is unique as other grafts must be deployed antegrade to perform modifications.

DEVICE IMPLANTATION

The correct implantation of the fenestrated device is paramount. Errors in implantation can result in significant morbidity and mortality. Percutaneous femoral access is obtained in the typical fashion. A large bore sheath is placed into the femoral artery for which the target vessels will be cannulated; our preference is the Gore® DrySeal Flex Introducer Sheath (W.L. Gore & Associates), typically 16–20 F depending on iliac artery access.

The modified device is oriented outside the body, which will allow visualization of the fenestrations in relationship to the gold markers. This will help orient the graft from a rotational aspect. If an aorto-bi-iliac graft is being utilized, it is helpful to consider the contralateral gate markers as the fenestrations were created with the gate orientation in mind (Figure 11.5).

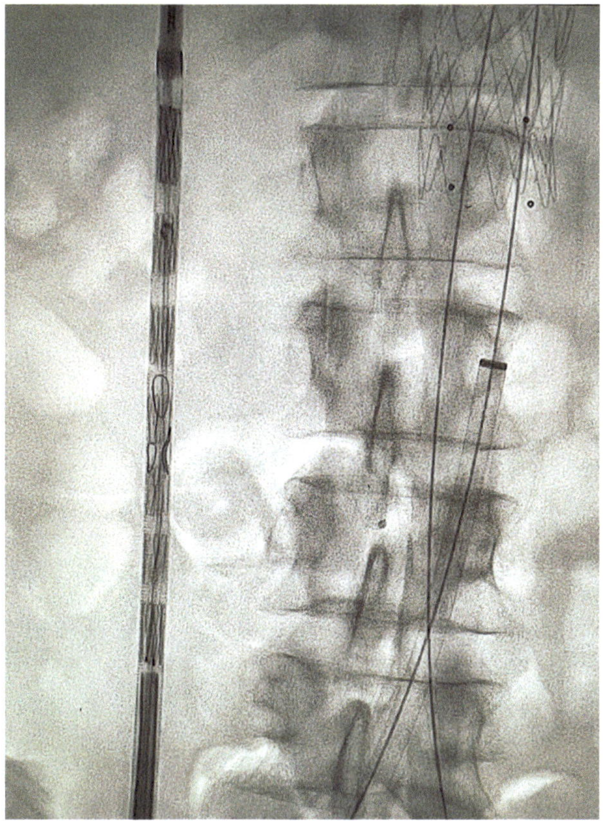

Figure 11.5 Gold markers at the 12 o'clock position as well as a single gold marker above the left renal artery fenestration.

The graft is then inserted via percutaneous access. Often, as the graft is advanced through the iliac system, the device will rotate; this behavior can be predicted by initially passing a dilator or sheath and paying attention to the flush port or markings. This will allow anticipation of inadvertent graft rotation as it is advanced through the aortoiliac segment.

The elevation of the graft is then oriented in relationship to the target vessels, typically one of the renal arteries. Our preference is to place a catheter/wire into the renal artery from the contralateral access to ensure proper elevation, though angiography with screen markings and 3D navigators can be utilized instead (Figure 11.6).

If rotation needs to be changed, the sheath and delivery catheter must be rotated as one unit with a gentle insertion and retraction of the device. This point must be emphasized as if the system is rotated separately, the trigger wires will wrap and make eventual deployment challenging. Once satisfied with the elevation and rotation, the graft is then segmentally deployed, making micro adjustments as needed for the gold markers. Once the graft is completely deployed, the wire in the renal artery is retracted and the caudal portion of the graft is cannulated. This cannulation is confirmed with catheter rotation or intravascular ultrasound. The large bore sheath is then advanced into the caudal portion of the graft or gate and sewn to the skin, ensuring that the sheath does not inadvertently migrate distally. Utilizing a 7F steerable sheath, crossing catheter, and glide wire, target vessels are then cannulated. It is not atypical for some difficulty with the initial cannulation as there might be device misalignment. Our preference is to cannulate the renal arteries, followed by the superior mesenteric artery, and finally the celiac artery. This allows for an efficient cranial to caudal bridging stent graft deployment utilizing the steerable sheath.

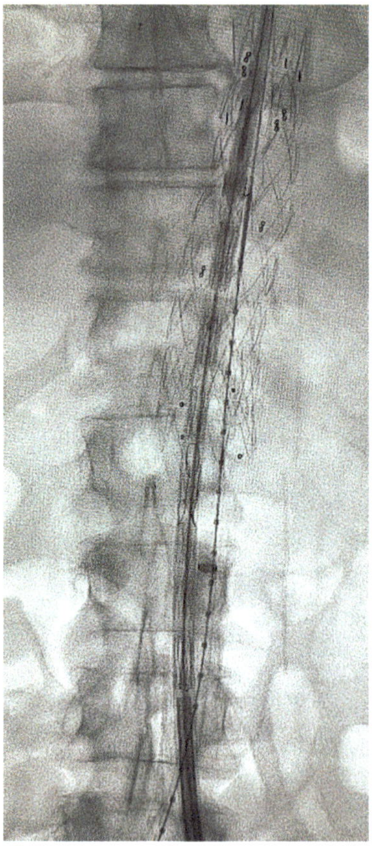

Figure 11.6 Graft within the aorta; proper alignment confirmed with the help of gold markers.

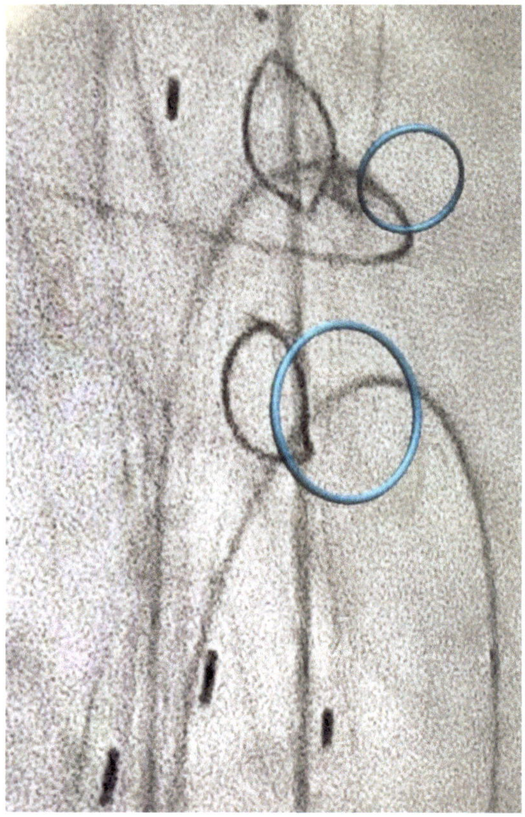

Figure 11.7 Celiac artery and superior mesenteric artery cannulation with the help of 3D navigators.

As vessels are cannulated, it is important to use proper endovascular technique with angiography and gentle wire and catheter manipulation as target vessels can be injured with dissections, perforations, and occlusions. It is important to perform selective angiography before placing a Rosen wire into the target vessel to ensure proper positioning of the wire, and that the intended vessel is truly cannulated (Figure 11.7).

After all the target vessels are cannulated, the physician-modified graft is completely deployed from the delivery system, and the diameter reduction is removed either with the trigger wire mechanism or utilizing a compliant balloon to disrupt the temporary chromic suture. This can be confirmed visually, and as the sutures are being disrupted, a vibration is felt within the balloon catheter. The delivery system is removed, and a smaller sheath can be replaced into the femoral access to promote pelvic and lower extremity perfusion by clinching on the Perclose Proglide (Abbott Cardiovascular, Redwood City, CA, USA) sutures if utilized [11].

Bridging stents are then implanted, typically balloon expandable stent grafts such as Gore® Viabahn® VBX (W.L. Gore & Associates) or iCAST (Getinge). These are sized to the target vessel diameter and placed into position minding early target branches. Approximately 5 mm of the stent is deployed into the aorta allowing subsequent flaring utilizing a larger angioplasty balloon. Selective angiography is then performed to ensure vessel patency and the lack of type 1 or 3 endoleak related to the bridging stent.

After the fenestrations and target vessels are stented, our preference is to perform an aortogram at this stage to ensure that there is a proper proximal seal and that all stented vessels are patent. After this is confirmed, visceral wires are removed and we proceed with the infra-renal graft implantation if utilizing a thoracic graft for the visceral repair; if an aorto-bi-iliac graft is utilized, then one can proceed with iliac limb deployment. This is done in the typical fashion. It is important to note, as these infra-renal devices are advanced and deployed, care must be taken to ensure bridging stents are not damaged. Concomitant iliac aneurysms or dissections should be treated based on preoperative imaging and case planning, and utilization of iliac branch devices should be planned and implanted.

Finally, completion angiography is performed, and the sheaths are removed. Patients are monitored for spinal cord injury with selective lumbar drain placement. Postoperative monitoring in the intensive care unit is critical to rescue issues related to bridging stents such as visceral ischemia, renal dysfunction, and lower extremity ischemia.

After discharge, patients are followed with surveillance protocols identical to that of infra-renal endovascular aortic aneurysm repair.

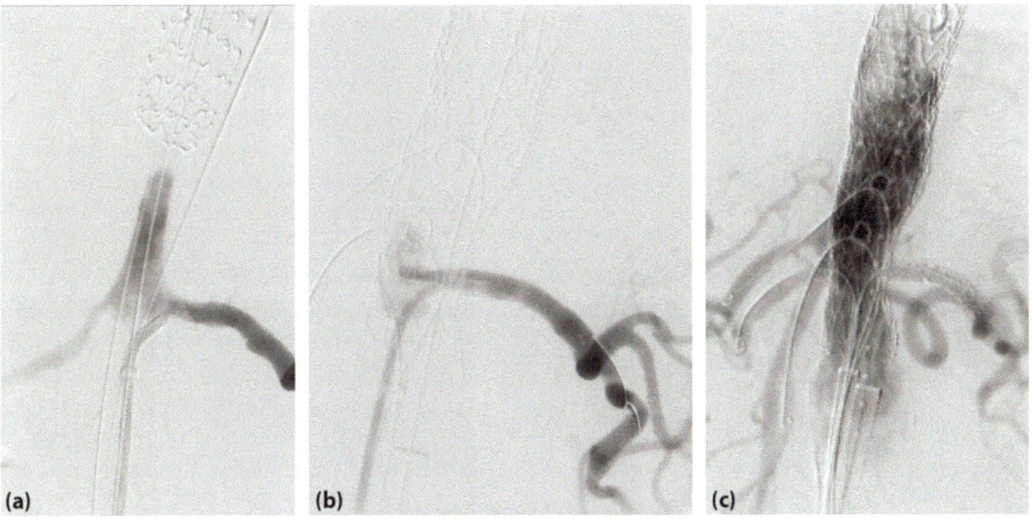

Figure 11.8 (a) True lumen significantly compressed. (b) Cannulation of the left renal artery through PMEG graft. (c) Target vessels cannulated with excellent expansion of PMEG graft due to septostomy.

CASE EXAMPLE CONTINUED

Based on the centerline reconstruction, a PMEG repair with a left-sided iliac branch device was offered with an effort to seal the false lumen. Due to the size of the true lumen, a thermal septostomy was performed. Successful aneurysm exclusion was achieved with false lumen thrombosis (Figures 11.8 and 11.9).

FUTURE DIRECTIONS

It must be noted that the contents of the chapter are investigational. At the time of the publication of this text, in the United States, we do not have an FDA-approved platform to perform these operations without physician modification. Some centers are involved in industry-sponsored trials that have access to custom-made devices, however, most surgeons do not and will not have access to this technology for the foreseeable future. For the patient with an emergency indication for surgery, transport to these centers is unlikely. PMEG offers a bridge in the gap for the treatment of patients with complex aortic pathology.

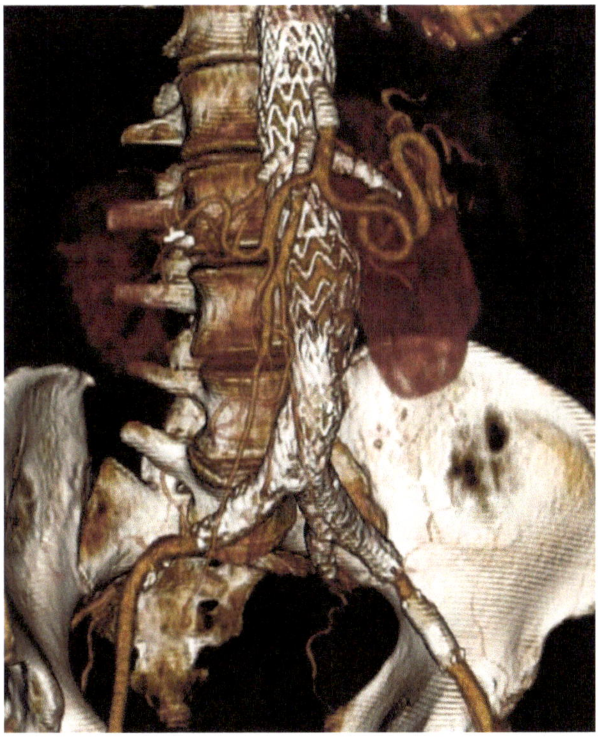

Figure 11.9 Postoperative 3D reconstruction demonstrating PMEG repair with visceral vessel incorporation and left-sided iliac branch device.

TRICKS AND TRAPS

1. Planning is paramount.
2. Build a program: teamwork and volume matter.
3. PMEG may appear like a minimally invasive procedure to patients, but it has multiple levels of error traps that require patience and finesse to navigate.
4. Try to modify the smallest diameter graft/taper in the largest delivery sheath based on the catalogs, this will make re-sheathing easier.
5. Intravascular ultrasound is mandatory for dissection aneurysms.
6. Do not underestimate access. Account for small, tortuous, and calcified iliac arteries. Adjunctive tools such as shockwave lithotripsy and external or endovascular conduits may be helpful.

QUESTIONS

1. While maximizing proximal seal with a physician-modified endograft, coverage of which arteries can result in spinal cord ischemia?
   a. Accessory renal arteries
   b. Phrenic arteries
   c. Replaced left gastric
   d. Lumbar/intercostal arteries
   e. Vertebral arteries

   Answer: d

2. Planning for a physician-modified endograft requires what type of preoperative imaging?
   a. MRI
   b. Ultrasound
   c. Catheter angiography
   d. Thin-cut CT angiography
   e. X-Ray

   Answer: d

3. Which device has provided a stable platform for target vessel cannulation and stenting?
   a. Vertebral catheter
   b. Steerable sheath
   c. Glide wire
   d. Rosen wire
   e. Angioplasty balloon

   Answer: b

4. Radiation exposure during complex endovascular aortic interventions can be minimized by utilizing?
   a. Digital subtraction angiography
   b. 3D overlay vessel navigator
   c. Cone beam CT

   Answer: b

REFERENCES

1. Suckow BD, Goodney PP, Columbo JA, et al. National trends in open surgical, endovascular, and branched-fenestrated endovascular aortic aneurysm repair in Medicare patients. *J Vasc Surg*. 2018;67(6):1690–1697.e1. doi:10.1016/j.jvs.2017.09.046
2. Prinssen M, Verhoeven ELG, Buth J, et al. A randomized trial comparing conventional and endovascular repair of abdominal aortic aneurysms. *N Engl J Med*. 2004;351(16):1607–1618.
3. O'Donnell TFX, McElroy IE, Boitano LT, et al. Comparison of treatment options for aortic necks outside standard endovascular aneurysm repair instructions for use. *J Vasc Surg*. Elsevier Inc. 2021;74:1548–1557. doi:10.1016/j.jvs.2021.04.052
4. Zettervall SL, Starnes BW. Planning and sizing of fenestrated/branched stent grafts. *Semin Vasc Surg*. 2022;35(3):252–258. doi:10.1053/j.semvascsurg.2022.07.006
5. Minion DJ, Davenport DL. Access techniques for EVAR: Percutaneous techniques and working with small arteries. *Semin Vasc Surg*. 2012;25(4):208–216. doi:10.1053/j.semvascsurg.2012.09.006
6. Mastracci TM, Eagleton MJ, Kuramochi Y, Bathurst S, Wolski K. Twelve-year results of fenestrated endografts for juxtarenal and group IV thoracoabdominal aneurysms. *J Vasc Surg*. 2015;61(2):355–364. doi:10.1016/j.jvs.2014.09.068
7. Oderich GS, Fatima J, Gloviczki P. Stent graft modification with mini-cuff reinforced fenestrations for urgent repair of thoracoabdominal aortic aneurysms. *J Vasc Surg*. 2011;54(5):1522–1526. doi:10.1016/j.jvs.2011.06.023
8. Kabbani L, Eng M, Onofrey K, Weaver M, Nypaver T. Novel technique to fenestrate an aortic dissection flap using electrocautery. *J Vasc Surg Cases Innov Tech*. Society for Vascular Surgery. 2023;9. doi:10.1016/j.jvscit.2023.101108
9. Baghbani-Oskouei A, Savadi S, Mesnard T, et al. Transcatheter electrosurgical septotomy technique for chronic post-dissection aortic aneurysms. *J Vasc Surg Cases Innov Tech*. Published online April 2023:101402. doi:10.1016/j.jvscit.2023.101402
10. Oderich GS. Technique of adding a diameter-reducing wire to the modified TX2 fenestrated stent graft. *Vascular*. 2010;18(6):350–355. doi:10.2310/6670.2010.00059
11. Melloni A, Grandi A, Melissano G, Chiesa R, Bertoglio L. Safety and feasibility of percutaneous purse-string-like downsizing for femoral access during complex endovascular aortic repair. *Cardiovasc Intervent Radiol*. 2020;43(7):1084–1090. doi:10.1007/s00270-020-02508-3

12

Endovascular repair of descending thoracic aortic aneurysms

LOAY S. KABBANI AND HAMZAH SALEEM

INTRODUCTION

Descending thoracic aortic aneurysms (DTAAs) are rare and comprise only 2–5% of all degenerative aneurysms. The first open repair of a DTAA was described by Lam and Aram in 1951, and the first DTAA repaired with a homemade "back-table" endograft was in 1994 [1]. The first commercially available thoracic endoprosthesis to treat DTAAs was approved by the Food and Drug Administration in 2005 [2]. Currently, thoracic endovascular aortic repair (TEVAR) for DTAAs has become the standard of care [3]. Compared with open repair, TEVAR is associated with decreased mortality, shorter length of stay, reduced blood transfusion, and earlier return to a baseline activity lifestyle. In addition, several studies have suggested that endoluminal grafting has an equal or lower incidence of neurologic complications [4].

INDICATIONS FOR TEVAR

Indications for the repair of DTAAs include a luminal diameter >5.5 cm in asymptomatic "low-risk" patients, saccular aneurysm, and postoperative pseudoaneurysm. Larger diameter thresholds are recommended for patients considered "high risk." Such patients include subjects who are at particularly high risk for mortality, renal failure, or spinal cord ischemia (SCI) based on their medical comorbidities and anatomical features. In current practice, all patients with suitable anatomy and acceptable access should be considered for TEVAR [3].

CONTRAINDICATIONS FOR TEVAR

An absolute contraindication for TEVAR is inadequate landing zones (see later in the chapter). There are a few relative contraindications as well, however, they can be resolved with proper preoperative planning. These include unsuitable access vessel anatomy such as a severe tortuous aorta that may not allow the stent graft to track into position, or small access vessels. TEVAR has a role in the emergent setting for patients with connective tissue disorders, however, it remains controversial in the elective treatment of such patients. Mycotic aneurysms are considered relative contraindication, but current guidelines suggest TEVAR as a temporary management option in symptomatic or ruptured mycotic aneurysms. Aorto-esophageal fistulas, however, do poorly with endovascular treatment. Data regarding long-term outcomes is lacking for TEVAR as the sole management option in infected cases [3].

PATIENTS WITH SPECIAL CONSIDERATIONS

Severe radiocontrast media allergy can usually be managed with premedication including steroids. In advanced renal insufficiency, the contrast dose should be minimized. Intravascular ultrasound (IVUS) may be used to help address anatomical variations and decrease the amount of contrast needed. Octogenarians with major comorbidities need to have a lengthy, honest discussion with their surgeon about the benefits of treating their aneurysm weighed against the risks of the procedure and long-term outcomes.

OPERATIVE PLANNING

The single most important task that determines the success of these operations is preoperative planning. Major considerations include poor access vessels, significant calcification, and arterial tortuosity.

DOI: 10.1201/9781003452096-12

Imaging

Computed tomography angiography (CTA) with centerline reconstruction is ideal for preoperative planning. Current recommendations suggest a thin slice CTA of the aorta that includes the thoracic branches and iliac and femoral arteries. Centerline images can accurately estimate the diameter and length of the landing zones. Magnetic resonance angiography may be used if the patient has renal insufficiency or a severe contrast allergy. A valuable tool that can be employed intraoperatively is IVUS. This can help in cases where preoperative imaging is of inadequate quality or judicious contrast usage is desired in the setting of poor renal function or severe contrast allergy.[3]

For reporting purposes, the aorta has been divided into 11 zones (Figure 12.1). This aortic zone classification has been supported by the Society for Vascular Surgery.

Sealing (landing) zones

The patient should have appropriate landing zones, or "necks," proximal and distal to the aneurysm, to have a "seal" between the aortic wall and the endoprosthesis. Ideally, the proximal landing zone should be sufficiently established beyond the origin of the subclavian artery (zones 3 or 4), and the distal landing zone should be proximal to the celiac artery (zone 5). Depending on device availability, the patient's landing zone diameter should be within the manufacturer's instructions for use (IFU). For example, the GORE® TAG® device IFU requires a landing zone length >20 mm and a sealing zone (aortic inner wall to inner wall) diameter ranging from 16 mm to 42 mm. When sizing an endograft, the graft is oversized compared with the landing zone diameter by 10–20%. Excessive oversizing can lead to infolding (Figure 12.2), gutter formation, poor sealing, and excessive radial force that may accelerate degeneration of the aortic neck. Placement of an undersized graft, on the other hand, increases the chance of endoleaks and migration.

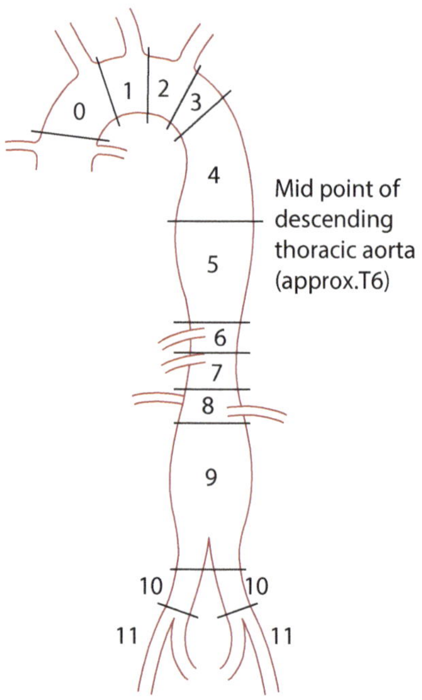

Figure 12.1 Zones of attachment in the aorta. (Adapted from Fillinger MF, Greenberg RK, McKinsey JF, et al. Reporting standards for thoracic endovascular aortic repair (TEVAR). *J Vasc Surg* 2010;52:1022–1033.)

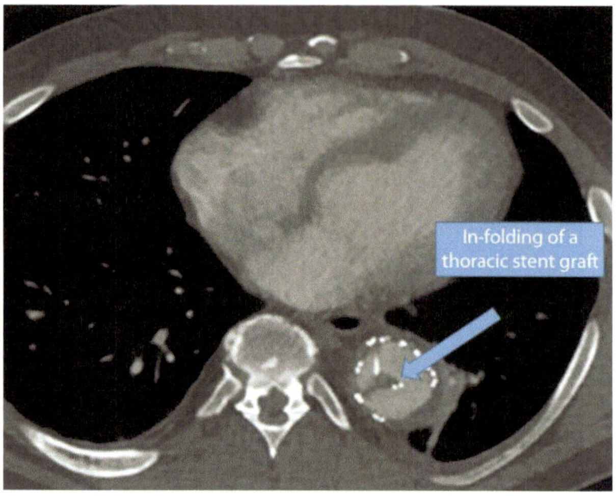

Figure 12.2 Coronal section from a computerized tomographic aortogram of a descending thoracic aortic aneurysm showing infolding of an oversized endograft (arrow).

Management of the arch and visceral arteries to extend the landing zones

Even though in an ideal setting the landing zone should be distal to the left subclavian artery, this is not always possible due to more proximal extension of aneurysmal disease. Among patients undergoing TEVAR, 17–43% need coverage of the left subclavian artery (LSA) (zone 2), the left common carotid artery (CCA) (zone 1), or even the brachiocephalic artery (zone 0), to achieve an adequate proximal seal (Figure 12.1). The left subclavian artery is an important vessel for perfusion of the brain and spinal cord, through the left vertebral artery and internal mammary artery, respectively. Furthermore, the internal mammary artery may have been used as a coronary conduit in patients who have undergone coronary artery bypass graft (CABG). Retrospective evidence suggests that covering the LSA increases the chance of periprocedural stroke and possibly SCI. Revascularization of the LSA is especially important when extensive coverage of the thoracic aorta is planned, or TEVAR is being performed in a patient with a prior infrarenal aortic replacement, occluded internal iliac arteries, a dominant left vertebral artery with a hypoplastic or absent right vertebral artery, or termination of the left vertebral artery into the posterior inferior cerebellar artery. These patients are

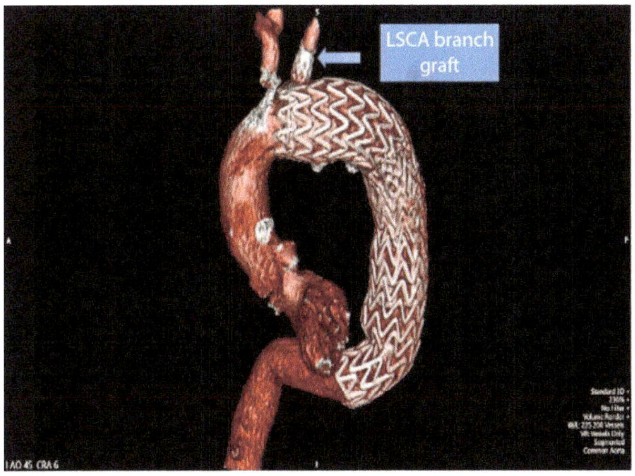

Figure 12.3 A GORE® TAG® Thoracic Branch Endoprosthesis endograft with a branch in the left subclavian artery (arrow).

at higher risk for SCI and posterior circulation strokes. Revascularization of the LSA is also crucial for patients with a patent LIMA graft post-CABG and in patients with functional AV dialysis access in the left arm.

Standard open surgical options for revascularizing the LSA include left CCA-to-LSA bypass grafting or LSA-to-left CCA transposition. The left CCA can be bypassed using an extra-anatomic carotid-carotid bypass if the thoracic endograft covers zone 1. For more proximal extension of the device, the brachiocephalic artery can be debranched via a median sternotomy, with arch debranching originating from the ascending aorta. For endovascular options, a thoracic branched endograft (GORE® TAG® Thoracic Branch Endoprosthesis) is currently available but has an IFU of a 2 cm landing zone between the LSCA and the LCA (Figure 12.3). Other options to bypass arch vessels are endovascular debranching with a chimney technique, laser fenestration of the thoracic endograft, or a physician-modified endograft (PMEG).

The celiac artery can be covered if there are adequate collaterals between the superior mesenteric artery and the celiac artery, via the gastroduodenal artery [5,6]. If revascularization is required, however, then options include open surgical revascularization or endovascular techniques (e.g., using a periscope graft, laser fenestration, or PMEG).

In dissected patients, there is increased interest in obtaining a distal seal zone with TEVAR. We have pioneered thermal septostomy with endovascular electrosurgical techniques. Please refer to the thoracic aortic dissection chapter for more discussion on this technique [7].

ACCESS SELECTION

The femoral artery is the most common access site for endograft insertion. The ideal size of the artery used for access is ≥7 mm, but this varies depending on the size of the endograft used (Table 12.1). Other than small luminal size, limitations can be due to extensive calcification and tortuosity of the access vessel. Conduits may be used if the femoral, external, or common iliac arteries (CIAs) are unsuitable. Traditional conduits entail sewing an 8–10-mm graft to the distal aorta or CIA through a suprainguinal oblique incision giving access to the retroperitoneal space. The conduit is tunneled out into the groin, the distal end is clamped, and a separate puncture is made in the conduit to introduce the sheath and endograft (Figure 12.4a). Direct puncture of the Iliac artery can also be performed, and a skin counter incision helps with the proper delivery angle. Endo conduits require accessing the femoral artery, followed by placement of a covered stent and dilating the artery to the appropriate size. This is technically considered a controlled rupture of the artery, but the covered stent prevents blood extravasation (Figure 12.4b). Caution must be taken to prevent the rupture from reaching a patent internal iliac origin. Other options include a transcaval approach or a transmediastinal approach.

With the availability of intravascular lithotripsy (IVL), calcified blood vessels can be angioplastied easily and safely to accommodate larger sheaths. Rarely have we needed to use endoconduits after the introduction of IVL [8].

When dealing with a very tortuous aorta or an arch with a small curvature radius, the "body floss" maneuver

Table 12.1 Types of available thoracic endografts

Graft	Diameter of endograft available (mm)	Sheath size (Fr)
Zenith Alpha™ (Cook Medical Inc.)	24–46	16–20 Fr
GORE® TAG® Device (W.L. Gore & Associates)	21–45	18–24 Fr
Valiant Thoracic Device (Medtronic)	22–46	22–25 Fr
RELAY® Device (Bolton Medical)	22–46	22–26 Fr

Cook Medical Inc., Bloomington, IN, USA; W.L. Gore & Associates, Inc., Newark, DE, USA; Medtronic, Minneapolis, MN, USA; Bolton Medical, Sunrise, FL, USA.

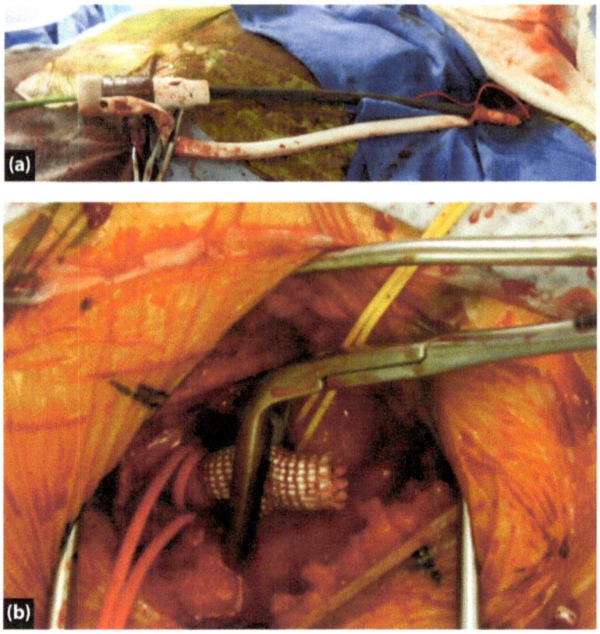

Figure 12.4 Conduits: (a) open: 10 mm PTFE graft anastomosed to the left common iliac artery and exited through a small groin incision; graft clamped distally and large sheath introduced proximally; (b) endoconduit: 8 mm covered stent exiting from right femoral artery; clamped distally.

may be helpful in advancing the device through the arch. This is accomplished by introducing a guidewire from the right brachial artery, which is then snared out through the femoral artery access site; the device may then be advanced over this guidewire (Figure 12.5). This is also a useful technique in cases involving a crumpled and distorted frozen elephant trunk (FET).

NEUROPROTECTION

Covering the intercostal arteries during the TEVAR procedure predisposes patients to the risk of SCI. This is important to consider when covering long segments of the descending thoracic aortic, especially covering the segments between T9 and L1 where the main spinal artery originates from the segmental arteries [9]. Hemodynamic stability for adequate perfusion of the spinal cord is important for these cases. Spinal drains work by decreasing intra-thecal pressure, thereby increasing spinal cord perfusion pressure. Cerebrospinal pressure is kept at 10 cm H_2O in prophylactic drain placements and down to 0 cm H_2O when placed for symptomatic SCI. The drain is kept for 48–72 hours and removed after clamping for 12–24 hours. Prophylactic spinal drains in TEVAR are controversial with an overall complication rate as high as 6% and severe complication rates such as intracranial hemorrhage as high as 2.6%. Since serial neurological exams can be performed after the procedure when the patient is awake, the placement of the spinal drain can be considered only in patients who develop SCI postoperatively [10]. In our practice, we still place a spinal drain prophylactically in elevated risk TEVAR patients, as "rescue" placement of a spinal drain in our institution is not guaranteed to be timely.

OPERATIVE TECHNIQUE

A hybrid operating room is the preferred location for the performance of this procedure. Surgery can be executed under local, regional, or spinal anesthesia. The author prefers general anesthesia to prevent patient movement during critical parts of the procedure and to hold respiration when needed for precise imaging.

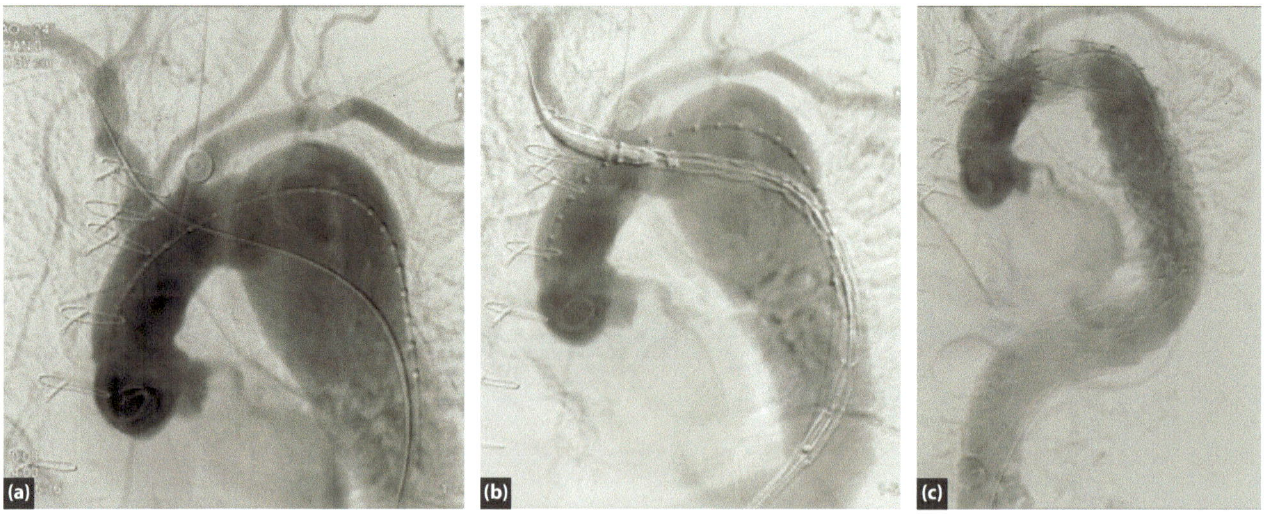

Figure 12.5 Endovascular deployment of a thoracic endograft. Note the placement of the stiff wire into the right subclavian artery to support advancement of the endograft ("body floss" maneuver): (a) predeployment angiogram; (b) endograft positioning; (c) postdeployment (completion) angiogram.

The patient is placed in a supine position. Bilateral groins are prepped. The left or right arm may be abducted and circumferentially prepped if the radial/brachial artery needs to be accessed as per preoperative planning. The iliofemoral circuit with less tortuosity is chosen, preferably for the introduction of the main device. The contralateral groin is used to place a marker pigtail catheter. Percutaneous access is usually chosen if femoral artery disease is absent or mild. A femoral artery angiogram is performed to confirm the access location (the common femoral artery) and rule out significant disease. Rarely, open exposure may be required if the artery is very calcified, or a femoral endarterectomy is needed. A 0.35-cm flexible tipped wire is then passed in a retrograde fashion under direct fluoroscopic guidance into the ascending aorta and exchanged for a stiff wire, such as a Lunderquist® Extra-Stiff Wire Guide (Cook Medical Inc., Bloomington, IN, USA) using a catheter. At this juncture, the patient is heparinized with approximately 100 IU/kg to maintain an activated clotting time of >250 seconds. If the iliofemoral artery is undiseased but small in caliber, serial dilators can be used to dilate the artery to the required size to accommodate the introducer sheath for device delivery. If the proximal inflow artery is calcified, we routinely use IVL to help expand the artery. Rarely do we need to cover the iliac arteries with a covered stent (endoconduit). The pigtail catheter from the contralateral side is used to perform an aortogram of the area of interest. An aortic image is then taken in a left anterior oblique projection, with the proximal landing zone in a perpendicular plane to the image intensifier. IVUS can also be used to locate important branches and evaluate the landing zone for size, length, and presence of a thrombus. The length and diameter of the proximal and distal landing zones may be measured using the preoperative CT scan, intraoperative IVUS, and/or angiogram. We believe centerline preoperative CTA is the most accurate imaging modality for measuring aortic diameter. The chosen stent graft is delivered under fluoroscopic guidance. Before deployment, blood pressure is reduced to below 100 mmHg systolic to decrease the chance of caudal migration of the endograft during deployment. This is less important with newer stent grafts that have tip-capture devices in place. The patient's respirations are held for stent graft deployment, which is carried out following the instructions for each device. Additional grafts may be required and should have an overlap of at least 5 cm to ensure adequate apposition and minimize the risk of a type III endoleak. Balloon molding may also be required and should be done in a proximal to distal sequence. Completion angiography is carried out to confirm placement and look for endoleaks. The stiff wire is then removed using a catheter and a soft tip wire is placed. The sheath is then removed over the wire. The arteriotomy is closed on both sides. Distal pulses are checked; if they correspond to the preoperative baseline, heparin is reversed. The patient is then extubated in the operating room, and a neurological assessment is made.

POSTOPERATIVE CARE

All patients with spinal drains are admitted to the intensive care unit postoperatively. Postoperative care includes spinal drain care, maintaining hemodynamics (MAP goal >90), and frequent neurologic assessments. A follow-up CTA is performed at one month, 12 months, and then yearly after that. Patients who are at low risk for expansion and have had stable CT findings for three years can have non-contrast CT imaging to follow the size. If any issues such as endoleaks are encountered at the one-month mark, then a repeat CTA can be performed earlier at six months [3].

COMPLICATIONS

Mortality is between 2% and 10%. Independent predictors of mortality include severe coronary artery disease, congestive heart failure, chronic kidney disease, and emergency procedures. The incidence of complications ranges widely. For SCI, the incidence varies from 0% to 6%, and for stroke, the incidence is between 2% and 5%. The reported overall incidence of primary endoleaks ranges from 3% to 10%. Most type II endoleaks appear to resolve without intervention. Type I endoleaks require treatment by extending the endograft. Retrograde type A thoracic aortic dissection after transfemoral TEVAR has a reported incidence of around 2% and is associated with increased morbidity and mortality. Several stent graft-related late complications have been reported, including graft migration, endoleaks, and stent graft fractures. It is important, therefore, to have periodic CT surveillance imaging to assess device integrity and positioning.

TRICKS AND TRAPS

- Achieving sufficient proximal and distal seal zones is crucial to prevent endoleaks and ensure the long-term durability of the repair. Inadequate sealing will lead to persistent flow into the aneurysm sac.
- Careful planning is necessary to preserve blood flow to important branch vessels. Branched or fenestrated endografts may be needed to achieve a good seal zone.
- Proper sizing and accurate positioning of the endograft are critical. Oversizing may cause device migration, enfolding, or endoleaks while undersizing can lead to incomplete sealing and continued aneurysm growth.
- The presence of severe aortic tortuosity or angulation can make delivery and deployment of the endograft challenging. Specialized techniques, such as through-and-through wire access from the arm to the groin may be needed.

- Postoperative surveillance is essential to detect and manage endoleaks promptly. Different types of endoleaks (e.g., type I, II, III) require specific approaches for intervention.
- Measures to minimize the risk of spinal cord ischemia and stroke include maintaining adequate perfusion pressures, cerebrospinal fluid drainage, and careful manipulation of the endograft around the thoracic aorta.
- Complications related to vascular access include access site hematoma, pseudoaneurysm formation, and arterial dissection. Close monitoring and prompt intervention are necessary to mitigate these risks.

QUESTIONS

1. A 69-year-old male is seen in the vascular surgery clinic after being referred by his primary care physician for a thoracic aortic aneurysm found incidentally on a screening CT chest given his extensive history of smoking. The aneurysm measures 6.2 cm in its maximum extent and is present in zone III, 3 mm from the left SCA take off. He has a history of hypertension, hyperlipidemia, diabetes, gout, and CABG with a LIMA graft. CTA of the chest, abdomen, and pelvis show iliac arteries measuring 8–9 mm bilaterally with mild calcification. In preparation for TEVAR, what aspect of case planning should the surgeon consider?
   a. Use of endoconduits for access
   b. Carotid subclavian bypass
   c. Preoperative placement of spinal drain
   d. No graft oversizing

   Answer: b

   Carotid subclavian bypass should be considered given the patient's history of CABG with a LIMA graft. In such cases, it is necessary to maintain perfusion through the subclavian artery to keep the LIMA graft patent. Endoconduits should be considered when iliac vessels are less than 7 mm and severely calcified. A spinal drain is an important consideration when lower thoracic level intercostal vessels will be covered by the endograft; typically, T9-L1 levels. One graft sizing is important when selecting an endograft for acute thoracic dissections, however, for thoracic aneurysms, the graft should be oversized 10–20%.

2. A 72-year-old female is undergoing endovascular repair of a zone IV-V thoracic aortic aneurysm. Deployment of the graft will necessitate celiac artery coverage to achieve adequate sealing zone. What anatomic considerations should be kept in mind while planning the repair in this situation?
   a. Celiac bypass must be performed
   b. Patency of GDA and PDA should be assessed preoperatively
   c. TEVAR is contraindicated in this case
   d. Both SMA and IMA should be patent if celiac is to be covered

   Answer: b

   Patency of GDA and PDA should be checked preoperatively as they provide an important collateral pathway for foregut circulation from the SMA. If these vessels are patent, the celiac artery can be covered to achieve adequate seal. Another option is to consider fenestrated or physician-modified endografts, especially if collateral flow is not satisfactory.

3. After undergoing a descending thoracic aortic aneurysm repair using an endograft, a 65-year-old male is recovering in the ICU. On POD 1, he is noted to have proximal thigh weakness bilaterally. He has 3/5 power on hip flexion bilaterally with intact sensations. He started vasopressor therapy and a spinal drain was placed. What is the basic principle of these interventions aimed at helping the patient's neurological status?
   a. Increasing perfusion pressure to the spinal cord
   b. Increasing CSF pressure
   c. Maintaining high cardiac output
   d. None of the above

   Answer: a

   Maintaining a MAP above 85–90 with CSF drainage aims at increasing the perfusion pressure to the spinal cord. A spinal drain lowers the CSF pressure, which, in turn, increases the spinal cord perfusion pressure (spinal cord perfusion pressure = MAP–CSF pressure). Since coverage of intercostals can result in decreased flow to the spinal cord resulting in ischemia, allowing higher perfusion pressure to the spinal cord from remaining patent vasculature helps mitigate this effect.

4. At the end of a TEVAR, final angiographic imaging shows contrast filling the aneurysmal sac from an intercostal vessel. What is the next step in management?
   a. Coil embolization of the intercostal vessel
   b. Thoracotomy with ligation of intercostal vessel
   c. CTA chest in one month
   d. Proximal and distal extension of endograft

   Answer: c

   Most type II endoleaks can be monitored with serial imaging as they tend to resolve on their own. A CTA should be performed in one month to assess for resolution or presence of any other endoleaks. If a type II leak is seen without any significant aneurysmal sac enlargement, CTA can be repeated in six months. If aneurysmal sac enlargement is seen, coil embolization can be performed. Type I and III endoleaks should be intervened on with placement of bridging stent grafts for type III leaks and extension of the endograft proximally and distally for type I leaks.

REFERENCES

1. Dake, M. D., Miller, D. C., Semba, C. P., Mitchell, R. S., Walker, P. J., & Liddell, R. P. (1994). Transluminal placement of endovascular stent-grafts for the treatment of descending thoracic aortic aneurysms. *N Engl J Med, 331*(26), 1729–1734. doi:10.1056/NEJM199412293312601
2. Kibbe, M. R., & Matsumura, J. S. (2003). The gore excluder US multi-center trial: analysis of adverse events at 2 years. *Semin Vasc Surg, 16*(2), 144–150. doi:10.1016/s0895-7967(03)00012-7
3. Upchurch, G. R., Jr., Escobar, G. A., Azizzadeh, A., Beck, A. W., Conrad, M. F., Matsumura, J. S., & Wang, G. J. (2021). Society for vascular surgery clinical practice guidelines of thoracic endovascular aortic repair for descending thoracic aortic aneurysms. *J Vasc Surg, 73*(1s), 55s–83s. doi:10.1016/j.jvs.2020.05.076
4. Alsawas, M., Zaiem, F., Larrea-Mantilla, L., Almasri, J., Erwin, P. J., Upchurch, G. R., Jr., & Murad, M. H. (2017). Effectiveness of surgical interventions for thoracic aortic aneurysms: A systematic review and meta-analysis. *J Vasc Surg, 66*(4), 1258–1268. e1258. doi:10.1016/j.jvs.2017.05.082
5. Mezzetto, L., Mastrorilli, D., Bravo, G., Scorsone, L., Gennai, S., Leone, N., . . . Veraldi, G. F. (2023). Celiac artery coverage after thoracic endovascular aortic procedure: a meta-analysis of early and late results. *J Endovasc Ther, 30*(4), 499–509. doi:10.1177/15266028221090443
6. Vaddineni, S. K., Taylor, S. M., Patterson, M. A., & Jordan, W. D., Jr. (2007). Outcome after celiac artery coverage during endovascular thoracic aortic aneurysm repair: preliminary results. *J Vasc Surg, 45*(3), 467–471. doi:10.1016/j.jvs.2006.11.040
7. Kabbani, L., Nadig, J., Ranjal, R. S., Rteil, A., Linchangco, R., Weaver, M., . . . Shepard, A. (2019). The level of persistent false lumen perfusion is associated with increased aortic size after thoracic endovascular aortic repair in patients with type B aortic dissection. *J Vasc Surg, 70*(3), e77–e78.
8. Ristalli, F., Dini, C. S., Stolcova, M., Nardi, G., Valente, S., Meucci, F., & Di Mario, C. (2019). Role of lithotripsy for small calcified iliacs in the era of big devices. *Curr Cardiol Rep, 21*(11), 143. doi:10.1007/s11886-019-1245-2
9. Saitoh, D., Yamazaki, Y., Tsuji, T., Sakoda, N., Yakuwa, K., Tabayashi, A., . . . Kin, H. (2024). Patterns of collateral arteries to the spinal cord after thoracoabdominal aortic aneurysm repair. *Interdiscip Cardiovasc Thorac Surg*. doi:10.1093/icvts/ivae087
10. Marcondes, G. B., Cirillo-Penn, N. C., Tenorio, E. R., Adam, D. J., Timaran, C., Austermann, M. J., . . . Oderich, G. S. (2023). Multicenter study to evaluate endovascular repair of extent I-III thoracoabdominal aneurysms without prophylactic cerebrospinal fluid drainage. *Ann Surg, 278*(2), e396–e404. doi:10.1097/sla.0000000000005653

13

Endovascular repair of type B aortic dissection

BRIAN SULLIVAN AND LOAY S. KABBANI

INTRODUCTION

The incidence of type B aortic dissection (TBAD) is three to five individuals/year per 100,000. As of 2020, a new classification system defines TBAD as hyperacute (symptom onset within 24 hours), acute (1–14 days), subacute (15–90 days), or chronic (>90 days) [1]. TBAD is further classified as "complicated" if there is rupture or malperfusion. Malperfusion itself can arise from either a static obstruction or dynamic obstruction of the branch vessels (Figure 13.1). Together, these classifications are used to assist decision-making regarding surgical intervention. Uncomplicated TBAD is principally managed with medical therapy, although some patients may ultimately require intervention. In this category, early mortality is reported to be 2–10%, stroke rate 1%, and spinal cord ischemia (SCI) 0.8% [2]. Complicated TBAD (rupture or malperfusion) occurs in 10% of patients who present with TBAD and often requires treatment with endovascular techniques. Clinical signs of malperfusion are listed in Table 13.1.

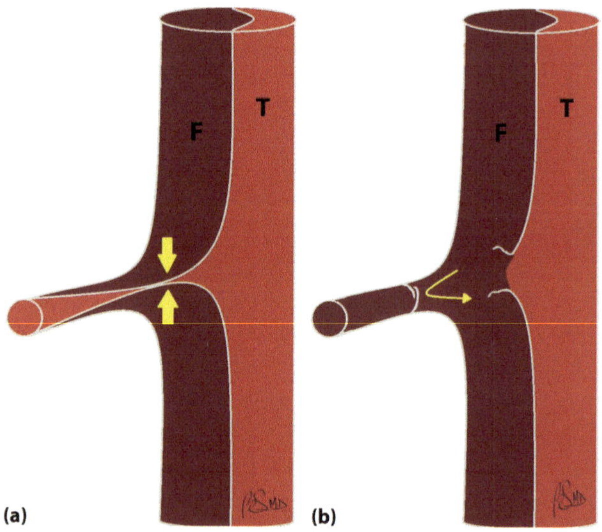

Figure 13.1 Dynamic (a) or static (b) branch vessel obstruction may occur in aortic dissection.

MANAGEMENT PRINCIPLES

The best therapy for any aortic dissection aims to start anti-impulse therapy and pain control as soon as possible. The theoretical aim of anti-impulse therapy is to reduce shear stress of the cardiac cycle on the aortic wall, while maintaining adequate visceral perfusion and limiting false lumen perfusion. Anti-impulse therapy goals are a heart rate of 60 beats per minute and a systolic blood pressure (BP) to below 120 mmHg [3]. This is achieved with titrated intravenous beta-blocking agents, with or without vasodilating drugs such as sodium nitroprusside. A calcium channel blocker may also be used to supplement beta blockade. Reducing cardiac contractility always takes precedence over lowering BP, so that beta blockade or a calcium channel blocker should be initiated prior to administering vasodilator therapy. It should be noted that decreasing the BP too fast in uncomplicated TBAD, especially in patients with chronic hypertension, may predispose to neurologic injury [4]. Once both a stable BP and symptom relief are obtained, a patient with uncomplicated type B aortic dissection can preferentially be discharged on oral medication, rather than receive surgical management within the acute period.

Clinical and imaging follow-up at one, three, and six months, and annually thereafter is essential to detect aneurysmal degeneration of the affected aortic segment, which affects about 30–40% of patients at five years [5]. During follow-up, patients with appropriate anti-hypertensive control have shown improved outcome with fewer aortic events including aortic expansion and rupture [6]. For TBAD transitioning to outpatient care, resting SBP

DOI: 10.1201/9781003452096-13

Table 13.1 Signs and symptoms of malperfusion

Organ	Presentation	Labs
Gut	Abdominal pain, nausea, bloody diarrhea	Rising lactate
Spinal cord	Paresis, paraplegia	
Lower extremities	Pain, paresthesia, paralysis, pulselessness	Elevated CPK
Renal	Refractory hypertension*	Rising Cr**

*Hypertension persisting despite >3 or more different classes of anti-hypertensive medication given at maximally recommended or tolerated doses has been suggested to reflect malperfusion of the kidneys.
**Cr, serum creatinine; other causes such as hyper/hypotension, or contrast induced nephropathy may also cause Cr to rise.
CPK, creatine phosphokinase.

should be kept at 130–150 mmHg, and the SBP during exercise should be kept below 180 mmHg [3], unless otherwise interdicted by return of symptoms.

There is evidence that the risks of perioperative complications such as rupture, retrograde type A dissection (rTAAD), and mortality are decreased if TEVAR is delayed until the subacute time frame [7, 8]. For this reason, it is our practice that patients with uncomplicated TBAD are treated medically for two to six weeks. After this period, if there are "high-risk features" (Table 13.2) on imaging, an informed discussion with the patient is held re: elective endovascular repair. Several studies have shown favorable aortic remodeling (increase in true lumen diameter and more false lumen thrombosis) after TEVAR for uncomplicated acute, subacute, and early chronic TBAD [7, 8]. This time interval may reflect a favorable window of plasticity in the tissues of the aortic wall after the immediate post-dissection inflammatory period has quieted. Within this range, early intervention has the additional benefit of preserving the full array of endovascular techniques, some of which may become infeasible once aneurysmal degeneration, septal "stiffening," or progressive dissection occurs.

Table 13.2 Risk factors for adverse long-term TBAD outcomes

Category	Predictor
History	Age <60 years
	Caucasian race
	Connective tissue disorder
Presentation	Refractory hypertension
	Refractory pain
Radiologic findings	Initial aortic diameter ≥40 mm
	Initial false lumen diameter ≥22 mm
	Partially thrombosed false lumen
	Sac formation in partially thrombosed false lumen
	Large entry tear >10 mm
	Entry tear on lesser curve
	Bloody pleural effusion

A number of studies have suggested prognostic factors for patients who will fare worse over time with aortic dissection (Table 13.2) and thus may benefit from more aggressive early management with TEVAR. These factors include patient characteristics such as younger age (≤60 years of age) and male gender [9]. Another high-risk subgroup is patients with refractory pain and hypertension despite medical therapy. Radiological predictors include an initial diameter ≥4 cm of the descending thoracic aorta (DTA), an initial false lumen diameter in the proximal descending aorta ≥22 mm, a fusiform aortic index of 0.64 or more, elliptical configuration of the true lumen in combination with a circular formation of the false lumen, proximal entry tear size >10 mm, or location of the tear on the inner curve of the arch [10]. The presence of only one entry tear, spiral configuration of the dissection, or partial false lumen thrombosis have also been suggested to be associated with an increased rate of aortic growth. On follow-up, computerized tomographic angiography (CTA), patency of the false lumen, developing an ulcer-like projection into the dissection, and saccular aneurysm formation are associated with higher aorta-related adverse events [9, 10]. On the other hand, complete false lumen thrombosis indicates aortic stability and portends fewer secondary events. TBAD patients with "borderline" malperfusion symptoms such as intermittent nausea and vomiting, prolonged ileus, or fluctuating pulse exams may also be more likely to benefit from TEVAR.

The vital step in TEVAR is coverage of the primary entry tear with a covered stent graft that results in predominant flow to the true lumen. This typically normalizes distal perfusion, restores branch vessel patency, and promotes false lumen thrombosis. Rates of false lumen thrombosis after TEVAR range between 60% and 90% for the proximal thoracic aorta, 30% and 60% for the distal thoracic aorta, and 3% and 20% for the abdominal aorta [11].

In a rupture scenario, the operator must go beyond sealing just the entry tear to fully isolate the flow lumen from the area of rupture, often necessitating extensive covered stent grafting, thus increasing the risk of morbidity.

TEVAR for complicated acute TBAD has a mortality of 7–16%, an SCI rate of 3%, and a stroke rate of 4%

[2]. Retrograde type A aortic dissection extension into the ascending aorta was reported in 0.4–2% [12] and is associated with >10% oversizing of the endograft in the proximal landing zone. Endoleaks, graft migration, renal failure, and device separation have also been reported. Performing a left carotid-subclavian bypass if the left subclavian artery is to be covered has shown decreased risks of neurologic complications with TEVAR in TBAD, especially stroke [13]. Some surgeons advocate covering the thoracic aorta down to the celiac artery in all cases of malperfusion and rupture; however, the risk of SCI increases with more extensive coverage, particularly zone 5. The Provisional Extension to Induce Complete Attachment (PETTICOAT) extends the stent-graft scaffold distally with open-cell bare metal stents; it may be most useful in cases of visceral malperfusion [12].

ENDOVASCULAR PROCEDURE

All patients with TBAD should undergo a dynamic 1 mm-cut CTA with phase delay imaging from the base of the skull to the femoral arteries. Phase delay imaging helps identify delayed filling of any branch vessels, which is common. The CTA gives important information about the type of dissection, proximal landing zones, true lumen compression, branch vessel obstruction, mechanism of obstruction (static vs. dynamic), access vessel size, and associated conditions such as aneurysmal disease. Reconstruction with centerline measurements, if available, can be very helpful in determining the suitability for TEVAR (Figure 13.2). Anatomic requirements for TEVAR include the presence of a 2-cm healthy landing zone at the proximal margin, a relatively non-angulated landing zone that is not tapered, and access vessels that are adequate in size, not too tortuous, and relatively free of atherosclerotic disease.

Preparation for surgery. All procedures are performed under general anesthesia for better control of hemodynamics and to limit respiratory motion during graft deployment. Radial artery catheter on the right is routine because of the frequent need to cover the origin of the left subclavian artery (LSCA). A lumbar drain is placed preoperatively whenever the TEVAR is to be extended to the distal DTA (eighth thoracic vertebra) or below.

Dual groin wire access is obtained and closure devices are deployed, if necessary, in the standard fashion. The main body side should be dilated to device size over a double-curved Lunderquist wire situated on the aortic valve; the contralateral side can be 5Fr to accommodate a long pigtail catheter, brought to rest on the aortic valve. Intravascular ultrasound (IVUS) is essential to document that the wires and grafts are in the true lumen prior to device passage and deployment, and can also assist in identifying entry tear location(s) (Figure 13.3). Covering the LSCA without bypassing it has been shown to increase the risk of stroke [13] and decrease collateral spinal cord perfusion. Bypassing the LSCA is especially important if the patient has a history of coronary artery bypass where the left internal mammary artery was used, if there is an inadequate right vertebral artery to compensate for the left, or the left vertebral artery terminates in the posterior inferior cerebellar artery. These anatomic constraints re-demonstrate the need for appropriate preoperative imaging.

The stent graft is deployed to cover the primary entry tear (Figure 13.4). The selected stent graft should have a diameter no more than 10% larger than the aortic diameter at the landing zone. As the true lumen expands, and

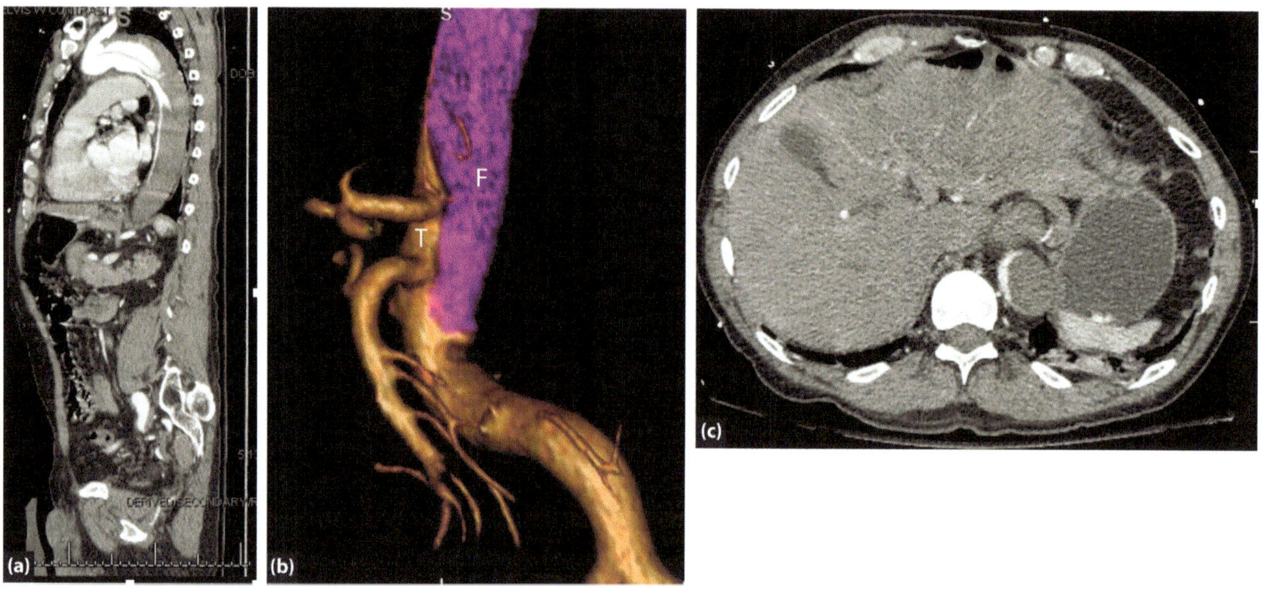

Figure 13.2 Computed tomography angiography of type B aortic dissection: (a) sagittal view; (b) three-dimensional reconstruction with true (T) and false (F) lumen; (c) axial view.

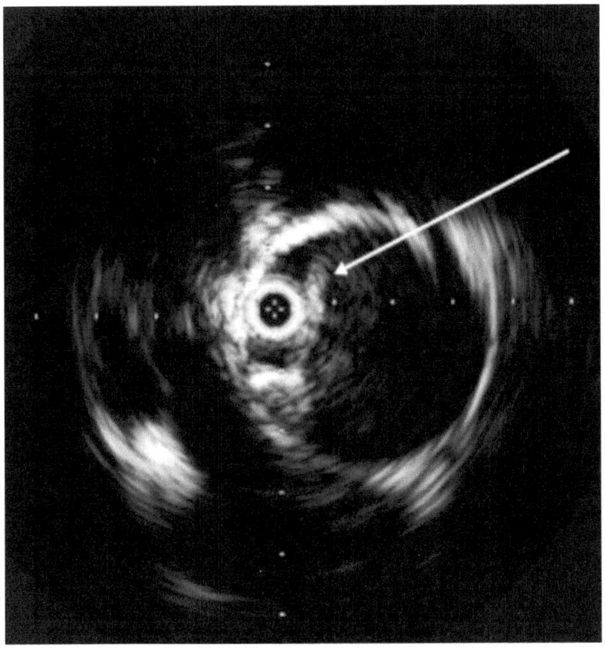

Figure 13.3 Intraoperative intravascular ultrasound image demonstrating that the probe and wire are within the severely compressed true lumen with the dissection flap (arrow) separating the true and false lumens. Note the visible entry tear near arrow.

flow through the false lumen is reduced or obliterated, any dynamic branch vessel compromise is ameliorated. After stent-graft deployment, molding of the graft to the aortic wall with a balloon should only be performed if absolutely needed, as this maneuver increases the risk of retrograde dissection or rupture. Completion angiogram and IVUS should be carried out routinely to make sure the dynamic obstruction(s) has resolved (Figure 13.5). If present, branch stenoses can be studied by measuring the pressure gradients across the area of narrowing. Significant stenosis is defined as a systolic gradient of >20 mmHg. A self-expanding stent can then be placed, oversized no more than 10% of the vessel diameter. When sizing such stents, it should be kept in mind that malperfused vessels in a patient with cardiovascular collapse (as in dissection) are undersized and may significantly enlarge once adequate perfusion is restored.

POSTOPERATIVE CARE AND FOLLOW-UP

Anti-impulse control should be optimized postoperatively with IV medications and rapidly transitioned to an oral regimen. Patients with preoperative malperfusion should be carefully monitored for the restoration of normal perfusion—visceral issues with serial abdominal exams, monitoring of lactate and liver function tests, and renal issues with urine output and serum Cr measurements. Worsening or failure to improve vital organ function warrants further investigation with imaging studies. Duplex scanning is sometimes sufficient, but in most circumstances, a repeat CTA will be necessary despite the need for administration of iodinated contrast in a short interval. Abnormalities should trigger prompt re-intervention.

Spinal cord function should be checked immediately postoperatively and hourly for the first 24 hours. A protocol for SCI should be in place and followed aggressively. This sometimes requires urgent return to the OR for LSCA revascularization. Patients should be maintained on lifelong antiplatelet therapy in addition to a statin.

Follow-up. Similar to preoperative imaging, a high-resolution CTA with reconstructions should be obtained at one-month follow-up to document proper stent positioning and aortic stability (Figure 13.6). Follow-up with a dedicated aortic team is important for long-term success. Expertise in the management of hypertension and

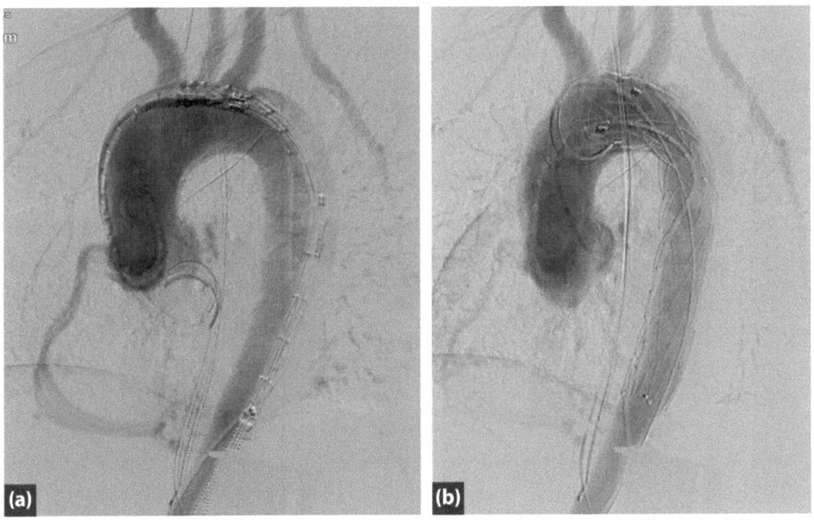

Figure 13.4 Intraoperative digital subtraction angiography images: (a) pre-deployment of stent graft; (b) post-deployment with complete coverage of entry tear.

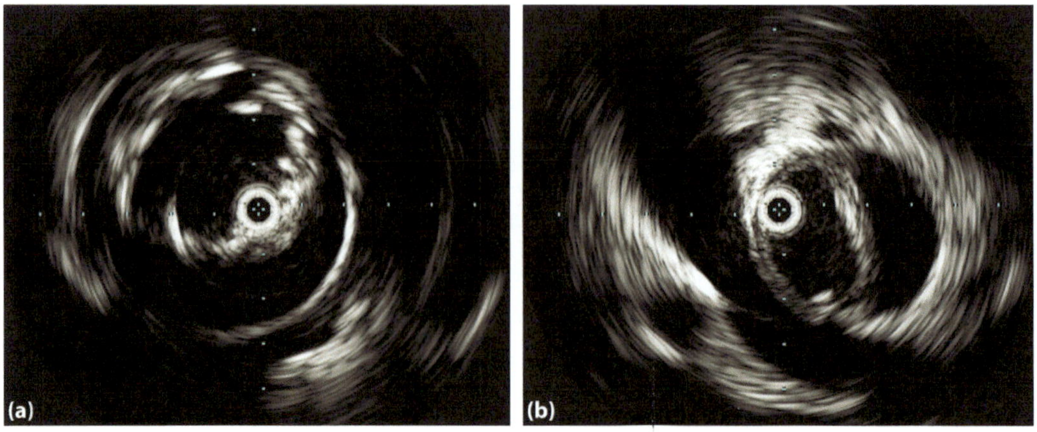

Figure 13.5 Intraoperative intravascular ultrasound images after placement of a thoracic endograft with expansion of the true lumen distally (same patient as in Figure 13.3). (a) Stent graft within true lumen. (b) Re-expanded true lumen in aorta below the stent graft.

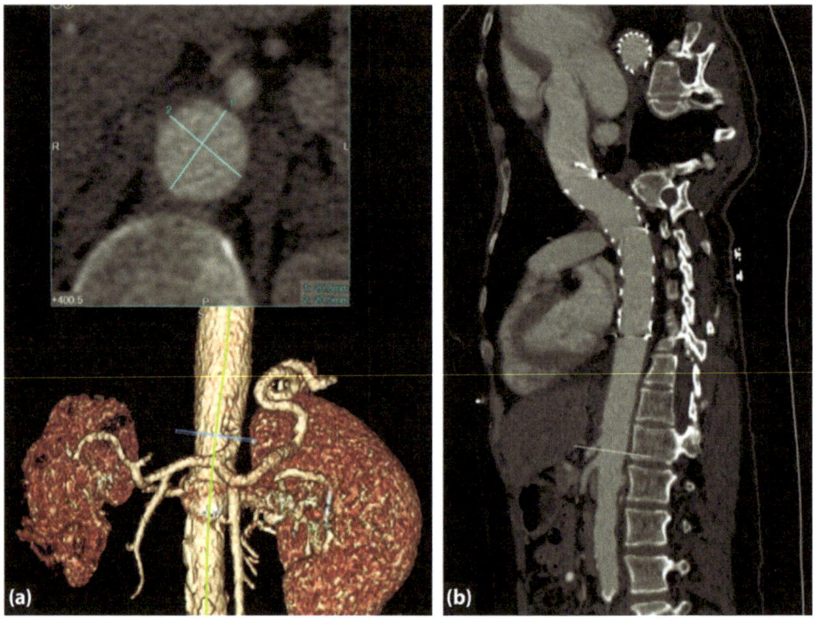

Figure 13.6 Six-month postoperative computed tomography angiography (CTA) images: (a) three-dimensional reconstruction with axial image (inset); (b) centerline image of CTA. Both images demonstrate a patent endograft with resolution of dissection.

other medical co-morbidities is a critical component of this team. Surveillance CTA monitoring should be performed at three months, six months, 12 months, and annual thereafter. Even with "successful" treatment of the acute issue, up to 30–40% of these patients will require additional aortic procedures in the future [1].

TRICKS AND TRAPS

- All patients benefit from initial medical management and impulse control.
- Carefully assess the patient's condition to determine the urgency of the procedure. Treat patients with malperfusion or rupture as an emergency.
- Inadequate imaging can lead to inappropriate decision-making and device selection and sizing.
- In patients with uncomplicated TBAD and high-risk features, we wait two to six weeks before discussing with the patient the benefits of TEVAR and balancing the risks of the dissection against the risks of perioperative complications.
- Stenting the true lumen with coverage of the primary entry tear is the principal goal in TEVAR for TBAD.
- To avoid retrograde dissection, oversizing of the TEVAR stent graft should be no more than 10% of the aortic diameter at the proximal landing zone.
- We do not routinely perform balloon expansion of the endograft in cases of TBAD.

- The proximal landing zone should be in an area of normal aorta that is unaffected by dissection or wall hematoma.
- In dynamic obstruction, it is our experience that true vessel thrombosis is uncommon, and restoration of proximal aortic flow to the true lumen relieves the obstruction.
- IVUS should be routinely employed when performing TEVAR for TBAD.
- Intensive care monitoring post-procedure is mandatory for signs of spinal cord ischemia, and a rescue protocol should be established ahead of time at the operating facility.

QUESTIONS

1. A 65-year-old woman presents to the ER with an aortic dissection. According to the SVS/STS guidelines for reporting, a type A aortic dissection is defined as having an entry tear in which of the following areas?
   a. Zone 0
   b. Zone 1
   c. Zone 2
   d. Zone 3

   Answer: a

2. A 49-year-old man is being followed in the intensive care unit two days after presenting with an acute, uncomplicated TBAD. What are the optimal goals for impulse control of TBAD for this patient?
   a. SBP <160, HR <100
   b. SBP <140, HR <80
   c. SBP <130, HR <70
   d. SBP <120, HR <60

   Answer: d

3. A 58-year-old man with chronic hypertension presents to the emergency room with tearing chest pain radiating to the back beginning four hours ago. On CTA, the patient is noted to have an uncomplicated TBAD with several high-risk features. He is a candidate for TEVAR. Which of the following time periods confers the best window for surgical management of this patient?
   a. Hyperacute: symptom onset within 24 hours
   b. Acute: 1–14 days
   c. Subacute: 15–90 days
   d. Chronic: >90 days

   Answer: c

4. A 74-year-old female presented to the emergency room with TBAD complicated by rupture and underwent successful stent-graft exclusion of aortic zones 2 through 5. In the recovery area, the patient is awake and stable with a blood pressure of 104/58 and a pulse of 87. She reports difficulty lifting her knees off the bed. What is the best next step in management?
   a. Impulse control
   b. Stat CTA
   c. Transfuse 1u packed red cells and re-evaluate
   d. Augment MAP >90, HGB >9, O2 >95%, and place a spinal drain

   Answer: d

REFERENCES

1. Lombardi JV, Hughes GC, Appoo JJ, et al. Society for Vascular Surgery (SVS) and Society of Thoracic Surgeons (STS) reporting standards for type B aortic dissections. *J Vasc Surg*. 2020 Mar;71(3):723–47.
2. Moulakakis KG, Mylonas SN, Dalainas I, et al. Management of complicated and uncomplicated acute type B dissection. A systematic review and meta-analysis. *Ann Cardiothorac Surg*. 2014 May;3(3):234–46.
3. Suzuki T, Eagle KA, Bossone E, et al. Medical management in type B aortic dissection. *Ann Cardiothorac Surg*. 2014 Jul;3(4):413–7.
4. Al Adas Z, Shepard AD, Weaver MR, et al. Cerebrovascular injuries found in acute type B aortic dissections are associated with blood pressure derangements and poor outcome. *J Vasc Surg*. 2018 Nov;68(5):1308–13.
5. Nienaber CA, Rousseau H, Eggebrecht H, et al. Randomized comparison of strategies for type B aortic dissection: The INvestigation of STEnt grafts in Aortic Dissection (INSTEAD) trial. *Circulation*. 2009 Dec 22;120(25):2519–28.
6. Kodama K, Nishigami K, Sakamoto T, et al. Tight heart rate control reduces secondary adverse events in patients with type B acute aortic dissection. *Circulation*. 2008 Sep 30;118(14 Suppl):S167–70.
7. Brunkwall J, Kasprzak P, Verhoeven E, et al. Endovascular repair of acute uncomplicated aortic type B dissection promotes aortic remodelling: 1 year results of the ADSORB trial. *Eur J Vasc Endovasc Surg*. 2014 Sep;48(3):285–91.
8. Nienaber CA, Kische S, Rousseau H, et al. Endovascular repair of type B aortic dissection: long-term results of the randomized investigation of stent grafts in aortic dissection trial. *Circ Cardiovasc Interv*. 2013 Aug;6(4):407–16.
9. Kitai T, Kaji S, Yamamuro A, et al. Impact of new development of ulcer-like projection on clinical outcomes in patients with type B aortic dissection with closed and thrombosed false lumen. *Circulation*. 2010 Sep 14;122(11 Suppl):S74–80.

10. Tolenaar JL, van Keulen JW, Jonker FH, et al. Morphologic predictors of aortic dilatation in type B aortic dissection. *J Vasc Surg*. 2013 Nov;58(5):1220–5.
11. Nienaber CA, Kische S, Skriabina V, et al. Noninvasive imaging approaches to evaluate the patient with known or suspected aortic disease. *Circ Cardiovasc Imaging*. 2009 Nov;2(6):499–506.
12. Lombardi JV, Cambria RP, Nienaber CA, et al. Aortic remodeling after endovascular treatment of complicated type B aortic dissection with the use of a composite device design. *J Vasc Surg*. 2014 Jun;59(6):1544–54.
13. Natour AK, Shepard A, Onofrey K, et al. Left subclavian artery revascularization is associated with less neurologic injury after endovascular repair of acute type B aortic dissection. *J Vasc Surg*. 2023 Nov;78(5):1170–9.e2.

14

Endovascular repair of splanchnic and renal artery aneurysms

WASIH KAMRAN AND NIK KOLICAJ

INTRODUCTION

In this chapter, a visceral artery aneurysm (VAA) is defined as fusiform or saccular dilatation of the celiac, superior mesenteric, inferior mesenteric, or renal arteries or their branches. Autopsy results indicate an incidence of up to 2–10%. Of note, some of the literature considers renal artery aneurysms distinct entities, thus the incidence of VAAs is underestimated in some studies.

Older data reported a majority (~60%) of VAAs are splenic artery aneurysms, with most others arising from the hepatic artery. Table 14.1 summarizes the more recently reported prevalence of VAAs. Around 30% of patients present with more than one aneurysm.

While most VAAs are asymptomatic and incidentally detected, up to 25% may present with rupture, which confers a mortality rate of up to 70%. The risk of rupture is especially high in women of childbearing age. The most common symptoms associated with VAAs include abdominal pain and intraabdominal or gastrointestinal bleeding. Major complications include rupture and acute mesenteric ischemia.

Table 14.1 Prevalence of visceral artery aneurysms in more recent studies

Artery of origin	Aneurysm prevalence
Splenic artery (SA)	30–64%
Celiac artery (CA)	2–46%
Hepatic artery (HA)	4–30%
Pancreaticoduodenal artery (PDA)	2–10%
Superior mesenteric artery (SMA)	1–9%
Gastroduodenal artery (GDA)	1–15%
Gastroepiploic artery (GEA)	2%
Inferior mesenteric artery (IMA)	1%

Based on Erben et al., Fankhauser et al., Corey et al., and Fargion et al.

The Society for Vascular Surgery (SVS) recommends initial evaluation of suspected VAAs with CT angiography; magnetic resonance angiography (MRA) is helpful in patients with contraindications to iodinated contrast material (e.g., renal insufficiency). Catheter angiography is reserved for preoperative planning and suspected ruptured aneurysms when emergent endovascular treatment is warranted.

Treatment options are based on the location of the aneurysm itself. As a convention, a grade 1B recommendation is made for emergent treatment of any patient who presents with aneurysm rupture.

Renal artery aneurysms. Grade 2 recommendation calls for treating uncomplicated aneurysms >3 cm in size. For patients of childbearing age and patients with medically consequential renal artery stenosis, intervention is recommended regardless of size. Open operative intervention is recommended as first line therapy, with endovascular intervention reserved for patients who are poor open operative candidates and/or have distal parenchymal aneurysms more amenable to coiling.

Splenic artery aneurysms. In the absence of rupture, elective treatment of any pseudoaneurysm is recommended due to the risk of rupture. True aneurysms in women of childbearing age should also be treated regardless of size. In patients with true aneurysms ≥3 cm in size, a grade 1 recommendation is given to treat electively. Aneurysms <3 cm in size can be monitored in patients with significant comorbidities. Endovascular treatment is recommended if anatomically feasible, with the main exception being aneurysms near the hilum due to the risk of splenic infarction and pancreatitis (grade 2B).

DOI: 10.1201/9781003452096-14

Celiac artery aneurysm. Treatment is recommended for non-ruptured pseudoaneurysms of any size and true aneurysms >2 cm due to the increased risk of rupture (grade 1B). Observation with annual CTAs can be considered in patients with aneurysms of <2 cm if significant comorbidities are present.

Gastric and gastroepiploic artery aneurysms. Grade 1B recommendations are made for endovascular treatment of all non-ruptured pseudoaneurysms and true aneurysms.

Hepatic artery aneurysms. Pseudoaneurysms and symptomatic true aneurysms should be repaired on diagnosis regardless of size due to the high risk of mortality. Asymptomatic patients without comorbidities should undergo repair if the aneurysm is >2 cm in size or increases by at least 0.5 cm per year. Patients with significant comorbidities should undergo repair if the aneurysm exceeds 5.0 cm. Endovascular techniques are the mainstay of treatment with the goal of maintaining arterial flow to the liver. Segmental resection may need to be considered in patients with large intrahepatic aneurysms to avoid necrosis.

Superior mesenteric artery aneurysms. A grade 1A recommendation is made to repair all true and pseudoaneurysms regardless of size.

Jejunal, ileal, and colic artery aneurysms. Elective intervention is recommended for aneurysms greater than 2 cm (grade 1B). Endovascular embolization is preferred, and further workup for vasculitis via inflammatory markers is recommended.

Pancreaticoduodenal and gastroduodenal artery aneurysms. Aneurysms of all sizes should undergo treatment due to the risk of rupture. Coil embolization is the treatment of choice in both intact and ruptured aneurysms (grade 1B). Grade 2C recommendations are given for covered stenting, stent-assisted coiling, and liquid embolic agents if coil embolization is not feasible.

PROCEDURE

The general principles of endovascular intervention can be broken down into four major steps: vascular access, vessel selection, embolization or stent-grafting, and closure. Each step has standard techniques, as well as variation based on clinical practice. Unique potential pitfalls also exist with each step warranting special attention.

ACCESS

Conventional arterial access is performed in the common femoral artery via ultrasound guidance. The authors opt for a micropuncture kit using a modified Seldinger technique, eventually upsizing to a 5Fr vascular sheath. Attention must be made to access the artery at a level overlying the femoral head to provide a good base to apply pressure if manual pressure is required during removal of the access system (Figure 14.1).

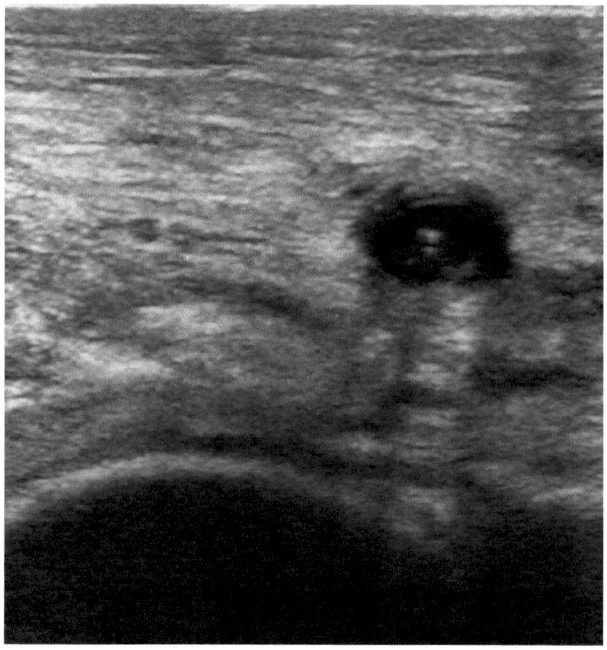

Figure 14.1 Ultrasound image of the right common femoral artery with an echogenic focus centrally within the lumen, delineating the micropuncture needle tip. Note the femoral head deep to the artery.

The common femoral artery is visualized in short axis, with the needle traversing it in short axis too. Before choosing an access site, the branch point of the profunda femoris artery and the inferior epigastric artery should be identified. Any large plaques should also be identified and avoided as these can embolize distally and render hemostatic devices less effective.

ANGIOGRAPHY AND SELECTION

A curved 5Fr catheter (e.g., Mikelson) is inserted over a J-wire and formed in the aorta. At this time, aortography can be performed if diagnostically indicated. The catheter is then manipulated to select for the desired first order branch of the abdominal aorta. Digital subtraction angiography of the first order branch can then be performed through the base catheter.

Further selection into second or third order branches can be performed using a triaxial system with a microcatheter and microwire placed through the base 5Fr catheter. Adequate advancement into the main branch with the base catheter is critical for maintaining stability while traversing smaller, more tortuous distal branches. The triaxial system also allows for greater control when anticipating difficult-to-select distal branches. Additionally, when using particle embolic agents, the microcatheter can be sacrificed without losing access to the culprit vessel.

EMBOLIZATION OR STENT-GRAFTING

This aspect of the procedure is the most variable based on the location of the aneurysm. Coils are the most commonly used embolic agent due to their variability in size, radio-opacity enabling proper visualization under fluoroscopy and ability to conform to tortuous or irregular arteries. They are also highly thrombogenic, particularly fibered coils. These are especially useful in smaller visceral arteries, as 0.018 microcoils can be used through microcatheters in a triaxial system. Both pushable and deployable coils are used in different aneurysms. Deployable coils confer the benefit of better control in placement, as they can be repositioned if not placed correctly within the vessel. These coils tend to be more expensive, so are used primarily when embolizing more proximal arteries where there is higher risk for distal off-target embolization. Coils should be 2–3 mm larger than the diameter of the target artery. In the case of saccular aneurysms, the target artery can often be spared from occlusion, as solely packing the aneurysm can provide durable treatment.

Stent-assisted coiling with an uncovered stent should be considered in larger vessels with wider-necked aneurysms where complete vessel sacrifice confers a higher risk of end-organ ischemia. After stent placement, a microcatheter and wire are placed within the aneurysm through the stent's interstices and the sac can be packed with embolic coils.

Covered stents have a limited utility in the treatment of VAAs as they confer specific limitations in vessel size, tortuosity, and location. The ideal vessel for a covered stent is large (>4 mm), has appropriate straight landing zones both proximally and distally, and is not too tortuous. Given the nature of VAAs, most aneurysms do not meet these criteria. Due to the risk of infection, the authors consider a suspected mycotic aneurysm a contraindication to covered stent placement. Antibiotic prophylaxis should be used in all cases of covered stent placement.

Covered stents can be split into two categories: self-expanding and balloon expandable. The enhanced flexibility of self-expanding stents compared with balloon expandable stents makes them more suitable for tortuous vessels and hence a better option for most VAAs when stent graft repair is considered.

Liquid adhesive embolics such as N-butyl-2-cyanoacrylate (NBMA) glue are less often used due to their unpredictable nature and potential for off-target embolization due to delayed polymerization.

Newer non-adhesive liquid embolic agents are seeing increased use. Products such as Onyx™ (Medtronic) and PHIL™ (precipitating hydrophobic injectable liquid) (Terumo) are increasingly coming to the market. These take longer to polymerize and do not adhere as much to catheter tips, making off-target embolization less likely. Their main disadvantage over other agents is cost and preparation time, as many require 20 minutes of shaking in dimethyl sulfoxide (DMSO).

Plugs such as Amplatzer vascular plugs (Abbott Cardiovascular) can also be used to block the afferent and efferent vessels to aneurysms but require relatively straight landing zones for the plug. Additionally, earlier versions of the plug require upsizing to larger base sheaths (up to 7Fr) and cannot be placed through microcatheters. Microvascular plugs are newer and can be used with microcatheters but have many of the same disadvantages as Amplatzer plugs and are typically reserved for arteries 7 mm or smaller.

CLOSURE

While manual pressure remains the gold standard for hemostasis in femoral artery puncture cases, its main disadvantage is the prolonged time needed to appropriately achieve hemostasis. Over the past few years, a myriad of closure devices have entered the market that significantly reduce the time to hemostasis. Multiple mechanisms of action exist but the main principle is the same, these devices either actively approximate the arteriotomy site or apply different inert plugs at the site using intraluminal anchors or a balloon to ensure placement. The authors' institution employs the use of three main devices.

Angio-Seal® (Terumo) uses an extraluminal collagen plug that covers the arteriotomy site. The plug expands as it is deployed over the site and triggers coagulation. Angio-Seal is approved for up to 8Fr sites.

MynxGrip™ (Cordis) is similar in that it contains a polyethylene hydrogel that covers the arteriotomy site. However, it contains an intravascular balloon that is inflated to ensure appropriate placement and anchor the gel. It is approved for use in up to 7Fr sites.

The Perclose™ device (Abbott Cardiovascular) percutaneously sutures the arteriotomy by deploying sutures on each side. The device contains a "footplate" that enters the vessel and opposes the wall. A suture needle is then deployed to approximate the arteriotomy. It is approved for sites up to 21Fr, making it ideal for larger arteriotomies.

CASE EXAMPLES

Case 1: Hepatic artery aneurysms

A 53-year-old male had a computerized tomographic angiogram (CTA) of the abdomen after undergoing a two vessel coronary artery bypass graft and aortic valve repair for endocarditis and CAD documenting completely normal hepatic circulation.

CTA of the chest, abdomen, and pelvis three months later revealed a 19 mm aneurysm arising from a branch of the right hepatic artery and a 3 mm aneurysm arising from a branch of the left hepatic artery. Given the patient's history, these were presumed to be mycotic. The patient was subsequently referred to interventional radiology for angiography and potential embolization therapy.

ANGIOGRAM

Conventional right common femoral artery access was performed with a micropuncture set as previously noted. The system was upsized to a 5Fr sheath, and the celiac trunk was selected using a Mikelson catheter. DSA revealed the two aneurysms in the right and left hepatic arteries. It was noted that the larger of the two (19 mm on CT) was arising from the main right hepatic artery, and the smaller of the two (3 mm on CT) was arising from a segment two branch of the left hepatic artery.

A triaxial system was then employed using a 2.4-French Progreat microcatheter with 0.018" Asahi Chikai microwire, both advanced through the 5Fr base catheter. The vascular sheath was advanced into the aorta for maximal purchase. Using the triaxial system, the right hepatic artery was selected, and DSA was performed that demonstrated filling of a lobular saccular aneurysm arising from a superior branch of the posterior division of the right hepatic artery (Figure 14.2a). Cone-beam CT was performed at this location to definitively determine the culprit branch. Three-dimensional reformatted images from the CT confirmed a 1.9 cm × 1.6 cm aneurysm arising from a branch of the posterior division of the right hepatic artery.

The microwire and microcatheter were then used to select this branch, and a DSA was performed at this location confirming the culprit branch. Using both Synchro and Asahi wires, the aneurysmal sac was accessed, and multiple large detachable coils were deployed in the aneurysmal sac. Afterward, the microcatheter and wire were advanced into the outflow branch of the aneurysm and multiple pushable coils were deployed. The system was then pulled back into the inflow tract and more pushable coils were used to embolize the inflow tract.

Follow-up DSA of the right hepatic artery showed no filling of the feeding branch of the right hepatic artery or the coiled aneurysm (Figure 14.2b). The hepatic parenchyma within the right liver lobe was fed with collaterals from adjacent branches of the right hepatic artery.

A similar procedure was performed for the tiny segment two branch aneurysm in the left hepatic artery with similar absence of flow on follow-up DSA.

After successful embolization of both branches, the system was removed and a 6-French Angio-Seal device was used for hemostasis, and the procedure was terminated. The patient was monitored in the interventional radiology postprocedural area for two hours and was subsequently discharged on the same day without complication.

Follow-up CT three months later showed coiled aneurysms without residual filling. Intrahepatic vasculature was grossly patent with no perfusion abnormalities within the liver parenchyma. The patient's LFTs remained within pre-procedural values at three- and six-month follow-up appointments. He continued doxycycline indefinitely under the guidance of infectious disease due to his infectious endocarditis.

Case 2: Gastroepiploic artery aneurysm

A 68-year-old female currently on dialysis secondary to end stage renal disease from long-standing hypertension was referred to interventional radiology by her transplant nephrologist for a fusiform aneurysm of her gastroepiploic artery of at least two years' duration. She was asymptomatic with a stable hemoglobin since discovery. Etiology was unclear.

A repeat CTA was performed that showed a slight increase in the size of an epiploic branch of her gastroduodenal artery (7 mm in diameter up from 5 mm two years prior). Her renal transplant team requested an embolization prior to listing her for a transplant.

The right groin was accessed in usual fashion under ultrasound guidance with a micropuncture set. The system was upsized over a 0.035 wire to a 5-French vascular sheath. A 5-French SOS 2 catheter was formed in the aorta and the celiac trunk was selected.

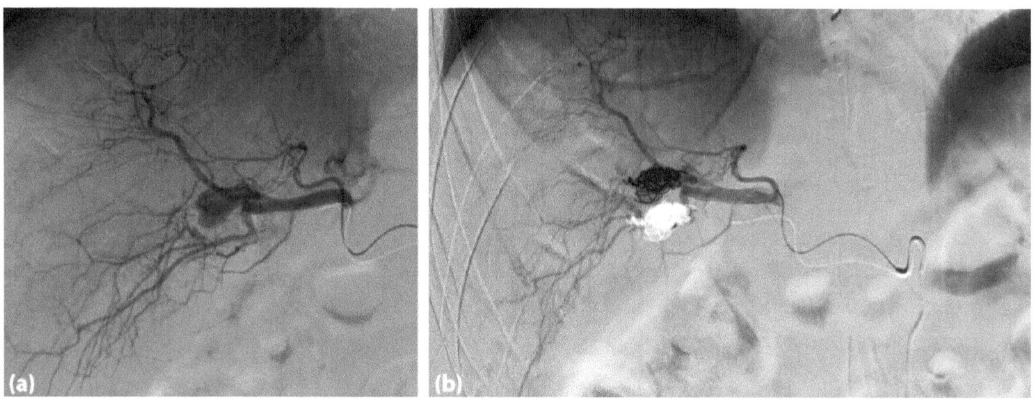

Figure 14.2 (a) Digital subtraction angiography of the right hepatic artery showing a lobular aneurysm arising from the posterior division of the right hepatic artery. (b) Post-embolization digital subtraction angiography of the right hepatic artery showing no filling of the coiled aneurysm or its feeding branch.

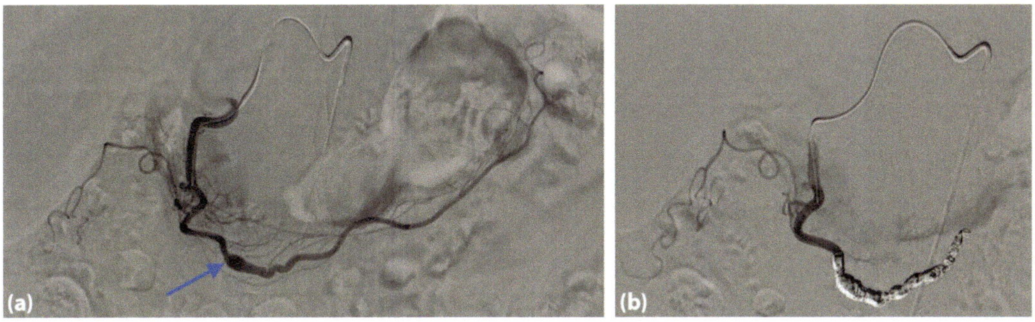

Figure 14.3 (a) Digital subtraction angiography of the gastroduodenal artery demonstrating fusiform aneurysmal dilatation of the gastroepiploic artery (blue arrow) without active contrast extravasation. (b) Post-embolization angiography of the gastroduodenal artery showing a coiled gastroepiploic artery without residual filling of the aneurysm.

A microwire and microcatheter were used to select the common hepatic and eventually the gastroduodenal artery. DSA was performed that showed fusiform dilatation of the proximal gastroepiploic artery with smooth distal tapering (Figure 14.3a).

The microwire was then used to select the artery beyond the aneurysm. DSA at this location showed normal caliber of the distal gastroepiploic artery. The decision was then made to coil embolize the artery from distal to proximal. In total, ten coils were used for the procedure. Post-embolization DSA showed no residual filling of the aneurysm (Figure 14.3b).

After successful embolization, the system was removed and a 6-French Angio-Seal device was used for hemostasis with no reported bleeding from the access site. The patient was discharged after being monitored in the interventional radiology recovery area for four hours and informed to follow-up in clinic in two to three months.

Two months later, she endorsed minimal groin pain for a few days after the procedure, but otherwise no residual symptoms. A follow-up CT angiogram did not show any residual filling of the gastroepiploic artery aneurysm.

FOLLOW-UP CARE AND SURVEILLANCE

The SVS recommends follow-up imaging for all cases of VAAs regardless of treatment due to the theoretical risk of reperfusion (9–15%). No strong guidelines have been described on specific imaging modalities or intervals due to the lack of overall data. At the author's institution, the convention is to perform a repeat CT angiogram two to three months after treatment to evaluate for any signs of reperfusion. Digital subtraction angiography follow-up is reserved for patients who remain symptomatic or exhibit CT findings suggesting reperfusion/expansion of the aneurysm.

Doppler and contrast-enhanced ultrasound has been described as a useful alternative to CTA in the follow-up of VAAs. However, due to operator variability of ultrasound and the relatively inaccessible nature of contrast-enhanced ultrasound, the authors still prefer the use of CTA for more definitive and consistent results. Once postoperative stability has been established two to three months after the initial intervention, the authors elect for annual surveillance with CTA. MRA is a reasonable alternative in younger patients or patients where ionizing radiation should be avoided.

Stent grafts pose more involved postprocedural management considerations, including anticoagulation. While no societal consensus has been established on anticoagulation/antiplatelet treatment, the authors suggest treatment with a direct oral anticoagulant and antiplatelet agent (e.g., apixaban and clopidogrel) for 90 days post-embolization.

In the specific event of a suspected or confirmed mycotic aneurysm, the authors prefer to discharge patients on six weeks of intravenous antibiotics under the guidance of an infectious disease specialist based off blood cultures and system-wide recommendations. In the event a covered stent graft is used, the duration of antibiotic treatment is usually extended, although a definitive endpoint has not been established and is typically determined on a case-by-case basis with guidance from our infectious disease colleagues.

TRICKS AND TRAPS

- The typical system used is a 5-Fr base catheter with a coaxial system of a microcatheter and microwire if second or third order branches are accessed.
- Embolization is typically performed with coils, however, other embolics like glue, particles, and vascular plugs can be used in specific scenarios.
- The primary approach to aneurysm embolization is to embolize the artery distal to the aneurysm, then access and embolize the aneurysm itself, and finally embolize the artery proximal to the aneurysm.
- Stent-assisted coiling is a viable option for larger vessels with wider-necked aneurysms where sacrificing the vessel is not feasible/desirable.

- Covered stents have limited utility in the treatment of VAAs as they confer specific limitations in vessel size, tortuosity, and location.
- Multiple closure devices are available to aid in hemostasis of the arteriotomy site. Operation instructions vary widely based on the manufacturer and mechanism of action.
- Ensuring no calcified plaques are present at the arteriotomy site at the time of access is important in aiding deployment of many vascular closure devices.

QUESTIONS

1. A 43-year-old female is being worked up for a renal artery aneurysm measuring 2.5 cm in size that was incidentally noted on a CT of the abdomen and pelvis done for an unrelated cause. What is the best next step in management?
   a. CTA surveillance at six months, then annually after if stable
   b. Emergent operative intervention
   c. Elective endovascular repair if feasible, otherwise open repair
   d. Further evaluation with MRA w/wo contrast

   Answer: c. Of these options, c is correct as any female patient of childbearing age with a renal aneurysm should undergo elective treatment.

2. A 65-year-old man presents to the emergency department with acute onset abdominal pain and syncope. His hemoglobin is 7.8 (baseline 10). CTA of the abdomen and pelvis shows a 3 mm pseudoaneurysm of a branch of the right renal artery and a moderate sized retroperitoneal hematoma. He has multiple comorbidities including CAD, ESRD, and COPD, making operative intervention riskier. The decision is made to undergo catheter embolization of the renal artery pseudoaneurysm. DSA of the right renal artery redemonstrated a 3 mm saccular aneurysm of a branch of the right renal artery that measures 6 mm in size. What embolic agent/technique would be least beneficial to use in this patient?
   a. Detachable coils
   b. Pushable coils
   c. Amplatzer plug
   d. Microvascular plug

   Answer: c. A feeder vessel of that size would be difficult to access with a system large enough to accommodate an Amplatzer plug. Likely, a triaxal system with a microcatheter would be needed, meaning a, b, and d could be used.

3. A 55-year-old man with a PMH of well-controlled hypertension and GERD presents to your clinic for evaluation of a proper hepatic artery aneurysm that was incidentally found on a CT performed for an unrelated reason six months ago. He says he experiences no pain, nausea, or vomiting, and has never had a hemoglobin level that was below normal. The aneurysm most recently measured 1.1 cm in diameter six months ago. What is the next best step in management?
   a. Call an ambulance and admit the patient for emergency aneurysm repair the next morning
   b. Dismiss the patient from the clinic and inform them to contact you if they ever develop symptoms
   c. Board the patient for elective open repair of the aneurysm
   d. Schedule a follow-up appointment in at least six months after getting a repeat CTA of the abdomen

   Answer: d. Given the artery's size (<2 cm), it falls into the category of hepatic artery aneurysms that can be monitored annually per the most recent Society of Vascular Surgery guidelines.

4. The same man from question 3 opts to undergo a repeat CT angiogram 12 months after his initial CT and returns to your clinic thereafter. He remains asymptomatic and otherwise healthy aside from his managed hypertension. The aneurysm now measures 1.8 cm on CT angiography. What is the next best step in management?
   a. Recommend elective endovascular aneurysm coiling
   b. Directly admit him for emergent open repair the next morning
   c. Continue annual CTA surveillance
   d. Discharge him from your clinic and inform him to call back if he has any new symptoms related to aneurysm growth (pain, nausea, vomiting, etc.)

   Answer: a. The patient does not meet absolute size criteria for hepatic artery aneurysm repair; however, his aneurysm grew by 0.7 cm in just 12 months. Society for Vascular Surgery guidelines suggest repair if an aneurysm grows by more than 0.5 cm per year.

5. You have been monitoring a patient in your clinic who has an aneurysm of her right hepatic artery that last measured 0.9 cm on CT angiogram one year ago. She calls your clinic prior to getting her annual CTA for further guidance. She recently discovered that she is nine weeks pregnant and read online that CT scans can produce harmful levels of radiation for developing fetuses. She would like to discuss any possible alternatives to her management that would be safe for her and her fetus. What would you advise?
   a. Proceed with regularly scheduled CT angiogram: she has been misinformed and CTs are completely safe for first trimester fetuses to readily undergo
   b. Cancel the CTA and obtain an MR angiogram with contrast: the exam itself will take longer but it is safe for both the expectant mother and fetus
   c. Cancel the CTA and obtain an MR angiogram without contrast
   d. Forgo this year's CTA and schedule one after she delivers, the chances the aneurysm grows during this period are negligible

   Answer: c. The exam is safe, but gadolinium has not been extensively studied in the pregnant population. MR without contrast is the safest of the listed answers, as it would not expose the fetus to ionizing radiation, nor would it delay any evaluation for the mother's aneurysm.

SUPPLEMENTAL READING

Chaer RA, Abularrage CJ, Coleman DM, Eslami MH, Kashyap VS, Rockman C, Murad MH. The society for vascular surgery clinical practice guidelines on the management of visceral aneurysms. *J Vasc Surg*, 2020;72(1):3S–39S.

Corey MR, Ergul EA, Cambria RP, English SJ, Patel VI, Lancaster RT, et al. The natural history of splanchnic artery aneurysms and outcomes after operative intervention. *J Vasc Surg*, 2016;63(4):949–957.

Deterling Jr, R. A. Aneurysm of the visceral arteries. *J Cardiovasc Surg*, 1992;164:215–219.

Erben Y, Brownstein AJ, Rajaee S, Li Y, Rizzo JA, Mojibian H, et al. Natural history and management of splanchnic artery aneurysms in a single tertiary referral center. *J Vasc Surg*, 2018;68(4):1079–1087.

Fankhauser GT, Stone WM, Naidu SG, Oderich GS, Ricotta JJ, Bjarnason H, et al. The minimally invasive management of visceral artery aneurysms and pseudoaneurysms. *J Vasc Surg*, 2011;53(4):966–970.

Fargion AT, Falso R, Speziali S, Biancofiore B, Esposito D, Giacomelli E, ... Pulli R. Results of current endovascular treatments for visceral artery aneurysms. *J Vasc Surg*, 2023;78(2):387–393.

Ibrahim F, Dunn J, Rundback J, Pellerito J, Galmer A. Visceral artery aneurysms: diagnosis, surveillance, and treatment. *Curr Treat Options Cardiovasc Med*, 2018;20(12):97.

Pasha SF, Gloviczki P, Stanson AW, Kamath PS. Splanchnic artery aneurysms. *Mayo Clinic Proceedings*, 2007;82(4):472–479.

Venturini M, Piacentino F, Coppola A, Bettoni V, Macchi E, De Marchi G, ... Fontana F. Visceral artery aneurysms embolization and other interventional options: state of the art and new perspectives. *J Clin Med*, 2021;10(11):2520.

15

Iliac vein stenting

MILES JACKSON, JACOB W. GUERRANT, AND ERIN PANG

INTRODUCTION

Chronic iliocaval venous obstruction is classified as primary (non-thrombotic iliac vein lesions) related to conditions such as May–Thurner syndrome [1], or secondary (post-thrombotic iliac vein stenosis [2]), which results from prior DVT. Secondary causes of iliac vein stenosis are more common. Non-thrombotic etiologies tend to affect more focal venous segments, whereas post-thrombotic venous disease manifests in longer distributions and may involve more than one venous segment [1]; post-thrombotic causes may also induce fibrous perivenous sheaths [2]. Venous collateralization is poorly understood; as large venous pathways become stenotic or occluded, increased pressure diverts venous return through pre-existing alternative pathways. It is uncommon for an occluded iliac vein to be adequately drained through collateral circuits given the exponential factors described by Poiseuille's law relating increased flow to larger veins. Clinical manifestations of chronic iliocaval venous obstruction include unilateral or bilateral edema, bursting pain known as venous claudication, skin changes (eczema, lipodermatosclerosis, dermatitis), and ulceration of the involved limbs.

DIAGNOSTICS

In addition to thorough history and physical examination including Doppler, diagnostic investigations should be focused on determining the etiology and extent of venous disease. These include venous Duplex ultrasound (VDU), air plethysmography, cross-sectional imaging such as CTV or MRV, and ascending venography including intravascular ultrasound (IVUS). VDU should be the first-line screening tool to evaluate for venous insufficiency, luminal obstruction, and flow patterns, and can also serve to identify the extent of involved venous segments. Air plethysmography, less commonly used in modern labs, provides information regarding the efficacy of calf muscle pump function. CTV or MRV can determine proximal venous anatomy, etiologies of compression or obstruction including abdominal or pelvic pathology, and identify important collateral circuits. Ascending venography, especially in conjunction with IVUS, can identify inflow and outflow segments and the severity of stenosis/obstruction.

CONSERVATIVE MANAGEMENT

All patients with symptomatic iliac venous disease should be treated with leg elevation (ideally to the level of the heart), graduated compression stockings, and local wound care as required. Conservative therapy fails in up to 50% of patients and can significantly impair quality of life [3]. Failure to improve or progression of symptoms should prompt evaluation for endovascular intervention. Generally, only patients with CEAP, C3 disease or greater should be considered for iliocaval intervention. In cases where a diagnosis of lymphedema is being considered, careful evaluation for iliac venous lesions should be performed. Associated venous reflux occurs commonly in iliac venous stenosis; if this is limited to the superficial venous system, catheter-based therapies may be employed at the same time as iliac vein endovascular intervention or may be performed in a staged fashion. Patients with deep venous reflux should undergo iliac vein stenting with subsequent re-evaluation of distal deep venous reflux disease.

ENDOVASCULAR TECHNIQUES

Endovascular treatment of iliocaval stenosis or obstruction requires stenting of the iliocaval segments and is the most commonly employed treatment for patients who are failing with conservative management.

Patients are placed under general anesthesia in a supine position with the affected extremity bent and externally rotated. Ultrasound guided access of the mid-thigh femoral vein is performed using either a MicroPuncture kit or

DOI: 10.1201/9781003452096-15

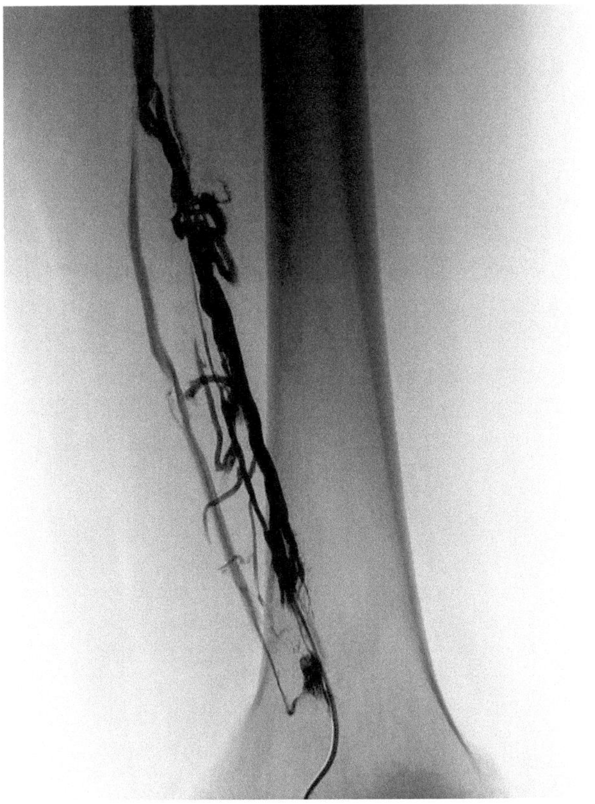

Figure 15.1 Access may be very difficult and requires several attempts at multiple locations if chronic venous thrombosis and residual scarring is present, which prevents wire advancement.

an 18-gauge needle. Access at superficial locations over bony points is not necessary given that low venous pressures facilitate deep venous access hemostasis with few hematomas (Figure 15.1).

A 0.035" J-wire or GLIDEWIRE (Terumo Medical Corporation, Somerset, NJ, USA) can be advanced into the IVC, or as proximally as possible, and a transverse skin incision should be made across using a #11 scalpel. A short, large diameter sheath—generally 11Fr 10 cm—is placed and flushed using a heparinized saline solution to confirm intraluminal access. Mid-thigh access allows enough room for the sheath to deploy stents below the inguinal ligament into the common femoral vein (CFV) if necessary. An on-table venogram should be performed in conjunction with IVUS (Volcano Corporation, San Diego, CA, USA) examinations of the IVC, common iliac vein (CIV), external iliac vein (EIV), and CFV to identify lesions and target landing sites; IVUS planimetry is also used to determine the diameter and area and these are compared with expected measurements (Table 15.1). In patients with renal impairment, the venogram can be skipped in favor of IVUS. Most symptomatic limbs will have >50% stenosis but any decreased diameter/area in a symptomatic patient warrants treatment (Figures 15.2 and 15.3).

Pre-dilation of the entire venous segment from CFV to the distal IVC with large caliber (14, 16, 18 mm)

Table 15.1 Expected luminal diameters for iliofemoral venous segments

Vein	Luminal area (mm^2)	Diameter (mm)
Common femoral vein	125	12
external iliac vein	150	14
common iliac vein	200	16

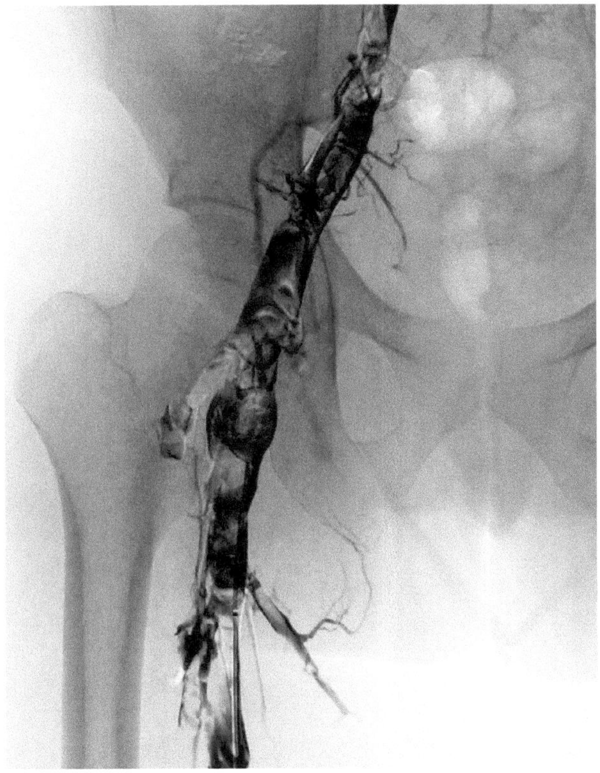

Figure 15.2 Ascending venogram demonstrating extensive left iliofemoral DVT

high-pressure or venous balloons such as ATLAS or VIDA PTA Dilation Balloon Catheter (BARD Peripheral Vascular Inc., Tempe, AZ, USA) is routine (Figure 15.4).

Unfortunately, isolated venoplasty is often insufficient treatment given the fibrotic recoil of iliocaval and femoral venous lesions. As such, large caliber stents reflecting the normal expected size of the iliofemoral vein are placed such as a 16 or 18 mm WALLSTENT Endoprostheses (Boston Scientific Corporation, Marlborough, MA, USA) with landing zones determined by IVUS; the proximal landing zones are usually 1–2 cm proximal to the iliac venous confluence and the distal landing zones are preferably placed in an healthy segment of EIV or CFV. The best upper and lower landing sites are chosen on IVUS views using the vertebral bodies and the femoral head as markers. Treating the entire diseased segment is essential for a successful result and most limbs with post-thrombotic venous disease require extension into the CFV. If necessary, this can be extended into the femoral or

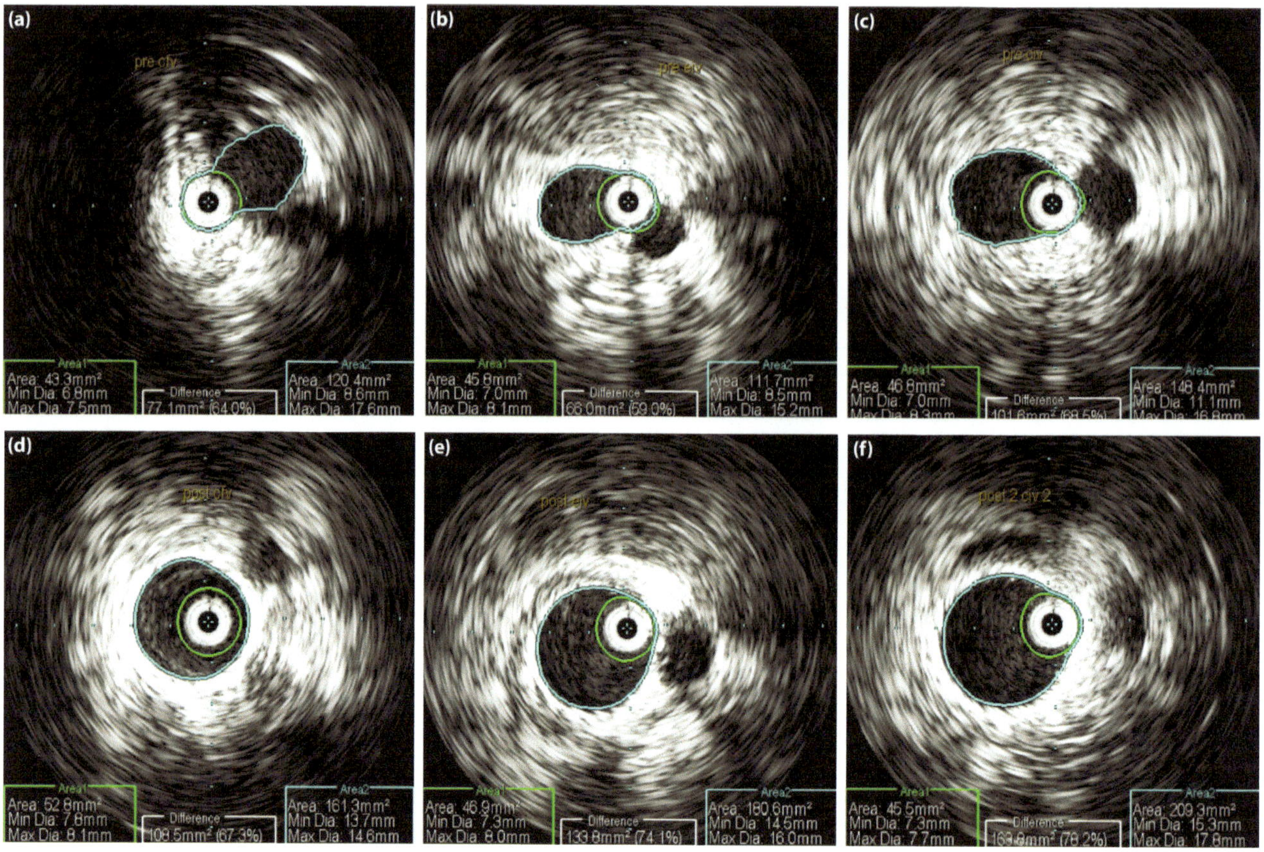

Figure 15.3 Intravascular ultrasound planimetry. Pre-dilation luminal areas of (a) common femoral (CFV), (b) external iliac (EIV), and (c) common iliac (CIV) veins. Postangioplasty and stenting luminal areas of (d) CFV, (e) EIV, and (f) CIV.

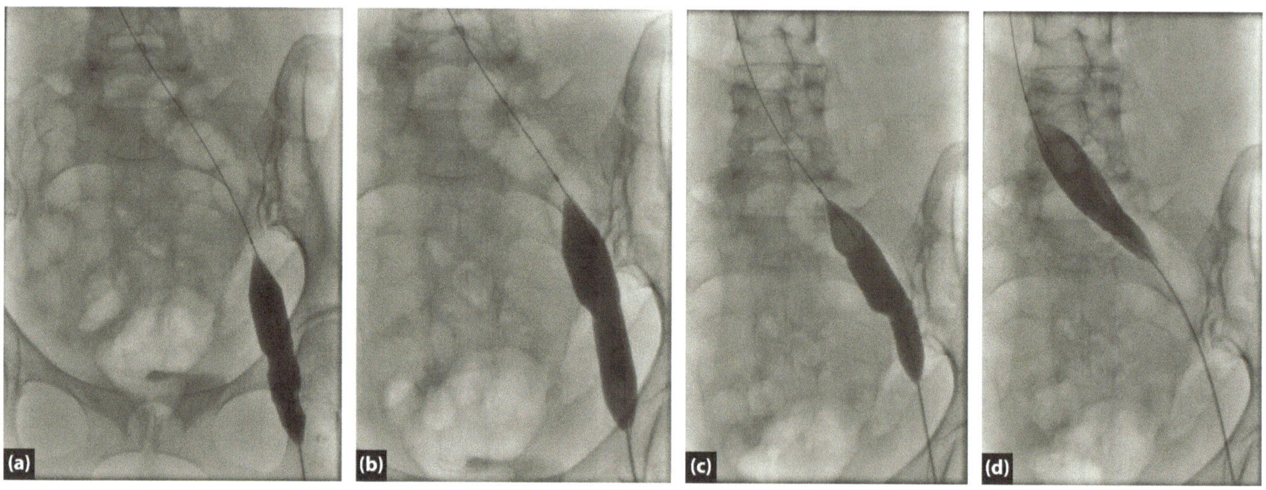

Figure 15.4 Sequential angioplasty of common femoral (CFV), external iliac (EIV), and common iliac (CIV) veins demonstrating multilevel disease suggestive of post-thrombotic syndrome: (a) CFV and EIV; (b) EIV; (c) EIV and distal CIV; and (d) CIV.

profunda femoris veins. Stent fractures for venous stents below the inguinal ligament are uncommon. Undersized stent placement is a very common cause of iatrogenic stenosis with recurrent/persistent symptoms. A Gianturco Z-stent (Cook Medical Inc., Bloomington, IN, USA) can be used to provide additional radial force at the level of the iliac confluence; this should have marginal extension of 5–10 mm proximally into the IVC. Adequate overlap of 2–3 cm in sequentially placed stents is necessary to account for length lost with post-dilation using large caliber venous balloons such as the ATLAS or VIDA PTA Dilation Balloon Catheter (BARD Peripheral Vascular Inc.). Completion IVUS (Volcano Corporation) is performed to ensure complete stent expansion and sufficient

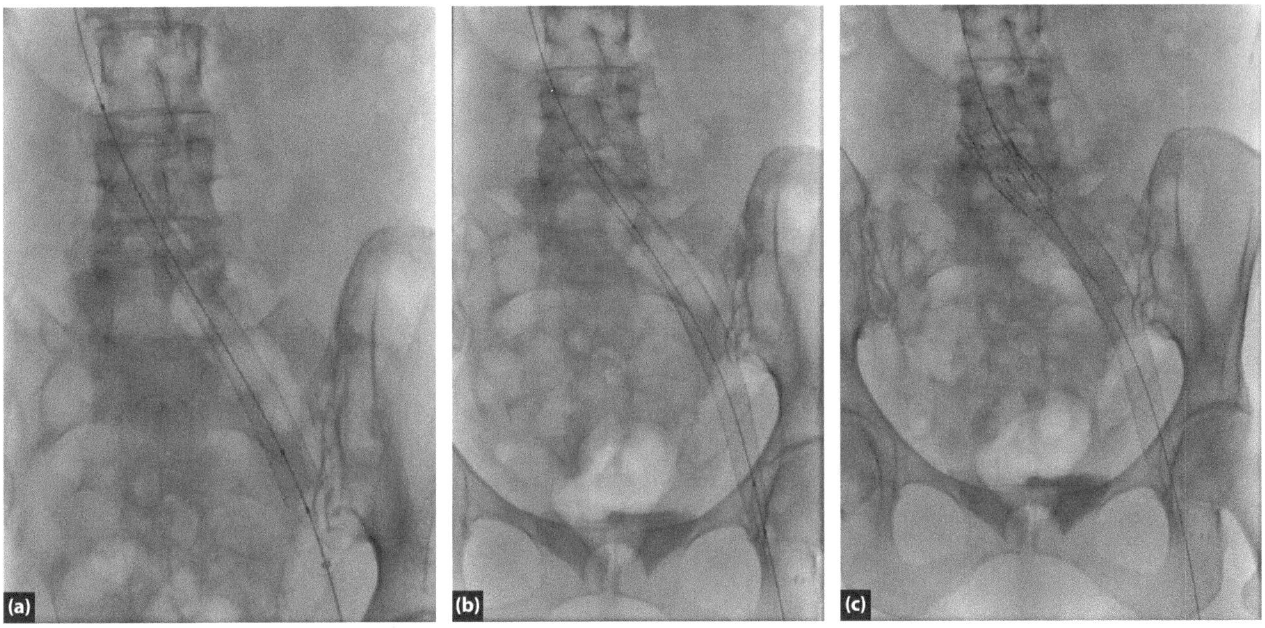

Figure 15.5 Stenting of the left distal femoro-ilio-caval tract: (a) Initial stent placement across iliocaval confluence; (b) stent extension distally; (c) stent stack post-deployment of Gianturco Z-stent across the confluence.

luminal area followed by venography to evaluate for adequate flow. Residual stenosis should be treated with repeat post-dilation using a larger caliber balloon (Figure 15.5).

Once completed, manual pressure is applied above and below the level of the access sheath, which is removed from the vein and left in the subcutaneous tissue. SURGICEL FIBRILLAR Absorbable Hemostat (Ethicon US, LLC, Somerville, NJ, USA) is then introduced through the sheath and the sheath is removed entirely. A 2-0 or 3-0 nylon suture (Ethicon US, LLC) can also be placed for additional hemostasis. Adequate manual pressure is held for 5–10 minutes, and a pressure dressing is applied (Figure 15.6).

Previously published results of almost 1,000 stents for non-malignant chronic obstructive femoral and iliocaval venous lesions demonstrated primary, primary-assisted, and secondary patency rates of 79%, 100%, and 100%, respectively, for non-thrombotic lesions. These outcomes for post-thrombotic lesions were 57%, 80%, and 86%, respectively [4] Post-thrombotic disease was a risk factor for in-stent restenosis (ISR) and stent occlusion [4,5].

Chronic total occlusion recanalization

Access is approached in an identical fashion as described earlier. Early venography can help to roadmap occlusive lesions and determine targeted wire paths that should correspond with native anatomical trajectories. Recanalization is best accomplished by careful passage of a 0.018" or 0.035" GLIDEWIRE (Terumo Medical Corporation) through the occluded segment without looping. Jugular access can be useful in some patients using a "body floss" technique. Careful advancement of straight or angled tip crossing catheters including NAVICROSS Support Catheter (Terumo Medical Corporation) is useful for step-wise progress. Wire advancement into collateral branches or extra-luminal planes should be apparent. Venoplasty can be performed with small caliber balloons to develop a flow lumen through the CTO while traversing the occlusion. Multiple re-entry or CTO catheters are now on the market; we have used the Quick-Cross Support Catheter (Spectranetics Corporation, Colorado Spring, CO, USA) with anecdotal success. Once the lesion is traversed, the wire is advanced into the IVC and confirmatory venography is performed. If passage is permitted, then immediate venoplasty to 18Fr is safe as venous ruptures are very rare. Stent placement is then performed in identical fashion as described previously. Notably, small perforations will often be self-limited once the large low resistance pathway is established. Inflow and outflow will determine stent patency; however, there is no reliable way to determine this intra-operatively. Some authors advise the creation of short-term AVF distal to the stented segment to promote flow.

In-stent restenosis

Stent compression in venous stents occurs from perivenous fibrosis. In-stent restenosis in symptomatic patients should be treated with standard distal venous access as described. Repeat venography and IVUS planimetry are performed to determine the degree of disease. Approaches are similar to those detailed above; the use of IVUS to confirm accurate wire passage through the stent lumen instead of stent interstices is critical to prevent damage to previously placed stents with venoplasty.

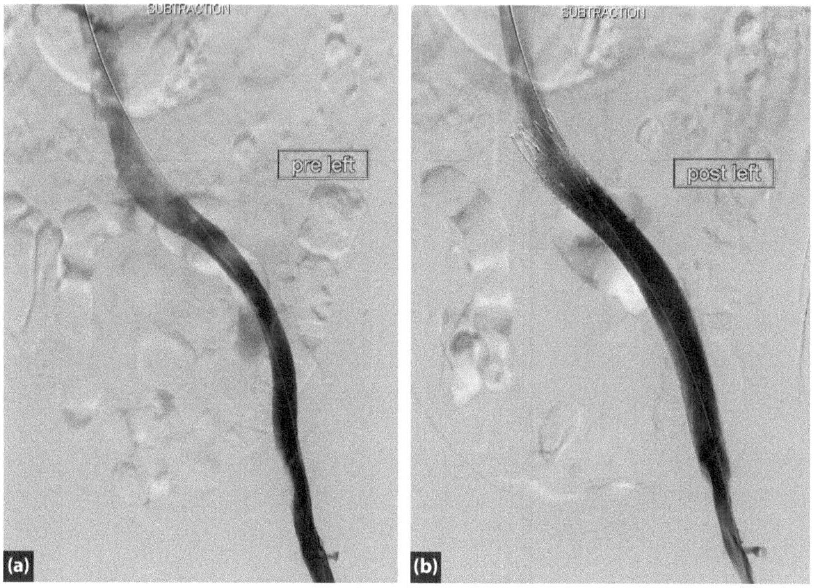

Figure 15.6 Ascending venogram: (a) baseline and (b) postangioplasty and stenting.

Review of prior operative documentation is essential to determine stent diameters if placed at outside institutions. Previously placed stents should be dilated beyond their nominal diameter using large caliber high-pressure balloons to ensure complete re-expansion.

Stent occlusion

Management of stent occlusions is determined by the acuity of the occlusion. Acute occlusions are often amenable to standard access techniques with thrombolytic administration with catheters such as the EKOS Endovascular System (Boston Scientific Corporation) with post-thrombolysis management of in-stent restenosis as identified by IVUS and venography. Chronic occlusions generally require recanalization using the techniques detailed previously. Newer mechanical thrombectomy devices such as the RevCore Thrombectomy Catheter (Inari Medical Inc., Irvine, CA, USA) can yield excellent results in re-establishing a flow channel and reducing chronic thrombotic burden (Figure 15.7).

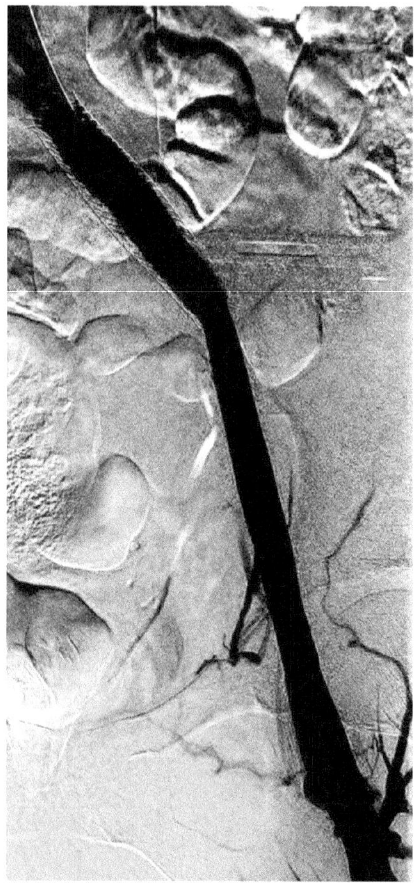

Figure 15.7 Post-treatment results of prior stent recanalization following recurrent thrombosis requiring thrombectomy and repeat venoplasty.

COMPLICATIONS

Hematoma

Clinically significant groin hematomas from venous access occur in <1% of patients. These are easily managed with adequate compression (approximately 1–2 minutes per French size) and a brief delay or interruption of anticoagulation or antiplatelet therapy.

Vein perforation/rupture

As previously mentioned, free venous perforation or rupture are very uncommon in low pressure venous systems. Perivenous fibrosis will also minimize the likelihood of this injury. If identified intra-operative, sustained balloon inflation or covered stent placement can be employed for control in unstable patients.

Stent thrombosis

Thrombosis develops based on inflow, outflow, and conduit selection. Contributing factors include adequate stent oversizing, length, peri-operative anticoagulation, and thrombophilia. These are managed by treating the major underlying contributing factor with stent extension or angioplasty as indicated.

Stent migration

This may occur secondary to the "watermelon seeding" effect of stent deployment into the distal IVC. It can be prevented with the use of the Gianturco Z-stent (Cook Medical Inc.) for increased radial force along the proximal stent in at the caval confluence.

ANTICOAGULATION AND ANTIPLATELET THERAPY

Peri-operative use of weight-based heparin is standard during venous interventions and endothelial injury should be treated with anticoagulation for a minimum of six weeks. There is broad variation in accepted anticoagulation protocols, but we recommend Plavix 75 mg daily at a minimum following stent placement for a minimum of six weeks. Long-term anticoagulation can be employed in patients with thrombophilia and/or recurrent thrombosis, ISR, or extensive stenting.

ONGOING MANAGEMENT AND FOLLOW-UP

All patients should continue with compression therapy and leg elevation at rest as previously established. Surveillance should be established early and regularly, and patients should undergo venous Duplex imaging at one week, four to six weeks, then every six months for stent malfunction. May–Thurner stents have lower rates of occlusion, whereas post-thrombotic veins should be monitored every three months to detect early in-stent restenosis prior to occlusion. Symptomatic change should prompt earlier evaluation.

TRICKS AND TRAPS

- Mid-thigh femoral vein access and large sheaths allow for good pushability and working length.
- A 0.035" GLIDEWIRE is often a great wire for identifying a lumen through a trabeculated vein; the majority of lesions can be traversed using this wire and a low-profile crossing catheter in step-wise fashion with a sheath being progressively advanced into the occluded segment.
- Several attempts may be required in order to traverse a difficult lesion which may end in perforation or impassable portions of the occlusion; you may have to pull back and start again multiple times to find a true path.
- The use of IVUS is imperative in all iliac vein cases and is superior to isolated venography for the determination of appropriate stent size and length for adequate lesion coverage.
- Always post-dilate iliac vein stents to at least their nominal diameter or higher and confirm adequate expansion using post-dilation IVUS and venography.
- Difficult lesions may require antegrade access from the ipsilateral CFV and retrograde access using the right internal jugular vein with a looped snare to establish the "body floss" technique.
- Some venous lesions may not be traversable, and these patients should be considered for open venous bypass if necessary; this is especially true in patients with recurrent in-stent restenosis and occlusion.

QUESTIONS

1. TRUE/FALSE: All symptomatic venous patients should undergo venous stenting as first-line therapy.

   Answer: FALSE—Conservative measures are universally employed first and generally only patients with C3 disease or greater are considered for intervention, which is primarily endovascular in nature.

2. What common diameters reflect common femoral vein, external iliac vein, and common iliac vein, respectively?
   a. 8, 12, 18
   b. 12, 14, 16
   c. 6, 8, 10
   d. 16, 18, 20

   Answer: b

3. TRUE/FALSE: Accurate venous sizing and landing site determination can be performed without IVUS.

   Answer: FALSE—The VIDIO trial has demonstrated superiority of IVUS planimetry in accurate vessel sizing and stent selection for occlusive iliac venous disease compared with isolated venography.

4. Proximal extension of iliac stenting should ideally land:
   a. At the proximal margin of venous disease
   b. 5–10 mm into the IVC
   c. 1–2 cm into the IVC
   d. To the level of the renal veins

   Answer: c

REFERENCES

1. May R, Thurner J. The cause of the predominantly sinistral occurrence of thrombosis of the pelvic veins. *Angiology*. 1957;8(5):419–427. PMID: 13478912.
2. Kahn S, Comerota A, Cushman M, et al. The post-thrombotic syndrome: evidence-based prevention, diagnosis, and treatment strategies: a scientific statement from the American heart association. *Circulation*. 2014;130:1636–1661.
3. Raju S, Hollis K, Neglen P. Use of compression stockings in chronic venous disease: patient compliance and efficacy. *Ann Vasc Surg*. 2007;21(6):790–795. PMID: 17980798.
4. Neglén P, Hollis KC, Olivier J, Raju S. Stenting of the venous outflow in chronic venous disease: long-term stent-related outcome, clinical, and hemodynamic result. *J Vasc Surg*. 2007;46(5):979–990. PMID: 17980284.
5. Murphy EH, Johns B, Varney E, Raju S. Endovascular management of chronic total occlusions of the inferior vena cava and iliac veins. *J Vasc Surg Venous Lymphat Disord*. 2017;5(1):47–59. PMID: 27987609.

16

Mechanicopharmacological thrombolysis for acute deep vein thrombosis

ALEXANDER K. LU, MICHAEL P. TRPKOWSKI, AND SACHINDER S. HANS

INTRODUCTION

Despite the number of affected patients with millions at risk due to immobility, trauma, surgery, and hypercoagulable states, studies have only recently addressed invasive therapies for the treatment of venous thromboembolism (VTE). Published guidelines have focused on acute and chronic medical therapies but do not address the use of invasive, catheter-driven therapies and thrombolysis, which has been shown to reduce the incidence of post-thrombotic syndrome (PTS) [1,2]. The most recent guidelines published by the American College of Chest Physicians proposed anticoagulant therapy alone over invasive therapy [3]. However, anticoagulants alone do not dissolve the occluding thrombus, decrease the venous outflow obstruction, or have any impact on the inflammatory reaction caused by persistent thrombus that is also believed to contribute to PTS. Removal of the thrombus alleviates the acute symptoms of VTE, improves venous patency, and reduces PTS rates [3,4]. This can be achieved much more reliably using catheter-directed thrombolysis (CDT) or pharmacomechanical CDT.

CDT uses fluoroscopy and image guidance to place a multiple side hole catheter directly into the thrombosed venous segment to infuse thrombolytic agents (Table 16.1), allowing for a higher local drug concentration. The most commonly used fibrinolytic drug is recombinant tissue plasminogen activator (rtPA), infused continuously at a low dose (typically 0.5–1.0 mg/hour), along with intravenous (IV) infusion of unfractionated heparin at subtherapeutic levels, ideally infused into the affected venous segment. CDT has been shown to be more effective at restoring iliofemoral vein patency versus anticoagulation alone, with some studies showing that CDT can also reduce the risk of PTS [1,2]. Reducing the thrombolytic dose decreases the risk of serious bleeding but requires longer infusion times with the need for specialized monitoring in the intensive care unit (ICU), adding to the burden of hospital resources. Pharmacomechanical CDT was developed to address these limitations by the addition of a mechanical device to break apart the thrombus and increase the surface area while delivering the thrombolytic agent. Several devices are available on the market, but the mechanisms of action remain the same: rotational or hydrodynamic thrombus fragmentation.

Table 16.1 Commonly used thrombolytic agents in the treatment of acute deep vein thrombosis

Thrombolytic agent	Infusion dose
Tissue plasminogen activator (tPA) Recombinant	0.5–1.0 mg/hr 0.01 mg/kg/hr
Urokinase	120,000–180 000 IU/hr 100,000 IU/hr 4400 IU/kg IV at a rate of 90 ml/hr
Streptokinase	100,000 IU/hr (maintenance)

Rotational (or microfragmentation) thrombectomy devices employ a high-speed rotating basket or impeller to break apart the thrombus. Examples include ArrowTrerotola™ Percutaneous Thrombolytic Device (Teleflex Medical Europe Ltd, Athlone, Ireland) and CLEANER15™ Rotational Thrombectomy System (Argon Medical Devices Inc., Plano, TX, USA).

Hydrodynamic (or rheolytic) devices employ high-speed saline jets in a retrograde direction, using recirculation and the Venturi effect to fragment the thrombus. The most widely used example is AngioJet™ Peripheral Thrombectomy System (Boston Scientific Corporation, Marlborough, MA, USA) (Figure 16.1). Balloon angioplasty can also be performed to macerate organized thrombus. The Indigo® Mechanical Thrombectomy

DOI: 10.1201/9781003452096-16

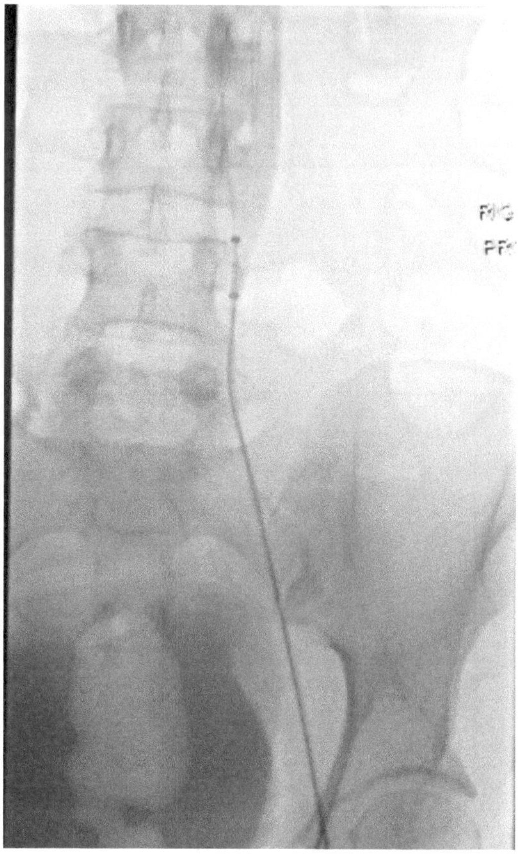

Figure 16.1 Mechanical thrombectomy device. The AngioJet™ Peripheral Thrombectomy System (Boston Scientific Corporation, Marlborough, MA, USA) is positioned just caudad to the IVC filter.

System (Penumbra, Inc., Alameda, CA, USA), initially used in stroke treatment, has been adapted for use throughout the body and employs a catheter/guidewire combined with a high-power aspiration pump. The EndoWave™ Infusion System drug delivery catheter (EKOS Corporation, Bothell, WA, USA) consists of an infusion catheter and a core wire with ultrasound (US) transducers. The US energy transmitted accelerates dispersion of the lytic agent and increases contact with thrombus-bound plasminogen receptors as it penetrates the clot. The Clot Triever system is a mechanical thrombectomy device specifically designed for the treatment of acute deep vein thrombosis (Inari Medical, Irvine, CA, USA).

PREPROCEDURE

There are no established criteria for which patients benefit most from CDT or pharmacomechanical CDT. Patients with limb-threatening phlegmasia cerulea dolens or young patients with significant symptoms from a proximal deep vein thrombosis (DVT) should be considered if they are not at an increased risk for bleeding complications. Additionally, involvement of the common femoral (CFV) or iliac veins should point toward endovascular therapy, because this level of involvement is associated with a much higher risk of PTS and recurrent DVT.[5] Otherwise, patient selection for intervention occurs on a case-by-case basis, with the clinical picture, concurrent medical comorbidities, risk of bleeding, patient desire, and ability to tolerate this procedure being the determining factors. The results of the ATTRACT trial among 692 patients with acute proximal deep vein thrombosis to receive anticoagulation alone (control group) or anticoagulation versus pharmacomechanical thrombolysis (catheter or device intrathrombus delivery of tPA [recombinant]) and thrombus aspiration or maceration with stenting showed that between six and 24 months [6] there was no significant difference in the percentage of patients with PTS between the two groups. However, there was a higher risk of major bleeding in patients in pharmacomechanical catheter-directed thrombolysis compared with anticoagulation alone [6].

Patients on long-term oral anticoagulation should be managed with unfractionated or low-molecular-weight heparin (LMWH) for more reliable periprocedural control. If there are no contraindications to hydration, aggressive IV fluids should be administered to reduce the risk of contrast-induced nephropathy and the possibility of acute tubular necrosis from intravascular hemolysis. Duplex ultrasound (US) of the other extremity should also be done to rule out contralateral involvement. Computed tomography venography (CTV) of the abdomen/pelvis should be considered in selected patients to assess proximal extension and associated anatomic pathologies.

EQUIPMENT AND PROCEDURE

The preferred access site for iliofemoral lysis is the popliteal vein in the popliteal fossa. The patient is positioned prone, with standard sterile prepping and draping. If the popliteal vein is not patent, the tibial veins can be accessed if they are patent. In the authors' experience, a non-thrombosed point of access is a critical element for success in lower limb thrombolysis; this ensures that there is some blood flow cephalad to maintain patency once the affected venous segments start to lyse.

US-guided access skills are a must; if lytics are being administered, the goal should be single-wall access with a single puncture access to the vein. Blind puncture is not feasible and carries a high risk of subsequent hemorrhage.

A 21-G access system ("micropuncture set") should be used. The ability to image the tip of the needle inside the lumen of the vein is key; if the access point is thrombosed, the needle should be stabilized and a 0.018-inch guidewire (such as the stainless Cope Mandril Wire Guide [Cook Medical Inc., Bloomington, IN, USA] or a floppy tip nitinol wire) is carefully advanced under fluoroscopy. Once access has been obtained and the microwire has been upsized to a 0.035-inch J wire, a sheath should be placed. An 8-Fr sheath is typically used at the authors' institution because it allows follow-up contrast injection around any lysis catheter, accommodates most available mechanical devices and angioplasty balloon catheters, and allows coadministration of heparin (through the sheath) around the infusion catheter.

Imaging is then performed, with contrast injection in small amounts to outline the thrombus and determine the extent. Digital subtraction is not typically used at this point because of a lack of flow. Images are saved for documentation. A 0.035-inch hydrophilic directional wire (e.g., stiff-angled GLIDEWIRE® Hydrophilic Coated Guidewire; Terumo Medical Corporation, Somerset, NJ, USA) may be used along with an angled-tip 4- or 5-Fr catheter (the authors prefer the GLIDECATH* Hydrophilic Coated Catheter; Terumo Medical Corporation) to access the iliac veins and the inferior vena cava (IVC). Digital subtraction inferior vena cavagram should be performed using a flush catheter with graduated markers to ascertain the level of caval thrombosis. Typically, contrast is power injected at 15 mL/second for two seconds at 500 psi through a flush catheter to study the IVC. Power injection of contrast should not be performed until after a test injection with a 10 mL syringe to verify that the catheter tip is in a patent IVC segment. The hydrophilic wire and angled catheter combination is useful to cross anatomic lesions (e.g., a May–Thurner stenosis). Once such a lesion has been crossed, avoid uncrossing it for the duration of the treatment. For eventual placement of a lysis catheter, the authors recommend exchanging for a stiff, nonhydrophilic 0.035-inch guidewire such as an Amplatz Super Stiff™ Guidewire (Boston Scientific Corporation). A 180 cm wire or even a 260 cm wire (if using the EKOS delivery system) will be needed because of the length of the infusion catheters.

Once the extent of the thrombus is documented, the operator must decide on the method of lysis. The simplest technique is CDT, which only requires placement of a multiside hole catheter (e.g., the Cragg-McNamara® Valved Infusion Catheter; Medtronic, Minneapolis, MN, USA; or the Uni-Fuse™ infusion catheter; AngioDynamics, Latham, NY, USA) with an infusion segment that spans all or at least most of the thrombosed segment. Avoid having too much infusion length of the catheter in a patent vein segment; this will increase systemic administration of rtPA without the benefit of thrombus lysis. In a thrombosed lower extremity, the typical length used is 50 cm, which may be too short to cover the entire thrombosed segment. The authors typically cover the distal part initially and leave the central thrombosed segment uncovered, changing the catheter out and placing the infusion segment more centrally once the distal thrombus is lysed. Lysing from distal to proximal is always a sound idea. Accelerated lysis is possible via bolus administration of rtPA into the infusion catheter, or a pulse spray technique. To accomplish this, the authors use rtPA in a concentration of 1 mg/mL of normal saline (the dose is dependent on the length of the thrombosed segment; up to 10 mg is typically used) administered by forceful pushes of a 1 mL syringe attached to a stopcock. This technique disperses rtPA into the thrombus and fills the catheter dead space with the lytic agent. After bolus administration, the stopcock should be closed until the rtPA pump infusion is ready. Infusion rates of 0.50–1.0 mg/hour of rtPA into the catheter are typically used, chosen by the operator with consideration of the amount of thrombus and individual patient risk factors for bleeding. In patients undergoing bilateral lower extremity and distal IVC lysis, the right- and left-sided catheters typically overlap in the IVC, resulting in a doubling of the rtPA dose in this largest venous segment. Another method of accelerating lysis is using a pharmacomechanical system such as the EndoWave™ system (EKOS Corporation) (Figure 16.2). Use of the EndoWave™ system requires the administration of a coolant fluid; the authors typically infuse normal saline at 35–70 mL/hour via the coolant port for this purpose. With any rtPA infusion system, concomitant infusion of heparin or other anticoagulant (Table 16.2) is usually performed via the access point sheath (popliteal, or in the case of an isolated iliac venous thrombus,

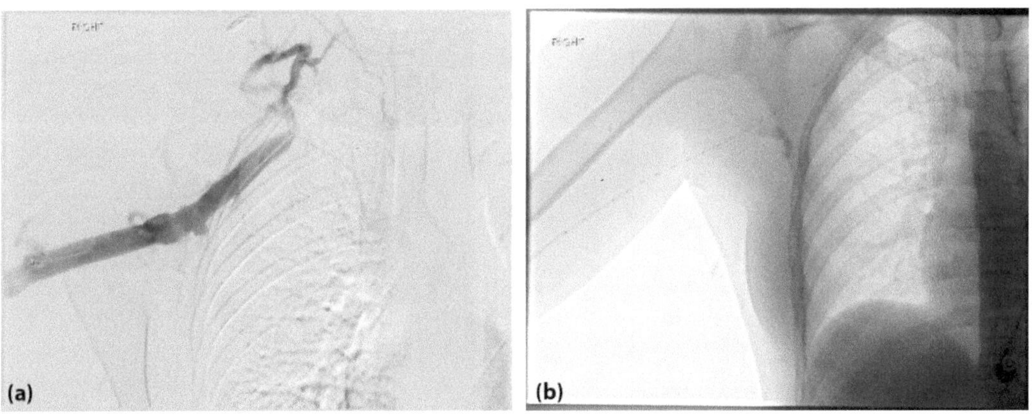

Figure 16.2 (a) Venogram performed through right brachial vein access shows complete occlusion of axillary vein with chronic thrombus in central basilic/peripheral axillary vein. There is a lack of any proximal filling. (b) Placement of 30 cm treatment zone EKOS thrombolysis catheter (EKOS Corporation, Bothell, WA, USA).

Table 16.2 Heparin and other anticoagulant drugs used concomitantly with a recombinant tissue plasminogen activator infusion system

Anticoagulant drug	Dosing
Unfractionated heparin	80 IU/kg bolus; 18 IU/kg/hour infusion for 5–7 days
Enoxaparin sodium	1 mg/kg twice daily or 1.5 mg/kg daily
Dalteparin sodium	100 IU/kg twice daily or 200 IU/kg daily
Argatroban monohydrate	2–10 pg/kg/minute infusion
Fondaparinux sodium	5 mg <50 kg, 7.5 mg 50–100 kg, 10 mg >100 kg

a femoral sheath). The usual dose at the authors' institution is 500 IU/hour heparin in total, divided between one or two sheaths if both extremities are being lysed. In the case of documented heparin-induced thrombocytopenia, heparin should be switched to argatroban monohydrate and titrated to a low therapeutic partial thromboplastin time (PTT) [7].

Placement of a retrievable IVC filter in the infrarenal IVC is an important consideration. If the thrombosis is due to an IVC filter already in place, or an anatomic lesion such as May–Thurner, the likelihood of pulmonary embolism (PE) because of lysis is very low. If there is no identified anatomic lesion, the PE risk is higher and the operator should consider placing a filter. This should be of a retrievable variety to be removed as soon as possible after the lysis procedure is complete and venous patency is restored to reduce the risk of recurrent DVT or caval thrombosis. Before leaving the interventional suite, all patients should undergo placement of a peripherally inserted central catheter to aid in the frequent laboratory monitoring necessary for the safe conduct of CDT. Venipuncture and arterial lines should be avoided after rtPA is started.

Once thrombolysis is initiated, the patient should return for follow-up imaging every 12–24 hours. Laboratory monitoring is discussed later in the chapter. Lysis of extensive thrombus, such as bilateral or even unilateral lower extremities, is not a speedy procedure; it is not uncommon for the entire process to run for 48 or 72 hours. Follow-up procedures may consist of simple repeat imaging, with return to the ICU for continued rtPA administration if the thrombus is still present, or an additional endoluminal intervention if adequate clot lysis has been achieved (Figure 16.3). "Adequate" lysis is determined by the operator, with the knowledge that an older thrombus will likely result in a slower and less complete lysis. The ability of the patient to tolerate a lengthy procedure, as well as bleeding and other problems, may limit the result that can be achieved.

Further interventions typically consist of balloon venoplasty to treat a significant stenosis or to macerate a thrombus that is resistant to rtPA after 24–48 hours of lysis (Figure 16.4). Lesions that demonstrate elastic recoil or otherwise inadequate response to venoplasty are stented with suitably sized metallic stents. May–Thurner lesions are primarily stented. To avoid PE, use caution when treating stenosis if the thrombus is still present. The authors strongly recommend deferring treatment of anatomic lesions until the end of the entire lysis procedure to avoid this risk. For example, dilating a May–Thurner lesion on the first day of treatment, before thrombus clearance, is a critical mistake to be avoided.

TREATMENT DURING LYSIS

Postprocedural orders require ICU monitoring and include strict bed rest and a clear liquid diet, with consideration of sequential compression device (SCD) sleeves

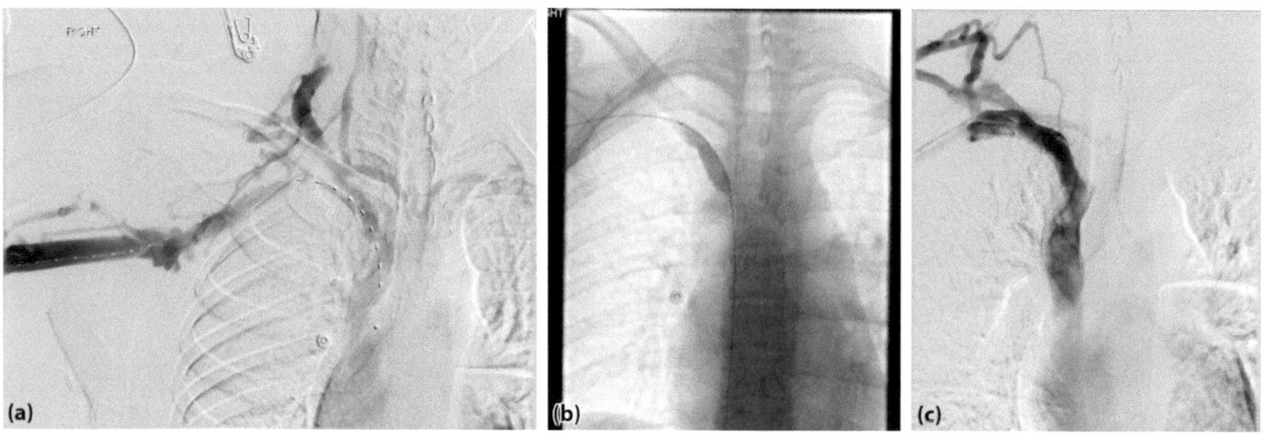

Figure 16.3 (a) Right upper extremity venogram 24 hours after lysis with EKOS catheter; (b) balloon venoplasty of brachiocephalic confluence; (c) after AngioJet suction thrombectomy of thrombus in right subclavian and brachiocephalic vein/SVC.

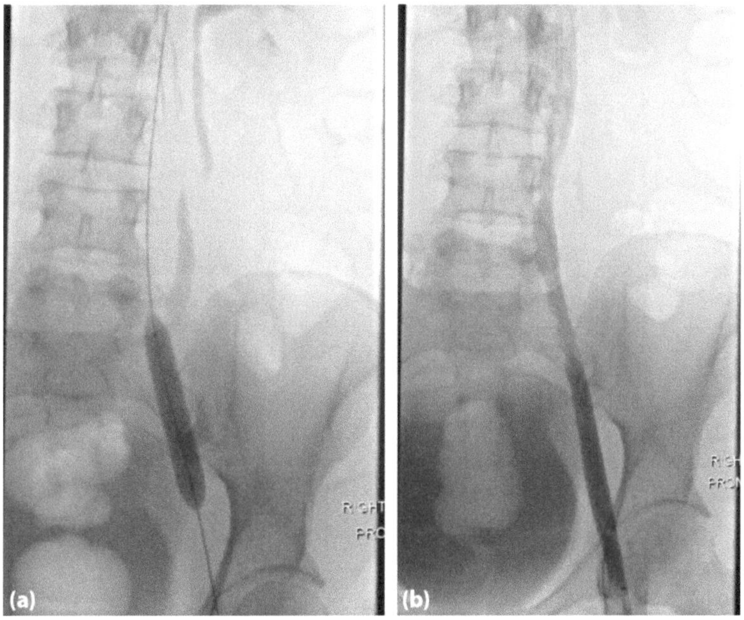

Figure 16.4 (a) Balloon venoplasty of right common iliac vein and (b) a digital subtraction angiogram demonstrates decreased thrombus burden and patency of the caval system.

on the lower extremities. Frequent puncture site checks for bleeding/hematoma are crucial, with avoidance of all intramuscular/intra-arterial injections/punctures. Simultaneous heparin (or argatroban monohydrate) infusions through the access sheath(s) must be used to prevent the opened venous segment from immediately reoccluding. Fibrinogen and PTTs are measured every four to six hours, with goals at the authors' institution of >100–150 mg/dL and 45–60 seconds, respectively. Additional laboratory testing includes hemoglobin, prothrombin time, and platelet count, which will reveal any ongoing bleeding or risk thereof. If there are abnormal bleeding parameters, rtPA is either held or stopped and the infusion is replaced with a similar volume of normal saline; fibrinogen level correction is typically done with cryoprecipitate. Ideally, the lytic agent infusion should be reduced, not stopped, while correction and laboratory retesting occur. The authors reduce the rtPA infusion to half if fibrinogen falls below 150 mg/dL, and hold it if <100 mg/dL, while infusing cryoprecipitate to augment levels. Red cell transfusion should be considered if hemoglobin falls below 8 mg/dL or anemia is symptomatic. The authors cannot stress enough that any correction must be timely and aggressive. Stopping rtPA administration for even a short period can result in loss of all gains achieved up to that point.

POSTPROCEDURE

After thrombolysis has been achieved and anatomic lesions have been treated, all catheters and sheaths are pulled while the patient is still in the interventional suite. Hemostasis is achieved with manual compression; closure devices are never used. Full-dose anticoagulation with heparin is started without a bolus to maintain the PTT at 70–90 seconds. After 18–24 hours, the authors transition to warfarin with LMWH bridging. Patients are maintained on bed rest for two hours and then allowed to ambulate with assistance as needed. Thigh-high SCDs are used throughout this period to optimize venous flow through the previously occluded venous segments.

Following observation for clinical signs and symptoms of complications, patients are discharged on LMWH until therapeutic levels can be reached with oral anticoagulants.

Ambulation is encouraged once the patient's condition permits. Clinical and sonographic evaluation is performed at follow-up visits at one, six, and 12 months after the procedure. Anticoagulation is maintained for a minimum of three to six months following thrombolysis in uncomplicated cases, with longer treatment regimens for those with a presumed hypercoagulable state.

COMPLICATIONS

The major complication with CDT is bleeding, with significant bleeding occurring in up to 9% of patients [1]. This is defined as intracranial bleeding, formation of a large hematoma requiring surgical evacuation, need for blood transfusion, and significant bleeding at the puncture site. Most bleeding is easily managed, although it may require cessation of the lysis procedure. Intracranial hemorrhage, while rare in the authors' experience, unfortunately may have devastating consequences. If significant bleeding occurs, the lytic agent should be stopped and hemostasis should be the goal with manual compression or sheath upsizing if at the access site. If major bleeding occurs elsewhere, thrombolysis should be stopped. Minor bleeding can manifest as pericatheter oozing, hematuria, or epistaxis. Physical inspection for bleeding and increased frequency of blood collection to monitor coagulation parameters are the reasons for patients requiring an ICU for periprocedure monitoring. The late complication of reocclusion can occur despite adequate anticoagulation therapy and compliance with DVT prevention strategies. In such cases, repeat thrombolysis can be considered.

TRICKS AND TRAPS

- Patients that benefit most from CDT or pharmacomechanical CDT are those presenting with phlegmasia cerulea dolens or young patients with proximal deep vein thrombosis.
- The preferred access site for iliofemoral lysis is the popliteal vein with the patient prone.
- A non-thrombosed point of access is an important factor for the success of lower limb thrombolysis, ensuring some blood flow cephalad to maintain patency once the affected venous segment begins to lyse.
- US-guided access is a must and blind puncture should be avoided.
- In patients with May–Thurner syndrome, the likelihood of PE as a result of lysis is low, therefore, placement of a retrievable IVC filter is not necessary at the time of the procedure.
- Older thrombus will result in a slower and incomplete lysis.
- The treatment of anatomic lesions should be deferred until the entire lysis procedure is completed.
- May–Thurner lesions should be primarily stented and venoplasty is not required.
- Significant bleeding during CDT often requires cessation of the procedure and hemostasis obtained by manual compression or upsizing the sheath at the access site.
- Periprocedure monitoring should be done in the ICU.

QUESTIONS

1. The major complication of CDT is significant bleeding that occurs in:
   a. Less than 5% of cases
   b. 5–7% of cases
   c. 8–10% of cases
   d. Greater than 10% of cases

   Answer: c

2. The patient least likely to require a retrievable IVC filter during CDT:
   a. Without identified anatomic lesion in the proximal venous system
   b. Thrombus in an already placed IVC filter
   c. May–Thurner syndrome
   d. A patient with duplicated IVC

   Answer: c

3. The results of the ATTRACT trial showed that among patients with acute proximal deep vein thrombosis, the addition of pharmacomechanical catheter-directed thrombolysis to anticoagulation resulted in a:
   a. Lower risk of PTS
   b. Lower risk of major bleeding
   c. Lower risk of major bleeding and lower risk of PTS
   d. Same risk of PTS but higher risk of major bleeding

   Answer: d

4. The preferred access site for iliofemoral thrombolysis is:
   a. Popliteal vein medically with the patient in the frog legs position
   b. Popliteal vein with the patient prone
   c. Post tibial vein at the ankle
   d. Femoral vein in distal thigh

   Answer: b

5. Serum fibrinogen levels during CDT should be maintained at:
   a. 50–75 mg/dl
   b. 76–100 mg/dl
   c. 101–150 mg/dl
   d. Greater than 150 mg/dl

   Answer: c

REFERENCES

1. Haig, Y., Enden, T., Grøtta, O., et al. (2016). Post-thrombotic syndrome after catheter-directed thrombolysis for deep vein thrombosis (CaVenT): 5-year follow-up results of an open-label, randomised controlled trial. *Lancet Haematol.*, *3*, e64–71.
2. Enden, T., Haig, Y., Kløw, N. E., et al. (2012). Long-term outcome after additional catheter-directed thrombolysis versus standard treatment for acute iliofemoral deep vein thrombosis (the CaVenT study): a randomised controlled trial. *Lancet*, *379*(9810), 31–38. https://doi.org/10.1016/s0140-6736(11)61753-4
3. Kearon, C., Akl, E. A., Ornelas, J., et al. (2016). Antithrombotic therapy for VTE disease: CHEST Guideline and Expert Panel Report. *Chest.*, *149*, 315–352.
4. Haig, Y., Enden, T., Slagsvold, C. E., et al. (2013). Determinants of early and long-term efficacy of catheter-directed thrombolysis in proximal deep vein thrombosis. *J Vasc Interv Radiol.*, *24*, 17–24.

5. Meissner, M. H., Manzo, R. A., Bergelin, R. O., et al. (1993). Deep venous insufficiency: the relationship between lysis and subsequent reflux. *J Vasc Surg.*, *18*, 596–605.
6. Vedantham, S., Goldhaber, S. Z., Julian, J. A., et al. (2017). Pharmacomechanical Catheter-Directed Thrombolysis for Deep-Vein Thrombosis. *N Engl J Med.*, 377(23), 2240–2252. https://doi.org/10.1056/NEJMoa1615066
7. Sharifi, M., Bay, C., Nowroozi, S., et al. (2013). Catheter-directed thrombolysis with argatroban and tPA for massive iliac and femoropopliteal vein thrombosis. *Cardiovasc Intervent Radiol.*, *36*, 1586–1590.

17

Inferior vena cava filter placement

GUILLERMO P. SERRA AND KAITLYN M. ROUNTREE

INTRODUCTION

Venous thromboembolism (VTE), encompassing deep venous thrombosis (DVT) and pulmonary embolism (PE), is one of the most common preventable causes of hospital death in both surgical and medical patients. The incidence of VTE has been estimated to be as high as 600,000 individuals per year [1], with the most common risk factor reported to be venous stasis [2]. Interruption of the inferior vena cava (IVC) has been used since 1960s [3] as a way to prevent lower extremity DVT from causing lethal PE. IVC filters provide a less invasive way to prevent PE in highly selected patients. The indications for IVC filter placement, relevant anatomy, filter types, procedural techniques, and complications are discussed in this chapter.

INDICATIONS

Several societies have issued guidelines on the management of VTE and highlight indications for the placement of IVC filters, each with slight variations. It is our practice to be selective of patients who receive IVC filters given the procedural risk involved in placement, the high incidence of loss-to-follow-up for retrieval, and the potential for long-term filter-associated complications [4]. Classic indications for IVC filters include patients with acute DVT or PE and absolute contraindication to anticoagulation, failure of anticoagulation, complications resulting from anticoagulation, or progression of DVT despite adequate anticoagulation [5]. For patients who are temporarily unable to tolerate anticoagulation (e.g., active bleed, concern for hemorrhage), IVC filter placement is indicated, with the caveat of initiating systemic anticoagulation as soon as the patient can safely tolerate treatment, even if an IVC filter is present. It must be remembered that IVC filters do not treat the underlying VTE but merely offer a mechanical barrier for deadly PE. As such, patients need to be regularly reassessed for their ability to tolerate anticoagulation and retrieval of the IVC filter (Table 17.1).

Physician discretion and discussion of risk should guide the use of extended criteria for IVC filter placement. These softer indications include patients with iliofemoral DVT with a time-limited indication for an IVC filter (e.g., a short-term contraindication to anticoagulant therapy). For example, in patients with a newly diagnosed VTE and need for surgery within one month of diagnosis, a retrievable filter would be reasonable as the anticoagulation would be interrupted for the perioperative period. For pregnant women with diagnosed VTE and contradiction to anticoagulation or delivery estimated within two weeks, placement of a retrievable IVC filter is also reasonable. Free-floating thrombus is a controversial indication, with some societies indicating it as an acceptable reason for IVC filter placement, and others arguing against this concept in those that can tolerate anticoagulation [5].

Prophylactic IVC filter placement is occasionally performed for patients who have not been diagnosed with VTE but are at elevated risk of developing VTE and cannot receive anticoagulation or cannot be monitored for the development or progression of VTE. Retrospective studies have demonstrated potential benefits in subsets of severely injured trauma patients including those with spinal cord injury with paralysis, complex pelvic fractures, multiple long bone fractures, and with contraindications to DVT chemoprophylaxis expected to persist beyond 72 hours [6]. Another select population includes patients scheduled for major spinal reconstruction surgery with high-risk profiles for developing VTE; small-sized studies have demonstrated a potential benefit with a decrease in postoperative PE and high filter retrieval rates [6]. There are currently no randomized control trials demonstrating the benefit of prophylactic IVC filters.

Contraindications to IVC filter placement include bacteremia and severe coagulopathy.

DOI: 10.1201/9781003452096-17

Table 17.1 Commercially available IVCFs

Filter	Manufacturer	Permanent or retrievable	Approved cabal diameter
Bird's Nest	Cook Medical	Permanent	40 mm
Simon Nitinol	Bard	Permanent	28 mm
Vena Tech LGM filter	B. Braun	Permanent/convertible	<28 mm
Vena Tech LP	B. Braun	Permanent/convertible	28 mm
Titanium Greenfield filter	Boston Scientific	Permanent	28 mm
TRAPEASE filter	Cordis	Permanent	30 mm
Recovery	Bard	Retrievable	28 mm
G2	Bard	Retrievable	28 mm
G2 Express and G2X	Bard	Retrievable	28 mm
Eclipse	Bard	Retrievable	28 mm
Meridian	Bard	Retrievable	28 mm
Denali	Bard	Retrievable	28 mm
Gunther Tulip	Cook Medical	Retrievable	28 mm
Celect	Cook Medical	Retrievable	28 mm
Option/Option elite	Rex Medical	Retrievable	28 mm

ANATOMY

The IVC originates at the level of the fourth or fifth lumbar vertebral body where the common iliac veins converge. The renal veins join at the level of the first or second lumbar vertebral body and the hepatic veins join just below the diaphragm. The typical infrarenal IVC measures 23 mm [7]. The operator should be familiar with anatomic variants of the IVC to appropriately place the IVC filter and apply a modified approach when needed.

A mega vena cava is described when the IVC measures >28 mm, which must be promptly identified to modify your approach for filter placement. The only commercially available filter indicated for IVC measuring greater than 30 mm is the Bird's Nest filter. Figure 17.1 demonstrates a megacava with undersized IVCF; this was removed and replaced with the Bird's Nest filter. Another variant to be mindful of is a retroaortic left renal vein, since it will generally drain into the IVC more caudally than the typical renal veins. It is important to note the possibility of having a left inferior vena cava draining into the azygos veins, which can make access difficult via a transjugular approach. A left IVC can persist when the right supracardinal vein regresses and the left supracardinal vein persists; it is common for the left IVC to drain into the left renal vein and then give a normal right IVC [7]. A duplicated IVC can occur if the bilateral supracardinal veins persist. In this configuration, the iliac veins will drain into their respective ipsilateral IVC, and due to its rarity, there has been debate on the best approach for filter placement (whether it is to place filters on the bilateral IVCs or to place one in the normal suprarenal IVC, as demonstrated in Figure 17.2).

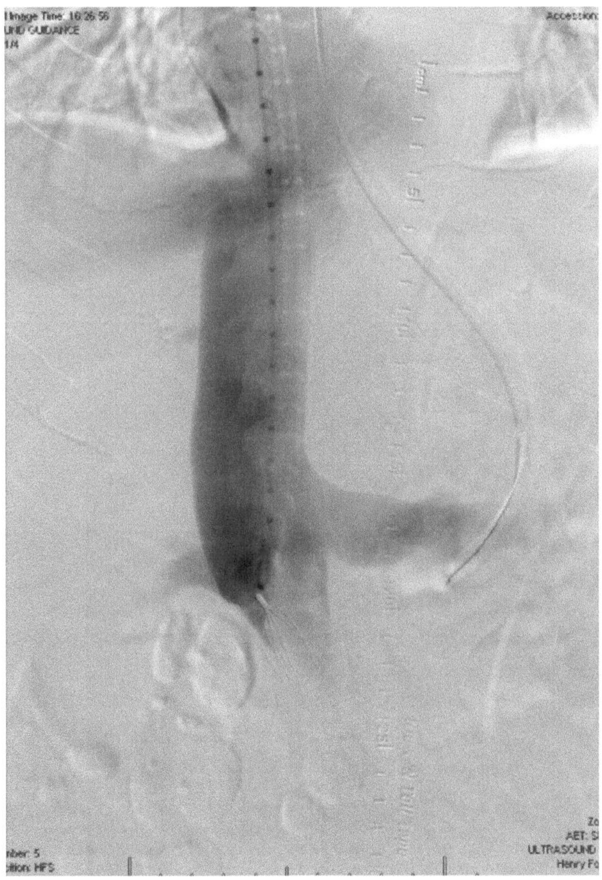

Figure 17.1 A mega vena cava with an infrarenal undersized IVCF. This filter was subsequently removed and replaced with a Bird's Nest filter.

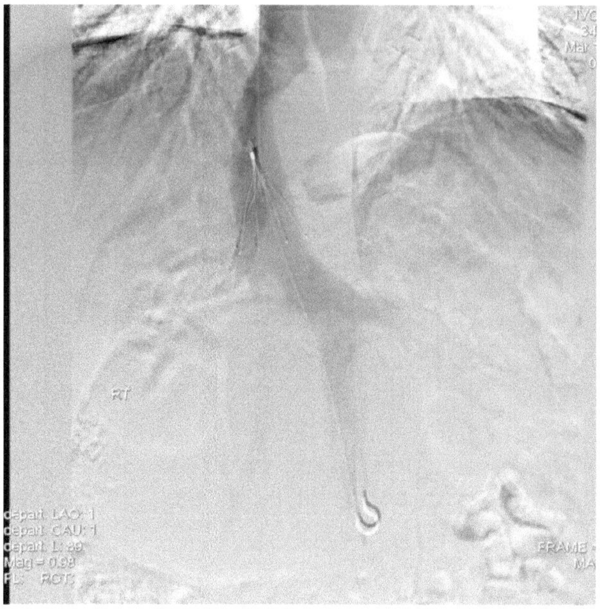

Figure 17.2 Duplicated IVC with an IVCF placed in the normal suprarenal IVC. The catheter is in the right infrarenal IVC from an internal jugular approach.

FILTER TYPES

There are three major types of IVC filters: permanent, convertible, and retrievable. While temporary filters are commercially procured, they are not available in the USA.

Permanent filters are made to be left in place for the patient's lifespan. Convertible filters are designed to function for a designated period of time and then "deactivate." A bioabsorable filament holds the cone-shaped filter in position within the canal lumen, and after a fixed period, the filament hydrolyzes, releasing the arms against the wall of the IVC where they are no longer functional.

Retrievable filters are similar to permanent filters, but within a certain timeframe they are intended to be removed in their entirety when no longer needed. The retrieval process can be more challenging depending on the duration that the filter has been in place. However, it has been reported that even filters with a prolonged dwell time can be safely removed, although there is an overall decreased retrieval rate with dwell times beyond six months [8].

TECHNIQUE

At our institution, patients are diagnosed with DVT by venous duplex ultrasound. In those with PE diagnosed on CT, a venous duplex is obtained reflexively. Evaluation by ultrasound spares the patient exposure to ionizing radiation while defining the characteristics of the thrombus such as chronicity, location, extent, and progression. Lower extremity venous duplex exams must include the contralateral common femoral vein for completeness and can identify those patients that require more proximal imaging. It is our practice to obtain an abdominal-pelvic CT venogram for patients with acute thrombus identified in the common femoral vein to further interrogate the iliac veins and IVC prior to IVC filter placement. This axial imaging also allows for clear identification of aberrant anatomy, accurate caval diameter measurement, and thrombus burden.

We perform IVC filter insertion under sterile conditions in the angiography suite with a fixed c-arm or in the operating room with fixed or mobile c-arms when necessary. The patient is placed supine on the table and the bilateral groins are prepped and draped with the pannus taped as needed. Ultrasound-guided common femoral venipuncture with micro introducer access is our standard, although not necessary. For operator comfort, the right side is preferred. In cases with iliofemoral thrombus inhibiting groin access, the right internal jugular vein is the preferred access site. The brachial vein is an alternative approach for certain filters such as the Simon Nitinol (Bard Peripheral Vascular, Inc., Tempe, AZ, USA), and the TRAPEASE Permanent Vena Cava Filter and OPTEASE Retrievable Vena Cava Filter (Cordis Corporation, Milpitas, CA, USA).

Once the initial 5F introducer sheath has been placed, a semi-stiff introducer wire is guided into the vena. Various methods can be used to delineate the venous anatomy including venogram with marker pigtail for measurement, intravascular ultrasound (IVUS), or iliocaval venogram with external radiopaque marker tape. Once the anatomy has been marked either on the screen with a marker, noted at the vertebral body level, or roadmap obtained, the introducer sheath is exchanged for the delivery system over stiff guide wire. Each commercially available IVC filter comes with its own delivery system, mostly consisting of a simple "push-pull" delivery method or a button sequence and are approved for use in caval diameters up to 28 mm. The exception is the Cook Medical Bird's Nest Filter, which has a 40 mm upper limit. The filter is positioned with the apex just below the most inferior renal vein with the base of the filter above the iliac vein confluence. A completion cavogram is required to demonstrate appropriate deployment in the infrarenal IVC with appropriate wall apposition of the limbs. Alternatively, post-procedure IVUS combined with plain fluoroscopy can be utilized for those with anaphylactic contrast allergy or severe renal insufficiency not yet on dialysis.

Special considerations include duplicated IVC, which is either identified on pre-procedure axial imaging or suspected with a smaller than expected cabal diameter. In this case, a contralateral ultrasound-guided femoral vein puncture and venogram should be performed to check for aberrant anatomy. In the case of duplicated IVC, bilateral filters are considered.

COMPLICATIONS

The most common immediate complications of IVC filter placement include bleeding and hematoma at the puncture site, arterial puncture, air embolus, and allergic reactions to contrast media or other medications that are used during the procedure. Additionally, malpositioning of the filter (1.3%) and entrapment of the guidewire within the filter may occur.

Long-term complications include thrombosis and occlusion of the IVC at the filter site, erosion through the vessel wall and into adjacent organs or the spine, and fracture of the IVC filter, as well as filter till and migration (1.0%).

TRICKS AND TRAPS

- The typical infrarenal IVC measures 23 mm.
- The Bird's Nest filter is the only commercially available device indicated for IVC measuring greater than 30 mm.
- Retrievable filters have an overall decreased retrieval rate with dwell times beyond six months.
- A CT venogram is useful to delineate duplicate cava systems, IVC dimensions, and clot burden prior to filter placement.
- IVC filters can be placed without the use of contrast with IVUS and plain fluoroscopy.

QUESTIONS

1. A trauma patient with bilateral femur fractures, AKI, and intracranial hematoma among other injuries is diagnosed with right leg DVT involving the common femoral and femoral veins. A CT venogram is obtained demonstrating an IVC diameter of 34 mm at the renal veins with no thrombus in the iliac system. What is the best approach to the management of this patient?
   a. Immediate systemic anticoagulation
   b. Percutaneous mechanical thrombectomy from the popliteal approach
   c. Placement of infrarenal IVC Bird's Nest IVC filter with IVUS
   d. Chemoprophylaxis dosing anticoagulation for 72 hours

   Answer: c

2. The largest commercially available IVC filter can accommodate up to what diameter IVC?
   a. 30 mm
   b. 28 mm
   c. 50 mm
   d. 40 mm

   Answer: d

3. Contraindications to IVC filter placement include:
   a. Severe coagulopathy
   b. Free-floating thrombus burden
   c. Pregnancy
   d. Anaphylactic allergy to contrast

   Answer: a

4. Which of the statements below is correct?
   a. IVC filter dwell time longer than six months indicates an increased retrieval rate
   b. All spinal surgeries should have prophylactic IVC filters placed two weeks pre-op
   c. In patients with duplicated IVC, placing bilateral common iliac vein filters is an acceptable approach
   d. There is no indication for a pre-procedure CT venogram for patients with common femoral DVT involvement on duplex imaging

   Answer: c

REFERENCES

1. Beckman MG, Hooper WC, Critchley SE, Ortel TL. Venous thromboembolism: a public health concern. *Am J Prev Med*. 2010;38(4 Suppl):S495–501. doi:10.1016/j.amepre.2009.12.017
2. Badireddy M, Mudipalli VR. Deep venous thrombosis prophylaxis. In: *StatPearls*. StatPearls Publishing; 2023. Accessed September 2, 2023. http://www.ncbi.nlm.nih.gov/books/NBK534865/
3. Kaufman JA, Barnes GD, Chaer RA, et al. Society of interventional radiology clinical practice guideline for inferior vena cava filters in the treatment of patients with venous thromboembolic disease: developed in collaboration with the American college of cardiology, American college of chest physicians, American college of surgeons committee on trauma, American heart association, society for vascular surgery, and society for vascular medicine. *J Vasc Interv Radiol JVIR*. 2020;31(10):1529–1544. doi:10.1016/j.jvir.2020.06.014
4. Sadri L, Rogers A, Sharma D, Tunis J, Sullivan T, Pineda DM. A survey of patients lost to follow-up after inferior vena cava filter placement. *J Vasc Surg Venous Lymphat Disord*. 2020;8(3):365–370. doi:10.1016/j.jvsv.2019.11.011
5. DeYoung E, Minocha J. Inferior vena cava filters: guidelines, best practice, and expanding indications. *Semin Interv Radiol*. 2016;33(2):65–70. doi:10.1055/s-0036-1581088
6. Rosner MK, Kuklo TR, Tawk R, Moquin R, Ondra SL. Prophylactic placement of an inferior vena cava filter in high-risk patients undergoing spinal reconstruction. *Neurosurg Focus*. 2004;17(4):E6. doi:10.3171/foc.2004.17.4.6

7. Doe C, Ryu RK. Anatomic and technical considerations: inferior vena cava filter placement. *Semin Interv Radiol.* 2016;33(2):88–92. doi:10.1055/s-0036-1581089

8. Garcia-Godoy F, Collins T, Sacks D, Vasas S, Sarani B. Retrieval of inferior vena cava filters after prolonged indwelling time. *Arch Intern Med.* 2011;171(21):1953–1956. doi:10.1001/archinternmed.2011.526

18

Endovascular techniques for retrieval of inferior vena cava filters and intravascular foreign bodies

PHILIP S. CHACKO, MICHAEL P. TRPKOWSKI, AND SACHINDER S. HANS

INTRODUCTION

Venous thromboembolism (VTE), a condition categorized into deep venous thrombosis (DVT) and pulmonary embolism (PE), affects 900,000 people annually in the USA with a 15% mortality from PE [1]. First-line treatment for VTE is systemic anticoagulation with a treatment length ranging between three and six months [2]. Depending on the extent and severity of the disease process, a small subset will require lifelong anticoagulation due to significant risk factors for hypercoagulability. In patients with contraindications to anticoagulation, the placement of an inferior vena cava (IVC) filter can be considered. Inferior vena cava thrombosis after IVC filter placement occurs in 2–30% of patients. The cause of filter thrombosis may be related to the patient's initial risk factors for thrombosis or the presence of foreign material within the body with progressive accumulation of thrombosis in the stents. Despite the advent of retrievable filters, the vast majority are never removed. Retrievable filters within a certain time interval can be removed once they are no longer needed. The duration of the filter that has been in place must be considered before removal. The less time it has been in place, the easier it is to remove because there is less endothelialization and incorporation into the arterial wall. Endovascular techniques in challenging cases of IVC filter retrieval can be applied to remove other foreign bodies (central venous catheter [CVC] and wire fragments) as well, which will be covered in this chapter.

IVC FILTER RETRIEVAL

Retrievable filters are generally removed through the IJV under fluoroscopic guidance using a coaxial system and snare catheter. After US-guided access and sheath placement, catheter and wire access to the IVC is obtained. An inferior vena cavagram is performed to determine IVC patency and the lack of thrombus within the filter. If the IVC is thrombosed up to the filter, or if there is significant thrombus within the filter, attempts at removal should be abandoned. Systemic anticoagulation is continued and, in the case of thrombus within the filter, the patient is re-evaluated for clearance of this thrombus in four to six weeks. After obtaining the inferior vena cavagram, the pigtail catheter is removed over a stiff wire.

A long, 12-Fr sheath is placed into the IVC over the stiff wire. A coaxial system with an inner sheath and snare is used to encircle the hook on the top of the filter. The filter is recaptured by keeping tension on the snare-filter combination while advancing the sheath over the filter. There should be no net upward or downward force during the recapture phase. The most difficult part of the procedure is the dislodgement of the hooks from the IVC wall (Figure 18.1). Operator judgment is required as to how long to persist and how hard to pull on the retrieval system, as these factors influence the risk of a tear in the IVC. No effort should be made to remove the coaxial system from the patient before the entire filter is within the sheath.

DOI: 10.1201/9781003452096-18

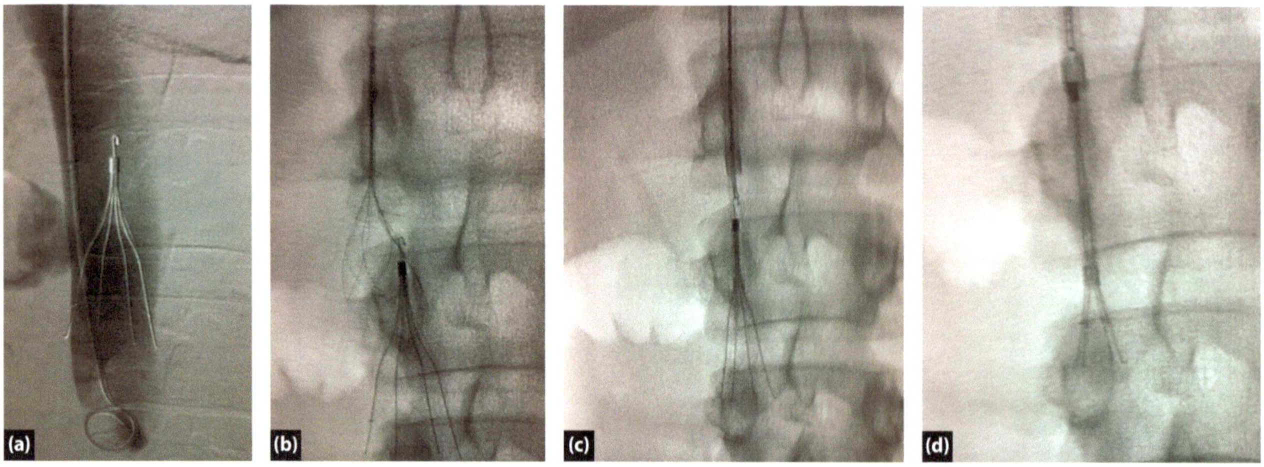

Figure 18.1 Images demonstrating the sequence for inferior vena cava (IVC) filter retrieval: (a) cavagram demonstrating patent IVC without filter thrombus; (b) snare capture of the filter apical hook; (c) advancement of the sheath over the apex of the filter; (d) release of the hooks from the IVC wall to complete recapture of the entire filter within the 12-Fr sheath.

Additional endovascular devices and strategies for challenging cases include the use of rigid forceps, modified loop snares, double loop techniques, balloon displacement, the Excimer laser, and open surgical removal. The use of these techniques can be extrapolated for the removal of intravascular foreign bodies in general.

INTRAVASCULAR FOREIGN BODIES

Intravascular foreign bodies (IFB) are a rare but serious and sometimes fatal complication. Multiple therapeutic interventions, such as placement of stents, inferior vena cava filters, venous catheters, and coil embolization, can lead to fragmentation of the instrument, with subsequent embolization, migration, or deployment of the fragment into an undesired location. Embolization of foreign body fragments can lead to sepsis, bacterial endocarditis, cardiac arrhythmias, or myocardial injury, all carrying reported mortality rates ranging from 24–60% [3]. Due to this high mortality rate, removal of a foreign body is almost always recommended, even in asymptomatic patients, with a percutaneous technique being the gold standard.

SOURCE OF IFBs: CENTRAL VENOUS CATHETERS

Central venous catheter (CVC) placement is a commonly performed procedure with an overall complication rate of approximately 15%, mainly due to hematoma formation, pneumothorax, infection, or arterial injury. Less commonly, with an incidence of 1%, embolization of a fragment of the catheter can occur [4].

The diagnosis can be challenging, as some patients may not manifest any symptoms. Surov et al. reported the signs associated with fragment embolization, which include the following in order of decreasing incidence: catheter malfunction, cardiac arrhythmia, shortness of breath, and signs of sepsis. If clinical suspicion is high, an upright chest x-ray should be obtained to confirm the location of the catheter, to ensure the catheter is intact, and to rule out any embolized fragments (Figure 18.2) and other post-procedural complications such as pneumothorax.

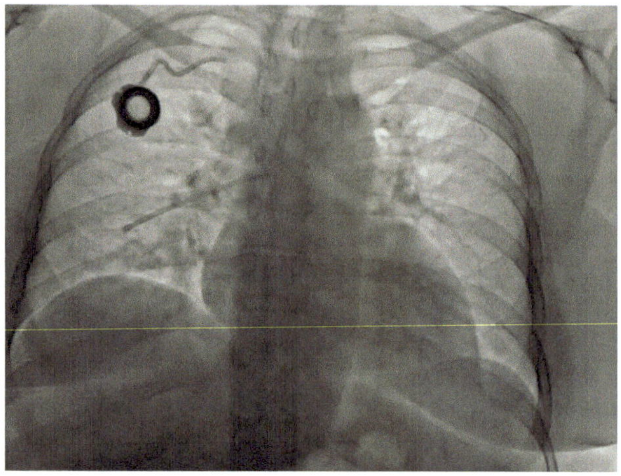

Figure 18.2 A patient with a fragmented mediport lodged in the right pulmonary artery.

The location of the fractured or migrated catheter is dependent on the following: the original vein it was placed in, catheter flexibility and length, patient positioning, and blood flow within the vessel and/or heart. Common locations of embolized material include the right atrium, pulmonary artery, right ventricle, superior vena cava, and subclavian vein.

SOURCES OF IFBs: WIRES

The evolution of percutaneous interventions over the past decade has led to an increasing incidence of wire-related complications. Wires can splinter and embolize or the entire wire can be lost in the vascular system, which may be rarely seen when losing wire access during CVC placement. Wires are subjected to stress with repetitive attempts to cross a narrowed, heavily calcified lesion, leading to weakening and eventual fracturing. This is a well-known phenomenon seen in percutaneous coronary intervention with a reported incidence of 0.2–0.8% [5]. Although less commonly reported in the literature, the same theory applies for broken wires during peripheral vascular interventions.

A foreign body in the arterial system can lead to thrombosis, ischemia, and/or infection. If identified during an intervention, it should be addressed immediately, but compared with venous foreign bodies, foreign bodies located in the arterial system can be managed conservatively if the following criteria are met: a small fragment lodged in an artery with chronic occlusive disease and if there is a low probability of embolization in an asymptomatic patient. If these criteria are not met, endovascular retrieval should be performed.

RETRIEVAL TECHNIQUES: LOOP SNARE

The rapid growth of endovascular interventions has led to the development of multiple devices used for the retrieval of IFBs. The loop snare is the most widely used and versatile device when it comes to IFB retrieval. It is designed to be flexible, facilitating navigation through the vasculature to reach the right atrium or pulmonary arteries. A disadvantage to its use is its weak grip strength, making chronic, adherent IFBs difficult to remove. The snare can be a single loop like the Amplatz Gooseneck Nitinol Snare (Ev3 Inc., Plymouth, MN, USA) or multiple loops like the EN Snare (Merrit Medical, Jordan, UT, USA). When deployed, the loop emerges perpendicular to the catheter at a 90-degree angle, making placement of the loop around the IFB much more feasible. The loop snare's design permits its use for removing a variety of IFBs, including fragmented CVCs, wires, stents, and IVC filters.

Various techniques using the loop snare device have been described. The proximal capture technique is the most basic of the approaches. To use this method, there must be a free end of the IFB accessible (Figure 18.3). The vascular system is accessed through one of the major vessels, most commonly the right CFV.

In certain situations, such as patients with IVC filters or bilateral iliac thrombus, the IJV or subclavian vein is the preferred access site. The catheter is advanced under fluoroscopic guidance into the desired vessel to a point just before the IFB. Once in position, the outer catheter is withdrawn, deploying the snare. The entire system is advanced until the loop is around the free end of the IFB. Once the loop encompasses the IFB, the snare is tightened by advancing the catheter. The IFB should then be oriented parallel to the vessel, which reduces the likelihood of vessel damage during removal (Figure 18.4).

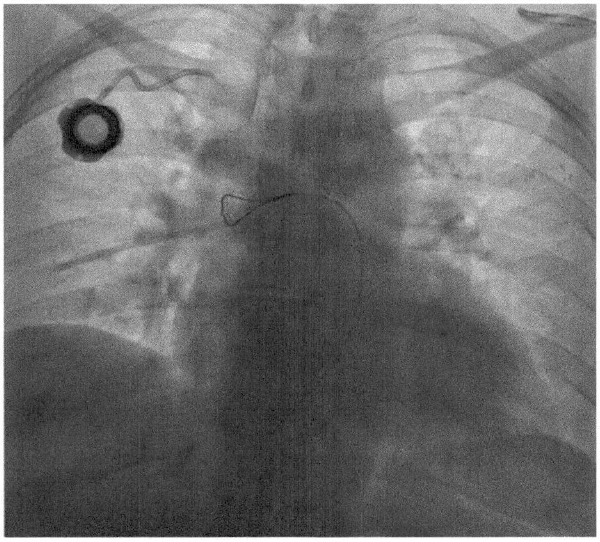

Figure 18.3 The gooseneck snare being used to retrieve an IFB. Note that the operator is attempting to grab the IFB at one of its free ends.

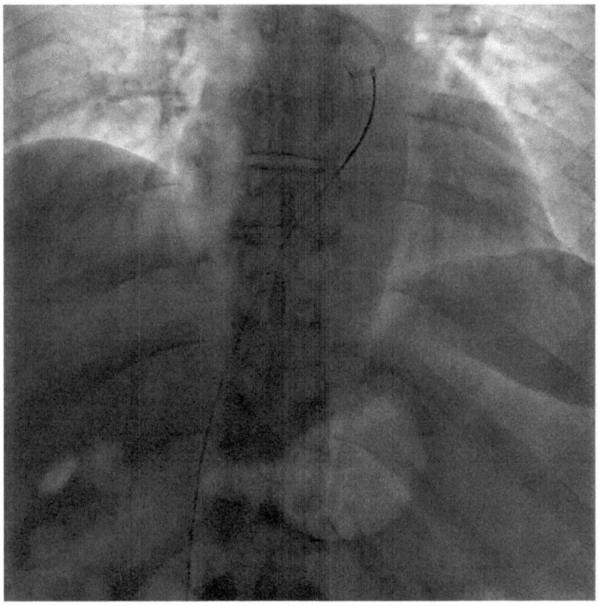

Figure 18.4 An IFB is grasped at its distal end and slowly removed. Note that the IFB is parallel to the vessel that it is traveling in.

The entire system, including the IFB, is then removed through an 8Fr sheath. Care must be taken to ensure that the loop is around the free end of the IFB. If the loop is in the middle, tightening of the snare will orient the IFB perpendicular to the catheter and vessel, which can ultimately lead to vessel wall damage and, in severe instances, laceration of the vessel wall. Using this technique, success rates have been reported to be more than 92%. Other techniques using the loop snare are primarily reserved for stent removal.

RETRIEVAL TECHNIQUES: ENDOVASCULAR RETRIEVAL FORCEPS

Endovascular forceps are not used as much as the loop snare for IFB retrieval. Their design typically employs side-opening jaws that allow for greater grip strength. Typically, it requires access through the IJV or CFV. They come in a variety of sizes ranging from 3Fr to 12Fr and can be passed through a guiding catheter. The vascular retrieval forceps (Cook Medical, Bloomington, IN, USA) are used in larger vessels and can be used to retrieve IFBs from central veins and the right atrium. The Alligator retrieval device (Covidien, Mansfield, MA, USA) can be used in small vessels and is used to remove coils from the cerebral circulation. Perhaps the greatest advantage of endovascular forceps is the ability to remove IFBs without having a free end. Drawbacks to using the forceps are their high risk of iatrogenic injuries and their rigid design leading to difficult navigation. Endovascular forceps have been used to facilitate the removal of stents, coils, and IFBs that adhere to the endothelium of the vessel. Caution should be used with the endovascular forceps given their risk for complications. IFBs that have been intravascular for more than 24 hours usually have some adherence to the vessel. If excessive force is used, the operator runs the risk of damaging the vessel lining and, in severe cases, perforating the vessel. Once access is obtained, the guiding catheter is directed to the desired location. Next, the forceps are passed through the catheter and gently advanced until the jaws emerge. The catheter and forceps are then manipulated to grasp the IFB. Once the IFB is in the jaws of the forceps, the guiding catheter and forceps are gently removed as a unit. Excessive force should be avoided to limit trauma to the vessel. Despite this risk, the advancement of endovascular retrieval options has decreased the morbidity associated with IFBs.

TRICKS AND TRAPS

- An inferior vena cavagram is obtained during the procedure to determine the patency of the IVC filter and the lack of thrombus in the filter. If there is significant thrombosis in the filter, the procedure should be abandoned.
- During retrieval of IVC filters, the most difficult part is the dislodgement of the hooks from the wall of the IVC. The entire filter should be within the sheath before the coaxial system is removed.
- Due to the high morbidity and mortality associated with intravascular foreign bodies, retrieval is recommended even in asymptomatic patients.
- The loop snare is the most widely used device for the retrieval of intravascular foreign bodies.
- Endovascular retrieval forceps are preferred in the removal of IFBs without a free end.
- Endovascular retrieval forceps are difficult to navigate and have a higher risk of iatrogenic injuries, but they are used to facilitate the removal of adherent IFBs.

QUESTIONS

1. An inferior vena cavagram is performed at the time of the retrieval of the IVC filter. A significant amount of thrombus is visualized within the filter. The next step in management should be:
   a. Continue IVC filter retrieval
   b. Administration of thrombolytic into the inferior vena cava with a catheter in the filter, wait for 30 minutes, and retrieve the filter if there is significant lysis of the thrombus
   c. The attempted retrieval should be discontinued and systemic anticoagulation continued for four to six weeks and the patient re-evaluated
   d. The attempted retrieval should be discontinued and systemic anticoagulation continued for 10–12 weeks followed by re-evaluation of the patient

   Answer: c

2. The embolization of a segment of catheter during coaxial venous catheter placement occurs in:
   a. 3%
   b. 2%
   c. 1%
   d. 0.5%

   Answer: b

3. Retrieval of intravascular foreign body with a free end is best achieved by a:
   a. Loop snare using distal capture
   b. Loop snare using proximal capture
   c. Endovascular retrieval forceps
   d. Open operation

   Answer: b

4. The use of endovascular retrieval forceps as compared to loop snare is associated with:
   a. Difficult navigation and a high risk of iatrogenic injuries
   b. Easy navigation and a high risk of iatrogenic injuries
   c. Difficult navigation and a low risk of iatrogenic injuries
   d. Easy navigation and a low risk of iatrogenic injuries

   Answer: a

5. The preferred venous access for removal of intravascular foreign bodies is:
   a. Right CFV
   b. Left CFV
   c. Right IJV
   d. Left IJV

   Answer: a

REFERENCES

1. Horlander, K, Mannino, D M, & Leeper, K V. (2003). Pulmonary embolism mortality in the United States, 1979–1998: an analysis using multiple-cause mortality data. *Arch Intern Med.*, 163, 1711–1717.
2. Ortel TL, Neumann I, Ageno W, Beyth R, Clark NP, Cuker A, Hutten BA, Jaff MR, Manja V, Schulman S, Thurston C, Vedantham S, Verhamme P, Witt DM, Florez ID, Izcovich A, Nieuwlaat R, Ross S, Schünemann HJ, Wiercioch W, Zhang Y, Zhang Y. American society of hematology 2020 guidelines for management of venous thromboembolism: treatment of deep vein thrombosis and pulmonary embolism. *Blood Adv.* 2020;4(19):4693–4738. https://doi.org/10.1182/bloodadvances.2020001830
3. Mitsopoulos G, Hanna RF, Brejt SZ, et al. Retrieval of a dislodged catheter using combined fluoroscopy and intracardiac echocardiography. *Case Rep Radiol.* 2015;2015:610362. doi:10.1155/2015/610362
4. Kumar Upadhyay A, Prakash B, Shekhar S, Kumar A, Prakash A. Embolization of a fractured peripherally inserted central catheter to pulmonary arteries: a sporadic life-threatening phenomenon. *Cureus.* 2023;15(8):e43044. Published 2023 Aug 6. doi:10.7759/cureus.43044
5. Datta G. Broken guidewire - A tale of three cases. *Indian Heart J.* 2015;67(Suppl 3):S49–S52. doi:10.1016/j.ihj.2015.07.025

19

Endovenous catheter ablation of the saphenous vein

JUDITH C. LIN, EVAN F. GUAY, AND YASAMAN KAVOUSI

INTRODUCTION

Chronic venous disease results in physical and mental suffering for millions of people each year, with the prevalence of C2 disease estimated at 21–23% in the Americas, and healthcare cost estimates of $3 billion in the United States alone each year [1]. Risk factors for developing chronic venous disease include increasing age, height, female sex, high parity, hormonal therapy, White identity, low activity level, BMI, history of DVT, and prolonged standing [2]. A recent study by Ragg and colleagues has also raised questions about congenital contributions to the development of venous incompetence [3].

Dating back to at least the 1960s, endovenous therapies for varicose veins emerged as an adjunct or alternative to conservative measures (e.g., compression garments) or open surgical interventions (e.g., vein stripping). First introduced in 2001 by Drs. Navarro and Min, endovenous laser ablation (EVLA) joined the longer-standing practice of radiofrequency ablation (RFA) to deliver electromagnetic or laser energy and obliterate the target vein in situ [4]. Numerous clinical trials have since been performed evaluating conservative interventions, sclerotherapy, surgical stripping, RFA, and EVLA for the great saphenous vein (GSV), showing similar primary failure and recurrence rates between the two endovascular techniques compared with standard stripping surgery [5–8]. Mounting evidence and improvements in techniques have made endovenous approaches the standard of care for treating chronic, superficial venous disease, leading the Society for Vascular Surgeons (SVS), the American Venous Forum (SVF), and the American Vein and Lymphatic Society (AVLS) to provide a grade 1 recommendation (with weak evidence) for endovenous ablation over surgical vein stripping in their updated guidelines on the management of saphenous vein disease [9,10]. The advantages of a catheter-based intervention with tumescent anesthesia over conventional surgical stripping include the following: shorter convalescence; less postoperative pain; greater quality of life; improved cosmesis; and lower overall economic costs [11–14]. SVS, AVF, and AVLS now recommend endovenous interventions in an ambulatory setting as the gold standard for treating incompetent superficial veins.

PROCEDURE

In the authors' practice, patients take diazepam 5–10 mg by mouth an hour before the procedure. If needed, patients may also apply topical anesthetics (2.5% lidocaine, 2.5% prilocaine cream, 30 g tube) over the saphenous vein and bulging varicosities at home two hours before the procedure to minimize the pain perception of normal intact skin from needle injection of local anesthesia and tumescent anesthesia during the procedure. Ablation procedures may be performed on the GSV and any truncal veins, such as the small saphenous vein (SSV), anterior accessory saphenous vein, and intersaphenous vein.

The procedural table set-up requires the following: microaccess needle; 0.018-inch microaccess wire; 4-Fr or 7-Fr sheath; 25-G needle; 1% lidocaine for local anesthesia (some have suggested inclusion of bicarbonate in the anesthetic); syringes (5, 20, and 30 mL); normal saline; gauze; three mosquito clamps; tumescent tubing; acoustic coupling gel; marking pen; and labels (Figure 19.1) [15]. A portable ultrasound (US) system should be available in the room.

The patient's GSV is mapped the day before the procedure and any bulging tributary varicose veins are marked the same day with a skin marker. After obtaining informed consent, the patient is placed supine on the procedure table, which is positioned in reverse Trendelenburg to distend the veins in the lower extremities. The entire lower extremity is prepped and draped in sterile fashion.

DOI: 10.1201/9781003452096-19

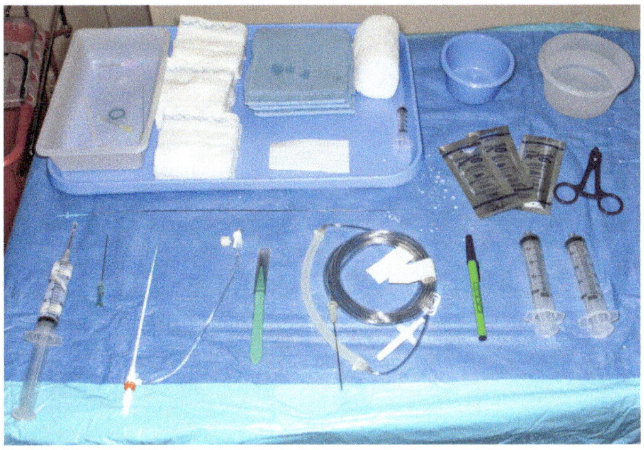

Figure 19.1 Procedural table set-up.

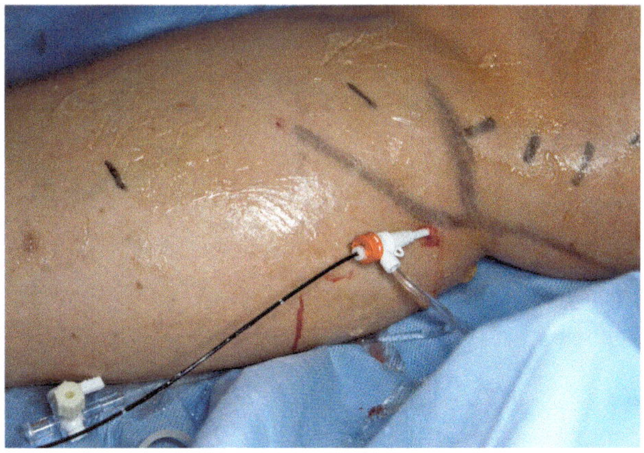

Figure 19.3 Insertion of sheath and catheter for radiofrequency ablation.

For veins <2 mm, nitroglycerine paste may be applied to the primary insertion site to dilate the vein and prevent venospasm before gaining intravascular access. Blood pressure, heart rate, and oxygen saturation are monitored intraoperatively.

A rapid US scan of the medial leg is performed to assess for areas of tortuosity and the location of tributaries and perforators. Under US guidance, 1% lidocaine is used to infiltrate the skin; percutaneous access to the GSV just below the knee is obtained with a micropuncture access needle (Figure 19.2). The authors use the VSI Micro-HV Introducer Kit (Vascular Solutions, Inc., Minneapolis, MN, USA) for RFA procedures or the VenaCure EVLA NeverTouch Direct Procedure Kit (AngioDynamics, Latham, NY, USA) for EVLA procedures. After needle cannulation of the GSV, a microaccess guidewire is introduced and the 6-Fr RFA or 4-Fr EVLA sheath is inserted (Figure 19.3).

An endovenous radiofrequency or laser catheter is advanced under US up to the saphenofemoral junction (SFJ) and the tip is withdrawn approximately 2 cm away from the saphenofemoral junction (Figure 19.4). Good

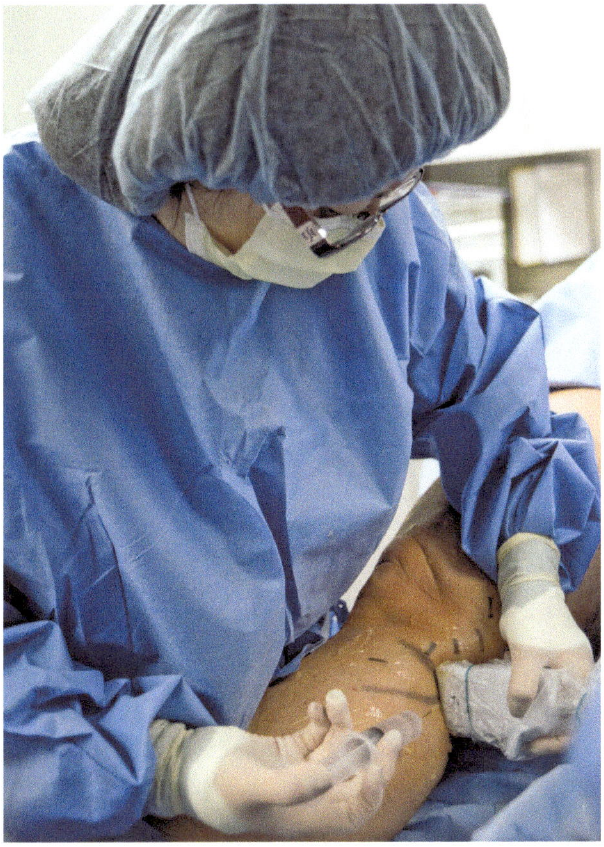

Figure 19.2 Ultrasound-guided percutaneous access of distal great saphenous vein.

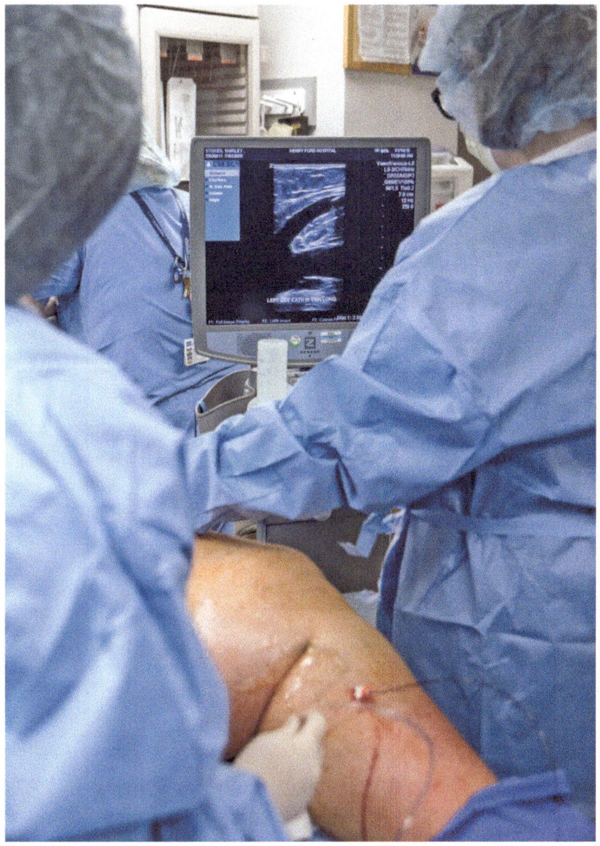

Figure 19.4 Confirmation of catheter tip placement via ultrasound.

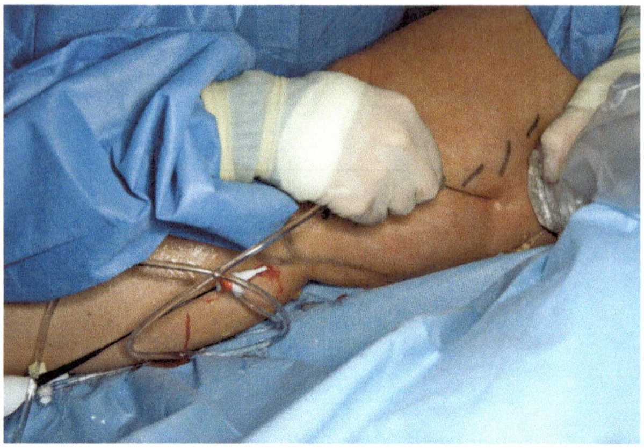

Figure 19.5 Ultrasound-guided injection of tumescent anesthesia.

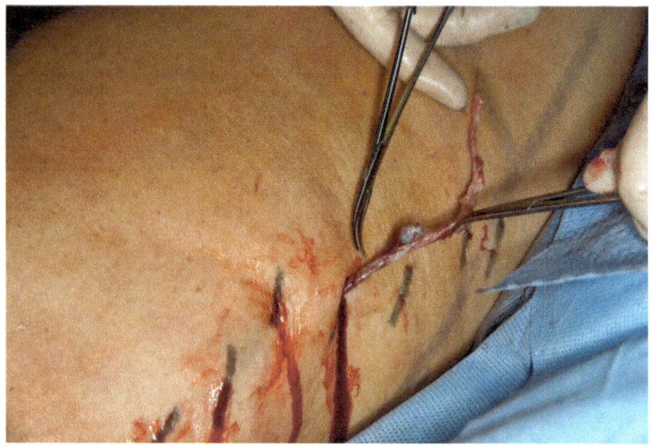

Figure 19.6 Extraction of varicosities for ambulatory phlebectomy.

positioning of the endovenous catheter distal to the SFJ must be obtained under US to reduce the incidence of heat-induced thrombus formation. The GSV below the calf is not routinely treated with thermal energy because of the increased risk of paresthesia from thermal injury to the saphenous nerve, which lies near the GSV.

Tumescent anesthesia is then injected into the perivenous space in the saphenous compartment using a 21-G spinal needle and tumescent pump under US guidance (Figure 19.5). The tumescent solution is composed of 1000 mL of 0.9% normal saline solution, 100 mL of 1% lidocaine with epinephrine, and 10 mL of 8.4% sodium bicarbonate. Tumescent anesthesia involves subcutaneous infiltration of this solution around the vein as a buffer from the thermal energy, deepening the truncal vein to >1 cm to reduce the risk of skin burn, and reducing GSV size so that vein ablation is more effective.

Following satisfactory tumescent anesthesia, endovenous ablation of the GSV is started. For RFA, the authors use a radiofrequency catheter via a 7-Fr sheath. The ClosureFast™ Endovenous Radiofrequency Ablation (RFA) Catheter (Medtronic, Minneapolis, MN, USA) heats the vein in 7-cm segments with 20-second treatment cycles. For EVLA, the authors use the VenaCure EVLA NeverTouch Direct system (AngioDynamics) with laser wavelengths of 980, 810, and 1470 nm via a 4-Fr sheath. Hemoglobin absorption does not play a role when using a wavelength >1320 nm, and water absorption is the dominant mechanism. Thus, the vein wall is gently heated and shrunk without perforations, translating into less pain, bruising, and paresthesia after EVLA at a higher wavelength, with no loss of efficacy [16,17]. The choice of thermal ablation mechanism depends on the operator and patient preference. On US, the GSV should be fully thrombosed and closed, and there should be no evidence of thrombus extending into the common femoral vein. The catheter is then removed with the sheath and hemostasis is obtained.

Removal of associated varicosities may be done concomitantly or as a staged procedure. The decision is based on the patient's choice and the surgeon's preference. Based on the authors' experience, there is a slightly increased risk of endovenous heat-induced thrombus with concomitant phlebectomy of varicosities. To perform ambulatory phlebectomy of varicosities, the skin is anesthetized with 1% lidocaine and small skin incisions are made over the bulging veins. Varady or Mueller phlebectomy hooks are used to extract the veins. Gentle traction is used to extract vein segments with mosquito clamps. Additional tumescent anesthesia may be used to further numb the area (Figure 19.6).

Hemostasis is obtained with direct pressure over the incision sites, which are closed with gauze bandage rolls. Suture is not generally required; if needed, 4-0 nylon suture may be used to obtain hemostasis. Gauze bandage rolls and compression elastic wrap bandages are applied from the foot to the upper thigh. Patients can ambulate immediately after the procedure. After two days, they may remove the gauze and bandage, shower, and wear thigh-high, elastic compression stockings (30-40 mmHg compression level) for an additional two weeks. Patients are followed with a venous duplex US and clinic appointment within one week of the procedure.

HAZARDS AND ADVERSE EVENTS

In addition to technical challenges associated with any endovenous procedure—including cannulation, guidewire placement, or catheter advancement—complications more specific to endovenous ablations include endovenous heat-induced thrombosis (EHIT), de novo deep vein thrombosis (DVT), superficial thrombophlebitis, nerve injury, ecchymosis, hematoma, thermal skin burn, persistent pain, and hyperpigmentation. Advanced age, female sex, more advanced CEAP, and a history of superficial thrombophlebitis are significant predictors of DVT after EVLA [18,19].

Mechanisms of EHIT and DVT are not entirely understood at this time, and ultrasound findings can appear from days to months following intervention. It is generally thought that a thrombus originating from the superficial vein extends into the deep venous system—termed postablation superficial thrombus extension—with the DVT generally resolving more quickly and decreased subsequent risk as compared with classic DVTs. A recent systematic review by Healy and colleagues containing 16,398 patients undergoing EVLA or RFA showed similar rates of complications between RFA and EVLA [19]. A study of National Surgical Quality Improvement Program data showed that patients undergoing endovenous ablation have higher odds of postoperative DVT, with the prevalence of DVT after RFA ranging from 0.2–1.2%.[4] That said, RFA in this subset of patients remains a safe approach with continuation or preprocedural anticoagulation [19]. Evidence from Chong and colleagues suggests that endovenous ablation of the superficial venous system is safe and effective in patients with deep venous reflux (DVR), even improving DVR on follow-up if DVR is limited to a single vessel [20]. If patients have a history of thrombosis or other clotting disorder, literature suggests that therapeutic anticoagulation—coumadin or DOAC—should be continued throughout the perioperative period [21,22].

A vein diameter of >8 mm, operative time >40 minutes, and male sex are predictive factors for EHIT following RFA [11]. Successful treatment of veins >12 mm carries a slightly higher risk of EHIT formation after ablation of larger truncal veins. The frequency of EHIT has been reported as 0–8% and it has been shown to decrease with ablation distance >2.5cm from the saphenofemoral junction. SVS and SVF 2021 guidelines for the management of EHIT depend on the grade (I–IV) of EHIT and patient-specific factors. In general, grade I may be observed; grade II may be observed or treated with antiplatelet or anticoagulation; grade III may be therapeutically anticoagulated until the thrombus regresses; and grade IV should be treated with therapeutic anticoagulation or thrombectomy [23].

Superficial thrombophlebitis often presents several days after the procedure, with a risk of phlebitis approximately 2.9% [24]. This condition is often self-limiting and treated with conservative management, including compression and nonsteroidal anti-inflammatory drugs.

Although the potential for nerve injury is greatly reduced in endovenous ablation as compared with conventional surgery, the risk of neurologic damage caused by thermal conduction to adjacent tissues remains a clinically important complication of thermal ablation. Paresthesia is seen in 19.6% of patients after surgery versus 9.7% after RFA and 4.8% after EVLA [24]. Nerve injury following endovenous ablation usually involves small cutaneous nerves in close anatomic proximity to the treated veins; however, larger nerves may be injured if aberrant veinous or neural anatomy is present. The SSV courses closely with the sural nerve, whereas the GSV is associated with the saphenous nerve. Because of the very close proximity of SSV and sural nerve from the distal calf to the ankle, puncturing the SSV at mid-calf may decrease postoperative paresthesia. Depending on the extent of injury, nerves may recover on their own, or surgical grafting or neuroma excision may be needed. Preoperative vein and nerve mapping, particularly in the popliteal region, may be helpful for minimizing such complications [25,26].

Skin burns are a well-documented complication of endovascular ablation techniques, with an incidence of around 1.2%. In EVLA, optimization of energy delivery and pullback speed, as well as administration of ample tumescent anesthesia, may reduce the frequency and intensity of skin burns and ecchymosis. Experimental data suggests that pullback speed should be aligned with depth of vein from skin, with 1 mm/s corresponding to 15 mm below skin, 2 mm/s corresponding to 10 mm below skin, and 4mm/s corresponding to 5 mm below skin [27]. Additionally, sufficient tumescent anesthesia helps to both create more distance between the vein and skin and provide thermal insulation.

Ecchymosis and hematoma are minor complications. Ecchymosis is self-limiting and can last approximately ten days. The rate of ecchymosis is unchanged between endovenous and conventional surgery groups. However, endovenous catheter ablation has shown reduced rates of hematoma by approximately 50–60% when compared with conventional surgery [10,18].

Overall, endovenous ablation in an ambulatory setting is a very safe, effective, and well-tolerated procedure. It is associated with lower postoperative complications, faster recovery time, and improved quality of life compared with standard surgery.

TRICKS AND TRAPS

- Keeping the procedure room warm, placing the patient in reverse Trendelenburg, and use of topical nitroglycerine are techniques that can dilate the vein and improve the ability to access the vein.
- Avoid ablation of GSV below the calf to decrease the risk of thermal injury to the saphenous nerve.
- Use tumescence fluid to deepen the vein to >1 cm to reduce the risk of skin burn.
- The SSV courses closely with the sural nerve, from the distal calf to the ankle; puncturing the SSV at mid-calf may decrease postoperative paresthesia.
- Beware that large vein size, longer procedural times, and male sex are predictive factors for EHIT.
- Superficial thrombophlebitis often presents several days after the procedure but is often self-limiting and treated with conservative management, including compression and nonsteroidal anti-inflammatory drugs.
- Skin burns: in EVLA, optimize energy delivery and pullback speed and tumescence to decrease risk.
- Beware of the area around the head and neck of the fibula when performing stab phlebectomy as the peroneal nerve is very superficial in this area and can be easily injured.

QUESTIONS

1. Proper positioning of the catheter tip is?
   a. 2–3 cm above the SFJ
   b. Within 2 cm of the SFJ
   c. 2–3 cm below the SFJ
   d. >3 cm below from the SFJ

   Answer: c

2. Which is the laser wavelength that has been shown to reduce pain, bruising, and paresthesia following EVLA?
   a. 360 nm
   b. 810 nm
   c. 1240 nm
   d. 1470 nm

   Answer: d

3. Operative planning for EVLA for patients with a history of DVT should entail:
   a. Holding anticoagulants for two to five days before the procedure
   b. Holding antiplatelet medications but continuing anticoagulants
   c. Continuing antiplatelet medications and anticoagulants
   d. Continuing antiplatelet medications but holding anticoagulants for two days preoperatively

   Answer: c

4. Proper pullback speed during EVLA is?
   a. 10 mm/s at 10 mm below the skin level
   b. 10 mm/s at 5 mm below the skin level
   c. 2 mm/s at 1 mm below the skin level
   d. 2 mm/s at 10 mm below the skin level

   Answer: d

REFERENCES

1. Salim, S., Machin, M., Patterson, B. O., *et al.* (2021). Global epidemiology of chronic venous disease: a systemic review of pooled prevalence analysis. *Annals of Surg*, *274*(6), 971–976.
2. Lin, J. C., Nerenz, D. R., Migliore, P., *et al.* (2014). Cost analysis of endovenous catheter ablation versus surgical stripping for treatment of superficial venous insufficiency and varicose vein disease. *J Vasc Surg Ven Lymph Disord*, *2*, 98–103.
3. Ragg, J., & Kuhlmann, N. (2022). Venous insufficiency in children and adolescents: progression over 4 years. *J Vasc Surg Ven Lymph Disord*, *11*(2), 470.
4. Benarroch-Gampel, J., Sheffield, K. M., Boyd, C. A., Riall, T. S., Killewich, L. A. (2013). Analysis of venous thromboembolic events after saphenous ablation. *J Vasc Surg Venous Lymphat Disord*, *1*(1):26–32.
5. Michaels, J. A., Campbell, W. B., Brazier, J. E., *et al.* (2006). Randomised clinical trial, observational study and assessment of cost-effectiveness of the treatment of varicose veins (REACTIV trial). *Health Technol Assess*, *10*(13).
6. Ratcliffe, J., Brazier, J. E., Campbell, W. B., *et al.* (2006). Cost-effectiveness analysis of surgery *versus* conservative treatment for uncomplicated varicose veins in a randomized clinical trial, *Br J Surg*, *I*(2), 182–186.
7. Lawson, J. A., Gauw, S. A., van Vlijmen, C. J., *et al.* (2018). Prospective comparative cohort study evaluating incompetent great saphenous vein closure using radiofrequency-powered segmental ablation or 1470-nm endovenous laser ablation with radial-tip fibers (Varico 2 study). *J Vasc Surg Ven Lymph Disord*, *6*(1), 31–40.
8. Siribumrungwong, B., Noorit, P., Wilasrusmee, C., *et al.* (2012). A systematic review and meta-analysis of randomised controlled trials comparing endovenous ablation and surgical intervention in patients with varicose vein. *Eur J Vasc Endovasc Surg*, *44*, 214–223.
9. De Maeseneer, M. G., Kakkos, S. K., Aherne, T., *et al.* (2023). Editor's choice – European society for vascular surgery (ESVS) clinical practice guidelines on the management of chronic venous disease of the lower limbs. *Eur J Vasc Endovasc Surg*, *63*(2), 184–267.
10. Gloviczki, P., Lawrence, P., Wasan, S., *et al.* (2022). The 2022 Society for vascular surgery, American venous forum, and American vein and lymphatic society clinical practice guidelines for the management of varicose veins of the lower extremities. Part I. duplex scanning and treatment of superficial truncal reflux. *J Vasc Surg Ven Lymph Disord*, *11*(2), 231–261.
11. Carruthers, T. N., Farber, A., Rybin, D., *et al.* (2014). Interventions on the superficial venous system for chronic venous insufficiency by surgeons in the modern era: an analysis of ACS-NSQIP. *Vasc Endovascular Surg*, 48, 482–490.
12. Boersma, D., Kornmann, V. N., van Eekeren, R. R., *et al.* (2016). Treatment modalities for small saphenous vein insufficiency: systematic review and meta-analysis. *J Endovasc Ther*, *23*, 199–211.
13. Marsden, G., Perry, M., Bradbury, A., Hickey, N., *et al.* (2015). A cost-effectiveness analysis of surgery, endothermal ablation, ultrasound-guided foam sclerotherapy and compression stockings for symptomatic varicose veins. *Eur J Vasc Endovasc Surg*, *50*(6), 794–801.

14. Rasmussen, L. H., Lawaetz, M., Lawaetz, B., Bjoern, L., *et al.* (2011). Randomized clinical trial comparing endovenous laser ablation, radiofrequency ablation, foam sclerotherapy and surgical stripping for great saphenous varicose veins. *J Br Surg, 98*(8), 1079–1087.
15. De Hert, S., De Baerdemaeker, L., & De Maeseneer, M. (2014). What the phlebologist should know about local anesthetics. *Phlebology, 29*(7), 428–441.
16. Arslan, Ü., Çalık, E., Tort, M., *et al.* (2017). More successful results with less energy in endovenous laser ablation treatment: long-term comparison of bare-tip fiber 980 nm laser and radial-tip fiber 1470 nm laser application. *Ann Vasc Surg, 45*, 166–172.
17. Malskat, W. S., Engels, L. K., Hollestein, L. M., *et al.* (2019). Commonly used endovenous laser ablation (EVLA) parameters do not influence efficacy: results of a systematic review and meta-analysis. *Eur J Vasc Endovasc Surg, 58*(2), 230–242.
18. Christenson, J. T., Gueddi, S., Gemayel, G., *et al.* (2010). Prospective randomized trial comparing endovenous laser ablation and surgery for treatment of primary great saphenous varicose veins with a 2-year follow-up. *J Vasc Surg, 52*, 1234–1241.
19. Healy, D. A., Kimura, S., Power, D., *et al.* (2018). A systematic review and meta-analysis of thrombotic events following endovenous thermal ablation of the great saphenous vein. *Eur J Vasc Endovasc Surg, 56*(3), 410–424.
20. Chi, Y. W., & Woods, T. C. (2014). Clinical risk factors to predict deep venous thrombosis post-endovenous laser ablation of saphenous veins. *Phlebology, 29*, 150–153.
21. Li, C., Jacobowitz, G. R., Rockman, C. B., *et al.* (2023). Superficial venous procedures can be performed safely and effectively in patients with deep venous reflux, *J Vasc Surg Ven Lymph Disord, 11*(2), 281–292.
22. Westin, G. G., Neal, S. C., Lee, V., *et al.* (2020). Radiofrequency and laser vein ablation of patients receiving warfarin anticoagulation is safe, effective, and durable. *J Vasc Surg Ven Lymph Disord, 8*(4), 610–616.
23. Chang, H., Sadek, M., Barfield, M. E., *et al.* (2023). Direct oral anticoagulant agents might be safe for patients undergoing endovenous radiofrequency and laser ablation. *J Vasc Surg Ven Lymph Disord, 11*(1), 25–30.
24. Kabnick, L. S., Sadek, M., Bjarnason, H., *et al.* (2021). Classification and treatment of endothermal heat-induced thrombosis: recommendations from the American venous forum and the society for vascular surgery. *J Vasc Surg Ven Lymph Disord, 9*(1), 6–22.
25. Merchant, R. F., & Pichot, O. (2005). Long-term outcomes of endovenous radiofrequency obliteration of saphenous reflux as a treatment for superficial venous insufficiency. *J Vasc Surg, 42*, 502–509.
26. Ahuja, A., Grant, T., Dumanian, G., *et al.* (2021). Development of traumatic neuromas in a patient following endovenous laser ablation and microphlebectomy procedures: a rare complication from the removal of varicose veins. *Cureus, 13*(6), e15830.
27. Shahid, K. R., Dellon, A. L., Amrami, K. K., *et al.* (2015). Sciatic and peroneal nerve injuries after endovascular ablation of lower extremity varicosities: case reports and review of the literature. *Annals of Plastic Surg, 74*(1), 64–68.

20

Renal artery revascularization

KAITLYN D. DOBESH AND ALEXANDER D. SHEPARD

INTRODUCTION

Advanced endovascular techniques—such as stenting and balloon angioplasty of the renal artery (RA) and fenestrated aortic endografts—have largely replaced open operative intervention for renal artery disease. Although many patients undergoing RA bypass are in the context of an open aortic aneurysm repair, some may still have need of an open operation for RA atherosclerotic disease, fibromuscular dysplasia, aneurysmal disease, mid-aortic syndrome, some complex suprarenal aneurysms (debranching), and failed prior endoluminal interventions.

INDICATIONS

Open aortic aneurysm repair patients can present with the need to undergo renal revascularization, including those where significant RA occlusive disease is present. Prophylactic revascularization has previously been investigated and found to have no benefit for patients with asymptomatic or severe unilateral renovascular disease. Only those with symptoms, including medically uncontrolled hypertension or rapidly deteriorating renal function, should be considered for renal artery revascularization. Patients who have demonstrated the most favorable renal recovery outcomes include those with severe hypertension, bilateral stenosis >90% or occlusion, or rapidly deteriorating renal function. When renal revascularization is done concomitantly with open reconstruction for aortic aneurysmal or occlusive disease, higher morbidity and post-operative dialysis rates have been demonstrated.

RENAL ARTERY EXPOSURE

There are several approaches utilized for exposure of the RAs—celiotomy with inframesocolic exposure or medial visceral rotation (MVR) from either side, and left flank retroperitoneal exposure. Celiotomy can be accomplished through a variety of incisions, the most versatile being an upper midline incision. However, with a unilateral procedure, most extra-aortic bypasses, or in the very obese, a subcostal or transverse incision may be advantageous. The most appropriate approach will be decided by the level of access needed to the suprarenal aorta, as well as whether a unilateral or bilateral exposure of the renal arteries is necessary and whether concomitant aortic reconstruction will be performed.

Inframesocolic

An inframesocolic approach provides good exposure of the proximal RAs bilaterally (Figure 20.1). The inframesocolic approach is a transperitoneal approach that starts with a midline celiotomy incision. The small bowel is retracted to the right and the transverse colon is reflected cephalad to expose the midline retroperitoneum. The posterior peritoneum is lifted and incised longitudinally directly over the infrarenal aorta. After entering the retroperitoneum, the fourth portion of the duodenum is dissected out and retracted to the right after dividing the ligament of Treitz. The left renal vein (RV) should now be identified crossing over the aorta and mobilized by dividing its adrenal, gonadal, and lumbar branches. Passing a large Penrose drain around the RV allows it to be reflected superiorly or inferiorly to expose the underlying renal arteries. Partially incising the left crus of the diaphragm may gain additional exposure of the proximal-most left RA. From this view, the proximal right RA can also be exposed with mobilization of the inferior vena cava (IVC) and left RV. This step sometimes requires ligation of a pair of lumbar veins that should be suture ligated on the IVC side to prevent possible suture dislodgement during subsequent manipulation with consequent bleeding. Overlying lymphatics should be divided with an ultrasonic scalpel or ligatures to prevent chyle leaks. Like the left side, partial division of the right diaphragmatic crus may provide additional exposure.

DOI: 10.1201/9781003452096-20

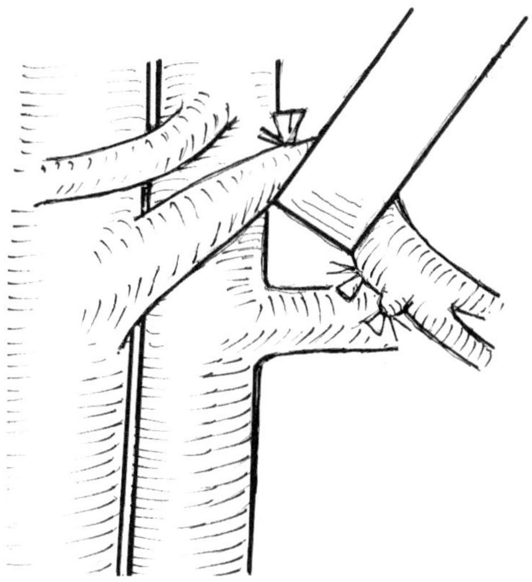

(a)

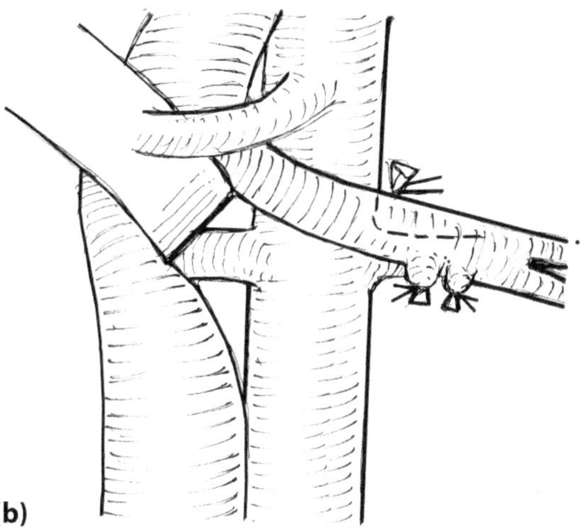

(b)

Figure 20.1 Transperitoneal, inframesocolic approach to pararenal aorta: (a) exposure of proximal left renal artery after extensive mobilization of left renal vein, including ligation and division of its adrenal, lumbar, and gonadal branches; (b) exposure of proximal right renal artery after mobilization of left renal vein and renal vein-caval junction.

Medial visceral rotation

If there is a need to access the aorta more proximally or to expose the RAs more distally, left or right medial visceral rotation (MVR) should be used. It is also a transperitoneal approach starting with a midline or transverse celiotomy. On the left side, the white line of Toldt of the descending colon is incised so that the colon can be reflected anteromedially allowing the creation of a retroperitoneal plane via blunt dissection lifting the spleen, tail of the pancreas (with the colonic flexure) to the patient's right. (See Figure 39.3 in Chapter 39.) This maneuver should expose the left kidney (which should remain down). Then the left renal vein can be mobilized from its position anterior to the artery by reflecting it either superiorly or inferiorly after dividing the adrenal, gonadal, and lumbar branches. This approach can also be used to expose the proximal

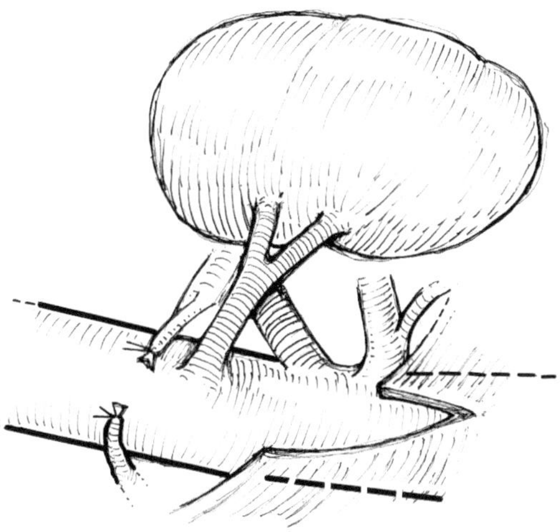

Figure 20.2 Oblique left flank retroperitoneal approach to the pararenal aorta and left renal artery. The left renal artery is identified just proximal to crossing lumbar branch of the left renal vein which has been ligated and divided. The left diaphragmatic crus has been divided longitudinally to expose the supraceliac aorta.

abdominal aorta by carrying the incision in the peritoneal reflection around the spleen toward the aortic hiatus. To expose the more distal right RA, the white line of Toldt is taken down to mobilize the right colon medially (partial right MVR). (See Figure 39.2 in Chapter 39.) The underlying duodenum is kocherized to expose the IVC and right RV. The right RV is carefully mobilized off the adjacent RA, dissecting it from the IVC junction distally, including ligation of any crossing branches.

Left flank retroperitoneal approach

The entire left renal artery and the ostial right renal artery can also be approached by a left flank retroperitoneal approach. An oblique left flank incision is made from the lateral edge of the rectus back into the tenth interspace for 10–15 cm. After dividing the abdominal wall and intercostal musculature, the retroperitoneal space is entered at the tip of the tenth rib and a plane created by sweeping the peritoneal sac and contents to the right. Using either a posterior to the kidney plane (easier) or an anterior plane, the entire left RA can be exposed. From a retrorenal plane, the left RA can be reliably identified as arising from the aorta just below a crossing lumbar branch of the left RV (Figure 20.2). It should be noted that when approached posteriorly, anteromedial retraction of the left kidney puts the left RA on considerable "stretch." Therefore, bypasses to the left RA in this position should always be performed under tension to avoid graft redundancy/kinking when the kidney is returned to its normal anatomic position. Left RA exposure through a plane anterior to the kidney leaves the kidney in its normal anatomic position but like left MVR requires mobilization of the left RV. Only the proximal-most right RA can be exposed through this flank approach and requires a dissection plane anterior to the left kidney, leaving the left kidney in place. So this approach is useful only for transaortic endarterectomy of the right RA as opposed to bypass. The left RA is amenable to either procedure from the flank.

AORTORENAL BYPASS

When performed from an inframesocolic approach, the infrarenal aorta just below the RAs is exposed through the same midline retroperitoneal incision used to expose the RAs. Several centimeters of undiseased aorta are mobilized in preparation for clamping and the creation of a proximal graft to aorta anastomosis. With aneurysmal or occlusive disease of the aorta, graft replacement of the aorta may be necessary to create a suitable inflow site. After systemic anticoagulation, the aorta is clamped proximally and distally, taking care to control any intervening lumbar arteries. Some authors have described using a side-biting, partially occluding clamp but this can sometimes be cumbersome unless the aorta is completely normal. An aortotomy is created with a #11 blade on the lateral aspect of the aorta a few centimeters below the RAs and enlarged with an appropriately sized aortic punch or by removing a small ellipse of the aortic wall. The resulting aortic opening should be a bit larger in diameter than the chosen graft. The graft is trimmed with a slightly upward bevel and sewn to the aorta with a running 5-0 Prolene suture using the parachute technique. After ensuring a hemostatic anastomosis, attention is directed to the target RA, which is clamped distally. The proximal RA is then suture ligated with a 4-0 Prolene. Care should be taken not to place this stitch through a calcified segment of artery or risk it falling apart. The artery is transected distally at the site of the proposed anastomosis and the end is spatulated in preparation for an end-to-end graft anastomosis with 5-0 Prolene (Figure 20.3). For more distal right RA bypasses, the graft should be tunneled retrocaval if possible [1].

The saphenous vein has historically been the recommended conduit, though in young patients and

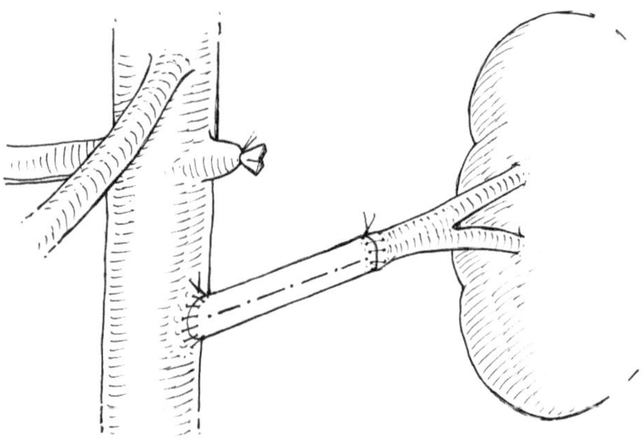

Figure 20.3 Aortorenal bypass with end-to-side proximal aortic anastomosis and end-to-end anastomosis to the left renal artery.

adolescents, there is a very real risk of aneurysmal degeneration over 20 years. In older patients, polytetrafluoroethylene (6–7 mm in diameter) is acceptable. The hypogastric artery has been used for pediatric patients with good results. When the patient is undergoing concomitant aortic reconstruction, a small caliber side-arm graft should be sewn on to the aortic prosthesis after careful consideration of graft orientation and configuration.

TRANSAORTIC RENAL ENDARTERECTOMY

Transaortic renal endarterectomy is a good technique for patients with bilateral ostial stenoses, particularly when associated with significant pararenal aortic plaque. Such stenoses essentially represent overflow disease of the aortic wall. Short-segment atherosclerotic disease within 1–1.5 cm of the origin of the RAs is amenable to this approach, especially if associated with post-stenotic dilatation, a marker of focal disease with a clear endpoint. This technique is particularly helpful with multiple RAs. It requires extensive mobilization of the pararenal aorta and the two (or more) RAs as well as the left RV. If plaque extends to involve the paravisceral aorta, then consideration of endarterectomy of this segment should be given. Similarly, infrarenal disease may require concomitant endarterectomy, or more commonly, prosthetic grafting. The necessary exposure usually requires a full left MVR or a left flank retroperitoneal approach, though an inframesocolic approach is suitable if there is at least 4 cm between the SMA and the most proximal RA. It is important to control lumbar arteries in the intervening segment as back bleeding from these branches can be a major impediment during endarterectomy. Because of the need for suprarenal aortic cross-clamping, good communication with the anesthesia team is critical.

After systemic anticoagulation, the aorta is clamped proximal and distal to the renal arteries and a longitudinal aortotomy extending 3 cm proximal and distal to the RAs is made. A cleavage plane is established in the aortic wall in the outer layers of the media and aortic plaque is separated circumferentially around the two renal ostia. Plaque extending into the RAs is carefully removed via eversion endarterectomy into the aortic lumen after transecting the aortic plaque both proximally and distally (Figure 20.4). The endpoints in both RAs and the distal aorta are carefully inspected to ensure that there is no potential for significant flap formation. The aortotomy is then closed with a running 4-0 Prolene suture. Patch angioplasty can also be utilized if necessary to avoid narrowing the lumen of a small aorta. If a concomitant infrarenal aortic reconstruction is to be performed for occlusive disease, the aorta can be transected a few centimeters distal to the longitudinal aortotomy and the intervening segment endarterectomized prior to aortotomy closure.

Alternatively, when an infrarenal aortic reconstruction is planned, the infrarenal aorta can be transected 1–2 cm below the RAs and the endarterectomy performed

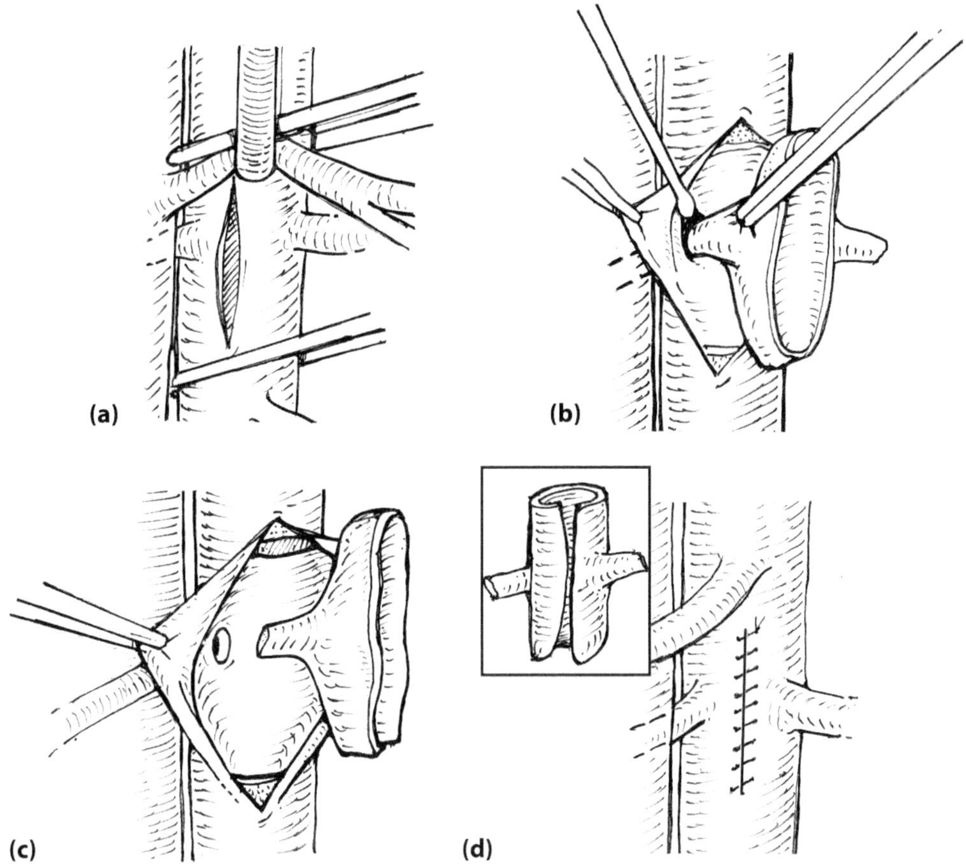

Figure 20.4 Transaortic endarterectomy of proximal renal arteries: (a) longitudinal aortotomy from just below the SMA to just below the renal arteries; (b) endarterectomy of pararenal aorta with circumferential mobilization of plaque in right renal artery origin prior to eversion endarterectomy; (c) tail of aortic plaque being removed from right renal artery. Note that aortic plaque has been transected proximally and distally; (d) aortotomy closure; inset shows sleeve of aortic wall plaque including origins of both renal arteries.

through the transected aorta (Figure 20.5) [2]. Following completion of the endarterectomy, a prosthetic aortic graft is sewn end-to-end to the endarterectomized cuff of the aorta using a 4-0 Prolene on a smaller needle given the thinned-out nature of the aorta. Full thickness circumferential aortic endarterectomy should be avoided in aneurysmal aorta. We routinely check the RA endarterectomy site with intraoperative duplex to ensure a good result.

EXTRA-ANATOMIC BYPASS

Extra-anatomic bypass is an option for those patients who either cannot tolerate an aortic cross clamp to create an aorto-renal bypass or whose aorta is too calcified for an anastomosis. Prior to considering an extra-anatomic bypass from the hepatic or splenic artery, it is necessary to rule out a celiac artery stenosis.

Hepatorenal bypass

If a hepatorenal bypass to the right renal artery is anticipated, an extended right transverse or vertical upper midline incision can be used. During positioning, use

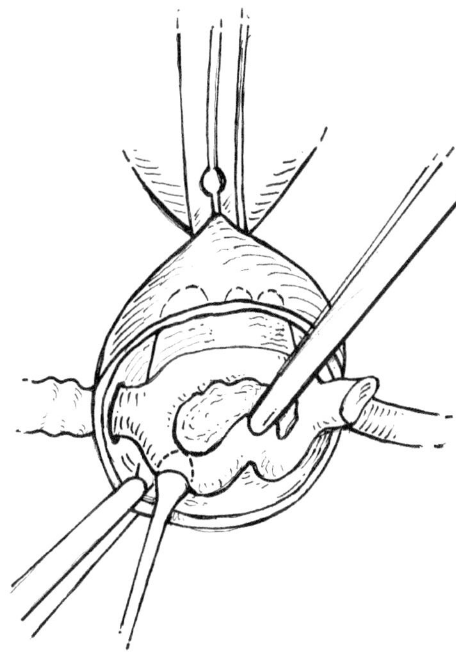

Figure 20.5 Transaortic endarterectomy of proximal renal arteries along with adjacent cuff of aorta performed through transected aorta just below the renal arteries.

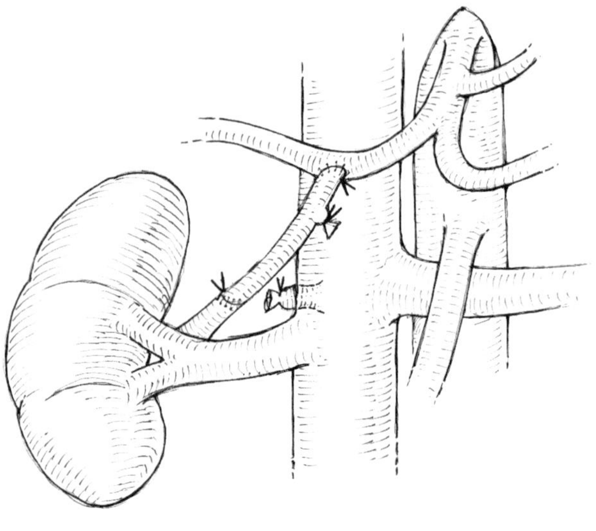

Figure 20.6 Hepatorenal bypass with a saphenous vein graft anastomosed end-to-side to common hepatic artery proximally (at the site of gastroduodenal artery takeoff) and end-to-end to right renal artery.

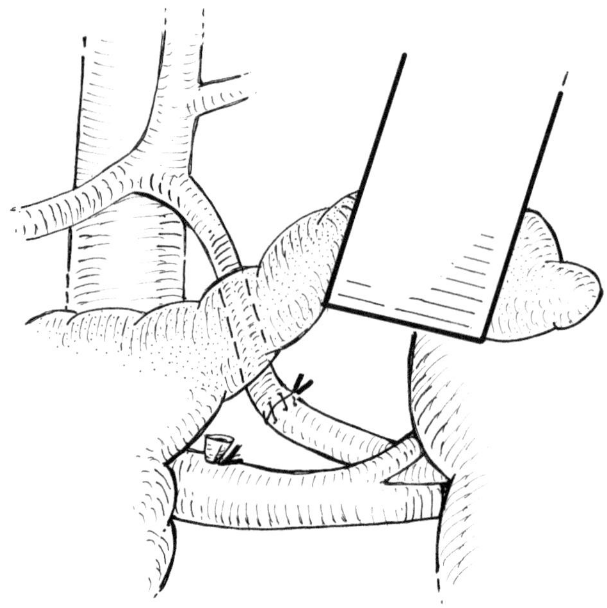

Figure 20.7 Splenorenal bypass with mobilized splenic artery anastomosed end-to-end to the left renal artery; the distal splenic artery is ligated.

of a right flank roll may be helpful. The hepatic artery is accessed by retracting the bowel inferiorly and the liver superiorly to expose the gastrohepatic ligament. The ligament should be palpated and inspected for a replaced left hepatic artery before entering the lesser sac. The common hepatic artery is dissected out along its course anterior to the pancreas until the gastroduodenal branch and proper hepatic are identified. An interposition saphenous vein graft is anastomosed end-to-side to the common hepatic artery often incorporating the stump of the gastroduodenal artery that has been ligated distally. The typical path of the graft runs anterior to the inferior vena cava. The distal anastomosis is then created in an end-to-end fashion with the spatulated right renal artery (Figure 20.6) [3].

Splenorenal bypass

If a splenorenal bypass for the left renal artery is anticipated, an extended left transverse or vertical upper midline incision can be used. Improved exposure of the splenic artery can be achieved with mobilization of the splenic flexure of the colon by taking down the white line of Toldt of the flexure and reflecting it down and medially. The gastrosplenic ligament can be incised partially, as well, but with care taken, as the left gastroepiploic artery collaterals will be present in this plane. The splenic artery is carefully mobilized from the superior margin of the pancreas toward the splenic hilum. Splenorenal bypass has two options for anastomosis. If the splenic artery is sufficiently redundant, it may be ligated distally and anastomosed in an end-to-end fashion with the renal artery to create a direct bypass (Figure 20.7). Splenic perfusion is maintained through collateral supply from the short gastrics and left gastroepiploic artery. If there is not sufficient length, then an interposition bypass can be created with either vein or a PTFE conduit.

Iliorenal bypass

Another option for patients who are not candidates for aortorenal bypass is to originate a renal bypass from the ipsilateral iliac artery. There should be no hemodynamically significant aortoiliac disease in this situation and the iliac (proximal) anastomotic site should be disease free. The iliac is exposed by reflecting the cecum and ascending colon medially on the right and the sigmoid and descending colon on the left. A retroperitoneal tunnel to the ipsilateral RA can be easily created before construction of anastomoses with 5-0 Prolene (Figure 20.8).

INTRAOPERATIVE RENAL PROTECTION

With an obligatory period of renal ischemia, care should be taken to minimize renal injury. Stopping potentially nephrotoxic drugs preoperatively, ensuring good hydration, and avoiding intraoperative hypotension seem obvious. Maintaining a good urine output prior to clamping is also obvious but frequently forgotten and requires good communication with the anesthesia team. Administration of mannitol is controversial but if nothing else, can boost urine output. We routinely administer 25 g 20 minutes prior to anticipated clamp time. Infusion of a cold renal protection solution (4° heparinized Ringers' lactate + mannitol + methylprednisolone) directly into the RA(s) is beneficial when clamp times are anticipated to exceed 25 minutes or when baseline chronic kidney disease (serum Cr $\geq$1.3 mg/dL) is present. We typically infuse through

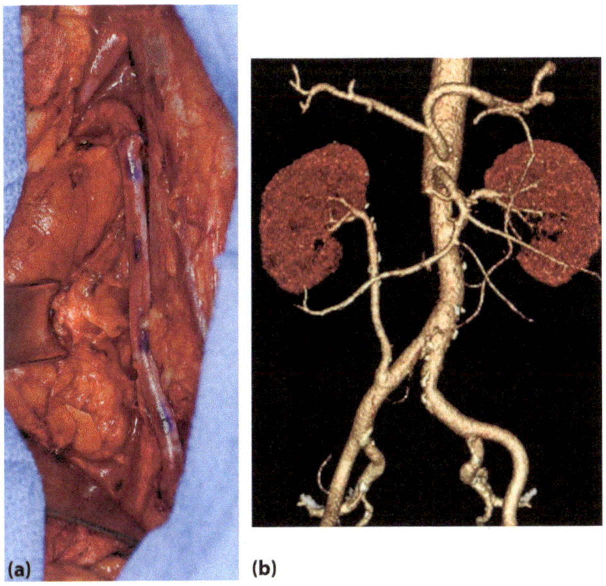

Figure 20.8 (a) Right iliorenal bypass with reversed saphenous vein graft. (b) Post-op CT angiogram showing patent right iliorenal bypass. (Courtesy TJ Nypaver.)

a small pediatric feeding tube (8 Fr) or a 9 Fr Pruitt balloon tipped infusion catheter (LeMaitre Vascular, Inc., Burlington, MA, USA) [4].

POST-OPERATIVE CARE

All patients should be closely observed post-operatively, usually in a critical care unit where hourly urine output can be monitored for the first 24 hours. Post-ischemic acute kidney injury can sometimes manifest as a brisk diuresis for the first 12 hours, which should be treated with appropriate fluid and electrolyte replacement. Hypokalemia and hypomagnesiumia are the most common findings when this occurs. Post-operative complications are all those of a major abdominal operation. A sudden drop in urine output might herald graft occlusion and should be investigated with a renal duplex. Patients should be maintained on an aspirin and statin post-operatively, usually for life. Renal artery duplexes should be performed at first follow-up, every six months for the first two years and then annually. Serum creatinine and GFR should also be monitored at regular intervals as a possible indicator of stenosis.

OUTCOMES

The goals of RA reconstruction are to improve hypertension control and preserve/improve renal function. In appropriately selected patients, all these goals can be met, though outright cure of hypertension is rare. The mortality of isolated RA bypass is low, approaching 1–2%, but when combined with aortic reconstruction can be considerably higher (5%).

TRICKS AND TRAPS

- Midline celiotomy with a transperitoneal, inframesocolic approach is the most used exposure of the proximal renal arteries.
- Distal renal artery exposure is accomplished by medial visceral rotation–on the right, this involves mobilization/reflection of the ascending colon and a Kocher maneuver, and on the left, mobilization of the splenic flexure, spleen, and pancreas.
- Mobilization of the renal vein is necessary to expose the underlying renal artery. On the left, this usually requires division of its adrenal, gonadal, and lumbar branches.
- If a left flank approach to left renal bypass is performed, it should be under slight tension, as the left renal artery is usually on "stretch" when approached posteriorly. This decreases the risk of redundancy or kinking when the left kidney is returned to its normal anatomic position.
- When performing a transaortic eversion endarterectomy of the RAs, look for native vessel dilatation just beyond the stenosis, which is usually an indicator of a clean endpoint.
- With transaortic endarterectomy of the RAs, extensive mobilization of the pararenal aorta is necessary, including control of lumbar arteries in the intervening aortic segment.
- When the aorta is too calcified for safe clamping or the patient too high-risk for aortic clamping, alternative inflow sites for RA bypass should be considered.

QUESTIONS

1. Exposure of bilateral proximal RAs is best accomplished through which approach?
   a. Right medial visceral rotation
   b. Left flank retroperitoneal approach
   c. Midline, transperitoneal with inframesocolic approach
   d. Left subcostal with medial visceral rotation
   e. Midline, transperitoneal with approach through the lesser sac

   Answer: c

2. The best method of renal protection during renal revascularization is:
   a. Good hydration preoperatively
   b. Administration of mannitol prior to clamping the RA
   c. Infusion of cold preservation solution
   d. Passive hypothermia
   e. There is no single "best" method of renal protection that applies in all situations of renal revascularization

   Answer: e

3. Transaortic RA endarterectomy is most appropriate for:
   a. Bilateral, long-segment RA stenoses
   b. Unilateral RA disease
   c. Bilateral, proximal RA stenoses
   d. Bilateral, proximal RA stenoses with post-stenotic dilatation
   e. Bilateral, proximal RA occlusions

   Answer: d

4. With a "porcelain" aorta unsuitable for clamping, the best approach for right RA revascularization may be:
   a. Supraceliac aorta to RA bypass
   b. Transaortic RA endarterectomy
   c. Superior mesenteric artery to RA bypass
   d. Hepatorenal bypass
   e. Left iliorenal bypass

   Answer: d

REFERENCES

1. Benjamin ME, Dean RH. Techniques in renal artery reconstruction: Part I. *Ann Vasc Surg.* 1996;10(3):306–314.
2. Stoney RJ, Messina LM, Goldstone J, Reilly LM. Renal endarterectomy through the transected aorta: A new technique for combined aortorenal atherosclerosis. *J Vasc Surg.* 1989;9(2): 224–233.
3. Benjamin ME, Dean RH. Techniques in renal artery reconstruction: Part II. *Ann Vasc Surg.* 1996;10(4):409–414.
4. Grab J, Krzyzaniak H, Devrome A, Moore R. Efficacy of cold renal perfusion protection for open complex aortic aneurysm repair: a metaanalysis. *Can J Surg.* 2022;65(6):805–815.

21

Carotid endarterectomy

SACHINDER S. HANS

INTRODUCTION

Carotid endarterectomy (CEA) is one of the most common arterial reconstructions performed by vascular surgeons. Technical aspects of the operation and appropriate patient selection are key to achieving satisfactory outcomes because a slight technical imperfection may result in a serious postoperative complication, for example, stroke. The primary indications for CEA are patients with:

- Recent mild-to-moderate stroke in the distribution of the middle cerebral artery (MCA) (and occasionally in the anterior cerebral artery) with good recovery.
- Transient contralateral motor or sensory deficits or ipsilateral amaurosis fugax (transient loss of vision; this may be either partial or complete and usually lasts for less than one hour).
- Symptomatic high-grade internal carotid artery (ICA) stenosis (>80% stenosis) in selected patients who are otherwise good risk and have at least five years of life expectancy.

Following clinical evaluation, carotid duplex imaging is performed. Imaging studies, such as computed tomography angiography (CTA) of the carotid artery, are often necessary to further evaluate the cervical carotid artery, for example, when the distal end of the plaque is not visualized by the duplex scan or when disease proximal and/or distal to the bifurcation is suspected. CT scans or magnetic resonance imaging (MRI) and magnetic resonance angiography (MRA) of the brain are performed in patients who exhibit focal neurologic symptoms and positive neurologic findings. MRA tends to overestimate the degree of stenosis by 15–20%.

Anesthetic choice (regional versus general) has been a matter of considerable debate over many years. Although the General Anaesthesia versus Local Anaesthesia for Carotid Surgery (GALA) trial showed no difference in the outcomes of patients undergoing CEA, under either cervical block anesthesia (CBA) or general anesthesia (GA), the author prefers CBA in most patients [1]. However, in patients with plaque extending cephalad, thereby requiring more extensive dissection (determined by preoperative imaging studies), those with extreme anxiety, and patients who are hearing impaired and/or have poor command of the language, GA is preferred.

SHUNT PLACEMENT DURING CEA

Most surgeons favor either routine or selective use of a carotid shunt. Selective shunting is based on intraoperative monitoring with ICA stump pressure (SP) (back pressure), electroencephalography, or transcranial Doppler monitoring under GA *or* continuous neurologic assessment when CEA is performed in awake patients under CBA. There have been a few case series, mostly historical, reporting satisfactory outcomes without shunt placement under GA. The rate of shunt placement for CEA in awake patients is 8–12% and in patients under GA (with neurologic monitoring) 15–18% [2–5]. In the presence of contralateral ICA/common carotid artery (CCA) occlusion, the rate of shunt use increases up to 20% under CBA [2].

POSITIONING

The neck is hyperextended by a roll behind the scapulae and an occipital support. The neck is turned toward the contralateral site. Incision options include either a transverse (skin fold) or oblique (anterior sternocleidomastoid) incision; the latter is often preferable because of better cosmesis, however, exposure can be limited. If the plaque extends considerably distally into the ICA or proximally into the CCA, an oblique incision provides better exposure. In patients with short necks, adhesive tape is applied to the shoulder, pulled downward, and attached to the operating table to improve access to the space between the clavicle and mandible.

DOI: 10.1201/9781003452096-21

Duplex imaging with evaluation of the carotid bifurcation in relation to the angle of the mandible and CTA (carotid bifurcation in relation to the level of the cervical vertebral bodies) are good guides for the length of the incision and its extension proximally or distally.

TECHNIQUE

An oblique incision is made, with the lower end of the incision 2 cm anterior to the anterior border of sternocleidomastoid muscle (SCM) and the upper end of the incision 2 cm posterior to the anterior border of the SCM (Figure 21.1). The platysma muscle is incised and the transverse cutaneous nerve is divided with scissors after infiltrating local anesthesia (LA); this is because when electrocautery is used to divide the nerve in awake patients, it leads to considerable discomfort. Any crossing external jugular vein and branches are ligated and divided. The greater auricular nerve is seen in the superior aspect of the incision; usually, it can be preserved.

Two toothed forceps are used to lift the skin and platysma (medial flap) superiorly. With Metzenbaum scissors, the dissection plane is developed along the anterior border of the SCM.

Two blunt Weitlaner retractors are placed superiorly and inferiorly, and a dissection plane is developed along the medial border of the internal jugular vein (IJV) in the lower part of the exposure. As the dissection proceeds cephalad along the medial border of the IJV, the common facial vein and its branches are individually ligated and divided. Superior to the common facial vein, deep cervical lymph nodes and fascia are carefully dissected and mobilized laterally. In the lower portion of the incision, the middle thyroid vein is ligated and divided as needed.

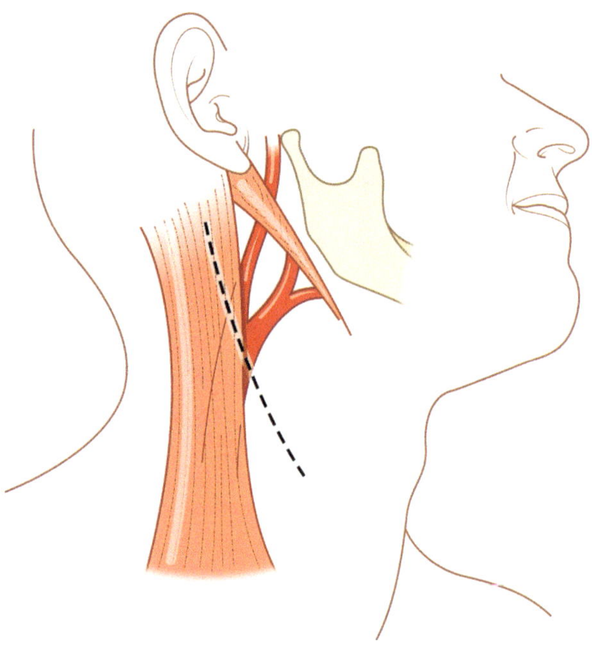

Figure 21.1 Line of skin incision.

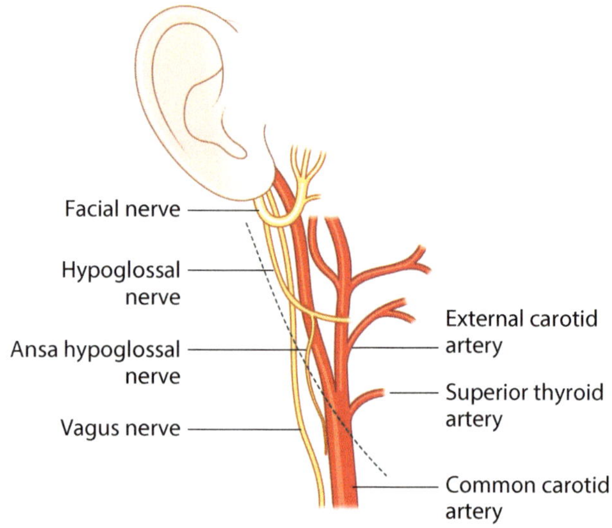

Figure 21.2 Anatomical relationship of the carotid bifurcation.

The carotid sheath is opened. The CCA is double-looped with a silastic vessel loop. The entire premise of the dissection is that both CCAs and ICAs are left in their bed and the patient is dissected away from the artery rather than performing extensive mobilization of the carotid artery, which can lead to embolization of intraluminal debris with serious consequences.

The external carotid artery (ECA) is double-looped with a silastic loop; tension is put on the loop caudally with a straight hemostat to get better distal exposure of the ICA above the bifurcation. The ansa cervicalis is seen anteriorly in the carotid sheath and is mobilized anteriorly. The vagus nerve is seen posteriorly between the IJV and the CCA; however, in the lower portion of the incision, the nerve can be seen lying in a more anterolateral plane and is carefully preserved (Figure 21.2). In the superior aspect of the exposure, small veins draining into the IJV are ligated and divided along with the sternocleidomastoid artery branch (sometimes two branches) off the occipital artery or ECA. The hypoglossal nerve (HGN) is visualized just below the posterior belly of the digastric muscle, with the superior end of the vagus nerve, which is closely related to the HGN about 3–4 cm beyond the origin of the ICA. Lidocaine 1% is infiltrated into the carotid body region to prevent bradycardia. Intravenous heparin (100 IU/kg) is given by the anesthesia team and the activated clotting time is monitored (250–300 seconds).

STUMP PRESSURE

A mean SP of 40 mmHg is considered a reasonable cutoff as a guide to shunt placement. In general, patients with SP >40 mmHg can tolerate carotid clamping provided systemic pressure does not decrease during the performance of CEA. Various types of shunts are available and include the Javid™ Peripheral Carotid Bypass Shunt

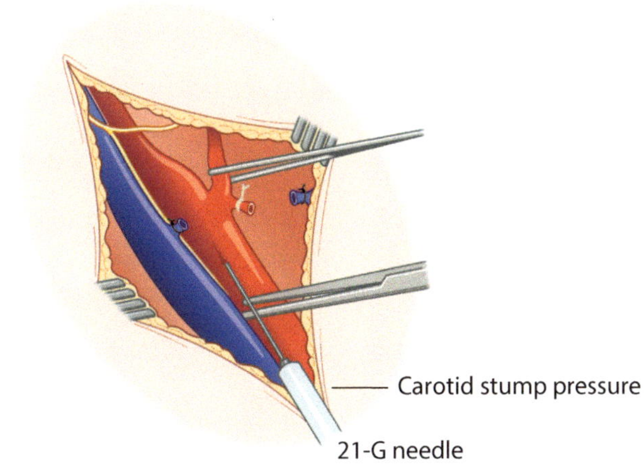

Figure 21.3 Measurement of carotid stump pressure.

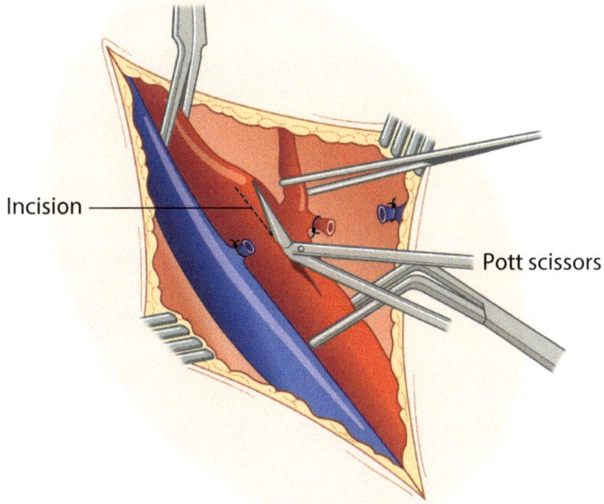

Figure 21.4 Arteriotomy incision in the distal common carotid artery and proximal internal carotid artery showing proximal and distal clamping.

(BARD Peripheral Vascular, Inc., Tempe, AZ, USA), the Argyle™ Carotid Artery Shunt (Medtronic, Minneapolis, MN, USA), the Pruitt-Inahara® Carotid Shunt (LeMaitre Vascular, Inc., Burlington, MA, USA), and the Sundt™ Carotid Endarterectomy Shunt (Integra LifeSciences Corporation, Plainsboro, NJ, USA). Surgeons should use the shunt they are most comfortable with during CEA. The author prefers the Sundt™ Shunt because of its relative ease of insertion and its flexibility. SP is measured by inserting a 21-G needle into the CCA after the proximal CCA and ECA have been clamped, and pressure tubing is connected to a recording monitor (Figure 21.3).

After applying an angled proximal vascular clamp to the CCA, the distal ICA is occluded with a Micro Kitzmiller clamp (Scanlan International, Inc., St. Paul, MN, USA) or a Yasergil clip (Aesculap Central Valley, PA, USA) and the double vessel loop is tightened and pulled caudally around the ECA. An arteriotomy is made in the distal CCA with a #11 blade and extended into the ICA and more proximally into CCA beyond all significant plaque with angled Potts scissors (Figure 21.4). In patients undergoing CEA for stroke, the ICA is not clamped because a recent thrombus may be present in the distal ICA and retrograde bleeding from the ICA will aid in extrusion of the thrombus, following which, the distal vascular clamp is applied to the ICA.

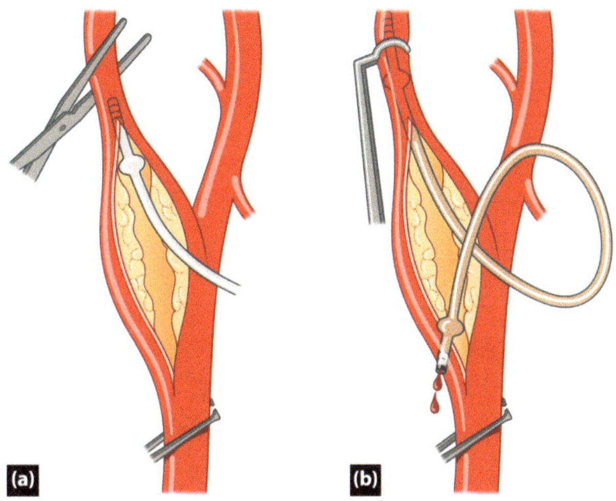

Figure 21.5 Endarterectomy technique. (a) Insertion of the distal end of the shunt. (b) Back-bleeding from the proximal end of the shunt.

TECHNIQUE OF SHUNT PLACEMENT

The smaller end of the Sundt™ Carotid Endarterectomy Shunt is inserted into the ICA and held in place with the smaller-size Javid shunt clamp. Retrograde bleeding occurs from the proximal end of the shunt, which is inserted into the CCA and held in place with the large Javid shunt clamp along with cinching down the proximal double vessel loop so that the shunt does not accidentally dislodge from the proximal end (Figures 21.5–21.8). In patients with soft plaque in the middle segment of the CCA, it may be preferable to insert the proximal end of the shunt to extrude any embolic plaque and then clamp the shunt with a Fogarty soft jaw clamp before inserting the distal end of the shunt into the ICA to prevent plaque emboli migrating into the brain. Shunt flow should be checked with a Doppler flow probe.

Plaque dissection is started with a Freer-Type elevator at the thickest portion of the plaque and then continued distally into the ICA until the plaque tapers smoothly like an onion peel. Plaque is removed from the ECA with an eversion technique and the carotid bifurcation plaque is then dissected proximally and sharply divided with Potts scissors (Figure 21.8). Irrigation of the endarterectomy site is performed with heparinized saline, removing loose

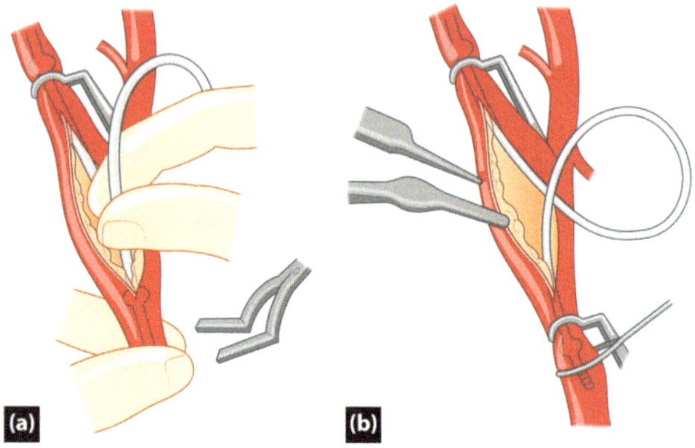

Figure 21.6 Endarterectomy technique. (a) Proximal insertion of the shunt into the common carotid artery. (b) Plaque dissection with the shunt in place.

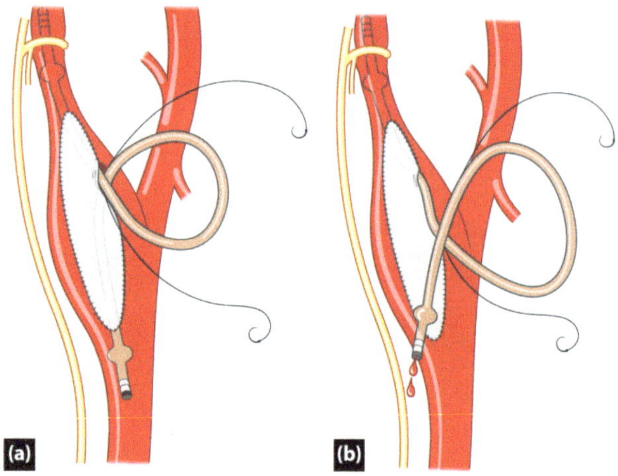

Figure 21.7 Endarterectomy technique. (a) Shunt with closure of endarterectomy with patch. (b) Removal of shunt from the common carotid artery

fibers of the media or any flimsy tissue debris. When a perfectly feathered distal breakoff point of the plaque cannot be obtained, tacking stitches should be placed to prevent dissection of the distal artery. This can be accomplished with U-shaped stitches of 7-0 polypropylene. The U-shaped stitches are placed parallel to the flow of blood in the artery, with one side of the stitch about 2 mm distal to the end point of the endarterectomy on one side and 2 mm proximal to the end point on the other. Stitches are placed across the back wall of the artery (Figure 21.9).

The author routinely patches all carotid artery closures unless the arteries are of extremely generous size (ICA diameter ≥6 mm) where patching would result in an aneurysmal artery. Patch selection is up to the individual surgeon, with no study demonstrating the superiority of one material over another. Bovine pericardium, PTFE, Dacron, and vein are all acceptable materials. Suturing is started distally in the ICA with a continuous 7-0 polypropylene suture and continued proximally. At the proximal end, the patch is divided and sutured to the CCA with a

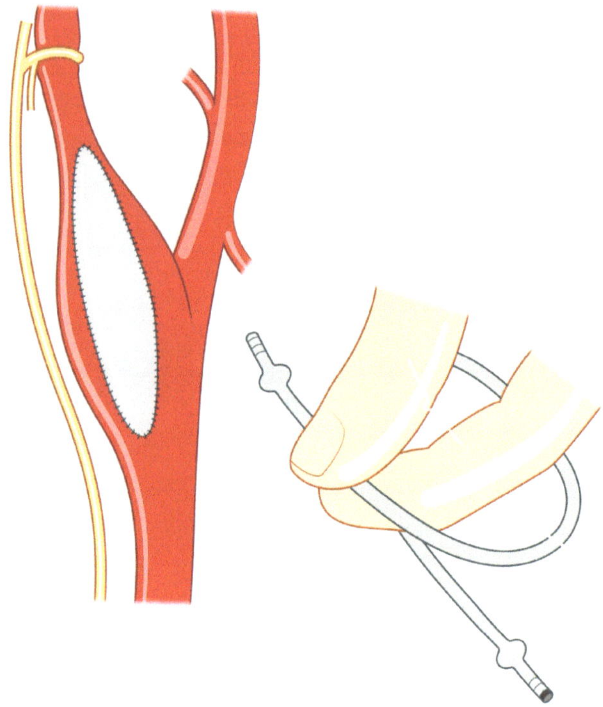

Figure 21.8 Removal of shunt; completion of patch closure.

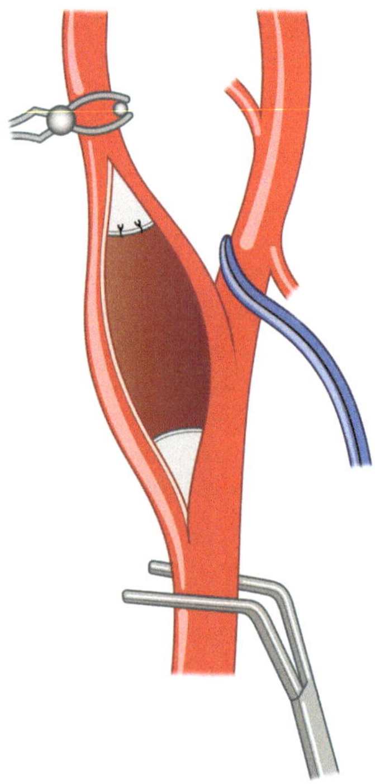

Figure 21.9 Endarterectomy site with tacking sutures.

6-0 polypropylene suture and the suturing is continued distally. On the medial side, suturing is completed; on the lateral side of the arteriotomy, the shunt protruding out of the artery prevents further closure. The shunt is first removed from the CCA. A proximal vascular clamp is applied, the shunt is removed from the ICA, and the ICA is clamped. The remaining suture line closure is rapidly completed. After the suture line closure is completed, the clamp is removed from the ECA first, the CCA second, and the ICA last to minimize the risk of cerebral embolism of any remaining debris/clot, and so on. Heparin is reversed with protamine sulfate; Protamine decreases serious bleeding complications at the time of CEA without increasing the risk of MI, stroke, or death.

COMPLICATIONS: NECK HEMATOMA

Neck hematoma is usually secondary to venous bleeding but can also result from unsatisfactory closure of the arteriotomy. Reactive airway edema can result from even small hematomas and result in upper airway compromise mandating intubation and hematoma evacuation.

Large, tense hematomas can cause compression of the airway and esophagus. They are considered an emergency and should be evacuated in the operating room immediately. It can be difficult to perform oral tracheal intubation in a patient with a large neck hematoma; therefore, it is preferable to evacuate the hematoma by removing the sutures under LA, which relieves pressure on the airway, and continue the procedure either under LA or subsequent maintenance of the airway by the anesthesiologist and GA, if necessary.

HEMODYNAMIC INSTABILITY

Patients undergoing CEA may develop hypotension associated with bradycardia during and in the first six hours after CEA. This is the result of carotid sinus nerve (CSN) stimulation and can be prevented in most instances by blocking the CSN during CEA with an injection of LA. Hypertension during and immediately after CEA occurs frequently and is more common in patients with uncontrolled blood pressure before the procedure. Hypertension during and following CEA needs immediate control with intravenous antihypertensive medication like labetalol hydrochloride, hydralazine hydrochloride, sodium nitroprusside, or nitroglycerine. The author and others have reported less hemodynamic lability in patients undergoing CEA under CBA.

CRANIAL NERVE PALSY

The HGN is the most common cranial nerve injured during CEA. Temporary HGN palsy (tongue deviation to the ipsilateral side) and vagal paresis (hoarseness) are not uncommon following CEA. Permanent nerve damage is suspected if there is no recovery of nerve function in three months. The transverse cutaneous nerve must be divided during neck incision, resulting in temporary loss of sensation anterior to the incision. Glossopharyngeal nerve injuries can occur in patients undergoing CEA for high plaque. Injury to the ramus mandibularis (mandibular nerve) can occur if dissection is done too close to the angle of the mandible, resulting in flattening of the lower lip. If a contralateral CEA is planned, a vocal cord functional assessment by an ear, nose, and throat surgeon is necessary before the procedure is contemplated, even in the absence of discernible hoarseness, because bilateral vagal nerve injury may necessitate a tracheostomy. Injury to the external laryngeal nerve resulting in loss of pitch of the voice can occur during mobilization of the superior thyroid artery. Injury to the spinal accessory nerve is uncommon.

POSTOPERATIVE STROKE

This is the second most dreaded complication of CEA [6]. Most post-CEA strokes are embolic, and in these patients, further surgical intervention may not be helpful. However, in patients with embolic occlusion of the main trunk of the MCA or its superior or inferior branches, neurovascular intervention with the Solitaire™ revascularization device (Medtronic, Minneapolis, MN, USA) can achieve successful recanalization and neurologic recovery if performed within eight hours of neurologic deficit. In patients, stroke can also develop secondary to cerebral ischemia because of a lack of shunt placement or the malfunction of a shunt in patients who do not tolerate carotid clamping. If a patient has a new neurologic deficit (minutes-to-hours) post-CEA, thrombosis should be suspected; the patient should undergo an immediate head CT (usually negative) to rule out a bleed and should be taken back to the operating room for carotid re-exploration and thrombectomy. There may be a distal intimal flap causing the thrombosis. Flap removal, use of tacking sutures, and a completion arteriogram should be performed. Given the widespread availability and speed of obtaining a high-quality CTA, such imaging can often be performed before a possible return to the OR and can help plan intervention. Intracerebral hemorrhage is a rare complication that may occur (usually between two and five days) in patients with uncontrolled hypertension and severe contralateral ICA disease, high-grade stenosis/occlusion; this is the result of hyperperfusion syndrome. Hyperperfusion syndrome in its mild form may manifest as post-CEA headache (common) that should resolve in a few days, or post-CEA seizures and intracerebral hemorrhage in its most severe form. Postoperative seizures are more common in patients undergoing CEA for stroke and usually respond to antiseizure medication but may be associated with postictal paralysis.

POSTOPERATIVE MYOCARDIAL INFARCTION AND CARDIAC ARRHYTHMIAS

The incidence of postoperative myocardial infarction should be less than 1% and is diagnosed by elevated serum troponin levels; an electrocardiogram and cardiology consult should be obtained. The patient may not experience classic chest pain or the typical symptoms of myocardial infarction following CEA.

PATCH GRAFT INFECTION

Synthetic patch graft infection, though rare, can be a very serious complication of CEA and requires removal of the patch with autogenous reconstruction using saphenous vein graft for patching or as an interposition graft. With an extensive infection within the cutaneous sinus, a myocutaneous flap by a plastic reconstructive surgeon may become necessary.

CAROTID ENDARTERECTOMY FOR HIGH PLAQUE

CEA for high plaque within the distal ICA can be an extremely challenging operation. High plaque is defined as plaque within the ICA that extends cephalad to the inferior border of the C2 vertebral body. Difficulty with CEA for high plaque is exacerbated in patients who have short necks or high carotid bifurcations. In most patients, high plaque can be anticipated by preoperative imaging studies (carotid duplex exam, CTA, or conventional digital subtraction angiography). However, in some patients, distally extending plaque is an unexpected finding at the time of CEA.

Additional exposure of the distal portion of the cervical ICA may be obtained by extending the skin incision cephalad and posteriorly behind the ear. Other aids in exposure include removal of the carotid sinus nerve branches at the carotid bifurcation and placing a double vessel loop around the external carotid artery with caudal traction using a hemostat at the end of the loop to the drape on the chest wall. As the dissection proceeds distally, the sternocleidomastoid branch of the occipital artery and the veins crossing the hypoglossal nerve are carefully ligated and divided. Division of the occipital artery helps in cephalad mobilization of the hypoglossal nerve, which can be looped carefully with a silastic loop. The posterior belly of the digastric muscle should be mobilized and divided if necessary. Similarly, the stylohyoid muscle may also be transected [7].

If further exposure is required, the styloid process can be carefully removed with a rongeur. In this maneuver, care should be taken to prevent injury to the glossopharyngeal nerve. In most instances, distal control can be obtained with a balloon occlusion catheter or a 4 mm or 4.5 mm Pilling dilator. After, plaque removal patch closure is started at the distal apex of the arteriotomy. Suturing is continued caudally on the artery; when the hypoglossal nerve is encountered, the patch and suture are passed under the nerve and suturing is completed in the standard fashion (Figures 21.10–21.12).

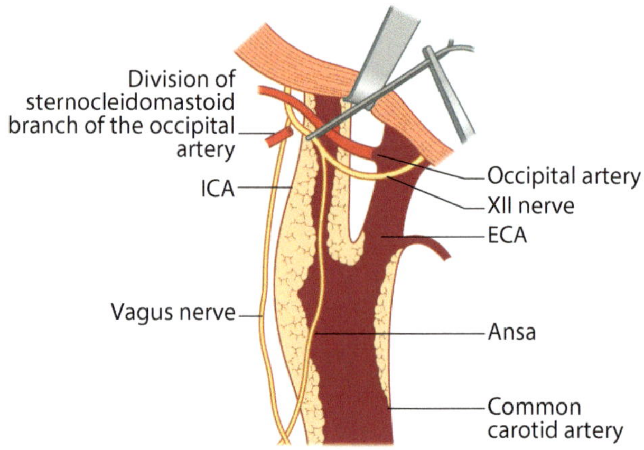

Figure 21.10 Exposure of common carotid artery and distal internal carotid artery for high plaque with upward retraction on the posterior belly of the digastric muscle and a silastic vessel loop around the hypoglossal nerve.

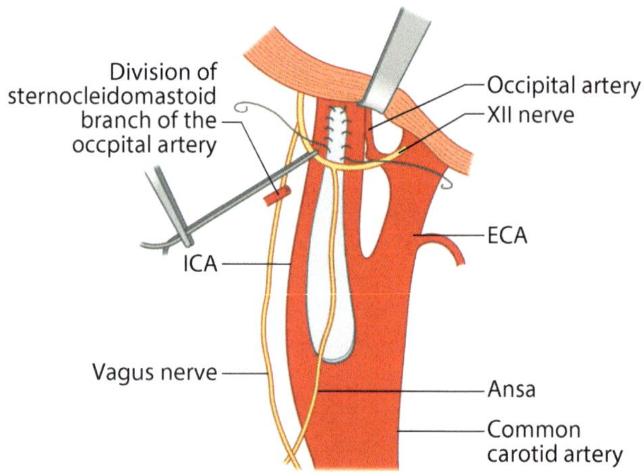

Figure 21.11 Upper end of the patch being sutured to the internal carotid artery above the hypoglossal nerve.

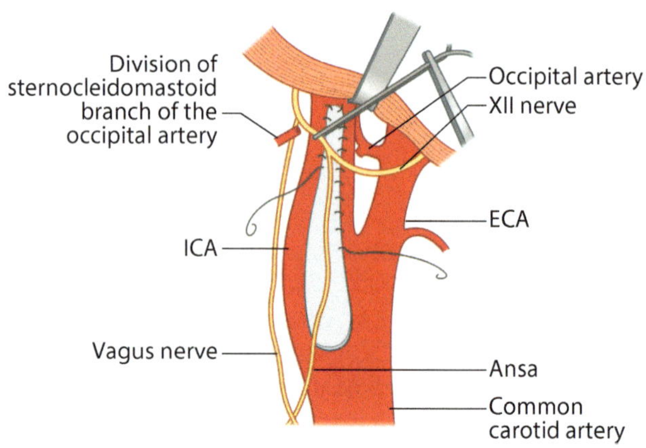

Figure 21.12 The patch is being sutured inferior to the hypoglossal nerve, which is retracted cephalad.

However, if the cephalad extent of the plaque is above the level of the C2 vertebral body, nasotracheal intubation should be considered with pre-incision mandibular subluxation carried out by an oral/maxillofacial surgeon. In rare instances, mandibular osteotomy or resection of the tip of the mastoid process may be needed but these are highly morbid alternatives to mandibular subluxation [3].

If the operating surgeon is uncertain about the end point of the CEA, intraoperative carotid angiography and stenting can be considered [4]. After closing the arteriotomy incision with patch grafting, the lower end of the incision is extended toward the base of the neck, dividing the inferior belly of the omohyoid muscle and the loop of the ansa cervicalis. Micropuncture of the CCA just above the base of the neck is performed and a 7-Fr sheath is inserted. A carotid/cerebral arteriogram is performed on the operating table by injecting 8–10 cc of diluted contrast through the sheath. If a significant endpoint defect is demonstrated, a 0.014 mm guidewire (Choice™ PT, Boston Scientific Corporation, Marlborough, MA, USA) is advanced under fluoroscopy into the intracranial portion of the ICA, and a 6 mm × 4 cm long, self-expanding PRECISE PRO RX Nitinol Stent System (Cordis Corporation, Baar, Switzerland) is deployed; post-deployment angioplasty is performed with a 5 mm angioplasty catheter at the superior end and a 6 mm balloon angioplasty catheter at the inferior end of the stent.

CAROTID INTERPOSITION GRAFTING

Compared to CEA, carotid interposition grafting (CIG) is infrequently performed. The main indications for CIG include: (1) failed endovascular therapy for restenosis following carotid artery stenting (CAS); (2) locally advanced head and neck cancer involving the carotid artery; (3) infected patch graft following CEA; (4) malignant carotid body tumor; (5) resection of a large extracranial carotid aneurysm; and (6) carotid artery trauma when primary repair is not feasible. In most patients, CIG can be performed without the need for an indwelling shunt. If, however, the EEG and monitoring show cerebral ischemia, or the SP is <40 mmHg, an indwelling shunt should be placed. The distal end of the shunt is first advanced into the divided ICA; after back-bleeding fills the shunt, the proximal end of the shunt is inserted into the CCA. The interposition graft is then passed over a second shunt, the first shunt is removed and the second shunt within the interposition graft is inserted (Figure 21.13). Distal end-to-end anastomosis is performed first followed by proximal anastomosis to the divided CCA. Before proximal anastomosis is completed, the shunt is removed, and suturing is completed. Sizing the graft length appropriately is *critical* to avoid redundancy and potential kinking.

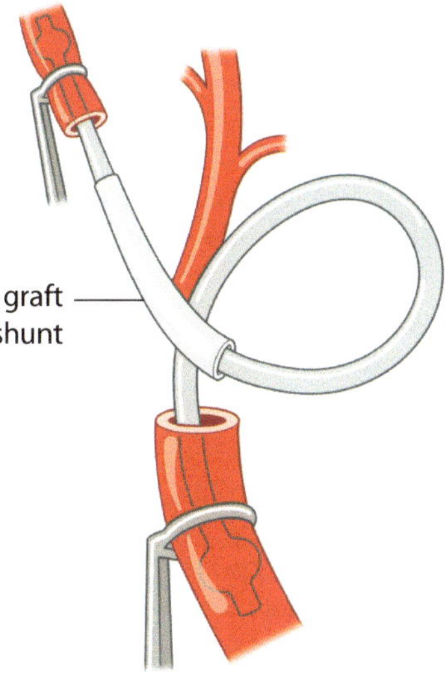

Figure 21.13 Polytetrafluoroethylene graft passed over the shunt with insertion of the distal and proximal ends of the shunt into the internal and common carotid arteries.

CAROTID ENDARTERECTOMY FOR RECURRENT STENOSIS

Indirect laryngoscopy should routinely be performed preoperatively to evaluate vocal fold function. This is especially important in patients who have had previous cranial nerve injury, preoperative neck radiation, previous neck surgery including CEA, and in patients with known head and neck cancers.

The author prefers a standard oblique incision, anterior to the sternocleidomastoid muscle. Pre-existing transverse incisions are modified to gain more distal exposure; otherwise, the previous neck incision is reopened in its entirety. Excessive "Weitlaner" retraction can cause a traction injury to the vagus nerve and should be avoided. Dissection should be carried out directly on the anterior surfaces of the arteries to avoid nerve injury. The vagus nerve and jugular vein are carefully dissected free from the carotid artery to avoid clamp and retractor injury. Distal dissection of the ICA needs to proceed cautiously. The hypoglossal nerve is frequently indistinguishable from surrounding scar tissue crossing the ICA. Dissection in unusual planes and increased retraction for "better exposure" may result in nerve trauma. Injury to the vagus, superior laryngeal, glossopharyngeal, recurrent laryngeal, and hypoglossal nerves are more common following re-do CEA than primary CEA and are to be avoided.

Distal control of the ICA should be obtained above the previous endarterectomy site. The posterior belly of the digastric muscle is divided over a right-angle clamp with electrocautery. Dissection along the lateral aspect of the hypoglossal nerve may provide additional mobility and allow for gentle vessel loop retraction of the nerve. Vigorous retraction of the mandible is occasionally necessary and can result in a marginal mandibular nerve injury. Fortunately, this usually resolves within six months. If preoperative assessment suggests that distal exposure will be problematic, nasotracheal intubation should be used along with all the steps previously described for dealing with high plaque. The placement of a Jackson Pratt drain should be considered in all re-do carotid operations.

TRICKS AND TRAPS

1. Carotid duplex imaging and high-quality CTA of the neck and brain are essential for planning CEA in symptomatic patients. In asymptomatic patients, CEA can be performed based on high-quality carotid duplex imaging. In patients with acute stroke symptoms, MRI of the brain is necessary.
2. Patients with minor to moderate stroke in the distribution of MCA with moderate to severe ipsilateral carotid stenosis should undergo early carotid intervention, i.e., within two weeks; emergent endarterectomy is rarely indicated.
3. Choice of anesthesia depends on surgeon expertise, distal extent of plaque, and the patient's cooperativeness.
4. Selective shunting based on ischemic EEG changes under GA or continuous neurological monitoring under CBA are satisfactory alternatives to routine shunting.
5. The distal end of the plaque usually feathers at its termination and should not be divided as this may result in flap formation. Tacking sutures (distally) is only necessary in patients in whom the distal intima is not well adherent to the arterial wall.
6. Patch graft closure of the endarterectomy site is preferred in almost all cases.
7. Patients with high plaque often need division of the sternocleidomastoid branch of the occipital artery (to mobilize the hypoglossal nerve cephalad) and of the posterior belly of the digastric muscle. Occasionally, the styloid process may need to be divided carefully, preserving the glossopharyngeal nerve.
8. Cervical hematoma is a well-recognized complication with significant hematomas causing airway compromise and difficulty in swallowing. Urgent/emergent re-exploration of the neck in the OR should be performed.
9. The most common cause of perioperative stroke is plaque embolization; cerebral ischemia (shunt malfunction), CEA site thrombosis, and intracerebral hemorrhage are less common causes of perioperative stroke.

QUESTIONS

1. The incidence of MI following CEA is:
    a. Less than 1%
    b. 1–1.5%
    c. 1.6–2.0%
    d. Greater than 2%

    Answer: a

2. The shunt requirement during CEA performed under CBA:
    a. Less than 5%
    b. 8–10%
    c. 11–15%
    d. 16–20%

    Answer: b

3. The peak incidence of hyperperfusion syndrome following CEA is:
    a. 0–2 days
    b. 3–6 days
    c. 7–9 days
    d. 10–12 days

    Answer: b

4. The cranial nerve at most risk during distal ICA exposure requiring resection of the styloid process is:
    a. Hypoglossal
    b. Spinal accessory
    c. Glossopharyngeal
    d. Vagus

    Answer: c

REFERENCES

1. Lewis, S. C., Warlow, C. P., Bodenham, A. R., et al. General anesthesia versus local anesthesia for carotid surgery (GALA): a multicentre, randomised controlled trial. *Lancet*, 2008;372:2132–2142.
2. Hans, S. S. & Jareunpoon, O. Prospective evaluation of electroencephalography, carotid artery stump pressure, and neurologic changes during 314 consecutive carotid endarterectomies performed in awake patients. *J Vasc Surg.*, 2007;45:511–515.
3. Schneider, J. R., Droste, J. S., Schindler, N., et al. Carotid endarterectomy with routine electroencephalography and selective shunting: influence of contralateral internal carotid artery occlusion and utility in prevention of perioperative strokes. *J Vasc Surg.*, 2002;35:1114–1122.

4. Calligaro, K. D., & Dougherty, M. J. Correlation of carotid artery stump pressure and neurologic changes during 474 carotid endarterectomies performed in awake patients. *J Vasc Surg.*, 2005;42:684–689.
5. Stone, D. H., Giles, K. A., Kubilis, P., et al. Protamine reduces serious bleeding complications associated with carotid endarterectomy in asymptomatic patients without increasing the risk of stroke, myocardial infarction, or death in a large national analysis. *Eur J Vasc Endovasc Surg.*, 2020;60:800–807.
6. Goodney, P. P., Likosky, D. S., & Cronenwett, J. L. Factors associated with stroke or death after carotid endarterectomy in Northern New England. *J Vasc Surg.*, 2008;48:1139–1145.
7. Vang, S., & Hans, S. S. Carotid endarterectomy in patients with high plaque. *Surgery,* 2019;166:601–606.
8. de Borst, G. J., Zanen, P., de Vries, J. P., et al. Durability of surgery for restenosis after carotid endarterectomy. *J Vasc Surg.*, 2008;47:363–371.

22

Eversion carotid endarterectomy

EVAN F. GUAY AND JUDITH C. LIN

INTRODUCTION

As of 2023, an estimated 795,000 people have a stroke each year in the United States, with around 87% of those being ischemic strokes. An estimated 2.8% of American adults have already experienced a stroke, and that number is expected to climb to 3.9% by 2030. Interventions on carotid arteries remain the main surgical prophylaxis for strokes, with 115,000 carotid endarterectomies (CEA) or carotid stenting (CAS) procedures performed in the United States in 2018 [1]. Despite recent advances in endovascular carotid revascularization (e.g., transcarotid artery revascularization [TCAR]) and changes in medical management, CEA has remained the standard of care since its introduction by Michael DeBakey 75 years ago, with few technical modifications [2,3]. Eversion CEA (ECEA) is an alternative endarterectomy technique used to remove plaque isolated to the carotid bulb and proximal internal carotid artery (ICA). Advantages of ECEA over standard CEA include the following: the ability to shorten/straighten a redundant/kinked ICA; better-visualized end point and easier detection of intimal flaps; faster closure by simple anastomosis of the ICA to the carotid bulb; autogenous reconstruction (no foreign bodies); and decreased restenosis rates in women. In the authors' practice, most patients undergo standard CEA with bovine or vein patch angioplasty or undergo TCAR; only a small minority of patients undergo ECEA. Candidates for ECEA must have relatively localized (to the carotid bulb and proximal-most ICA) plaque. Patients with long-segment CCA or ICA disease are not candidates for this technique.

TECHNIQUE

Anesthetic choice, cerebral monitoring, and neuroprotection are identical for standard CEA. During the case, neurologic monitoring is routine. Electroencephalographic monitoring is used for patients undergoing general anesthesia (more common in the authors' practice), while continuous neurologic assessment is used for patients undergoing CEA under cervical block anesthesia. Most patients undergoing CEA do not require intraoperative shunt placement. If shunting is needed during ECEA, it is performed after everting and removing the bulk of the ICA plaque with the shunt held in place with shunt clamps. An extension of the common carotid artery (CCA), arteriotomy may be needed to expose the open lumen before a shunt is inserted into the CCA. The authors prefer to use the short Sundt™ internal shunt (Integra LifeSciences Corporation, Plainsboro, NJ, USA) with a nonreinforced segment (3 × 4 mm).

For the procedure, the patient is placed supine on the operating table with a shoulder roll to slightly extend the neck and the head rotated to the opposite side. The neck is prepped and draped to expose the mastoid process, angle of the mandible, and sternal notch. An incision is made along the anterior border of the sternocleidomastoid muscle (SCM) over the carotid bifurcation. Some surgeons mark the level of the carotid bulb with ultrasound before incising the skin to minimize the length of the incision. The authors prefer a longitudinal (rather than transverse) incision because of better exposure of the distal ICA, and the ability to extend as necessary. After the platysma is divided, dissection is made along the anterior border of the SCM to identify the confluence of the internal jugular (IJV) and facial veins. The gatekeeping facial vein is suture-ligated and divided to expose the underlying carotid artery medially. The carotid artery is exposed circumferentially to isolate the ICA and the carotid bulb. Care should be taken to identify and protect the hypoglossal nerve, which may run directly over the carotid bulb. Within the carotid sheath, the vagus nerve lies posteriorly between the CCA medially and IJV laterally. If sinus bradycardia occurs, 1–2 mL of 1% lidocaine without preservatives may be administered topically between the ICA and external carotid artery (ECA) to block nerve conduction from the carotid sinus. Dissection

DOI: 10.1201/9781003452096-22

and circumferential mobilization of the carotid bulb and proximal ICA are much more extensive with ECEA than standard CEA, especially if the plan is to straighten a redundant carotid artery.

After dissection of the CCA, ICA, and ECA, intravenous heparin is administered to achieve an activated clotting time of >250 seconds. The ICA, CCA, and then ECA are clamped in series to mitigate the chances of embolizing debris into the brain. The ICA is then transected obliquely by starting at the crotch of the carotid bulb and extending to a point more proximally on the lateral side of the CCA. An opening of 15–20 mm can be obtained without extending the arteriotomy at either end. If necessary for plaque removal or achieving adequate anastomotic luminal diameter, the arteriotomy on the lateral wall of the CCA may be extended caudally and the arteriotomy on the medial wall of the ICA extended cephalad to a similar length to facilitate later anastomosis of the arteries.

ECEA is performed by circumferentially elevating the plaque with a Penfield elevator from the arterial wall to remove both the intima and diseased media, with care to avoid creating multiple planes. The adventitia is grasped with two fine forceps and everted while an assistant holds the plaque under tension until it thins out distally and is dislodged (Figure 22.1). Any loose flaps are then removed (Figure 22.2). Only rarely is it necessary to tack down the endpoint with double arm 7-0 polypropylene sutures.

The ICA is unrolled and irrigated with heparinized saline, and the luminal surface is again inspected for loose debris. To shorten an elongated or kinked ICA, the transected ICA is then pulled down to straighten out the carotid kink, which must have been previously fully

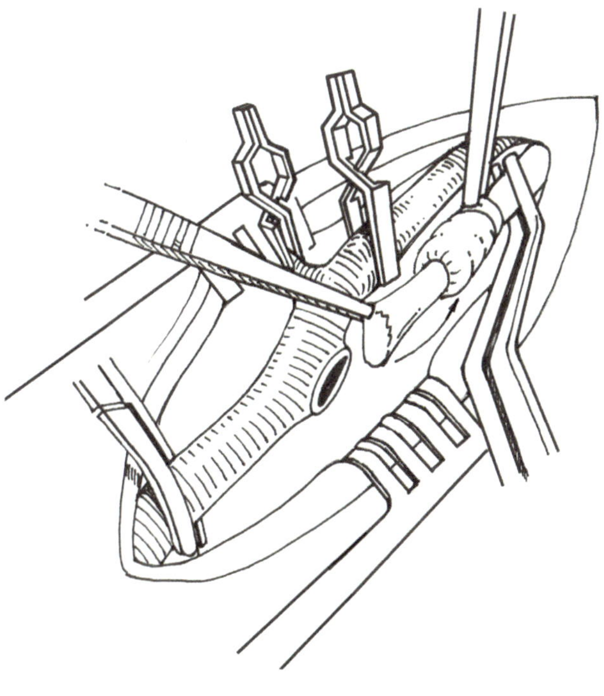

Figure 22.1 Oblique transection and circumferential elevation of plaque from the arterial wall.

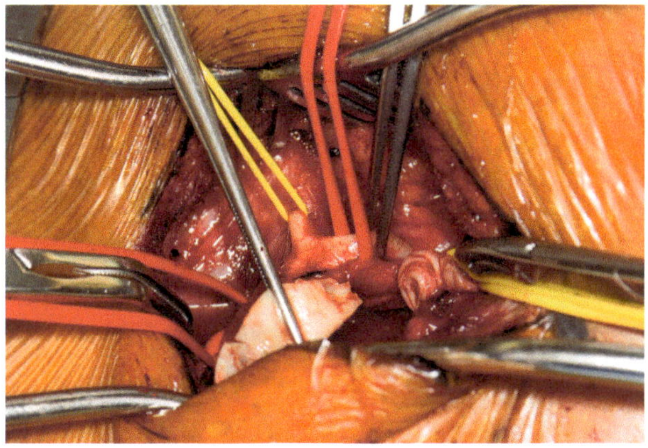

Figure 22.2 Inspection of distal intimal end point.

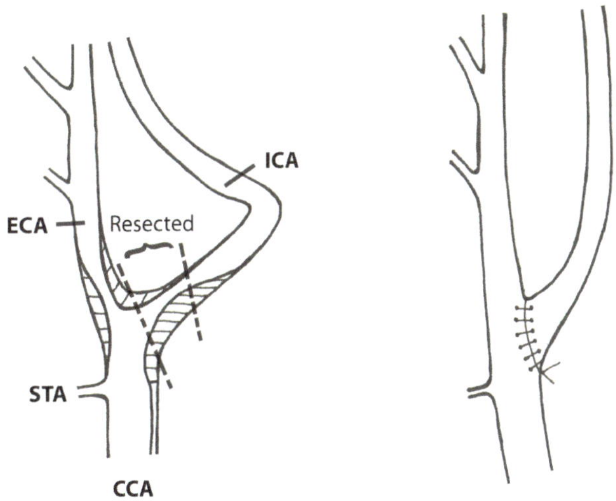

Figure 22.3 Shortening of an elongated internal carotid artery and straightening of the carotid kink by resecting a short segment of the internal carotid artery (ICA). CCA, common carotid artery; ECA, external carotid artery.

mobilized (Figure 22.3). A segment of redundant ICA is excised, taking care to transect the ICA on a slight bevel to match the length of the original arteriotomy at the bifurcation. The distal CCA and the ECA are inspected for plaque removal. The plaque in the bulb is then lifted with a Penfield elevator and an endarterectomy plane carried up the ECA and proximally into the CCA, with or without eversion. The arteriotomy is irrigated with heparinized saline, loose fragments are removed, and then the arteriotomy is irrigated with low-molecular-weight dextran to inhibit platelet adhesion (Figure 22.4). Another method of shortening a redundant ICA is to spatulate the two ends by opening the ICA and CCA longitudinally for a short distance.

Primary anastomosis between the ICA and CCA is performed with continuous 6-0 monofilament sutures, starting at the most cephalad portion of the ICA arteriotomy. The back wall of the anastomosis is usually sewn from the inside of the artery, which provides the best

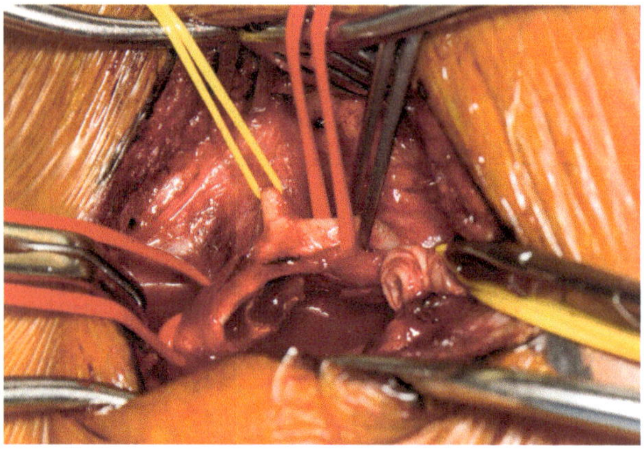

Figure 22.4 Irrigation to remove loose fragments and primary anastomosis.

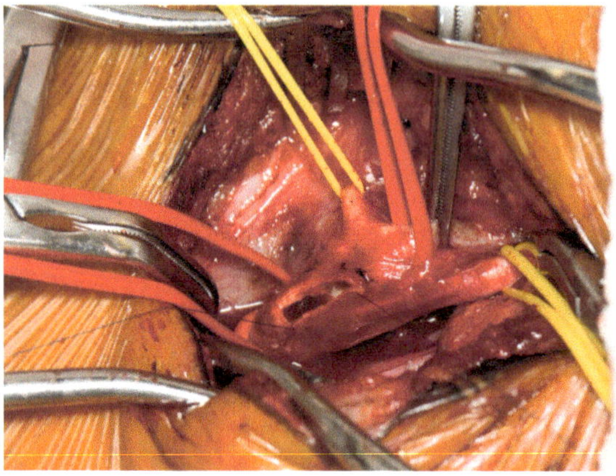

Figure 22.5 Continuous monofilament suture starting from the back wall and inside the artery.

visualization (Figure 22.5). The running suture is completed posteriorly, then brought anteriorly where it is tied to the other end after venting the arteries (Figure 22.6). After completion of the anastomosis, blood flow is restored in the usual sequence: (1) temporarily opening the ICA first to allow backfilling of the bulb; (2) unclamping the ECA to allow backfilling; (3) opening the CCA to allow forward blood flow into the ECA; and (4) finally opening the ICA. Hemostasis is then obtained.

Postoperative care is routine, with blood pressure control and assessment of neurologic deficits. Postoperative complications of ECEA are similar to standard CEA: stroke, transient ischemic attack (TIA), cranial nerve injury, neck hematoma, and cardiac morbidity. Cranial nerve injury includes the hypoglossal, vagus, pharyngeal, and laryngeal branches of the vagus and glossopharyngeal nerves.

LITERATURE REVIEW

Results of the Eversion Carotid Endarterectomy versus Standard Trial (EVEREST) validated the short- and

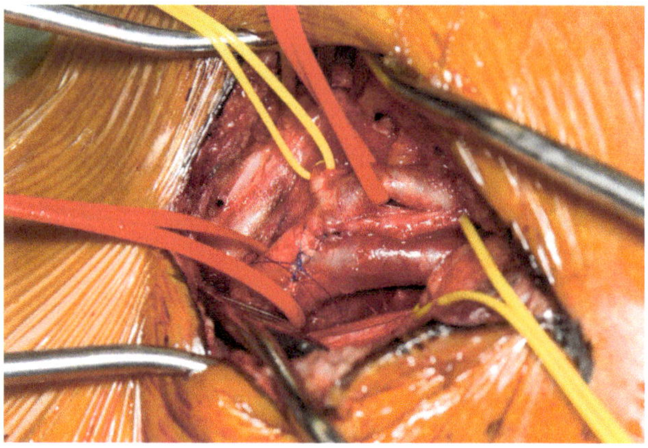

Figure 22.6 Completion of anastomosis and restoration of blood flow.

long-term safety and efficacy of ECEA for carotid atherosclerosis. This prospective, multicenter, randomized trial published in 2000 compared rates of carotid occlusion, restenosis, major stroke, and death among standard CEA ($n = 675$) and ECEA ($n = 678$) patients. Long-term results showed a significantly lower restenosis rate in the eversion group (2.7 versus 5.6%; $p = 0.01$) at a mean follow-up of 33 months. Eversion CEA was an independent predictor of carotid patency, in that the eversion population of patients was three times less likely to have restenosis than patients who had standard CEA. Subgroup analysis suggests that patched CEA and ECEA with primary closure have similar patency [4].

Several single-institution studies have provided a consensus that there is no significant difference between eversion and standard techniques in early (<30 days) postoperative complications [5]. Among its advantages, ECEA is associated with decreased operative times and shorter cross-clamp times due to a single anastomosis and the fact that most carotid disease suitable for ECEA are very localized. Conventional CEA is usually required for long segment and complicated carotid plaque treatment. Schneider and collaborators compared the results of 2,635 ECEAs and 17,155 standard CEAs [6]. Early perioperative morbidity, including ipsilateral stroke and TIA, were equivalent, although ECEA showed a significantly shorter operative time (median 99 versus 114 minutes; $p < 0.001$) but a higher incidence of return to the operating room for bleeding (1.4 versus 8%; $p = 0.002$). Chen and colleagues recently added to this discussion in their retrospective study of 441 patients over six years, which showed no difference in clinical outcomes between ECEA and standard CEA with patching; however, ECEA was associated with lower costs and short hospitalization, raising important points in this value-conscious era of healthcare [7].

Antonopoulos and collaborators pooled randomized and nonrandomized studies in a meta-analysis that favored ECEA in both short- and long-term outcomes in 16,251 CEA procedures [8]. Eversion CEA was associated with a significant reduction in perioperative stroke (odds ratio [OR] 0.46; 95% confidence interval [CI]: 0.35–0.62; number needed to treat [NNT] = 68; 95% CI: 56–96), death (OR 0.49; 95% CI: 0.34–0.69; NNT = 100; 95% CI: 85–185), and stroke-related death (OR 0.40; 95% CI: 0.23–0.67; NNT = 147; 95% CI: 115–270). Regarding long-term outcomes, ECEA was associated with a significant reduction in late carotid artery occlusion (OR 0.48; 95% CI: 0.25–0.90; NNT = 143; 95% CI: 100–769) and late mortality (OR 0.76; 95% CI: 0.61–0.94; NNT = 40; 95% CI: 25–167). Subgroup analysis of patched CEA replicated only the finding on late mortality. More recently, Jonsson and colleagues leveraged a Swedish database containing 2,496 ECEA and 6,710 conventional CEA (primary or patch closure) [9]. They found no significant difference in stroke or death rate between ECEA and patch CEA with median follow-up for 4.2 years, although primary closure CEA did have an elevated risk of stroke (OR 1.7, $p = 0.002$) within the first 30 days post-op.

In the longest follow-up published to date, Black and collaborators reported a restenosis rate of 4.1% ($n = 20/534$) within a mean follow-up period of 8.86 years (95% CI: 6.56–9.16) [10]. The mean time to recurrence was 4.4 years, suggesting these occurrences represent systemic atherosclerotic disease rather than neointimal hyperplasia of the single ECEA suture line.

Regarding complications more commonly associated with CEA versus ECEA, concerns have been raised about postoperative blood pressure regulation following carotid sinus disruption in ECEA. A meta-analysis from Demirel and colleagues examining blood pressure in the first postoperative week found that ECEA was more commonly associated with post-op hypertension (OR 2.75, $p < 0.0001$) and conventional CEA was more commonly associated with post-op hypotension (OR 11.37, $p = 0.0023$) [11]. Nolde and colleagues subsequently examined this subject over a longer follow-up period, comparing 615 CEA and 47 ECEA patients, and they found no significant differences in blood pressure or blood pressure medication adjustments following CEA or ECEA for up to three years post-op [12].

Current level I evidence studies and meta-analyses comparing ECEA and standard CEA have validated excellent results with both techniques. Although the eversion method has not shown superior results conclusively, ECEA provides another reliable technique that should be in every vascular surgeon's armamentarium for the treatment of high-grade COD, particularly when associated with a kinked or highly redundant ICA.

QUESTIONS

1. If shunting is needed, the optimal time for shunt placement is:
   a. Before the ICA is transected
   b. Before plaque removal
   c. After removing the bulk of the ICA plaque
   d. Once the back wall of the carotid re-anastomosis has been performed

   Answer: c

2. Carotid transection landmarks:
   a. Horizontally through the equator of the carotid bifurcation
   b. Longitudinally through the ICA and CCA
   c. Horizontally through the ICA takeoff
   d. Obliquely through the carotid bulb from the lateral aspect of the CCA to the bifurcation between the ICA and ECA.

   Answer: d

3. The EVEREST Trial showed ECEA provides:
   a. Lower restenosis rates
   b. Lower stroke rates
   c. Shorter length of hospitalization
   d. Shorter length of ICU stay

   Answer: a

4. Single-institution studies suggest that advantages of ECEA may include:
   a. Shorter operative times and lower infection rates
   b. Lower rates of vagus and glossopharyngeal nerve injury
   c. Expanded surgical indications and improved patency rates
   d. Greater technical ease and decreased need for shunting

   Answer: a

REFERENCES

1. Tsao, C. W., Aday, A. W., Almarzooq, Z. I., et al (2023). American Heart Association Council on Epidemiology and Prevention Statistics Committee and Stroke Statistics Subcommittee. Heart Diseases and Stroke Statistics, 2023 Update: A Report from the American Heart Association. *Circulation*, *147*(8), e93–e621.
2. Stonko, D. P., Goldsborough, B. S. III, Kibrik, P., et al (2022). Use of Transcarotid Artery Revascularization, Transfemoral Carotid Artery Stenting, and Carotid Endarterectomy in the US (United States) from 2015 to 2019. *JAMA Netw Open.*, *5*(9), e2231944.

3. Columbo, J. A., Stone, D. H., Martinez-Camblor, P., et al. (2023). Adoption and Diffusion of Transcarotid Artery Revascularization in Contemporary Practice. *Circ Cardiovasc Interv., 16*(9), e012805.
4. Cao, P., Giordano, G., De Rango, P., et al. (2000). Eversion Versus Conventional Carotid Endarterectomy: Late Results of a Prospective Multicenter Randomized Trial. *J Vasc Surg., 31*(1 Pt 1), 19–30.
5. Ben Ahmed, S., Daniel, G., Benezit, M., et al. (2017). Eversion Carotid Endarterectomy without Shunt: Concerning 1385 Consecutive Cases. *J Cardiovasc Surg (Torino)., 58*, 543–550.
6. Schneider, J. R., Helenowski, I. B., Jackson, C. R., et al. (2015). A Comparison of Results with Eversion Versus Conventional Carotid Endarterectomy from the Vascular Quality Initiative and the Mid-America Vascular Study Group. *J Vasc Surg., 61*, 1216–1222.
7. Chen, G. Z., Yuan, W. Z., Peng, D. Y., et al. (2018). Comparison of Eversion Carotid Endarterectomy and Patch Carotid Endarterectomy: A Retrospective Study of 6 Years of Experience. *Med Sci Monit.*, 24, 5820–5825.
8. Antonopoulos, C. N., Kakisis, J. D., Sergentanis, T. N., et al. (2011). Eversion Versus Conventional Carotid Endarterectomy: A Meta-Analysis of Randomised and Non-Randomised Studies. *Eur J Vasc Endovasc Surg., 42*, 751–765.
9. Jonsson, M., Hammer, K., Lindberg, M., et al. (2023). Nationwide Outcomes Analysis of Primary Carotid Endarterectomy in Symptomatic Patients Depending on Closure Technique and Patch Type. *Eur J Endovasc Surg., 65*, 467–473.
10. Black, J. H., Ricotta, J. J., & Jones, C. E. (2010). Long-term Results of Eversion Carotid Endarterectomy. *Ann Vasc Surg., 24*, 92–99.
11. Demirel, S., Goosen, K., Bruijnen, H., et al. (2017). Systematic Review and Meta-Analysis of Post-Carotid Endarterectomy Hypertension after Eversion Versus Conventional Carotid Endarterectomy. *J Vasc Surg., 65*(3), 868–882.
12. Nolde, N. M., Cheng, S. F., & Richards, T. (2021). No Evidence for Long Term Blood Pressure Differences between Eversion and Conventional Carotid Endarterectomy in Two Independent Study Cohorts. *Eur J Vasc Endovasc Surg., 63*, 33–42.

23

Extracranial carotid artery aneurysms

SACHINDER S. HANS

INTRODUCTION

Aneurysms of the extracranial carotid artery are uncommon and account for less than 1% (0.3–0.6%) of all arterial aneurysms [1–5]. Aneurysms are either true aneurysms or false (pseudoaneurysms) [1–5]. Atherosclerosis is by far the most common cause of true aneurysms. Other less common etiologies are connective tissue disorders, fibromuscular dysplasia, post-radiation, arteritis, and cystic medial necrosis. True aneurysms can either be fusiform or saccular. Fusiform carotid aneurysms are usually bilateral, degenerative, and near the carotid bifurcation. Saccular aneurysms are unilateral and occur in the mid-segment of the ICA. Pseudoaneurysms result from disruption in the arterial wall and may occur anywhere in the cervical carotid artery [6]. Pseudoaneurysms may occur at the site of prosthetic patch grafting performed in conjunction with carotid endarterectomy or may result from infection in a prosthetic patch. Other causes include arterial dissection and trauma, both blunt and penetrating [2,4,6].

CLINICAL PRESENTATION

Patients with carotid artery aneurysms may present as an asymptomatic neck mass but more often present with symptoms of TIA or stroke due to embolization. The neck mass has expansile pulsation but can be incorrectly diagnosed as a carotid body tumor, enlarged cervical lymph node, or even as an abscess. Large carotid artery aneurysms may cause a local mass effect with the compression of adjacent cranial nerves and/or the aerodigestive tract resulting in dysphagia, cranial nerve deficits, and occipital or retro-orbital pain and headaches. Patients may present with Horner's syndrome. Rupture of a true carotid artery aneurysm in the neck is relatively uncommon; however, an expanding cervical hematoma in the neck may result in the airway comprised secondary to tracheal compression from a rupture. Many aneurysms are asymptomatic and detected during imaging for other problems.

DIAGNOSIS AND IMAGING

An expansile or pulsatile mass is usually palpable on physical examination of the neck. In the elderly, in thin individuals with a history of hypertension, an ectatic common carotid and/or subclavian artery just above the thoracic inlet can be mistaken for a carotid aneurysm. In patients with a mycotic carotid aneurysm, the neck mass is often tender with overlying erythema of the skin and can be incorrectly diagnosed as a neck abscess. Carotid duplex imaging is often the first study obtained for the diagnosis of carotid aneurysm. CT or MR angiography of the neck is extremely useful for diagnosis and treatment planning. The extent of the aneurysm and its relation to bony structures is best delineated by a thin-cut CTA of the neck (Figure 23.1). Catheter-based carotid/cerebral arteriography can help evaluate intracranial circulation in the event ICA ligation is required in patients with a surgically inaccessible aneurysm. Catheter-based angiography has a small risk of ischemic stroke due to embolization (Figure 23.2). In situations where ICA ligation is contemplated, a balloon occlusion test should be performed to ensure that this can be safely performed.

In an asymptomatic patient with a small extracranial carotid aneurysm, conservative management may be all that is required with antiplatelet agents, statins, and antihypertensives and surveillance by carotid duplex imaging at regular intervals. This approach is also appropriate in patients with a short life expectancy or with inoperable aneurysms near the skull base. Patients with symptomatic aneurysms are considered candidates for invasive treatment. The aim of treatment is to prevent thromboembolic complications from associated mural thrombus and/or to relieve symptoms and/or complications such as cranial nerve palsy or pharyngeal compression.

DOI: 10.1201/9781003452096-23

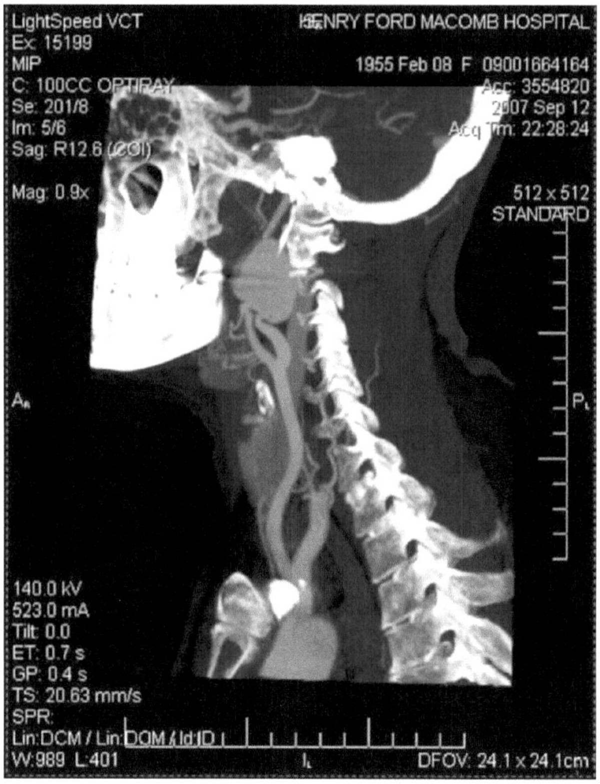

Figure 23.1 CTA showing aneurysm of the left mid-ICA.

SURGICAL MANAGEMENT

The primary treatment modality is resection of the carotid aneurysm and restoration of common carotid artery (CCA) and ICA continuity. Aneurysm resection should only be undertaken following a careful delineation of the size and location of the aneurysm, redundancy of the ICA, and the presence/absence of surrounding inflammation. A standard oblique surgical incision just anterior to the sternocleidomastoid provides good exposure. We use pre-incision ultrasound to identify the extent of the aneurysm and plan the incision accordingly. The internal jugular vein is reflected laterally and branches crossing the CCA/ICA are ligated and divided. The surrounding nerves—vagus, hypoglossal, and superiorly (if necessary), the glossopharyngeal nerves—should be identified and preserved. The posterior belly of the digastric muscle often requires division if there is cephalad extension of the aneurysm. The sternocleidomastoid branch of the occipital artery should be ligated and divided, and, in some cases, the occipital artery itself may need to be sacrificed to free up the hypoglossal nerve, which then can be mobilized cephalad to gain better exposure. Most patients do not require shunt placement. A stump pressure of greater than 40 mmHg and absent ischemic changes on EEG monitoring indicate satisfactory collateral circulation through the circle of Willis. Median nerve somatosensory evoked potential monitoring can also be helpful. If any difficulty in obtaining distal ICA control is anticipated, mandibular subluxation (by an oral-maxillofacial or ENT surgeon) following nasotracheal intubation should be considered. Mobilization of the aneurysm should be careful and deliberate to prevent embolization of contents *and/or* injury to surrounding nerves.

Heparin is administered (100 units per kilogram by anesthesia) prior to carotid clamping and the activated clotting time is maintained between 280 and 300 seconds. Small carotid aneurysms with a redundant ICA can be resected and the artery reconstructed with a primary repair using an end-to-end spatulated anastomosis with 6-0" or 7-0" CV polypropylene sutures. It may be preferable to leave the hypoglossal nerve posterior to the ICA during this reconstruction. (Figure 23.3). Transposition of distal ICA into the proximal external carotid artery after complete excision of the aneurysm has also been described. Saccular aneurysms can be treated with resection of the aneurysmal wall and patch angioplasty using a prosthetic patch and is a helpful option in patients with anatomically high aneurysms. All the thrombotic material should be removed prior to suturing the patch. In these cases, the posterior wall is left intact to avoid injury to the vagus nerve coursing posterior to the aneurysm.

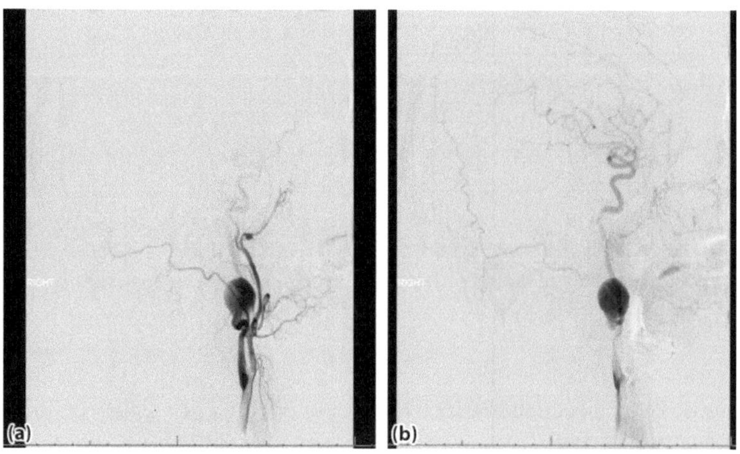

Figure 23.2 Carotid arteriograms showing an aneurysm in the mid-segment of the right ICA with associated tortuosity.

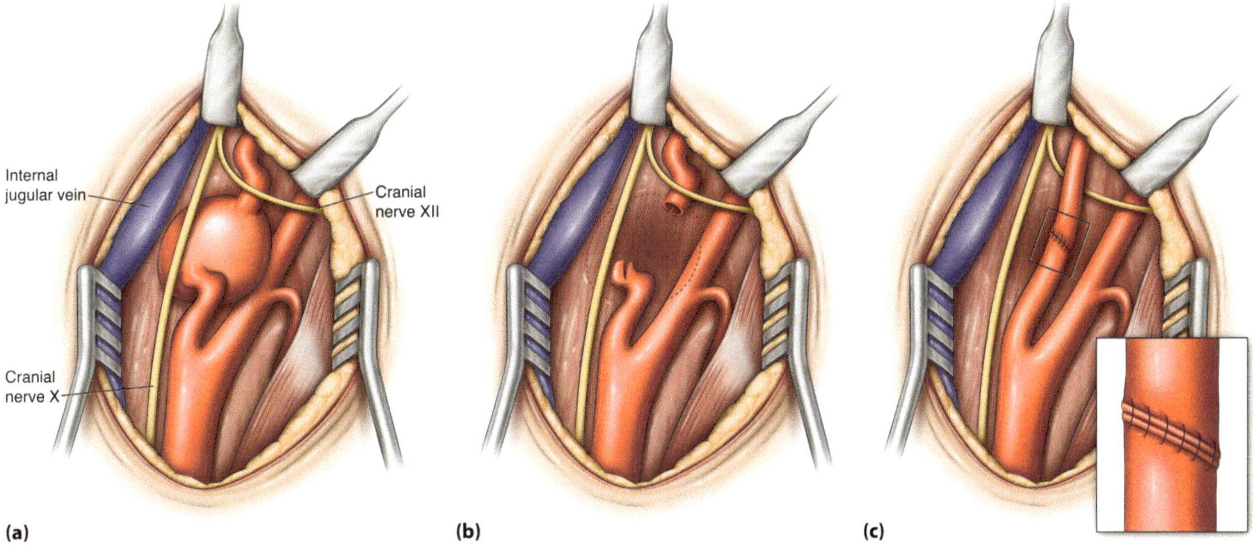

Figure 23.3 Repair of a right ICA aneurysm with primary end-to-end anastomosis of redundant ICA segments. In (c), note the transposition of the reconstructed artery anterior to the hypoglossal nerve.

Interposition grafting should be considered in patients where direct end-to-end anastomosis of the redundant artery is not feasible.

Choice of conduit depends on size of the vessel and the status of the surrounding operative field. In non-infected fields, the conduit is selected based on the diameter match and the length of the bypass needed. The patency of a prosthetic graft in this position is only slightly worse than a vein and the ease and time saved with a prosthetic justifies its use in high-risk patients. Tapered polytetrafluoroethylene grafts are useful when transitioning from a larger diameter CCA to a small diameter ICA. The length of the interposition conduit should be carefully measured to avoid kinking and redundancy. Vein bypasses distend in both diameter and length after establishment of arterial flow. In patients undergoing the repair of a mycotic carotid aneurysm, GSV or superficial femoral artery as a conduit for interposition graft are preferred. Post-reconstruction imaging with either duplex scanning or completion angiography is our practice. Placement of an external drain is preferable. In patients with an aneurysm in an inaccessible location (near the skull base), an extracranial to intracranial (EC-IC) carotid bypass with proximal ligation of the ICA should be considered.

Post-endarterectomy pseudoaneurysms can be particularly challenging since they are "re-do" operations. If not infected, the patch can sometimes be resected and replaced with another patch after vessel wall debridement. However, in the setting of possible infection, the new patch should be an autogenous vein. Often the artery is too destroyed by infection/inflammation and the only solution is an autologous interposition graft. In this setting, it is important that the aneurysm and any infected surrounding tissue be completely excised/debrided.

COMPLICATIONS

The most common postoperative complication of carotid artery aneurysm repair is cranial nerve injury, which ranges from 3–17%. The mortality and stroke rates are similar to that of standard carotid endarterectomy. The surgical repair of an extracranial carotid artery aneurysm is a safe procedure with good long-term results.

ENDOVASCULAR TREATMENT

During the past 15 years, endovascular therapy for extracranial carotid aneurysms has evolved into a feasible option. The placement of a covered stent using femoral access is a suitable option, particularly for ruptured aneurysms or those that are surgically difficult to access (e.g., near the skull base). In patients with a hostile neck due to prior neck radiation, tracheostomy following laryngectomy, or following radical neck dissection, endovascular techniques are a more suitable option. A few small case series of covered stents for pseudoaneurysms of the ICA in the neck have been reported; self-expanding covered stents are preferred. The potential for thromboembolic complications is high and patients should be treated with dual antiplatelet therapy. Coil embolization with thrombosis of the sac has been performed with mixed results and the potential risk of distal embolization. EC-IC carotid bypass following ligation of the ICA may be indicated in carefully selected patients who cannot be managed using ICA ligation because of poor collateral circulation in the brain. Clinical neurological monitoring, transcranial Doppler, and EEG monitoring are all helpful in assessing tolerance to angiographic balloon occlusion. An occlusion balloon (e.g., HyperGlide™ system, ev3 Endovascular Inc., Plymouth, MN, USA) is advanced into the ICA origin using femoral access and a 6F guiding catheter positioned in the proximal portion of the CCA. The balloon is inflated to occlude the ICA. A decrease in the peak systolic velocity (measured by duplex scanning) ≤30% relative to baseline during balloon occlusion is a consistent predictive value adequate for collateral flow.

Extracranial vertebral artery aneurysms are rare and are usually pseudoaneurysms resulting from trauma or dissection. Primary cervical vertebral aneurysms are due to connective tissue or hereditary disorders including Ehlers–Danlos syndrome, Marfan's syndrome, and neurofibromatosis. Morasch et al. documented successful treatment of nine extracranial vertebral artery aneurysms in seven patients with a variety of reconstruction techniques [7]. The natural history of vertebral artery aneurysms is not well-defined, as a result, repair should only be considered for large symptomatic aneurysms. A hybrid approach with detachable coils and balloons with associated open bypass may be required. Embolization without revascularization may result in posterior circulation stroke. In patients with Ehlers–Danlos syndrome, repair can be challenging due to tissue degeneration, and interrupted monofilament sutures using mini-pledgets are often necessary. However, in spite of all the necessary precautions, repair may not be successful and the vertebral artery may require ligation.

TRICKS AND TRAPS

1. Thin slice CTA of the neck and head is essential for the diagnosis and planning of carotid aneurysm repair. Catheter-based arteriography is not necessary except, possibly, for aneurysms near the skull base.
2. Most extracranial carotid aneurysms can be repaired using standard cervical incisions. For aneurysms located more cephalad, nasotracheal intubation and mandibular subluxation should be considered.
3. Intraoperative shunting is rarely necessary. EEG and somatosensory median nerve evoked potential monitoring is useful.
4. Injury to the hypoglossal, vagus, and (for more cephalad aneurysms) glossopharyngeal nerves should be avoided.
5. Associated redundancy of the ICA will frequently allow aneurysm resection followed by a primary end-to-end (spatulated) anastomosis.
6. If primary anastomosis is not feasible, interposition grafting with autologous GSV or a tapered PTFE graft is recommended.
7. Ligation of the ICA is rarely necessary except in inaccessible aneurysms near the skull base with adequate collateral circulation.

QUESTIONS

1. The incidence of extracranial carotid artery aneurysm is:
   a. Less than 1%
   b. 1–2%
   c. 2.1–3.1%
   d. 3.1–3.5%

   Answer: a

2. The best imaging modality for planning repair of a carotid aneurysm is:
   a. Carotid duplex study
   b. CT angiography
   c. MRA of the neck
   d. Catheter-based carotid/cerebral arteriography

   Answer: b

3. Most carotid aneurysms in the neck are repaired by:
   a. Endovascular techniques
   b. Carotid artery ligation
   c. Carotid aneurysm resection with re-establishment of arterial continuity by primary repair if remaining arterial segments redundant, and if not, by interposition grafting
   d. Ligation and bypass with a Dacron graft

   Answer: c

4. The most common complication of carotid artery aneurysm repair is:
   a. Stroke
   b. Cranial nerve injury
   c. Neck hematoma
   d. Pseudoaneurysm formation at the site of repair

   Answer: b

REFERENCES

1. Attigah N, Kulkens S, Zausig N, et al. Surgical therapy of extracranial carotid artery aneurysms: long-term results over a 24-year period. *Eur. J. Vasc and Endovasc. Surg.* 2009; 37(2): 127–133.
2. Srivastava SD, Eagleton MJ, O'Hara P, et al. Surgical repair of carotid artery aneurysms: a 10-year single centric experience. *Ann. Vasc. Surg.* 2010; 24: 100–105.
3. Frankenhauser GT, Stone WM, Fowl RJ, et al. Surgical and medical management of extracranial carotid aneurysms. *J. Vasc. Surg.* 2015; 61(2): 389–393.

4. El-Sabrout R, Cooley DA. Extracranial carotid artery aneurysms: Texas Heart Institute experience. *J. Vasc. Surg.* 2000; 31(4): 702–712.
5. Martins de Souza N, Vikatmaa P, Tulamo R, et al. Etiology and treatment patterns of ruptured extracranial carotid artery aneurysm. *J. Vasc. Surg.* 2021, 71(6): 2097–2113.
6. Garg K, Rockman CB, Lee V, et al. Presentation and management of carotid artery aneurysms and pseudoaneurysms. *J. Vasc. Surg.* 2012; 55: 1618–1622.
7. Morasch MD, Phade SV, Naugton P, et al. Primary extracranial vertebral artery aneurysms. *Ann. Vac. Surg.* 2013; 27(4): 418–423.

24

Resection of carotid body tumors

MITCHELL R. WEAVER AND DANIEL J. REDDY

INTRODUCTION

Carotid body tumors (CBTs), also referred to as chemodectomas or carotid body paragangliomas, are the most common head and neck paragangliomas. These tumors arise from paraganglionic cells that migrate from the neural crest, near the sympathetic ganglia. Usually benign and indolent, they often go undetected until they are large enough to be visible or palpable. Less commonly, CBTs present with symptoms secondary to mass effect, such as cranial nerve dysfunction or dysphagia. In recent years, with the increased use of cross-sectional imaging, they are more commonly diagnosed as incidental findings. They are most prevalent in patients in their fourth to sixth decades of life and are found in greater number in women than men [1–3].

A common presentation is that of a painless, slow growing, anterolateral neck mass that has been present from weeks to years. Most symptoms are secondary to local mass effect and compression on neighboring structures and include the following: neck pain; dysphonia; dysphagia; hoarseness; stridor; jaw pain; sore throat; odynophagia; amaurosis fugax; facial droop; and Horner syndrome. Along with a CBT, initial differential diagnosis includes an enlarged lymph node, carotid artery aneurysm, branchial cleft cyst, and neurilemmoma.

Larger tumors, especially if >3 cm in size, are usually palpable on physical examination. They are identified as a neck mass anterior to the sternocleidomastoid muscle and overlying the carotid bifurcation. These tumors are usually nontender and often appear pulsatile because of their proximity to the carotid artery. Typically, the tumor is mobile in a lateral or side-to-side fashion, but not in a vertical plane (Fontaine's sign) [2]. A thorough examination of the oral and nasal pharynx should be performed. Cranial nerve examination with special attention to the function of the facial, glossopharyngeal, vagus, and hypoglossal nerves should be carefully documented.

Tumor biopsy to confirm the diagnosis is not recommended because of the significant vascularity of these tumors. CBTs rarely produce neuroendocrine secretions or catecholamine-related symptoms, thus routine screening of urine catecholamines is not indicated. However, such screening should be considered in the rare case that the tumor is accompanied by paroxysmal hypertension, tachycardia, or palpitations. Likewise, metastatic disease is rare, but in those patients with additional systemic symptoms of weight loss and malaise, further workup should be considered [2, 3].

Although they are usually benign and indolent, once identified in acceptable-risk patients, CBT resection is indicated. If allowed to grow large enough to cause symptoms, such as a palpable mass or cranial nerve dysfunction, because of its significant vascularity and adherence to neurovascular structures, a CBT will present significantly greater technical challenges for surgical resection.

IMAGING AND PREOPERATIVE PLANNING

Several imaging studies are available to confirm the diagnosis and provide adequate information for surgical planning. These studies include color-flow duplex ultrasound (Figure 24.1), computed tomography (CT), magnetic resonance imaging (MRI) (Figure 24.2), conventional catheter-directed angiography with digital subtraction imaging (Figure 24.3), and positron emission tomography. Spiral CT technology with multiplanar reformatting has become the authors' diagnostic test of choice.

The diagnostic finding is that of a vascular mass at the carotid bifurcation displacing the internal (ICA) and external carotid (ECA) arteries. Adequate preoperative imaging must define the extent of the tumor, the presence of any synchronous ipsilateral or contralateral tumors, and any associated carotid artery occlusive disease. This information allows thc surgcon to plan the most appropriate surgical approach, being prepared for extended distal exposures and arterial reconstructions. In cases of

DOI: 10.1201/9781003452096-24

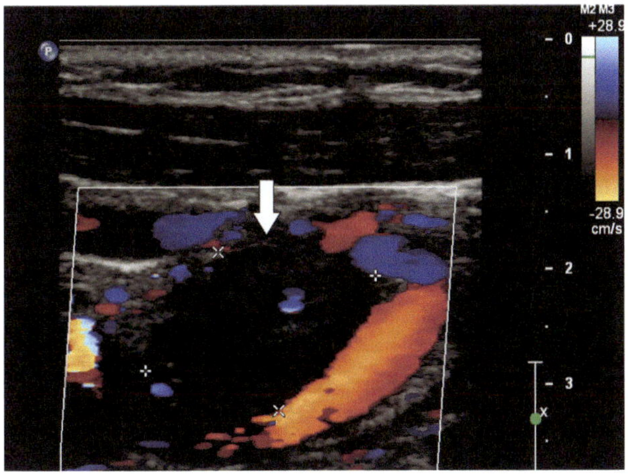

Figure 24.1 Carotid bifurcation duplex ultrasound demonstrating carotid body tumor splaying the carotid bifurcation (arrow).

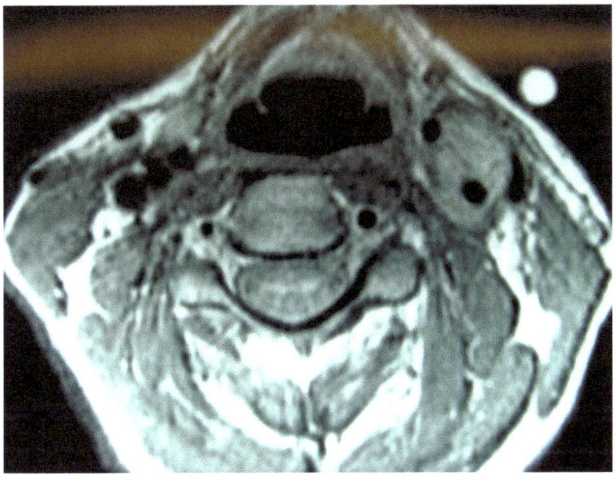

Figure 24.2 Magnetic resonance image demonstrating a left carotid body tumor. The external marker overlies the mass.

bilateral disease, the surgeon can determine the appropriate order of staged resections.

Traditionally, catheter-directed angiography has been the gold standard for the diagnosis of CBTs. However, this invasive imaging study is not necessary in most cases. In certain situations, angiography may provide clearer information regarding the blood supply to the tumor that may be of value in planning resection; in the same setting, this modality also offers the opportunity for embolization of the tumor when appropriate, with the hope of reducing perioperative blood loss [4]. In an effort to reduce intraoperative blood loss during the resection of these tumors, highly selective embolization of these tumors was introduced with reports of reduced blood loss; however, other series failed to demonstrate any significant benefit of this technique and questioned whether the benefits outweigh the risks, namely stroke or transient ischemic attack, as well as the additional cost of the procedure. Consideration

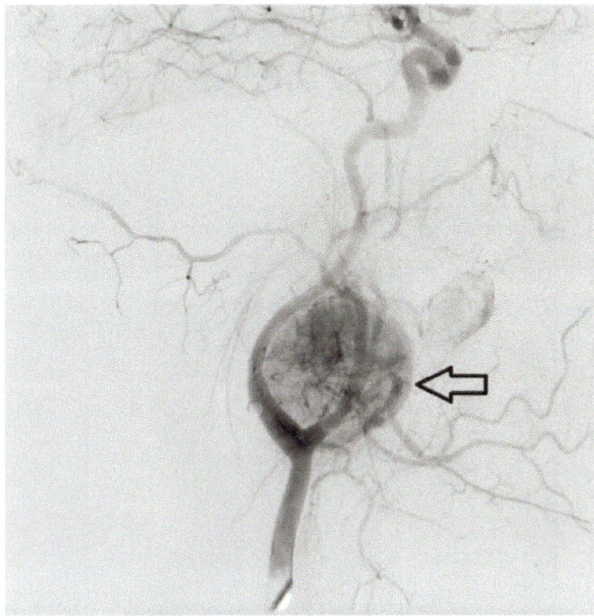

Figure 24.3 Digital subtraction angiography demonstrated significant vascularity of the carotid body tumor (arrow), which splayed the internal and external carotid arteries.

of performing preoperative embolization would typically be reserved for those tumors >5 cm that appear to pose a significant technical challenge [5,6].

More recently, the preoperative technique of direct percutaneous embolization of CBT with ethylene-vinyl alcohol copolymer (Onyx; ev3, Irvine, CA, USA) has been reported [7,8]. Over the last decade, the authors of this chapter have adopted this strategy for resection of all but the smallest of CBT and have found it to be beneficial. (Figure 24.4) When embolization is performed, surgical resection is recommended within the next 24–48 hours to avoid a postembolization inflammatory response in the surrounding tissue.

For tumors extending cranially, if the need for distal ICA exposure is anticipated by preoperative imaging, nasal intubation and mandibular subluxation should be strongly considered. Mandibular subluxation is performed by the authors' ear, nose, and throat colleagues after induction of anesthesia, but before prepping and draping for tumor resection. The desired result is that the ramus of the mandible is displaced forward; with this alteration in position of the mandible, the normal narrow triangular field is converted to a rectangular field. This increased width provides additional distal ICA exposure. However, the local anatomy becomes slightly distorted with this positioning. The posterior belly of the digastric muscle and the hypoglossal nerve are displaced anteriorly and superiorly, and the carotid bifurcation and ICA and ECA are rotated medially.

Other preparations for operation include the following: the availability of autotransfusion for larger tumors; intraoperative cerebral monitoring with electroencephalography

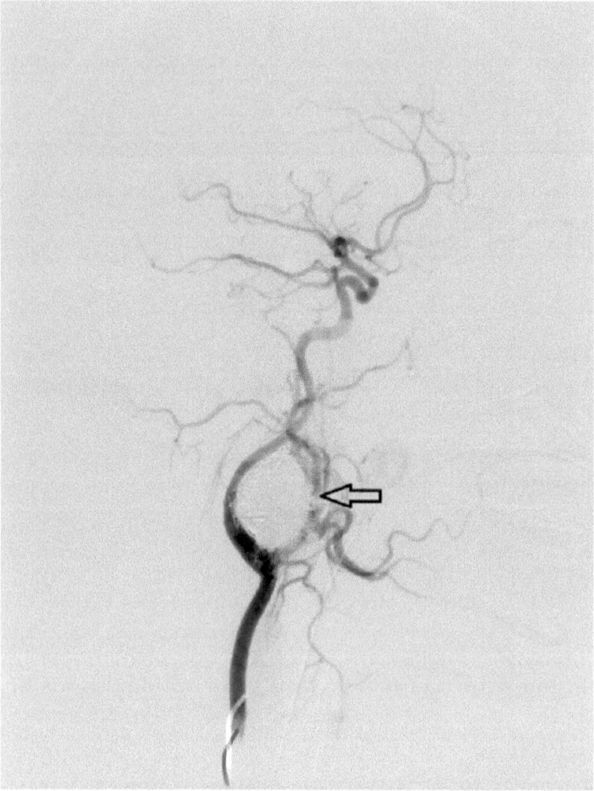

Figure 24.4 Digital subtraction angiography demonstrated lack of flow into the carotid body tumor following direct percutaneous embolization of CBT with Onyx. Pre-embolization imaging is demonstrated in Figure 24.3.

in cases that may require carotid artery clamping or reconstruction; vein mapping and preparation of a saphenous vein harvest site; and the use of bipolar cautery to avoid heat conduction injury to adjacent nerves.

SURGICAL MANAGEMENT

The procedure is performed under general anesthesia and once induced, if mandibular subluxation is planned, it is performed at this time. A roll is placed under the patient's shoulders and the neck is extended and rotated slightly to the contralateral side, before performing sterile prepping and draping of the skin. The authors' standard approach is through a longitudinal anterior sternocleidomastoid incision, like that for a carotid endarterectomy. Once the tumor is visualized, assessment of the carotid artery is performed, and dissection is typically directed to achieve control of the common carotid artery (CCA) proximally and then the ECA and ICA distal to the tumor. The vagus nerve should be identified proximally along the CCA and followed distally. The vagus nerve and adjacent uninvolved cranial nerves are separated from the tumor and protected by dissecting through the tumor pseudocapsule. Distal exposure can be facilitated with standard techniques, such as division of the posterior belly of the digastric muscle, taking care not to injure the glossopharyngeal nerve that is then mobilized. Ligation and division of the occipital artery will assist with this. The next maneuver is division of the stylohyoid muscle groups. If further exposure is required, styloidectomy and mastoidectomy are described but carry with them an increased risk of morbidity with cranial nerve injury. During dissection of the ECA, one needs to be aware of the hypoglossal nerve anteriorly and the superior laryngeal nerve posteriorly. In exposing the ICA, one must be aware of several nerves, including the mandibular branch of the facial nerve, proximal hypoglossal nerve, vagus nerve, pharyngeal branch of the vagus nerve, spinal accessory nerve, and glossopharyngeal nerve.

Having completed proximal and distal exposure of the arterial structures, further intervention is based on the extent of the tumor as described by the Shamblin classification system [9]. This system classifies tumors in relation to their involvement with the carotid artery and the subsequent difficulty in surgical resection. Group I tumors can be resected without significant trauma to the vessel wall or tumor capsule. Those in group II are more adherent to the adventitia and partially surround the artery, making their dissection more difficult, but can be excised without sacrificing the vessel. In group III, the artery is completely encased in the tumor and is best treated by resection of the involved artery with the tumor (Figures 24.5 and 24.6). Thus, for less advanced tumors, an attempt is made to create a periadventitial dissection plane between the tumor and the artery (white line of Gordon-Taylor) and resect the tumor in a caudal-to-cranial fashion, leaving the artery intact (Figures 24.7 and 24.8). The use of energy sealing and dissecting devices is helpful in performing a more hemostatic resection. The typical blood supply to the tumor originates from the ECA and these multiple feeding branches are sequentially ligated and divided. It is not unusual to also find branches originating from the ICA. For larger tumors, the ECA may be ligated and divided to assist with mobilization and resection. A minority of cases will require some type of arterial repair, such as lateral arteriorrhaphy, patch angioplasty, or bypass. In cases where the tumor completely encases the artery, the tumor and artery are resected en bloc, followed by arterial reconstruction, usually with saphenous vein. When carotid artery clamping and reconstruction are required, the authors recommend monitored anticoagulation, along with selective shunting, depending on the findings of intraoperative electroencephalography. An attempt should be made to remove the whole tumor since incomplete excision is associated with a high likelihood of local recurrence [5]. If suspicious lymph nodes are encountered, a biopsy should be performed; if nodal metastasis is present, a modified neck dissection should be performed. A closed suction drain is placed before closure and usually removed on postoperative day one or two.

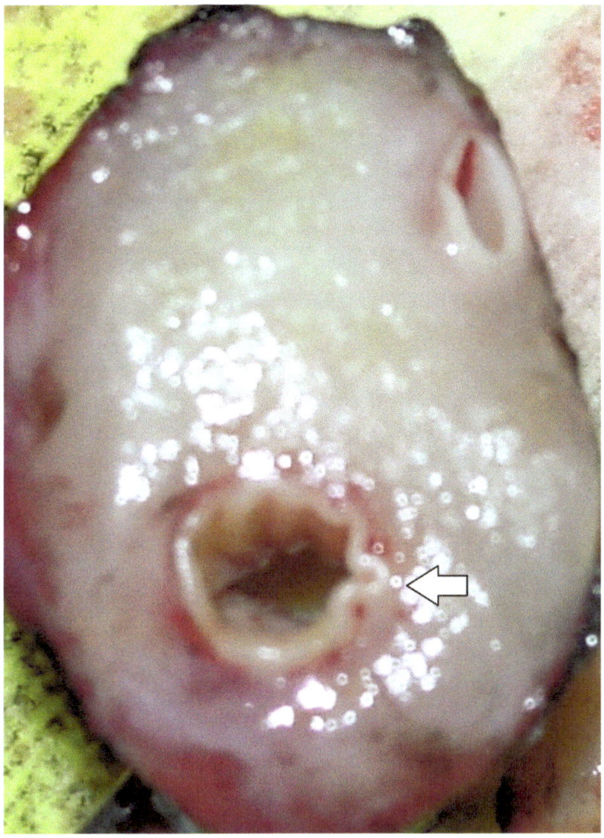

Figure 24.5 Transected gross specimen of a carotid body tumor, Shamblin classification group 3, demonstrating complete encasement of the internal carotid artery (arrow).

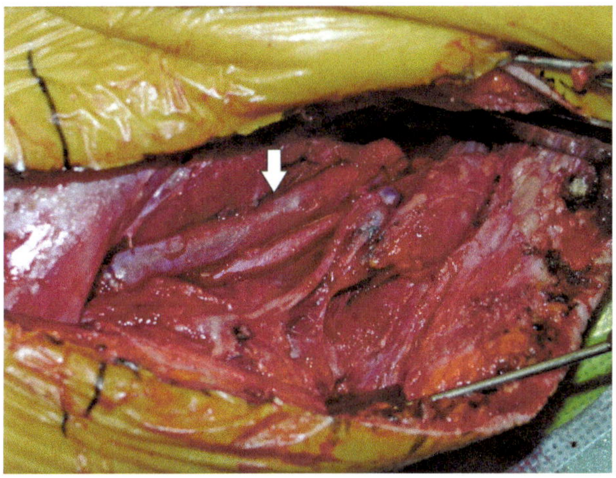

Figure 24.6 Intraoperative photograph demonstrating common carotid-to-internal carotid artery reconstruction with reversed great saphenous vein conduit (arrow), following en bloc resection of a carotid body tumor with carotid artery bifurcation.

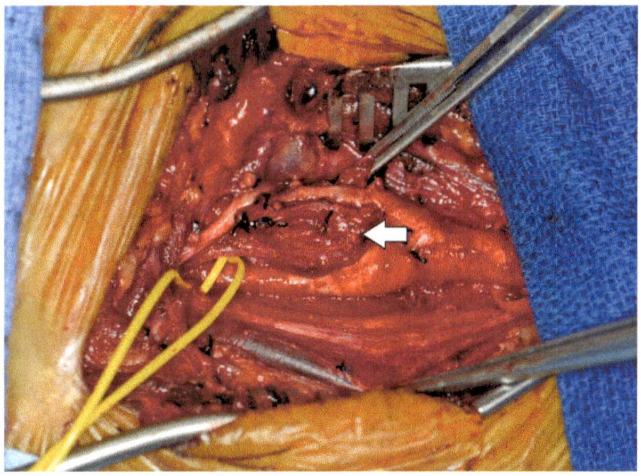

Figure 24.7 Intraoperative image of a Shamblin classification group I tumor (arrow) with several of the feeding branches ligated.

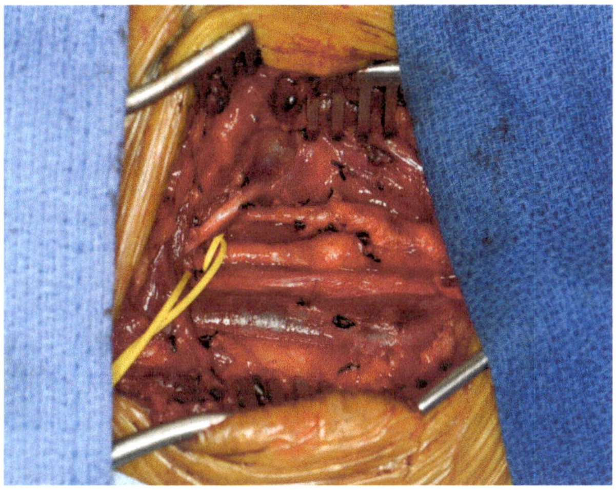

Figure 24.8 Operative image of carotid bifurcation following complete resection of a carotid body tumor (Figure 24.7).

OUTCOMES

Most current series report mortality for surgical resection of CBTs at <3%; however, it has been reported as high as 8.8% with more complex resections requiring arterial reconstruction [4,5,10,11]. Postoperative cranial nerve dysfunction remains significant, with an incidence of up to 40%, and permanent cranial nerve injuries occur in about 20% of patients with a range from 8% to 39% [2,4,11,12]. Perioperative stroke occurs in 0–16% of patients [1,4,13]. Mortality and morbidity have been reported more frequently in cases of advanced tumors and those requiring arterial reconstruction. Complete resection of CBTs can be accomplished in most patients; those patients with complete resection can expect a survival rate similar to that of their peers. Recurrence is rare, but does occur, suggesting the need for continued surveillance [1,3,4].

TRICKS AND TRAPS

- Obtain adequate preoperative imaging that defines the extent of the tumor.
- Be prepared for extended distal exposures (mandibular subluxation) and arterial reconstructions.
- Consider preoperative direct percutaneous embolization of the tumor with ethylene-vinyl alcohol copolymer (Onyx; ev3) for larger CBTs.
- Avoid delaying surgical resection more than 24–48 hours when embolization is performed due to the postembolization inflammatory response in the surrounding tissue that makes dissection more difficult.
- Identify cranial nerves prior to dissection of the tumor.
- Sample abnormal cervical lymph nodes when present to evaluate for metastatic disease and the need for concomitant modified neck dissection.
- Be aware that CBT can distort anatomy and be very adherent to adjacent structures.
- During dissection, stay in subadventitial plane, avoid performing an "exarterectomy" or risk having the artery fall apart.

QUESTIONS

1. The most common complication following resection of a carotid body tumor is:
   a. Cranial nerve injury
   b. Stroke
   c. Upper airway obstruction
   d. Hemorrhage requiring transfusion

   Answer: a

2. Carotid body tumors most commonly present with:
   a. Hoarseness
   b. Cranial nerve deficit
   c. Swallowing difficulty
   d. Horner's syndrome
   e. No symptoms

   Answer: e

3. Following preoperative embolization of a carotid body tumor, the most ideal time frame to perform resection of the tumor is within:
   a. Two days
   b. One week
   c. Two weeks
   d. Four weeks

   Answer: a

4. Extended distal exposure for resection of a carotid body tumor is best facilitated by:
   a. Excision under general anesthesia with orotracheal intubation
   b. Excision under general anesthesia with nasotracheal intubation
   c. Excision under general anesthesia with orotracheal intubation and mandibular subluxation
   d. Excision under general anesthesia with nasotracheal intubation and mandibular subluxation

   Answer: d

REFERENCES

1. Paris, J., Facon, F., Thomassin, J. M., et al. (2006). Cervical paragangliomas: neurovascular surgical risk and therapeutic management. *Eur Arch Otorhinolaryngol*, *263*, 860–865.
2. Patetsios, P., Gable, D. R., Garrett, W. V., et al. (2002). Management of carotid body paragangliomas and review of a 30-year experience. *Ann Vasc Surg.*, *16*, 331–338.
3. Papaspyrou, K., Mann, W. J., & Amedee, R. G. (2009). Management of head and neck paragangliomas: review of 120 patients. *Head Neck*, *31*, 381–387.
4. Kakkos, S. K., Reddy, D. J., Shepard, A. D., et al. (2009). Contemporary presentation and evolution of management of neck paragangliomas. *J Vasc Surg.*, *49*, 1365–1373.
5. Plukker, J. T., Brongers, E. P., Vermey, A., et al. (2001). Outcome of surgical treatment for carotid body paraganglioma. *Br J Surg.*, *88*, 1382–1386.
6. Smith, R. F., Shetty, P. C., & Reddy, D. J. (1988). Surgical treatment of carotid paragangliomas presenting unusual technical difficulties. The value of preoperative embolization. *J Vasc Surg.*, *7*, 631–637.
7. Elhammady, M. S., Farhat, H., Ziayee, H., & Aziz-Sultan, M. A. (2009). Direct percutaneous embolization of a carotid body tumor with Onyx. *J Neurosurg.*, *110*(1), 124–127. doi: 10.3171/2008.4.17513. PMID: 18847339.
8. Felbaum, D. R., Syed, H. R., McCullough, M. F., Armonda, R. A., Liu, A. H., & Bell, R. S. (2016). Embolization of carotid body tumors: revisiting direct puncture technique, preliminary experience and literature review. *Cureus*, *8*(2), e483. doi: 10.7759/cureus.483. PMID: 32175212; PMCID: PMC7053799.
9. Shamblin, W. R., ReMine, W. H., Sheps, S. G., et al. (1971). Carotid body tumor (chemodectoma). Clinicopathologic analysis of ninety cases. *Am J Surg.*, *122*, 732–739.

10. Wang, S. J., Wang, M. B., Barauskas, T. M., et al. (2000). Surgical management of carotid body tumors. *Otolaryngol Head Neck Surg., 123*, 202–206.
11. Maxwell, J. G., Jones, S. W., Wilson, E., et al. (2004). Carotid body tumor excisions: adverse outcomes of adding carotid endarterectomy. *J Am Coll Surg., 198*, 36–41.
12. Sajid, M. S., Hamilton, G., Baker, D. M., et al. (2007). A multicenter review of carotid body tumour management. *Eur J Vasc Endovasc Surg., 34*, 127–130.
13. Hallett, J. W., Jr, Nora, J. D., Hollier, L. H., et al. (1988). Trends in neurovascular complications of surgical management for carotid body and cervical paragangliomas: a fifty-year experience with 153 tumors. *JVasc Surg., 7*, 284–291.

25

Carotid-subclavian bypass and carotid-subclavian transposition

MITCHELL R. WEAVER

INTRODUCTION

Traditionally, nonanatomic arterial reconstructions between the major vessels of the aortic arch, such as carotid-subclavian bypass or transposition, have been performed for the treatment of symptomatic, proximal, occlusive disease in one of these vessels when there is a non-diseased vessel to serve as a donor. The most typical lesions treated have been those of the proximal left subclavian artery (SCA). More recently, the maturation of endovascular techniques has led to a decrease in the number of open arterial reconstructions required for this indication. However, the advent of endovascular means to treat aortic arch pathology has led to an increase in the number of these procedures being performed to "debranch" the aortic arch and thereby create a satisfactory proximal landing zone for a thoracic stent graft (Figures 25.1 and 25.2).

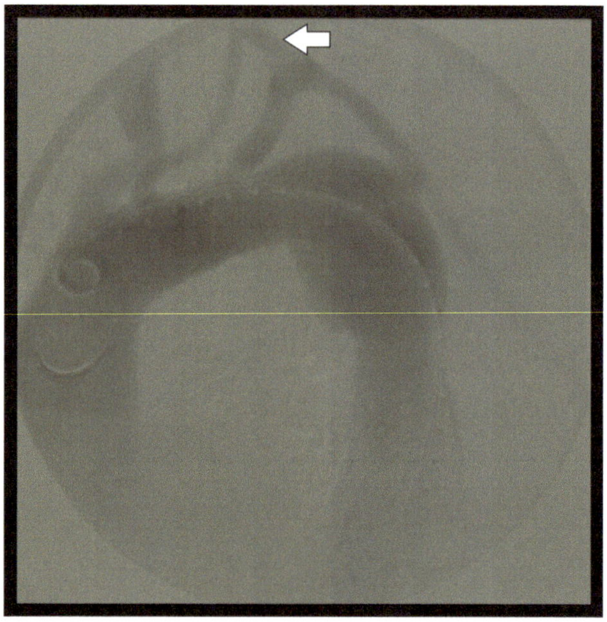

Figure 25.1 Left carotid-subclavian bypass before thoracic endografting (arrow) to treat a descending thoracic aortic aneurysm.

PREOPERATIVE CONSIDERATIONS

Carotid-subclavian transposition is technically more difficult than carotid-subclavian bypass because it requires a more extensive dissection, including identifying and isolating the internal thoracic and vertebral arteries. However, it has the advantage of avoiding the use of a prosthetic graft.

OPERATION

The operation is performed under general anesthesia with the patient in a supine, semi-Fowler's position with the head and torso raised approximately 30 degrees. A rolled-up sheet is placed underneath the patient's shoulder blades. The neck is extended and rotated slightly to the contralateral side. The ipsilateral arm is adducted with slight downward pull to depress the shoulder. Perioperative antibiotics, typically a first-generation cephalosporin, are administered before skin incision. The neck and chest are prepped in a sterile fashion.

A transverse incision is made, starting approximately 1 cm lateral to the midline and 1–2 cm above the clavicle. The incision is continued laterally approximately 6–8 cm. The platysma muscle is divided with cautery and flaps are developed superiorly, approximately 5 cm, and inferiorly to the clavicle. The sternocleidomastoid muscle (SCM) is mobilized along its lateral border, and if necessary, more often in the case of SCA transposition, the clavicular head

DOI: 10.1201/9781003452096-25

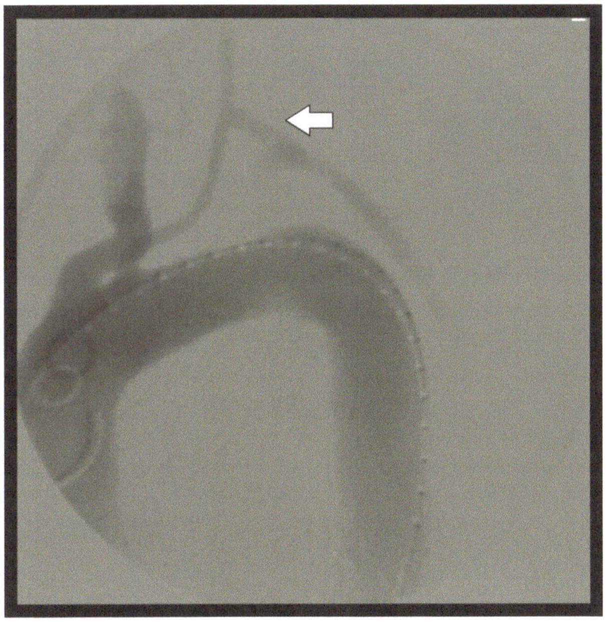

Figure 25.2 Angiogram following thoracic aortic endografting demonstrating the exclusion of the aneurysm and distal arterial flow maintained in the left subclavian artery via carotid-subclavian bypass (arrow).

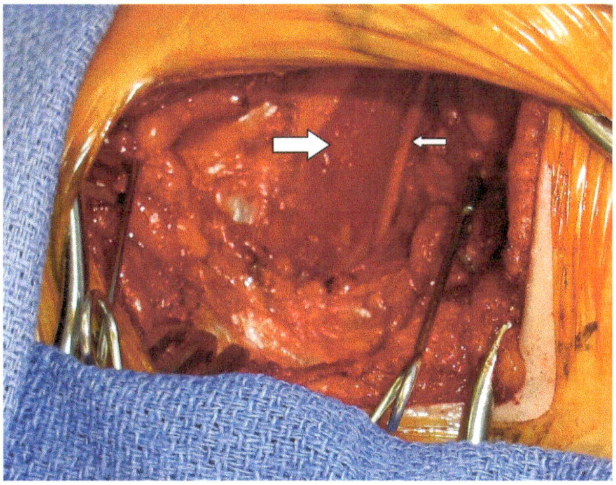

Figure 25.3 Left supraclavicular incision (top of the photo is cranial). Reflection of the anterior scalene fat pad exposes the anterior scalene muscle (large arrow) and overlying phrenic nerve (small arrow).

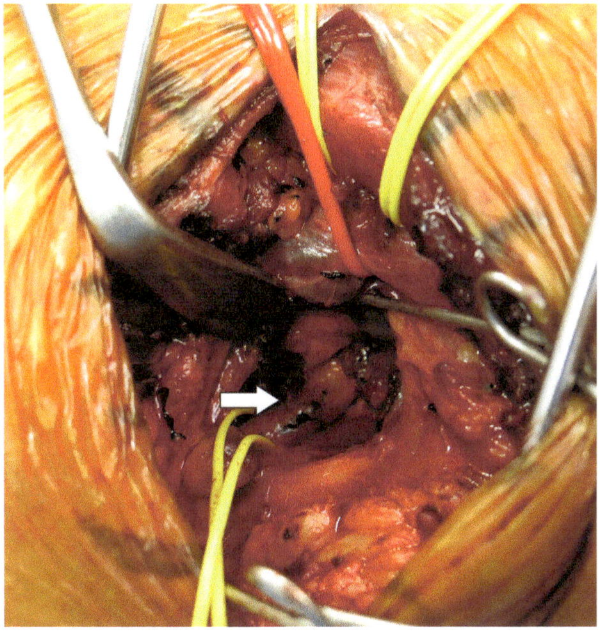

Figure 25.4 Left supraclavicular exposure (top of the photo is cranial). Division of the anterior scalene muscle reveals the left subclavian artery (arrow) with encircling yellow silastic loop to the right. Two yellow silastic loops to the left of the photo are around the left common carotid artery, which is covered by the left internal jugular vein encircled by the red silastic loop.

of the SCM is divided at the clavicle to allow for extended medial exposure.

Once the SCM has been mobilized medially and anteriorly, the carotid sheath is identified and incised, taking care not to injure the structures within it. The common carotid artery (CCA) is approached posterolaterally by mobilizing the internal jugular vein (IJV) and vagus nerve running parallel with it anteriorly and medially. This is also the pathway through which the transposed SCA or bypass graft will traverse. Approximately 5–6 cm of the CCA is exposed to allow for clamping and creating the anastomosis. In cases where the goal of the operation is to treat proximal disease of the left CCA (carotid-subclavian transposition), the artery is dissected proximally as far as possible to allow for adequate length to transpose to the SCA. If a concomitant procedure is planned for the more distal carotid artery (e.g., carotid endarterectomy), this portion of the artery may be exposed through a separate more distal incision along the anterior border of the SCM.

To approach the SCA, the omohyoid muscle is encountered and divided, furthering exposure of the anterior scalene fat pad. Starting on the medial edge of the anterior scalene, it is separated from the IJV; its inferior border is then mobilized. This allows for it to be retracted laterally and superiorly. During this dissection, all lymphatics are carefully ligated as they are divided. On the left side, care is taken not to injure the thoracic duct; however, if injured or divided, it is meticulously oversewn with fine monofilament polypropylene sutures.

The anterior scalene muscle (ASM) is then exposed along with the phrenic nerve that runs lateral to medial, anterior to, and within the investing fascia of the muscle (Figure 25.3). The nerve is carefully mobilized off the muscle by incising the fascia a few millimeters on either side of it. The edges of the ASM are then freed and the muscle is divided, exposing the SCA (Figure 25.4) and brachial plexus. For cases in which carotid to SCA bypass is planned, only enough of the SCA needs to be exposed to allow for the application of vascular clamps for proximal and distal control and to provide an area to perform the anastomosis. When carotid-subclavian transposition is planned, more proximal dissection of the SCA is required. This dissection is continued medially, identifying and mobilizing the internal mammary and vertebral arteries. Dividing the vertebral vein, which is often encountered in this dissection running anterior to the subclavian artery, facilitates this exposure of the proximal SCA. An adequate length of SCA proximal to the vertebral artery needs to be exposed to allow for safe clamping and oversewing of the proximal stump, as well as sufficient length to reach the CCA. Consideration may be made to ligating and dividing the internal mammary artery to allow for increased mobility of the SCA.

Having completed the dissection, the proximal SCA is palpated and assessed to ensure that it can be successfully clamped and oversewn, while still leaving adequate length for transposition to the carotid artery. If there is uncertainty, carotid-subclavian transposition should be abandoned in favor of performing a carotid-subclavian bypass.

Having made the decision to proceed with carotid-subclavian transposition, the patient is systemically anticoagulated with heparin (100 IU/kg), with its effect monitored using activated clotting time. After adequate anticoagulation is achieved, vascular clamps are applied to the SCA and its branches. The SCA is divided proximal to the vertebral artery, and the proximal stump is carefully oversewn with monofilament polypropylene sutures. Before cutting the sutures, the clamp is slowly released and the arterial closure is inspected for hemostasis. Once hemostasis is ensured with the clamp completely removed, the sutures are cut. This is a critical point because loss of control of the SCA as it retracts back into the chest after ligation may lead to catastrophic bleeding that is very difficult to control.

Having controlled the proximal stump, the distal end of the divided SCA is swung over to the adjacent CCA posterior to the IJV. The carotid artery is clamped proximally and distally with atraumatic vascular clamps. A No. 11 blade knife is used to create an arteriotomy that is lengthened in a longitudinal fashion on the lateral aspect of the carotid artery with Potts scissors to a size that will accept the SCA. An end of the SCA to the side of carotid artery anastomosis is then performed, typically with running 5-0 or 6-0 monofilament polypropylene sutures. Just before the completion of the anastomosis, the vessels are vented. The anastomosis is completed and flow is restored. Distal perfusion is assessed with pulse examination and continuous wave Doppler interrogation. If found to be satisfactory, the heparin effect is reversed with protamine sulfate. The author does not routinely monitor cerebral perfusion with electroencephalography during this procedure.

The wound is inspected for bleeding and any sign of lymphatic leak. Having ensured hemostasis and ligation of any possible lymphatic leaks, the anterior scalene fat pad is reapproximated to its original position. A closed suction drain is placed within the wound and taken out through the skin via a separate inferior stab incision. The platysma muscle is closed with interrupted 3-0 braided polyglactin sutures and the skin is closed with running 4-0 braided polyglactin sutures. The drain is removed only after the patient has resumed normal oral intake without signs of lymphatic leak.

When carotid-subclavian bypass is planned, having completed adequate dissection and initiated anticoagulation as described previously, one is ready to proceed with the bypass operation. Typically, a prosthetic graft is chosen. The author prefers a Dacron graft because of ease of handling and reduced needle hole bleeding. While the size of the graft is ultimately determined by the size of the donor and recipient vessels, a graft 6–8 mm in diameter is typically chosen.

Technically, it is easier to perform the SCA anastomosis first, followed by the carotid artery anastomosis. The mid and most apical portion of the SCA is typically the site chosen for the anastomosis. Atraumatic clamps are applied proximally and distally while allowing adequate space for the anastomosis. One should be aware that the SCA is more fragile than the typically encountered common femoral artery. Manipulation should be minimized, including clamping and unclamping of the artery; significant caution should be exercised if considering arterial endarterectomy. Clamps should be applied in a deliberate and gentle manner. Once the artery is controlled, an arteriotomy is created with a No. 11 blade scalpel on its superior surface and extended appropriately with Potts scissors. The end of the graft is cut in a beveled fashion and sewn end-to-side to the artery with running 5-0 or 6-0 monofilament polypropylene sutures. Once the anastomosis is completed, the proximal and distal arteries are vented through the graft and the anastomosis is tested for hemostasis. After ensuring hemostasis, the graft is brought over to the carotid artery posterior to the IJV. The graft is then cut so as not to be redundant or under tension when anastomosed to the carotid artery (Figure 25.5). The anastomosis is performed as described previously for the carotid-subclavian transposition as is closure of the wound. In operations when the carotid artery is transposed to the SCA (Figure 25.6), obtaining adequate proximal length of the CCA is essential. Also, the same care is required when ligating the proximal stump as with the proximal SCA.

When an additional carotid intervention is planned, such as carotid endarterectomy, the graft to the SCA anastomosis is performed first, followed by the endarterectomy. If a carotid shunt is required during the endarterectomy, it may be placed. The endarterectomy is then performed, and prior to patch closure of the artery, a second arteriotomy is created on the lateral aspect of the CCA for the bypass anastomosis. Once completed, patch closure of the artery may be performed and the shunt removed just before completion.

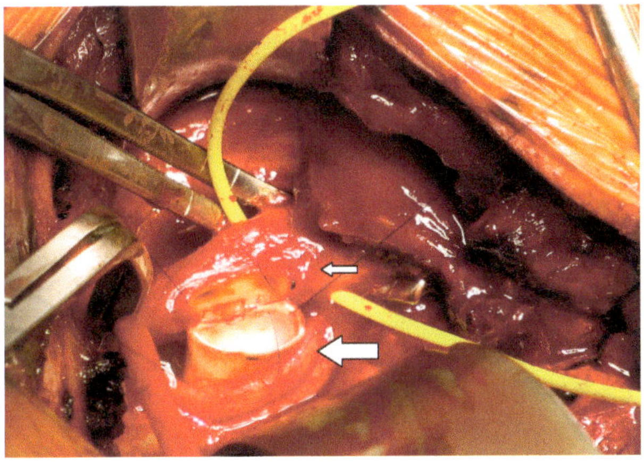

Figure 25.5 Left supraclavicular exposure (top of the photo is cranial). An arteriotomy is created in the lateral aspect of the left common carotid artery (small arrow) encircled distally with a yellow silastic loop. An end of the prosthetic graft tunneled under the jugular vein (large arrow) to the side of the artery anastomosis is performed with a running suture.

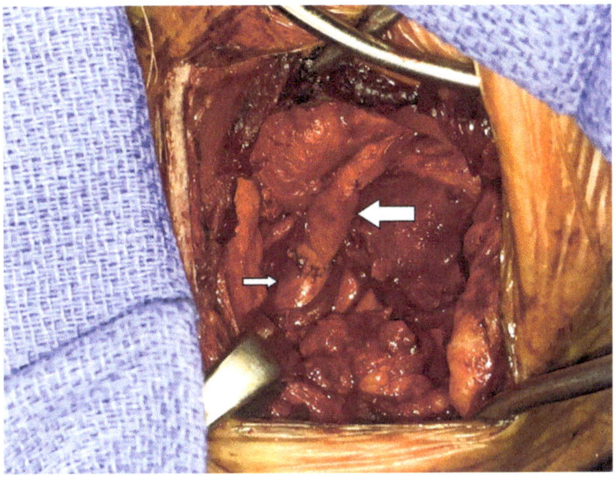

Figure 25.6 Operative image demonstrating a completed end of carotid artery (large arrow) to the side of subclavian artery transposition (small arrow).

Both carotid-subclavian bypass and carotid-subclavian transposition have low morbidity and excellent long-term patency (75–80% at five years for carotid-subclavian bypass and almost 100% for carotid-subclavian transposition) [1-5]. Complications include injury to adjacent nerves (brachial plexus, phrenic nerve, and sympathetic chain) and lymphatic structures (thoracic and accessory thoracic ducts). Nerve injuries are usually self-limited. Lymphatic injuries can be problematic and, if drainage is significant or persistent, early re-exploration and thoracic duct ligation are advised.

TRICKS AND TRAPS

- During exposure of the subclavian artery, the anterior scalene fat pad is mobilized superiorly and laterally with careful ligation/division of all lymphatics.
- The phrenic nerve is carefully mobilized after identifying it on the anterior surface of the anterior scalene muscle running lateral to medial.
- The subclavian artery is a more fragile artery than its more muscular cousin, the common femoral; manipulation should be minimized.
- For bypass, only the apex of the subclavian artery needs to be mobilized; for a transposition, more extensive dissection of the proximal subclavian is necessary along with its branches (the internal mammary and vertebral arteries). Ligation/division of the internal mammary artery is sometimes needed to prevent kinking of a transposed subclavian.
- A 7–8 mm prosthetic graft or the transposed subclavian artery is tunneled behind the internal jugular vein.
- With bypass, the subclavian anastomosis is performed first and the common carotid anastomosis last.
- Medium caliber (15 Fr) closed suction drains are used routinely and not removed until the patient has resumed a regular diet without drainage.
- Significant post-operative chyle leaks should prompt early return to the OR for wound exploration.

QUESTIONS

1. The most common indication for carotid-subclavian artery bypass in contemporary vascular surgery practice is:
   a. Arterial reconstruction in the treatment of a subclavian artery aneurysm
   b. Prior to TEVAR in a patient with a dominant left vertebral artery
   c. Vertebral basilar insufficiency
   d. Left arm ischemia secondary to left subclavian artery stenosis

   Answer: b

2. On post-operative day two following carotid-subclavian bypass, 500 mL of milky fluid is noted in the drain. Which of the following statements describes optimal management?
   a. Nothing by mouth and observation
   b. Coil embolization of thoracic duct
   c. Re-exploration of neck incision and ligation of thoracic duct leak
   d. Ligation of thoracic duct via thoracotomy

   Answer: c

3. Appropriate indications for carotid-subclavian bypass include all the following except:
   a. A patient with 75% stenosis of the proximal subclavian artery and vertebrobasilar symptoms with the use of the left upper extremity
   b. A patient with findings of left subclavian artery occlusion on work up for blood pressure discrepancy between arms
   c. A patient with a history of coronary artery bypass with a left internal mammary artery graft with recurrent angina and severe proximal left subclavian artery stenosis
   d. A patient with 90% left subclavian artery stenosis and left upper extremity lifestyle limiting effort fatigue

   Answer: b

REFERENCES

1. Aziz, F., Gravett, M. H., & Comerota, A. J. (2011). Endovascular and open surgical treatment of brachiocephalic arteries. *Ann Vasc Surg., 25*, 569–581.
2. Aiello, F., & Morrissey, N. J. (2011). Open and endovascular management of subclavian and innominate arterial pathology. *Semin Vasc Surg., 24*, 31–35.
3. Ziomek, S., Quiñones-Baldrich, W. J., Busuttil, R. W., et al. (1986). The superiority of synthetic arterial grafts over autologous veins in carotid-subclavian bypass. *J Vasc Surg., 3*, 140–145.
4. AbuRahma, A. F., Robinson, P. A., & Jennings, T. G. (2000). Carotidsubclavian bypass grafting with polytetrafluoroethylene grafts for symptomatic subclavian artery stenosis or occlusion: a 20-year experience. *J Vasc Surg., 32*, 411–418.
5. Law, M. M., Colburn, M. D., Moore, W. S., et al. (1995). Carotidsubclavian bypass for brachiocephalic occlusive disease: choice of conduit and long-term follow-up. *Stroke., 26*, 1565–1571.

26

Vertebral artery reconstruction

MARK D. MORASCH

INTRODUCTION

Atherosclerosis is the most common disease affecting the vertebral artery. Uncommon pathologic processes include trauma, fibromuscular dysplasia, Takayasu's arteritis, osteophyte compression, dissections, and aneurysms [1,2], all of which can lead to symptoms of posterior circulation ischemia. Approximately 25% of all ischemic strokes occur in the vertebrobasilar territory; 50% of patients present initially with stroke and 26% of patients present with transient ischemic symptoms rapidly followed by stroke [3]. For patients who experience vertebrobasilar transient ischemic attacks, disease in the vertebral arteries indicates a 22–35% risk of stroke over five years [4–6]. The mortality associated with a posterior circulation stroke is 20–30%; this is higher than that for an anterior circulation event [7–9].

Ischemia affecting the temporo-occipital areas of the cerebral hemispheres or segments of the brain stem and cerebellum characteristically produces bilateral symptoms. The classic symptoms of vertebrobasilar ischemia are as follows: dizziness; vertigo; drop attacks; diplopia; perioral numbness; alternating paresthesia; tinnitus; dysphasia; dysarthria; and ataxia.

In general, the ischemic mechanisms can be broken down into those that are hemodynamic and those that are embolic. Hemodynamic symptoms occur because of transient "end organ" (brain stem, cerebellum, occipital lobes) hypoperfusion and rarely result in infarction. Symptoms tend to be transient, repetitive, and more of a nuisance than a danger. For hemodynamic symptoms to occur, occlusive pathology must be present in both paired vertebral vessels or in the basilar artery. In addition, compensatory contribution from the carotid circulation via the circle of Willis must be incomplete. Alternatively, hemodynamic ischemic symptoms may follow proximal subclavian artery (SCA) occlusion and SCA/vertebral artery steal syndrome.

Up to one-third of vertebrobasilar ischemic episodes are caused by embolization from plaques or mural lesions of the SCA, vertebral, or basilar arteries [10]. Actual infarctions in the vertebrobasilar distribution are most often the result of embolic events.

Surgical reconstruction is not indicated in an asymptomatic patient with stenotic or occlusive vertebral lesions because these patients are well compensated from the carotid circulation through the posterior communicating vessels. The minimal anatomic requirement to justify vertebral artery reconstruction for patients with true hemodynamic symptoms is stenosis >60% diameter in both vertebral arteries if both are patent and complete, or the same degree of stenosis in the dominant vertebral artery if the opposite vertebral artery is hypoplastic, ends in a posteroinferior cerebellar artery, or is occluded. A single, normal vertebral artery is sufficient to adequately perfuse the basilar artery, regardless of the patency status of the contralateral vertebral artery. Conversely, patients with symptomatic vertebrobasilar ischemia due to emboli are candidates for surgical revascularization regardless of the condition of the contralateral vertebral artery.

Surgical intervention is not indicated in asymptomatic patients who harbor suspicious radiographic findings.

Duplex ultrasound (US) is an excellent tool for detecting lesions in the carotid artery, but it has significant limitations when used to detect vertebral artery pathology. The usefulness of duplex US lies in its ability to confirm reversal of flow within the vertebral arteries and detect flow velocity changes consistent with a proximal stenosis [11].

Contrast-enhanced magnetic resonance angiography (MRA) with three-dimensional reconstruction and maximum image intensity techniques provides full imaging of the vessels, including the supra-aortic trunks and the carotid and vertebral arteries. Better than computed tomography, transaxial magnetic resonance imaging can readily diagnose both acute and chronic posterior circulation infarcts.

The most common site of disease, the vertebral artery origin, may not be well imaged with US or MRA and often

DOI: 10.1201/9781003452096-26

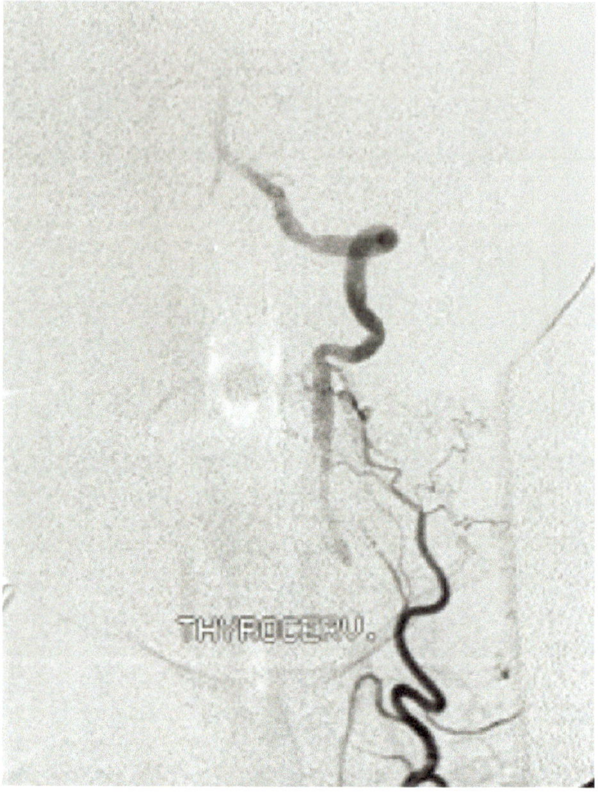

Figure 26.1 V3 segment reconstitution via thyrocervicalcollateral.

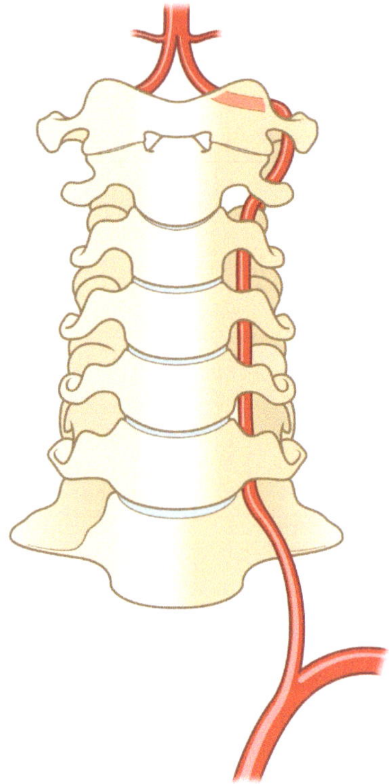

Figure 26.2 Vertebral artery anatomy: V1–V4 segments.

can only be displayed with catheter-based angiography that employs oblique projections, which may not be part of standard arch evaluation. Patients with suspected vertebral artery compression should also undergo dynamic angiography, which incorporates provocative positioning. Finally, delayed imaging should be performed to demonstrate reconstitution of the extracranial vertebral arteries through cervical collaterals, such as the occipital artery, or via collaterals from the ipsilateral SCA, such as branches of the thyrocervical trunk (Figure 26.1) [12].

OPERATIVE STRATEGY AND TECHNIQUE

Surgical anatomy of the vertebral artery

The surgical anatomy of the paired vertebral arteries is divided into four segments: (1) the V1 segment, the origin of the vertebral artery arising from the SCA to the point at which it enters the C6 transverse process; (2) V2, the segment of the artery buried deep within the intertransversarium muscle and the C6-C2 cervical transverse processes; (3) V3, the surgically accessible extracranial segment between the C2 transverse process and the base of the skull before it enters the foramen magnum; and (4) V4, the intracranial portion beginning at the atlantooccipital membrane and terminating as the two vertebral arteries converge to form the basilar artery (Figure 26.2).

Disease location dictates the type of surgical reconstruction that is required. With rare exceptions, most reconstructions of the vertebral artery are performed to relieve either an orificial stenosis (V1 segment), or stenosis, dissection, or occlusion of its intraspinal component (V2 and V3 segments).

Stenosing ostial lesions in the V1 segment [13] are best managed surgically with transposition of the proximal vertebral artery onto the adjacent carotid artery. More distal pathology usually requires bypass from the common carotid artery (CCA) to the V3 segment vertebral artery between Cl and C2.

EXPOSURE AND TRANSPOSITION OF THE VERTEBRAL ARTERY INTO THE CCA

The approach to the proximal vertebral artery is the same as the approach for a SCA-carotid transposition. The patient is positioned in a slight chair position to decrease venous pressure. The incision is made transversely just above the clavicle and directly over the two heads of the sternocleidomastoid muscle. Subplatysmal skin flaps are created to provide adequate exposure. Dissection follows between the two bellies of the sternocleidomastoid muscle after the omohyoid muscle is divided. The jugular vein is retracted laterally, and the carotid sheath is entered. The vagus nerve is retracted medially with the CCA (Figure 26.3). The remainder of the dissection is carried out between the jugular vein and the carotid artery at the base of the neck.

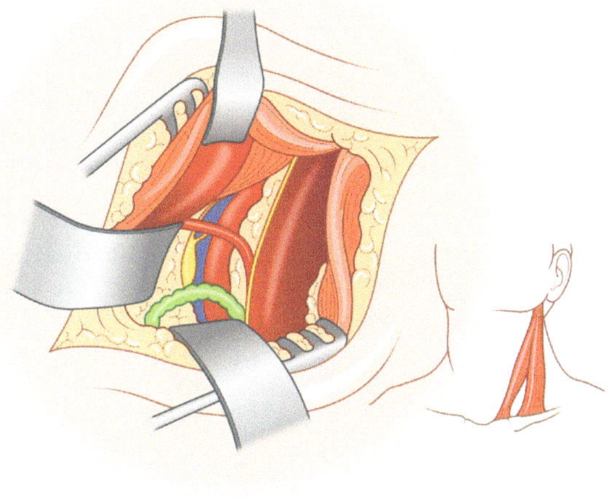

Figure 26.3 Surgical approach to the V1 segment of the vertebral artery. The jugular vein is retracted laterally and the carotid sheet is entered. The vagus nerve is retracted medially with the common carotid artery.

On the left side, the thoracic duct is encircled with a right-angled clamp and then divided between ligatures. Accessory lymph ducts, often seen on the right side of the neck, are also identified, ligated, and divided. The entire dissection is confined medial to the prescalene fat pad that covers the scalenus anticus muscle and phrenic nerve. These structures are left unexposed lateral to the field. The inferior thyroid artery runs transversely across the field, and it is ligated and divided.

The vertebral vein should be identified as it emerges from the angle formed by the longus colli and scalenus anticus muscles. The vein invariably overlies the proximal vertebral artery and, at the bottom of the field, the SCA. It is ligated and divided. The vertebral and subclavian vessels lie immediately deep to the vein. It is important to identify and avoid injury to the adjacent sympathetic chain. The vertebral artery is exposed from its origin at the posteromedial aspect of the SCA distally to the tendon of the longus colli muscle where it enters the transverse foramen of C6. The vertebral artery is freed from the sympathetic trunk resting on its anterior surface without damaging the trunk or the ganglionic rami.

Once the artery is fully exposed, an appropriate site for carotid reimplantation is identified. The patient is given systemic heparin. The distal portion of the V1 segment of the vertebral artery is clamped below the edge of the longus colli muscle with a microclip, avoiding any axial twisting. The proximal vertebral artery is ligated with a 5-0 cardiovascular polypropylene (Ethicon, Rariton, NJ, USA) transfixion suture immediately above its origin. The artery is divided, pulled from under the sympathetic chain, and brought over to the CCA. The free end is spatulated for anastomosis (Figure 26.4). The carotid artery is

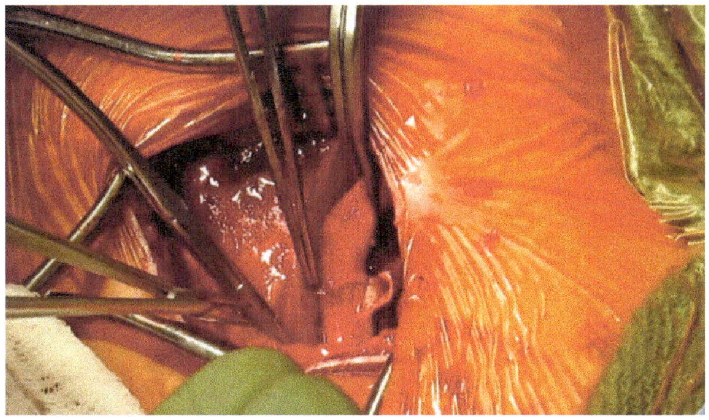

Figure 26.4 Surgical approach to the V1 segment of the vertebral artery. The distal portion of the V1 segment is clamped and the proximal vertebral artery is ligated immediately above its origin. The artery is then divided, pulled from under the sympathetic chain, and brought over the common carotid artery. The free end is spatulated for anastomosis.

cross-clamped. An elliptical 5–7 mm arteriotomy is created in the posterolateral wall of the CCA with an aortic punch. The anastomosis is performed in parachute fashion with continuous 7-0 polypropylene suture. On completion of the anastomosis, the suture slack is tightened, standard flushing maneuvers are performed, the suture is tied, the clamps are removed, and flow is reestablished (Figure 26.5). A drain is placed. This can be removed the following morning provided there is no chylous leak. The incision is then closed by reapproximating the platysma and closing the skin with a subcuticular stitch.

V3 SEGMENT EXPOSURE AND DISTAL VERTEBRAL ARTERY RECONSTRUCTION

Saphenous vein bypass from the CCA or SCA to the V3 vertebral segment is the technique most commonly used to perform a distal reconstruction [12]. Alternatively, the radial artery can be used as a conduit in the absence of a suitable vein. The distal portion of the reconstruction is generally completed at the C1-C2 spinal level.

The skin incision is placed anterior to the sternocleidomastoid muscle, the same as in a carotid operation, and is carried superiorly to immediately below the earlobe. The dissection proceeds in a retro-jugular plane between the vein and the anterior edge of the sternocleidomastoid muscle. The spinal accessory nerve will be encountered and should be dissected gently over a 5 cm length so that it can be retracted safely. The nerve is followed proximally as it crosses in front of the jugular vein and the C1 transverse process. The first cervical vertebrae can be easily felt with finger palpation.

The levator scapulae muscle is exposed by removing the fibroadipose tissue overlying it. Once the anterior edge of the levator scapulae muscle is identified, the anterior ramus of C2 becomes visible. With the ramus as a

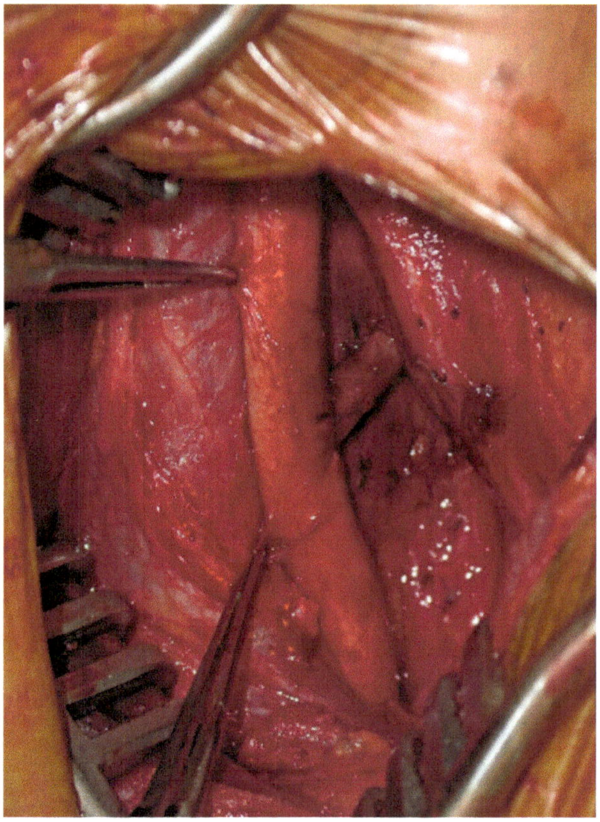

Figure 26.5 Completed proximal vertebral-to-common carotid artery transposition.

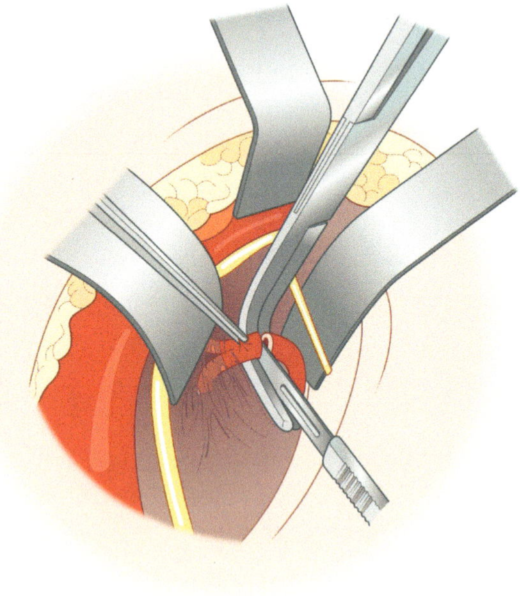

Figure 26.6 Transection of the C2 nerve root and the V3 segment of the vertebral artery, which lies just deep to this structure. The C2 ramus should be cut before it branches.

guide, a right-angle clamp is slid under the levator scapulae muscle and then divided. The C2 ramus divides into three branches after crossing the vertebral artery. The ramus should be cut (Figure 26.6) before it branches. This exposes the V3 segment of the vertebral artery that can then be freed from the surrounding venous plexus over a 1–2 cm length.

Once the vertebral artery is adequately exposed, the distal CCA should be prepared as inflow for the bypass graft. There is no need to dissect the carotid bifurcation; the location selected for the proximal anastomosis should not be too close to the bifurcation because cross-clamping at this level may fracture an underlying atheroma.

A suitable conduit of appropriate length is harvested and prepared. A valveless segment of vein facilitates back-bleeding of the vertebral artery after completion of the distal anastomosis. The patient is given intravenous heparin. The vertebral artery is elevated by gently pulling on an encircling vessel loop and is occluded with a small J clamp. This isolates a short segment for an end-to-side anastomosis. The vertebral artery is opened longitudinally over a short length adequate to accommodate the spatulated end of the vein graft. The end-to-side anastomosis is done with continuous 7-0 polypropylene suture and fine needles. A vascular clamp is placed in the vein graft proximal to the anastomosis and the vertebral J clamp is removed.

The proximal end of the graft is passed behind the jugular vein and in proximity to the side of the CCA. The CCA is then cross-clamped, an elliptical arteriotomy is made in its posterior wall with an aortic punch, and the proximal vein graft is anastomosed end-to-side to the CCA (Figure 26.7). Before the anastomosis is completed, standard flushing maneuvers are performed, the suture is tied, and flow is reestablished. The vertebral artery is occluded with a clip placed immediately below the anastomosis to create a functional end-to-end anastomosis and avoid competitive flow or the potential for recurrent emboli. The wound is closed without a drain by reapproximating the platysma muscle and closing the skin with a subcuticular stitch.

Intraoperative completion imaging with digital angiography is useful and should be considered for all types of vertebral artery reconstruction. Reparable technical flaws may be identified and repair can prevent reconstruction failure.

POTENTIAL POSTOPERATIVE COMPLICATIONS

The perioperative complication rates differ for proximal versus distal vertebral artery repairs. Perioperative complications that can follow any reconstruction include stroke, bleeding, thrombosis, and nerve injury.

Stroke is usually the result of prolonged clamp time or immediate postoperative thrombosis of vertebral arteries or conduits. Completion angiography may be helpful in preventing these complications. Distal reconstructions

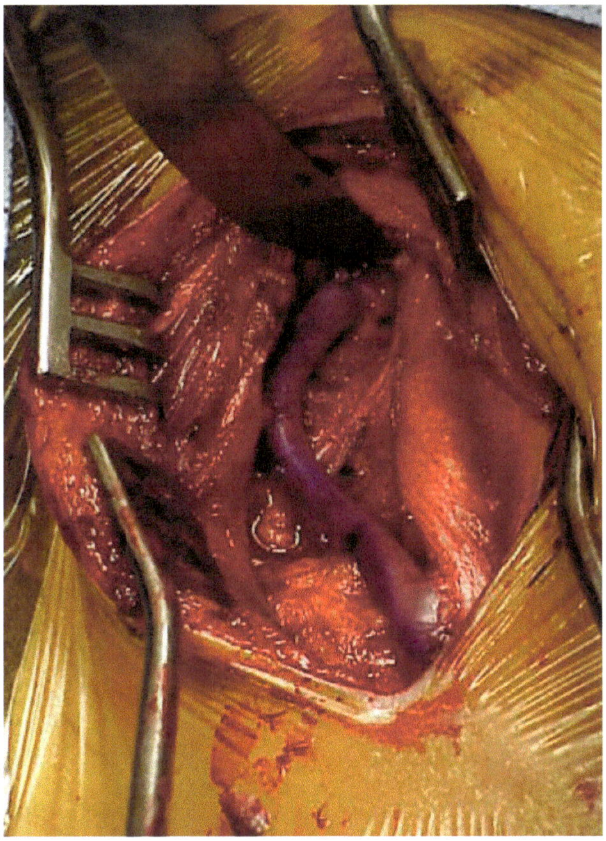

Figure 26.7 Completed common carotid artery-to-V3 segment vertebral artery bypass using reverse great saphenous vein as a conduit.

have a combined stroke and death rate of 3–4% and have higher stroke and death rates than operations on the proximal vertebral artery [12].

NERVE INJURY

Complications that are specific to proximal reconstruction include vagus and recurrent laryngeal nerve palsy (2%) and Horner syndrome (8.4–28%). Complications that may follow distal reconstruction include vagus (1%) and spinal accessory nerve (2%) injuries. Most patients who undergo proximal vertebral reconstruction experience at least a short-lived Horner syndrome. Often, it is not noticeable to the patient but can be seen by other observers. The treatment is expectant. Most, if not all, resolve in time. Vagus nerve injuries manifest as hoarseness and are most often the result of traction on the vagus nerve itself during exposure of the deep neck structures during proximal vertebral transposition or during mobilization of the CCA in a distal bypass. Because this is rarely the result of cutting the recurrent nerve, usually time and patience are all that are required. If vocal cord palsy persists beyond three months, cord medialization may be warranted. A spinal accessory nerve injury results from undo traction. Most neuropraxia-type injuries resolve in time.

Conservative management is appropriate initially for a chylous or significant lymphatic leak as most resolve in time. This includes local compression, dietary manipulation, and administration of octreotide. Leaks that persist beyond three days require re-exploration of the surgical wound; direct suture repair should be attempted. Purse-string placement of a small-gauge monofilament suture works best to control a large lymphatic or thoracic duct leak. If all else fails, ligation of the thoracic duct with video-assisted thoracotomy surgery can be considered.

CASE EXAMPLE

A 69-year-old man initially presented to an academic institution with symptoms of hemodynamic posterior circulation ischemia including vertigo, tinnitus, diplopia, and perioral numbness. An MRA demonstrated chronically occluded right internal carotid (ICA) and right vertebral arteries, a high-grade stenosis of the left vertebral artery, a patent left ICA, but an incomplete circle of Willis. He was managed at this institution with a left proximal vertebral angioplasty with stent placement. His symptoms resolved transiently, but after eight months he was referred to the author with recurrent symptoms. Angiography demonstrated vertebral stent fracture and recurrent high-grade vertebral artery stenosis at the site of the stent damage (Figure 26.8). Because the stent extended the full length of the V1 segment, proximal vertebral-carotid transposition was not feasible. Instead, he underwent a left CCA-to-V3 segment vertebral artery bypass. Six years later, he remains symptom-free.

TRICKS AND TRAPS

- The minimal anatomic requirement to justify vertebral artery reconstruction in patients with posterior circulation stroke or TIA symptoms is stenosis greater than 60% diameter in both vertebral arteries, if both are patent and complete or 60% stenosis in the dominant vertebral artery in the presence of a hypoplastic contralateral vertebral artery, or the contralateral vertebral artery is occluded or even in a posteroinferior cerebellar artery.
- The vertebral vein should be identified overlying the vertebral artery and the SCA at the inferior portion of the exposure during exposure of the vertebral artery for transposition into the CCA.
- On the left side, the thoracic duct is encircled with a right-angled clamp and divided between ligatures on the right side, accessory lymph ducts are identified, ligated, and divided.
- The vertebral artery is freed from the sympathetic trunk resting on its anterior surface without causing injury to the sympathetic trunk or its ganglion.
- An elliptical 5–7 mm arteriotomy is created in the posterolateral wall of the CCA with an aortic punch and anastomosis is performed in a parachute manner.

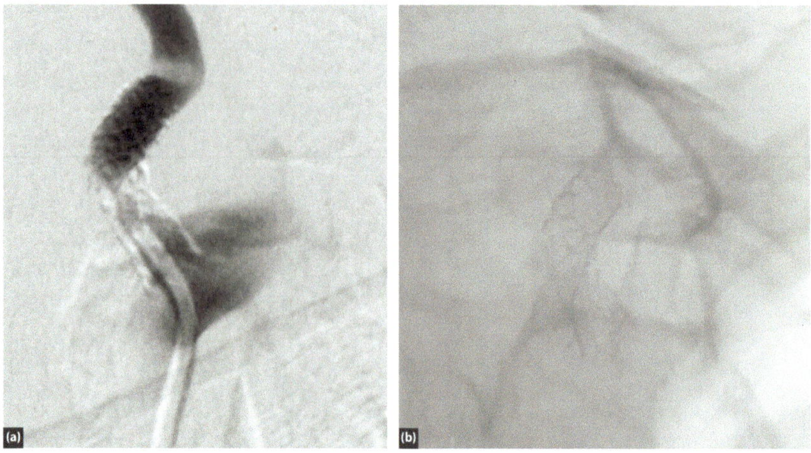

Figure 26.8 Angiography of a 69-year-old man (case example) showing vertebral stent fracture and recurrent high-grade vertebral artery stenosis at the site of the stent damage. (a,b) V1 segment stent fracture with symptomatic in-stent restenosis.

- A drain is placed and removed after 24–48 hours provided there is no chylous leak.
- The saphenous vein from the CCA or SCA to the V3 segment is most commonly used as a conduit. If a suitable vein is not available, the radial artery can be used.
- For V3 segment arterial reconstruction of the vertebral artery, the spinal accessory nerve is carefully mobilized and gently dissected for a distance of 5 cm. The anterior edge of the levator scapulae is identified with identification of C-2 ramus. The levator scapulae is divided under a right-angled clamp and the C-2 ramus is cut, thus exposing the V3 segment of the vertebral artery.

QUESTIONS

1. In patients experiencing TIA in the distribution of vertebrobasilar territory stroke risk over five years is:
   a. 5–15%
   b. 16–20%
   c. 21–33%
   d. >33%

   Answer: c

2. A patient develops a chylous leak following vertebral artery transposition into the common carotid artery. Initial management consists of:
   a. Dietary manipulation and octreotide
   b. Local operative exploration
   c. Thoracic duct embolization
   d. Video-assisted thoracotomy and thoracic duct ligation

   Answer: a

3. High-grade stenotic ostial lesion of the V1 segment of the vertebral artery in a symptomatic patient with contralateral vertebral occlusion should be treated with
   a. Balloon angioplasty
   b. Anticoagulation with Coumadin
   c. Vertebral artery endarterectomy
   d. Transposition of proximal vertebral artery into the common carotid artery

   Answer: d

4. Distal vertical artery (V3 segment) reconstruction has a confirmed stroke and death rate of:
   a. 1–2%
   b. 3–4%
   c. 4–5%
   d. >5%

   Answer: b

5. Which nerve is encountered during exposure of the V3 segment of the vertebral artery:
   a. Vagus
   b. Sympathetic trunk
   c. Spinal accessory
   d. Glossopharyngeal

   Answer: c

REFERENCES

1. Morasch, M. D., Phade, S. V., Naughton, P., et al. (2013). Primary extracranial vertebral artery aneurysms. *Ann Vasc Surg.*, *27*, 418–423.
2. Sultan, S., Morasch, M., Colgan, M. P., et al. (2002). Operative and endovascular management of extracranial vertebral artery aneurysm in Ehlers-Danlos syndrome: a clinical dilemma. Case report and literature review. *Vasc Endovascular Surg.*, *36*, 389–392.

3. Wityk, R. J., Chang, H. M., Rosengart, A., et al. (1998). Proximal extracranial vertebral artery disease in the New England medical center posterior circulation registry. *Arch Neurol.*, *55*, 470–478.
4. Cartlidge, N. E., Whisnant, J. P., & Elveback, L. R. (1977). Carotid and vertebral-basilar transient cerebral ischemic attacks. A community study, Rochester, Minnesota. *Mayo Clin Proc.*, *52*, 117–120.
5. Heyman, A., Wilkinson, W. E., Hurwitz, B. J., et al. (1984). Clinical and epidemiologic aspects of vertebrobasilar and nonfocal cerebral ischemia. In: R. Berguer & R. B. Bauer (Eds.), *Vertebrobasilar Arterial Occlusive Disease: Medical and Surgical Management*. New York, NY: Raven Press, pp. 27–36.
6. Whisnant, J. P., Cartlidge, N. E., & Elveback, L. R. (1978). Carotid and vertebral-basilar transient ischemic attacks: effect of anticoagulants, hypertension, and cardiac disorders on survival and stroke occurrence: a population study. *Ann Neurol.*, *3*, 107–115.
7. Jones, H. R., Jr, Millikan, C. H., & Sandok, B. A. (1980). Temporal profile (clinical course) of acute vertebrobasilar system cerebral infarction. *Stroke.*, *11*, 173–177.
8. McDowell, F. H., Potes, J., & Groch, S. (1961). The natural history of internal carotid and vertebral-basilar artery occlusion. *Neurology.*, *11*(Pt2), 153–157.
9. Patrick, B. K., Ramirez-Lassepas, M., & Synder, B. D. (1980). Temporal profile of vertebrobasilar territory infarction: prognostic implications. *Stroke.*, *11*, 643–648.
10. Caplan, L. R., Wityk, R. J., Glass, T. A., et al. (2004). New England medical center posterior circulation registry. *Ann Neurol.*, *56*, 389–398.
11. Berguer, R., Higgins, R., & Nelson, R. (1980). Noninvasive diagnosis of reversal of vertebral-artery blood flow. *N Engl J Med.*, *302*, 1349–1351.
12. Berguer, R. (1985). Distal vertebral artery bypass: technique, the "occipital connection," and potential uses. *J Vasc Surg.*, *2*, 621–626.
13. Edwards, W. H. & Mulherin, J. L., Jr (1980). The surgical approach to significant stenosis of vertebral and subclavian arteries. *Surgery.*, *87*, 20–28.

27

Upper extremity arterial occlusive disease

HISHAM BASSIOUNY AND AMR EL SHAFEI

INTRODUCTION

Distal to the axillary arteries, critical limb-threatening ischemia may result from a host of diverse pathologies. In contrast to the lower extremity arterial tree, atherosclerotic arterial occlusive disease is less common and may preferentially affect the forearm and digital vessels of patients with diabetes and end-stage renal disease. This chapter reviews contemporary revascularization techniques for managing upper extremity critical ischemia. Such techniques vary, by necessity, according to the type of pathology encountered.

ETIOLOGY

CLTI most commonly occurs from (a) thrombo-embolism of the axillary, brachial, and forearm arteries. Proximal sources of thromboembolism include atrial fibrillation, valvular heart disease or left ventricular aneurysm, subclavian ulcerative plaque or aneurysmal degeneration likely from thoracic outlet syndrome; (b) trauma related to orthopedic fractures, penetrating and blunt trauma, or iatrogenic cannulation; and (c) hand ischemic steal syndrome from high volume arteriovenous fistulae or grafts originating from proximal inflow such as the brachial artery.

Less commonly, the axillary artery and arterial segments beyond are afflicted by (a) repetitive extrinsic trauma as in high-performance athletes (e.g., baseball pitchers) (axillary artery) and in workers who employ jackhammers (ulnar artery hypothenar hammer syndrome) (Figure 27.1); (b) autoimmune vasculitides, radiation involving the axillary and brachial segments; and (c) digital vasospastic and collagen vascular diseases such as ergotism, Raynaud's disease or phenomena, and cold exposure. Such entities are unsuitable for open or endovascular revascularization techniques (Figure 27.2) and respond better to vasodilators or sympathectomy [1,2].

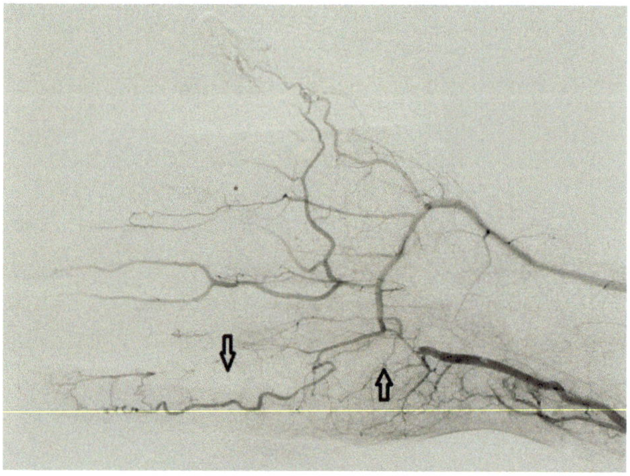

Figure 27.1 Angiography of hypothenar hammer syndrome of the right hand. The upward arrow points to distal ulnar artery occlusion as it traverses through the hypothenar region. The downward arrow points to embolic occlusion of one of the digital arteries of the little finger, resulting from clot in the thrombosed ulnar artery.

CLINICAL EVALUATION AND INITIAL MANAGEMENT

Initially, it should be determined if the clinical scenario is indicative of acute or chronic limb-threatening ischemia. An accurate history and physical examination, in most instances, will indicate the arterial segment involved and the severity of forearm and hand ischemia. The presence of classic symptoms and signs of acute ischemia, namely the six Ps (pulselessness, pallor, paralysis, paresthesia, pain, and poikilothermia) should prompt emergency evaluation and early revascularization for severe ischemia during the golden six-hour period from the onset of ischemia. Delay in reperfusion risks permanent extremity neuromuscular impairment. In acute thromboembolic occlusion, systemic anticoagulation should be

DOI: 10.1201/9781003452096-27

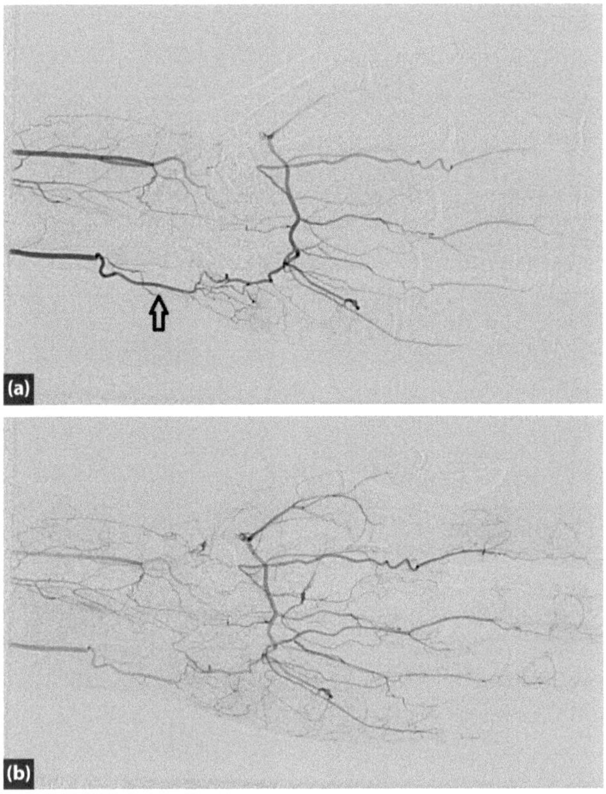

Figure 27.2 Angiography of non-reconstructible small artery occlusive disease of the left hand: (a) early phase demonstrating occlusion of the distal radial and ulnar arteries—the arrow points to a large collateral around the occluded ulnar artery; (b) later phase demonstrating occlusion of multiple digital arteries.

started promptly to minimize thrombus propagation and progressive ischemia. In patients suffering from joint or fracture dislocations, correction of the culprit orthopedic injury may restore distal arterial perfusion. Even if pulses distal to the injury are restored, it is imperative that the proximate artery be subjected to close surveillance by duplex ultrasound (US) or computed tomography (CT) angiography to identify a "silent" intimal injury, nonocclusive thrombus, or pseudoaneurysm.

In the intensive care unit setting, digital ischemia due to radial artery thrombosis from an indwelling catheter is commonly encountered. Initial management entails line removal, anticoagulation if feasible, and weaning of vasopressors to improve digital flow. Most of these patients are high risk and unfit for thrombectomy or lytic therapy. In select cases, surgical thrombectomy via a minimal cutdown overlying the occluded radial artery can be successful in instances when the radial artery is the dominant arterial supply to the hand and short segmental occlusion is present with a patent distal outflow.

NON-INVASIVE VASCULAR TESTING

As with lower extremity arterial occlusive disease, segmental pressure testing including selected digits is useful in determining the degree of extremity and digital ischemia as well as the level of the arterial occlusive pathology. Digital pressure measurements with cold immersion help diagnose suspect vasospastic disorders. Improvement in digital pressures during arteriovenous access compression substantiate the diagnosis of ischemic steal syndrome [3].

Duplex US is invaluable as a first-line, non-invasive test to define the nature and extent of arterial pathology. The examination should include imaging of the arterial tree from the proximal axillary artery to the wrist and hand. High-resolution B-mode imaging can readily distinguish acute thromboembolism, diffuse radiation-induced fibrotic stenosis or autoimmune vasculitis, aneurysmal degeneration, and any associated venous pathology. In suspected athletic injuries, positional shoulder maneuvers assist in detecting muscular entrapment of the axillobrachial artery or humeral head compression. In cases of isolated digital ischemia, patency of the palmar arch can be evaluated with duplex imaging; however, selective arteriography provides a more comprehensive and reliable assessment of palmar arch and digital artery patency.

INDICATIONS FOR UPPER EXTREMITY ARTERIOGRAPHY

In acute ischemic conditions, preoperative conventional or CT arteriography may add little to the physical examination and a high-quality arterial duplex evaluation. That said, intraoperative arteriography is essential to confirm outflow patency beyond the site of the arterial reconstruction. In the case of extensive forearm and hand arterial thrombosis, arteriography helps guide decision-making for thrombo-mechanical lysis and catheter placement for optimum drug delivery. In chronic arterial ischemia, CT arteriography provides sufficient information to formulate an intervention strategy for correcting the underlying ischemic condition. Suboptimal visualization of distal runoff arteries in the distal forearm and hand by CT arteriography should prompt further selective conventional arteriography to determine the feasibility of planned revascularization procedures.

OPEN SURGICAL REVASCULARIZATION

Open revascularization techniques vary according to the arterial pathology encountered. Figure 27.3 illustrates the preferred incisions for the operative exposure of various arterial segments.

THROMBOEMBOLECTOMY

Emboli of cardiac origin can be readily removed by exposure of the distal brachial artery and its bifurcation via a longitudinal skin incision just distal to the elbow crease in the proximal forearm. The median nerve is in close proximity and should be kept out of harm's way. Division

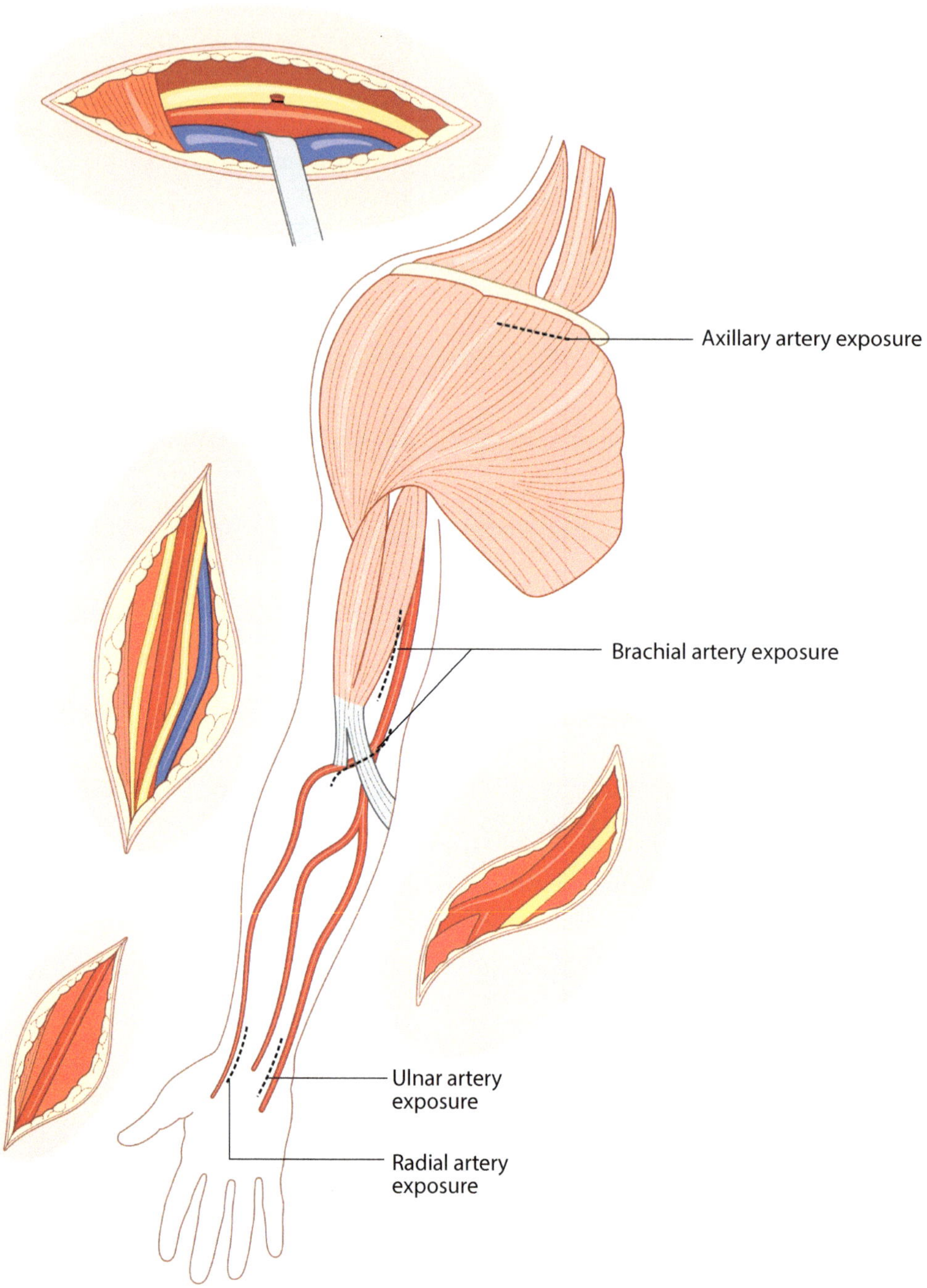

Figure 27.3 Surgical exposures of the axillary, brachial, and ulnar and radial arteries.

of the bicipital aponeurosis facilitates exposure. An adequate length (2–3 cm) of the artery is dissected and the vessel is looped to allow for proximal and distal control.

Before clamping, systemic anticoagulation with heparin is administered to achieve an activated clotting time of >200 seconds. Fine bulldog or pediatric arterial clamps are used for proximal and distal clamping. A 3 mm transverse arteriotomy is performed with a No. 11 scalpel blade on the brachial artery, just above its bifurcation, to allow selective catheterization of the radial and ulnar arteries as necessary. The thrombo-embolus is extracted with a 3- or 4-Fr Fogarty catheter introduced proximally and preferably a 2 Fr catheter in the forearm arteries distally. The catheter is advanced proximally to the subclavian artery to extract any residual proximal thrombus and to achieve brisk arterial inflow. While retrieving the thrombus from the distal arterial bed, it is crucial to avoid balloon overinflation and iatrogenic injury of the forearm outflow vessels. Complete removal of the occluding thrombo-embolus may require several catheter passages to accomplish satisfactory pulsatile inflow and back-bleeding. Completion arteriography is performed to document adequate distal thrombus extraction. The arteriotomy is repaired with an interrupted 6-0 polypropylene suture to avoid purse stringing and narrowing of the artery lumen. The artery is fore and back bled before complete arteriotomy closure.

Restoration of palpable radial and ulnar pulses indicates successful clot removal. Lack of a palpable distal pulse should prompt evaluation of the distal arterial tree with arteriography, if not already performed. Intraoperative fluoroscopy with roadmapping assists in the guidance of over-the-wire thrombectomy catheters in the forearm arteries. When available, over-the-wire coronary suction thrombectomy catheters assist in thrombus retrieval. Should arteriography demonstrate segmental vasospasm, intra-arterial infusion of a vasodilator (e.g., 30–60 mg of dilute papaverine or 100 mcg aliquots of nitroglycerin diluted in normal saline) should be considered. Additional cutdown on the distal radial and ulnar arteries at the wrist may be necessary to extract residual thrombus. In the forearm arteries, longitudinal vein patch closure minimizes the risk of iatrogenic stenosis associated with the primary repair of a transverse arteriotomy.

Intraoperative, catheter-directed thrombolysis is rarely necessary but should be considered to clear residual thrombus distal to the wrist. No more than 5–6 mg of tissue plasminogen activator should be given intraoperatively; the infusion can be continued at 1–2 mg per hour postoperatively. In this instance, the catheter is removed in the operating room following a satisfactory completion arteriogram.

ARTERIAL RECONSTRUCTION

Autogenous conduits, namely the greater saphenous vein and more recently the radial artery [4], are the conduits of choice for reconstruction of the axillary artery and beyond. The greater saphenous vein is preferred over the cephalic or basilic vein because of ease of handling and length requirements. The cephalic and basilic veins, however, should be preserved in traumatic injuries associated with deep vein injury to avoid venous outflow issues with venous hypertension and possible resulting compartment syndrome.

Interposition bypass grafting

Interposition bypass grafting is the technique of choice for traumatic injuries and aneurysmal degeneration of the axillary and brachial arteries (Figure 27.4). Transmural or significant intimal damage related to repetitive athletic or occupational trauma, orthopedic traction injury, and penetrating or blast injuries should be resected to healthy margins. While it is sometimes possible to mobilize the artery and perform an end-to-end arterial anastomosis with focal injuries, caution should be exercised to avoid undue tension as this may lead to subsequent suture line disruption and/or in situ thrombosis. With interposition bypass grafting, the proximal and distal anastomoses are performed in an end-to-end fashion with anterior and

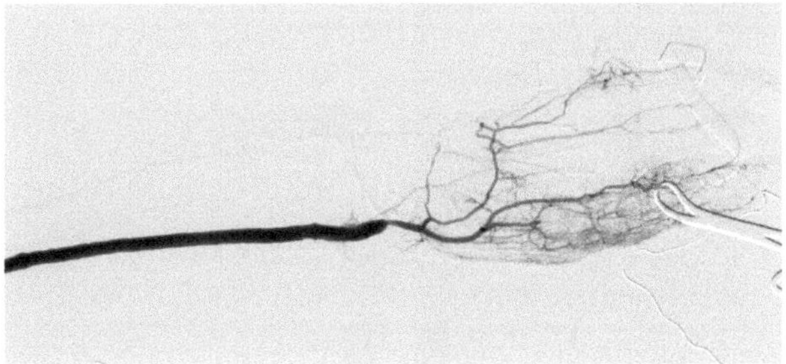

Figure 27.4 Upper extremity arterial interposition bypass graft from brachial artery to distal radial artery with a reversed greater saphenous vein conduit.

posterior spatulation of the artery and vein, respectively, to avoid suture line stenosis. For upper arm arteries, a running suture starting from both corners of the anastomosis is used, while interrupted sutures are advised for forearm anastomoses.

Careful attention is paid to conduit course and length to avoid musculofascial entrapment or repetitive trauma by a bony prominence. A subcutaneous course is preferred to facilitate conduit access for postoperative clinical and duplex surveillance and in the rare circumstance that a redo procedure becomes necessary. Conduits traversing the elbow joint should be of sufficient length to avoid tension on the anastomotic suture lines when the joint is fully extended. Reduction and fixation of fracture dislocation(s) in the arm and forearm may inadvertently alter conduit course or orientation. Hence, conduit integrity and patency must be verified before exiting the operating room after orthopedic manipulation and fixation.

For distal ulnar artery bypass, the conduit of choice is the contralateral radial artery because of a better size match and superior long-term performance. Continuity of the palmar arch is evaluated by an Allen test and duplex imaging before the radial artery is harvested.

Either end-to-side or end-to-end anastomosis is performed with an interrupted or running 7-0 polypropylene suture.

Endarterectomy and vein patch angioplasty

Endarterectomy is rarely used; the sole indication might be a focal stenosis at a joint line where balloon angioplasty has failed.

Ischemic hand secondary to steal-revascularization procedures

Patients with ischemic steal syndrome due to high-flow brachial arteriovenous procedures may be managed by a variety of open reconstructive techniques that include distal revascularization and interval ligation (DRIL) (Figure 27.5), revision using distal inflow, proximalization of arterial inflow, banding, or ligation. The DRIL

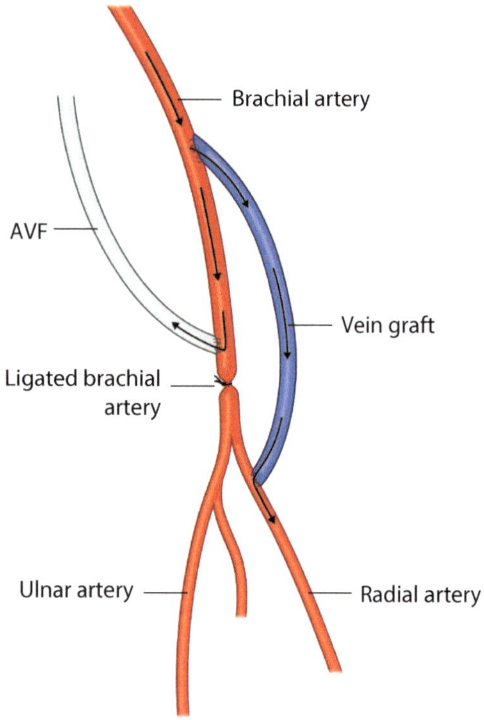

Figure 27.5 Distal revascularization and interval ligation procedure for steal syndrome in patients with upper extremity arteriovenous fistulae.

procedure is used in vascular practice to correct ischemic hand symptoms secondary to steal with preservation of functioning arteriovenous access. A disease-free brachial artery proximal to the arterial anastomosis, an adequate saphenous vein conduit, and reasonable forearm outflow are essential for a successful DRIL procedure [5].

Initially, the brachial artery is ligated just distal to the arteriovenous anastomosis above the elbow crease. This is followed by distal revascularization to restore arterial perfusion to the forearm and hand. The location of the proximal anastomosis of the distal revascularization bypass is the key variable for the hemodynamic success of this procedure. The proximal bypass anastomosis must be created 5–10 cm proximal to the arteriovenous anastomosis where there is normal systemic pressure to drive blood flow into the bypass *and* the arteriovenous communication. Intra-arterial pressure measurements help to select the optimum region for the proximal anastomosis. Distally, the bypass is anastomosed to the distal brachial artery or the proximal radial or ulnar arteries below the elbow crease.

ENDOVASCULAR INTERVENTIONS

1. *Pharmacologic thrombolysis* [6] for acute thrombotic occlusions that are inaccessible with surgical techniques; focal or diffuse arterial stenosis; and aneurysmal disease. The access site depends on the location of the lesion. Axillary or proximal brachial artery pathology requires either a transfemoral or retrograde transbrachial route. For forearm arterial pathology, antegrade brachial access is used. Access with low-profile sheaths (5 and 6 Fr) is advised. It remains debatable whether a percutaneous or open cutdown technique is safest. If a percutaneous technique is used, US-guided puncture is advised. The author prefers the open cutdown technique for several reasons: (a) relative ease in exposing the upper arm vessels with a limited incision; (b) direct closure of the puncture site, which avoids hematoma formation and allows for continuing systemic anticoagulation; and (c) primary closure, which minimizes the risk of in situ thrombosis from compression of the puncture site after percutaneous sheath removal.
2. *Mechanical thrombectomy* has gained increasing popularity for rapidly resolving lower extremity acute thrombi without the need for prolonged catheter-directed thrombolysis and required ICU admission. As such, successful outcomes have been achieved with the use of mechanical thrombectomy catheters such as Penumbra 3.4 and 6 Fr catheters (Penumbra Inc, Alameda, CA, USA) in isolated case reports; acute hand ischemia following COVID-19 infection in a young professional volleyball player after failed thrombolysis and in patients with middle cerebral artery embolism associated with uni or bilateral upper extremity ischemia [7,8]. However, the efficacy of mechanical suction devices in upper extremity thromboembolectomy deserves further study.
3. *Balloon angioplasty/stenting* is employed for stenotic lesions. As the advantage of drug-eluting balloons in upper extremity atherosclerotic or vasculitic stenosis is unknown, such balloons may be considered for off-label use in recurrent stenotic lesions. Stenting across joint lines is ill-advised to avoid stent compression and fracture. Treating the rare case of an axillobrachial artery aneurysm with a covered (self-expanding or balloon-mounted) stent is a reasonable option in patients deemed at high risk for surgery.

Catheter-directed interventions [9] may be more frequently employed as experience evolves; however, further studies examining the long-term efficacy of such interventions for upper extremity arterial occlusive disease are needed.

COMPLICATIONS

Because most patients who suffer from upper extremity acute thromboembolic occlusion have disease-free arteries, it is not uncommon to encounter segmental vasospasm of the forearm and hand arteries on completion arteriography after balloon catheter thrombus retrieval. The dictum "spasm is CLOT until proven otherwise" should be exercised with caution. Repeat arteriography after intra-arterial administration of papaverine or nitroglycerine should be undertaken to resolve this quandary. The operator must consider the risk of intimal damage with repetitive catheter passage. If there is adequate arterial continuity to the entire palmar arch, it is unnecessary to persist in recanalizing all forearm arteries to minimize the risk of iatrogenic arterial injury. In this scenario "the enemy of good is better."

Another potential complication is clamp injury to the forearm and hand arteries, which can be heavily calcified in patients with diabetes and those undergoing dialysis. Use of a tourniquet is highly advised to avoid clamping while creating arterial anastomoses to such a vessel, although sometimes proximal vessels are too calcified to be successfully occluded even in this fashion. Alternatively, intraluminal balloons can be used for inflow and outflow control.

TRICKS AND TRAPS

- Attention to occupational and athletic history and potential related injuries.
- Assessment of silent arterial pathology proximate to orthopedic injuries.
- In thromboembolic occlusion, evaluate for a proximal cardiac or subclavian source.
- Look for inflow stenosis in ischemic hand steal and reduced hemodialysis access flow.
- Avoid interventions for hand ischemia in hemodynamically unstable patients on vasopressor support.
- Vein patch angioplasty is advisable if there is concern for arterial stenosis following arteriotomy closure.
- Minimize use of Fogarty catheters greater than 2F in forearm arterial branches to avoid mural arterial injury.
- Intraoperative t-PA infusion to lyse inaccessible palmar arch and digital thrombus.
- If pharmacologic thrombolysis fails, consider mechanical thrombectomy.
- Intraoperative completion arteriography is imperative.
- Vasospasm is common in forearm arteries following endovascular intervention and responds to intra-arterial vasodilator administration.

QUESTIONS

1. Which of the following is not a cause of occlusive disease in the upper limb?
   a. Ischemic monomelic neuropathy
   b. Atrial fibrillation
   c. Thoracic outlet syndrome
   d. Hypothenar hummer syndrome

   Answer: a

2. In ICU-admitted patients, the most common cause of bluish discoloration of the index and thumb is
   a. Hypoperfusion
   b. Brachial artery embolus
   c. Thrombosed radial artery after arterial line insertion
   d. Vasculitis

   Answer: c

3. The only test that tests the palmar arch continuity is:
   a. Roos test
   b. Allen's test
   c. Elvey's test
   d. Adson's test

   Answer: b

4. The proper treatment of ischemic steal syndrome associated with low flow AV access is:
   a. DRIL
   b. RUDI
   c. Balloon angioplasty of possible stenotic lesions
   d. Banding of the veins

   Answer: c

5. The following is considered a sign of successful embolectomy:
   a. Completion angiogram revealing patent arterial tree
   b. Audible flow by Doppler signals over radial and ulnar arteries
   c. Back-bleeding before closure of arteriotomy
   d. Advancement of the Fogarty catheter down to the arch

   Answer: a

REFERENCES

1. Longo, G. M., Pearce, W. H., & Sumner, D. S. (2005). Evaluation of upper extremity ischemia. In R. B. Rutherford (Ed.), *Vascular Surgery* (6th ed., pp. 1274–1293). Philadelphia, PA: Elsevier/Saunders.
2. Herrick, A. L. (2013). Management of Raynaud's phenomenon and digital ischemia. *Curr Rheumatol Rep., 15*, 303.
3. Grasu, B. L., Jones, C. M., & Murphy, M. S. (2015). Use of diagnostic modalities for assessing upper extremity vascular pathology. *Hand Clin., 31*, 1–12.
4. Masden, D. L., Seruya, M., & Higgins, J. P. (2012). A systematic review of the outcomes of distal upper extremity bypass surgery with arterial and venous conduits. *J Hand Surg Am., 37*, 2362–2367.

5. Aimaq, R., & Katz, S. G. (2013). Using distal revascularization with interval ligation as the primary treatment of hand ischemia after dialysis access creation. *J Vasc Surg.*, *57*, 1073–1078.
6. Schrijver, A. M., De Borst, G. J., Van Herwaarden, J. A., et al. (2015). Catheter-directed thrombolysis for acute upper extremity ischemia. *J Cardiovasc Surg (Torino).*, *56*, 433–439.
7. Achim, A., Kákonyi, K., Jambrik, Z., & Ruzsa, Z. (2022). A case report of COVID-19-associated acute hand ischaemia in a young professional volleyball player. *Eur Heart J Case Rep.*, *6*(3), ytac099.
8. Katano, T., Suzuki, K., Kimura, R., Nakagami, T., Numao, S., Takeshi, Y., ... Kimura, K. (2020). Thrombectomy for upper extremity artery occlusion with major cerebral artery occlusion using mechanical thrombectomy devices for acute ischemic stroke. *J Neuroendovascular Ther.*, *14*(10), 454–460.
9. Tomoi, Y., Soga, Y., & Fujihara, M., et al. (2016). Outcomes of endovascular therapy for upper extremity peripheral artery disease with critical hand ischemia. *J Endovasc Ther.*, *23*, 717–722.

28

Open non-ruptured infrarenal abdominal aortic aneurysm repair

ALEXANDER D. SHEPARD

INTRODUCTION

Widespread adoption of endovascular repair has made open repair of infrarenal (IR) abdominal aortic aneurysms (AAA) an infrequent operation in the modern era. It is usually reserved for patients with complex aneurysm anatomy not amenable to stent grafting. Other indications include large size (>6.5 cm in diameter), young (≤65 years)/fit patients, associated renovascular anomalies, and concerns re: follow-up compliance. As a result, open repair has become more technically challenging than in the past.

APPROACHES

Transperitoneal (TP) exposure when performed through a midline incision is the most versatile approach allowing unlimited exposure of the IR aorta and its branches (Figure 28.1). Special positioning is not required, and aortic exposure is rapid, making this approach more suitable for emergencies than a left flank retroperitoneal (RP) approach. When combined with left medial visceral rotation, it can provide exposure of the suprarenal aorta to the level of the aortic hiatus. Drawbacks include the occurrence of adhesions and a high incidence (>25%) of incisional hernia. Transverse incisions are less painful and hence valuable for patients with pulmonary compromise. A supraumbilical ("frown") transverse incision is particularly helpful when contemplating concomitant distal renal artery reconstruction while an infraumbilical ("smile") incision is useful when needing good pelvic exposure for large iliac/hypogastric aneurysms. Exposure beyond the iliac bifurcations is harder with a supraumbilical incision, while exposure of the pararenal aorta is difficult through an infraumbilical transverse incision.

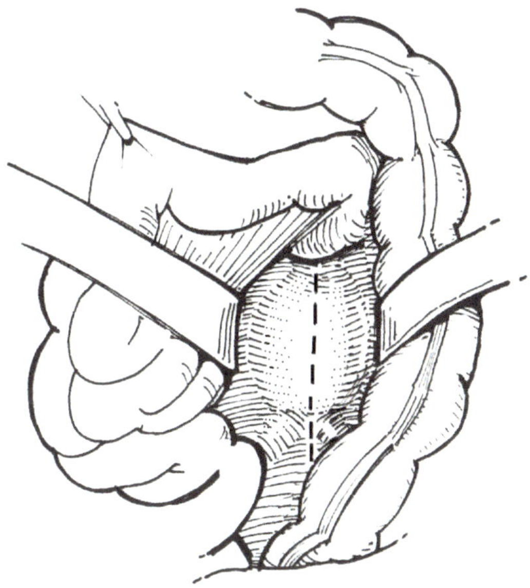

Figure 28.1 Initial inframesocolic exposure of infrarenal AAA with transverse colon reflected superiorly, small bowel retracted to the right, and descending/sigmoid colon retracted to the left.

A left flank RP approach is useful for complex open AAA repair with exposure of the entire abdominal aorta from diaphragm to the proximal iliacs. Visualization of the distal right iliac system and the right renal artery, however, is limited. This approach is helpful for exposure/control of the suprarenal aorta, re-do aortic operations, concomitant horseshoe kidney, large (>8 cm) or inflammatory AAA, "hostile" abdomen (multiple prior celiotomies or ostomy), morbid obesity, abdominal wall diastasis, and because of reduced pain compared with midline incisions, pulmonary compromise.

DOI: 10.1201/9781003452096-28

PREPARATION

Assuming normal cardiopulmonary risk and renal function, the most important preoperative test is a high-quality, thin-cut computerized tomographic angiogram (CTA). This study determines the type of reconstruction and suitable clamp sites in addition to identifying concomitant intraabdominal pathology and venous anomalies (e.g., retroaortic left renal vein [LRV]). An epidural catheter provides postoperative analgesia to decrease the surgical stress response and reduce pulmonary complications. Central line, arterial line, Foley catheter, and large bore IVs are standard, but pulmonary artery catheters are not. We rely on transesophageal echocardiography for cardiac monitoring when necessary. Cell saver, body warmers, and lower extremity sequential compression devices are also routine.

TRANSPERITONEAL APPROACH

The abdomen is opened through a long xiphoid to pubis incision. Abdominal exploration is unnecessary because of the accuracy of preoperative CTA. A mechanical retraction system (e.g., Omni Tract or Thompson) allows the procedure to be performed with only a first assistant. The IR aorta is exposed through an inframesocolic approach by reflecting the omentum and transverse colon superiorly out of the abdomen and retracting the small bowel to the right. When feasible, the small bowel is packed into the right side of the abdomen to reduce bowel edema. The ligament of Treitz is divided to retract the duodenum off the aortic neck (Figure 28.1).

The midline retroperitoneum overlying the aneurysm is incised from the proximal neck to the bifurcation with division of the overlying lymphoareolar tissue. The crossing LRV is identified proximally and for most infrarenal aneurysms marks the proximal extent of exposure (Figure 28.2). The much smaller inferior mesenteric vein is frequently encountered coursing obliquely, more superficially, and can be divided as necessary. A short segment of the LRV is cleared off to expose the underlying aorta, taking care to ligate any associated lymphatics to prevent a chyle leak. Subsequent dissection stays on the aorta and the non-aneurysmal aortic neck is cleaned off anteriorly, and on either side down to the lumbar spine, enough to allow the application of a vertically oriented aortic cross-clamp. An ultrasonic scalpel can be helpful; circumferential dissection of the aortic neck is usually unnecessary. If the posteriorly coursing lumbar branch of the LRV is encountered during this dissection, it may need to be ligated and divided to avoid injury.

For more proximal aortic exposure, the LRV may be either mobilized (our choice) or ligated/divided. With mobilization, the RV is skeletonized from close to the inferior vena cava (IVC) back toward the kidney with division of the three major branches distal to the kidney (lumbar branch, gonadal, and adrenal veins) (Figure 28.3).

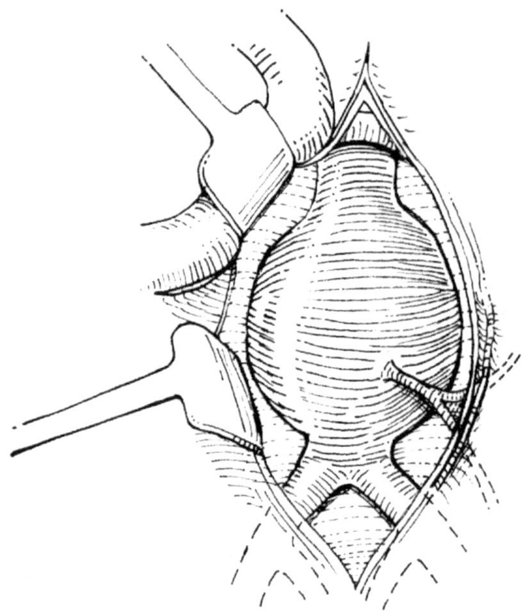

Figure 28.2 Incision through retroperitoneum to expose infrarenal aneurysm from crossing renal vein superiorly to bifurcation distally. The inferior mesenteric artery (IMA) is the only major branch originating anteriorly.

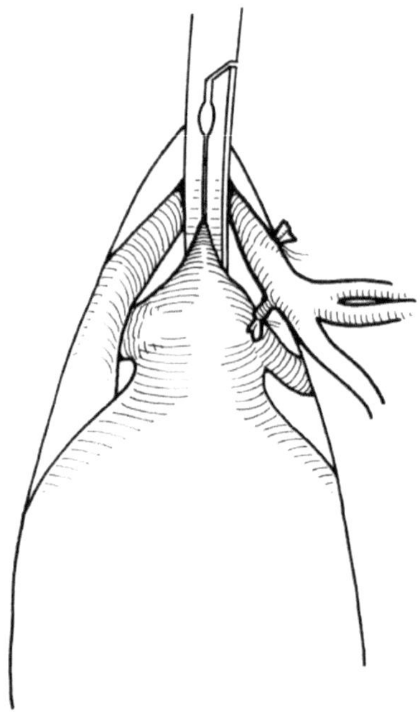

Figure 28.3 Mobilization of left renal vein following division of adrenal and lumbar branches to expose pararenal aorta and allow the placement of a suprarenal aortic cross-clamp.

It is important to decide which technique to use because preservation of these branches is critical to providing collateral outflow to the kidney if the LRV is divided.

If the inferior mesenteric artery (IMA) is patent, its origin should be identified and protected as dissection is carried distally down the aorta. The aortic bifurcation is identified, and special attention paid to preserving the parasympathetic nerve chain passing over the origin of the left common iliac artery (CIA). In younger patients in whom sexual function is a concern, a nerve-sparing dissection can be carried down the right side of the aorta, reflecting the nerve plexuses to the patient's left and specifically avoiding the inferior mesenteric plexus that surrounds the IMA [1]. This dissection is more time-consuming than standard midline dissection and precludes utilization of tube graft reconstruction, but it is associated with a higher degree of normal sexual function post-op.

The proximal CIAs are mobilized carefully to avoid injury to the caval confluence or iliac veins, which can be adherent posteriorly secondary to aneurysm and/or atherosclerosis-induced inflammation. Circumferential control is not always necessary and clamping the iliacs slightly more distally may be safer. Venous injuries in this area are very challenging and sometimes require aortic clamping and iliac artery division to repair!

The retroperitoneal incision can be extended along the right iliac for exposure. If only the distal right iliac (bifurcation or beyond) exposure is necessary, a second short retroperitoneal incision over the artery can be made, taking care to identify and protect the ureter as necessary. The proximal-most left CIA can be exposed from the midline retroperitoneal incision, but for distal left iliac exposure, the sigmoid colon is mobilized after dividing its lateral peritoneal reflection. If necessary, the femoral arteries can be exposed through standard groin incisions, although it is best to avoid distal anastomoses at the femoral level whenever possible because of the risk of infection.

Prior to clamping, patients are heparinized (100 units/kg to maintain activated clotting time >250 seconds). This test is repeated q30 min during clamping and additional heparin administered as necessary. Lower body warmers and sequential compression sleeves are turned off prior to clamping. Distal arteries are usually clamped prior to proximal arteries. The proximal aortic clamp site is chosen carefully. It is important to avoid multiple clamp applications with a diseased/calcified aorta or when clamping above the RAs. Occasionally, this requires clamping the supraceliac (SC) aorta, which is frequently the least diseased abdominal aortic segment. The Cherry clamp is our preferred clamp.

Intraluminal repair has supplanted resection of the aneurysm sac because of less bleeding, lower risk of injury to adjacent structures, speed, and the ability to use the aneurysm sac to provide graft coverage. Resection is still occasionally used for very small or infected AAA. Prior to clamping, a graft sizer can help decide on graft size; experience suggests that a graft one size smaller than measured by the sizer on the pressurized aorta (e.g., 18 mm when the sizer suggests 20 mm) usually gives the best match. Dacron grafts are preferred to polytetrafluoroethylene (PTFE) unless there is significant iliac occlusive disease because of the 20% risk for peri-graft seromas with PTFE [2].

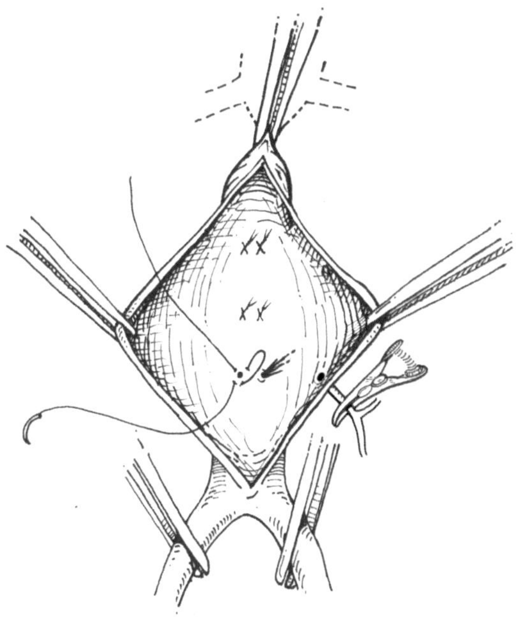

Figure 28.4 Aneurysm sac opened with oversewing of back bleeding lumbar arteries. The inferior mesenteric artery controlled with a small bulldog clamp.

After clamping, the aneurysm sac is opened longitudinally from a point just distal to the planned proximal anastomotic suture line to just above the aortic bifurcation, taking care to go to the right of the IMA and avoid the autonomic nerves crossing the left iliac origin. Intraluminal mural thrombus is bluntly removed and back bleeding lumbars identified and oversewn with 3-0 polypropylene sutures (Figure 28.4). If the aortic wall is heavily calcified, it is easier to perform an endarterectomy around the lumbars, which allows transfixing stitches to cinch down appropriately. If there is good back bleeding from a patent IMA, it can be suture-ligated from the inside; if back bleeding from a patent IMA appears questionable, then the IMA can be controlled by either placing a small clamp across its origin or inflating a 3Fr balloon catheter intraluminally.

Reconstruction proceeds with a tube or bifurcated graft. A tube graft is faster and is suitable when there is no significant iliac occlusive disease, and the CIAs are ≤16 mm in diameter unless the patient is very young or has a known connective tissue disorder. Tube grafts are avoided when the preservation of sexual function is a concern because it is difficult not to injure the parasympathetic plexus coursing over the left iliac artery when trying to create a distal sewing ring. In younger patients, avoiding injury to these "sex" nerves is most easily accomplished by tunneling the limbs of a bifurcated graft through the origins of the iliac arteries, leaving the aortic bifurcation intact. When sewing to the iliacs, one always tries to get beyond all aneurysmal disease *and* preserve flow to at least one hypogastric.

A proximal sewing ring is created by "T-ing" off the aortotomy at the junction between normal aorta and

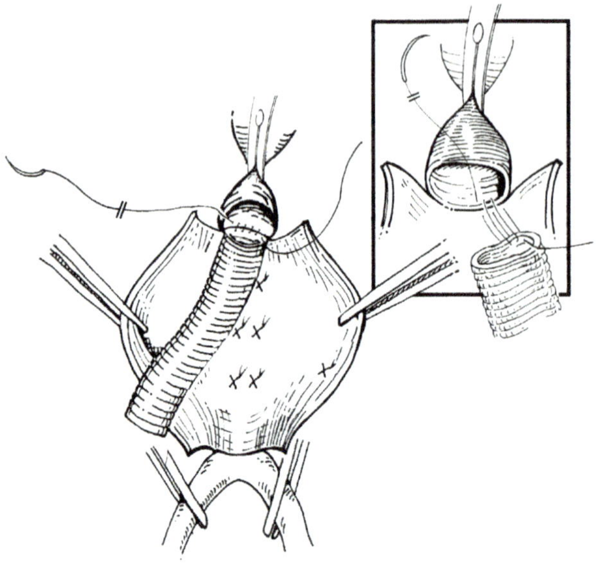

Figure 28.5 Aorta "T'd off" proximally and distally to create sewing rings for tube graft anastomoses. Inset shows proximal aorta-to-graft anastomosis being constructed via the "parachute" technique with double-thickness bites through non-transected posterior wall.

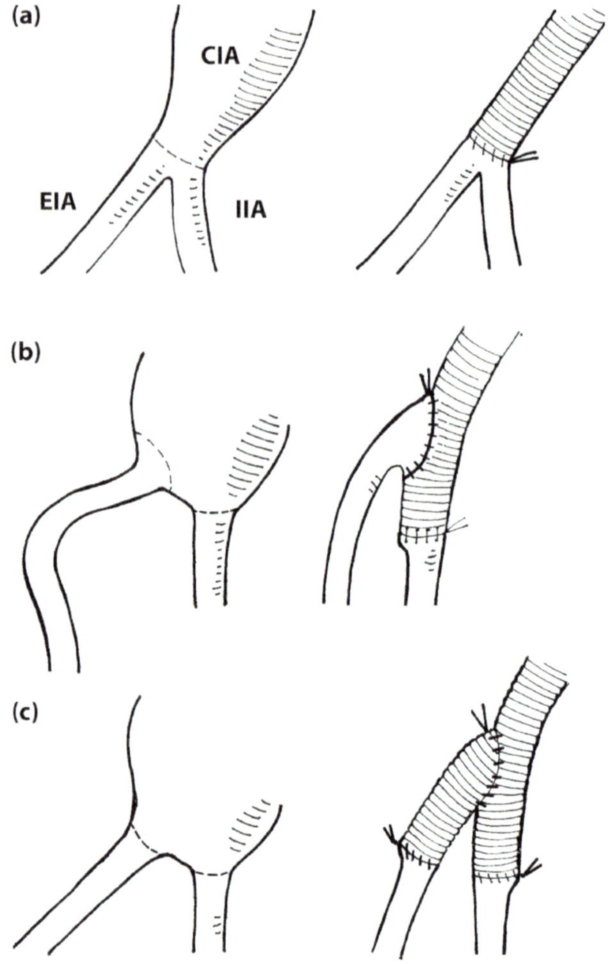

Figure 28.6 Iliac artery bifurcation reconstruction techniques: (a) limb sewn to bifurcation; (b) limb sewn to the hypogastric artery with re-implantation of the end of the redundant external iliac into the side of the graft; (c) limb sewn to the internal iliac artery with jump graft to external iliac. CIAA, common iliac artery aneurysm; EIA, external iliac artery; IIA, internal iliac (or hypogastric) artery.

aneurysm sac and incising the lateral walls of the aorta to leave only the posterior third of the wall intact (Figure 28.5). Avoid sewing to aneurysmal aorta except in extenuating circumstances. Extensive, full-thickness endarterectomy of a calcified aorta is also avoided because of the risk of further weakening already abnormal aortic wall. If a bifurcated graft is chosen, the main shaft is trimmed to leave no more than a few centimeters. The proximal anastomosis is created with a running stitch of 3-0 polypropylene on an SH needle beginning at one corner of the posterior wall and incorporating double-thickness bites of the back wall before transitioning to single-layer bites for the remainder of the anastomosis. After securing and testing this anastomosis, attention is directed to the distal anastomosis(es). A distal aortic sewing ring can be created at the bifurcation by "T-ing" off the aorta in identical fashion to proximally. After pressurizing the graft, it is trimmed to an appropriate length and the distal anastomosis is performed like the proximal. The posterior wall at the bifurcation can be quite calcified, making needle passage challenging. Local endarterectomy is usually not possible without the risk of creating a flap in one or both iliacs. Creating a track for needle passage with a penetrating towel clip is a useful maneuver for traversing a short segment of such a calcified wall. Iliac anastomoses are usually easier because there is less disease. When constructing these end-to-end anastomoses, we usually transect the artery completely after dissecting the posterior artery wall off the adjacent vein, which is much easier with a non-pressurized artery. It is important to get full-thickness bites as the adventitia has a tendency to peel away from the media on the iliac arteries.

With CIA aneurysms, it is sometimes difficult to preserve flow into the hypogastrics if the origins of the external iliac and hypogastric arise at some distance from each other. A variety of reconstruction techniques are available but the easiest to perform is an end-to-end anastomosis of the graft limb to the hypogastric followed by re-implantation of the external iliac end-to-side to the graft limb; if there is not enough external iliac redundancy, then an interposition jump graft is performed to the external iliac (Figure 28.6). This is easier than trying to reimplant the hypogastric into the side of a graft limb that has been sewn to the external iliac. After reconstructing one hypogastric in this fashion, the contralateral one may be safely ligated. When going to the iliacs, it is important to tunnel the graft limbs *posterior* to the ureters to avoid entrapping them in scar tissue which frequently forms between the graft limb and native artery.

Prior to completing a distal anastomosis, the graft and distal vessel(s) should be vented to remove any atherothrombotic material that could embolize distally. Once the anastomosis is secured, flow is restored to the lower extremity(ies)—carefully communicating this step to the anesthesia team. One leg is unclamped at a time and the femoral artery on that side is compressed to direct any loose debris into the ipsilateral hypogastric *and* reduce the hemodynamic alterations caused by reperfusion. A drop in pressure of at least 20 mmHg is expected when the first leg is opened; anything less may be a sign of inadequate flow restoration to that extremity. Following return of flow to both legs, distal perfusion is verified by checking pedal pulses/Doppler flow signals.

If there was concern over back bleeding from a patent IMA previously, it should be rechecked at this point, making sure to remove any retractor blades that may be compressing the meandering mesenteric or other collaterals. If back bleeding remains poor, implanting the IMA into the graft may be necessary. The IMA is excised along with a small button of adjacent aorta. It is usually necessary to endarectomize this button and great care should be taken to not raise a flap into the proximal IMA. While it is possible to place a "deep" partially occluding clamp on an aortic tube graft, we have found it much easier to implant the IMA into the left limb of a bifurcated graft after occluding it proximally and distally (Figure 28.7). In this situation, it is important to anticipate this eventuality so that the main shaft of the graft is not left too long. A small disc of graft wall is excised to allow an end-to-side anastomosis with 5-0 polypropylene. After restoration of IMA flow, heparin anticoagulation is reversed, and the hemostatic profile corrected as necessary. Following hemostasis, the aneurysm sac is closed over the graft with absorbable sutures and the edges of the retroperitoneal incision re-approximated (Figure 28.8). Great care should be taken during fascial closure because of the documented high incidence of incisional hernias in this population. Placement of prophylactic mesh has been advocated by some authorities to reduce this complication [3].

RETROPERITONEAL APPROACH [4]

Proper patient positioning is key—the patient is placed in a modified right lateral decubitus position with the shoulders positioned at 70° to the table and the hips rotated as far posteriorly as possible. Such axial rotation is important when groin incisions for femoral exposure are anticipated (Figure 28.9). A vacuum "beanbag" is helpful in maintaining this alignment. The midpoint between the patient's right costal margin and right iliac crest is centered over the break in the table and the table can be "jackknifed" to open up the left flank if desired. The primary operator stands on the patient's left, and the

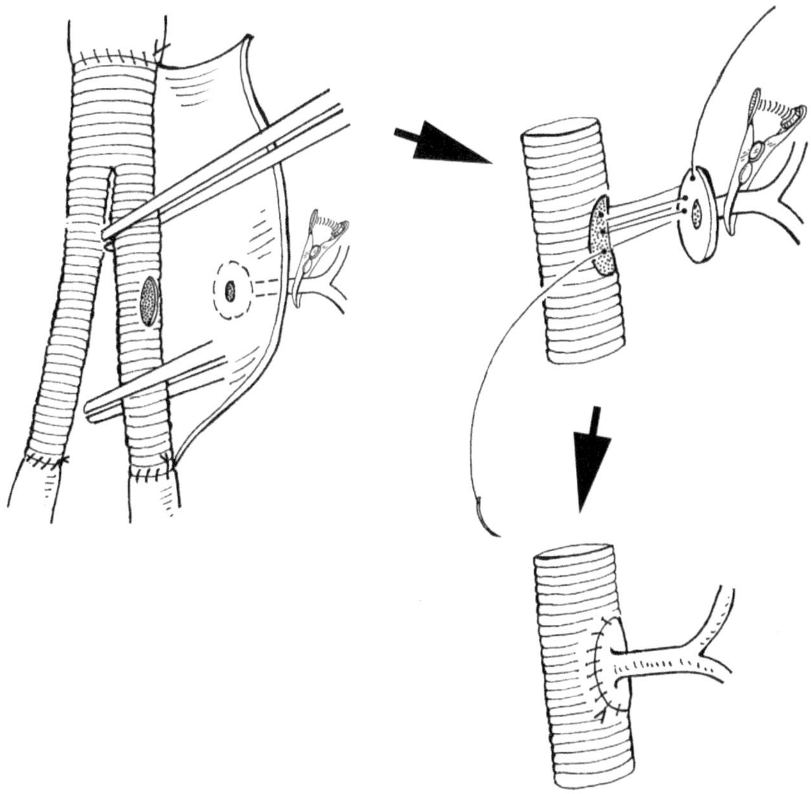

Figure 28.7 Inferior mesenteric artery reconstruction. The left limb of an aortoiliac graft occluded proximally and distally with the creation of a small graftotomy to which a Carrel patch containing the inferior mesenteric artery is sewn.

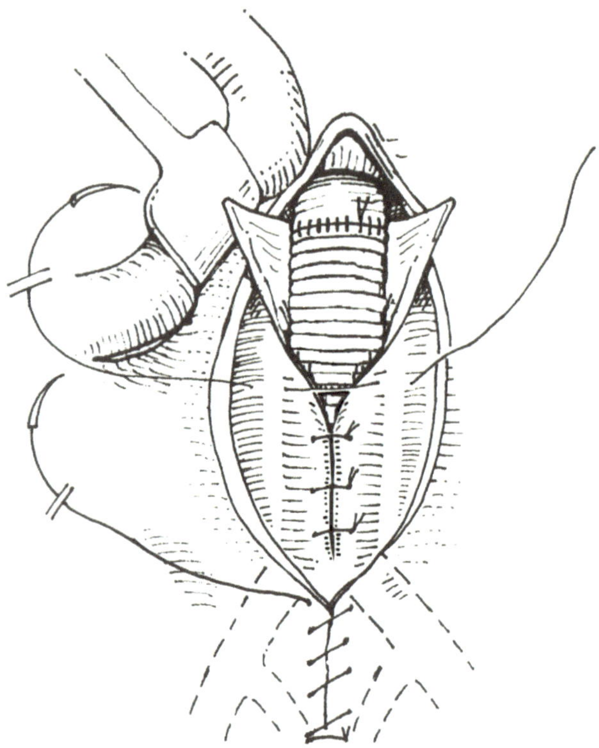

Figure 28.8 The aneurysm sac wall is closed over the graft followed by re-approximation of the edges of the retroperitoneal opening to prevent bowel adhesion to the prosthetic graft.

table rotated to the right during abdominal incision and exposure, and all the way back to the left to flatten out the hips as much as possible if groin incisions are required.

For IR aortic procedures, the standard flank incision extends from the lateral margin of the left rectus sheath, just below the umbilicus laterally into the 11th intercostal space for 8–10 cm. When exposure of the pararenal aorta is necessary, a 10th interspace incision is more suitable. The abdominal wall and intercostal musculature are divided in the line of the incision and the extraperitoneal space entered at the tip of the 11th or 12th rib. The peritoneum, often with the overlying transversalis fascia, is stripped away from the abdominal wall musculature anteriorly as far as the rectus sheath. Posterolaterally, the plane of the flank musculature and psoas are followed as the peritoneal sac and its contents are retracted anteriorly. This plane is developed superficial to the lumbodorsal fascia (the posterior extension of the transversalis fascia) behind the left kidney so that the left ureter and kidney are also reflected anteriorly (Figure 28.10). Small bridging veins should be carefully cauterized when identified prior to division to avoid troublesome bleeding. The abdominal aorta and more caudally the left iliac artery are exposed in the base of the wound. The left RA is the only significant structure that can now be injured so it is critical to identify and protect this vessel during the early stages of dissection. In thin patients, this artery is usually easy to palpate as it courses anteriorly off the left lateral wall of the aorta to the retracted left kidney. In individuals with more abundant retroperitoneal fat, some dissection is usually necessary. The lumbar branch of the left RV coursing across the aorta proximally is a reliable landmark to this artery, which is found just above and proximally. This vein usually requires ligation/division to adequately expose the IR aortic neck. If the lumbar branch is much larger than normal, then the preop CTA should be re-examined to ensure that the patient does not have a retroaortic left RV. In this situation, it is necessary to expose the aorta anterior to the kidney to avoid ligating the left RV. Once the left RA has been identified, the left posterolateral wall of the aorta can be safely exposed by

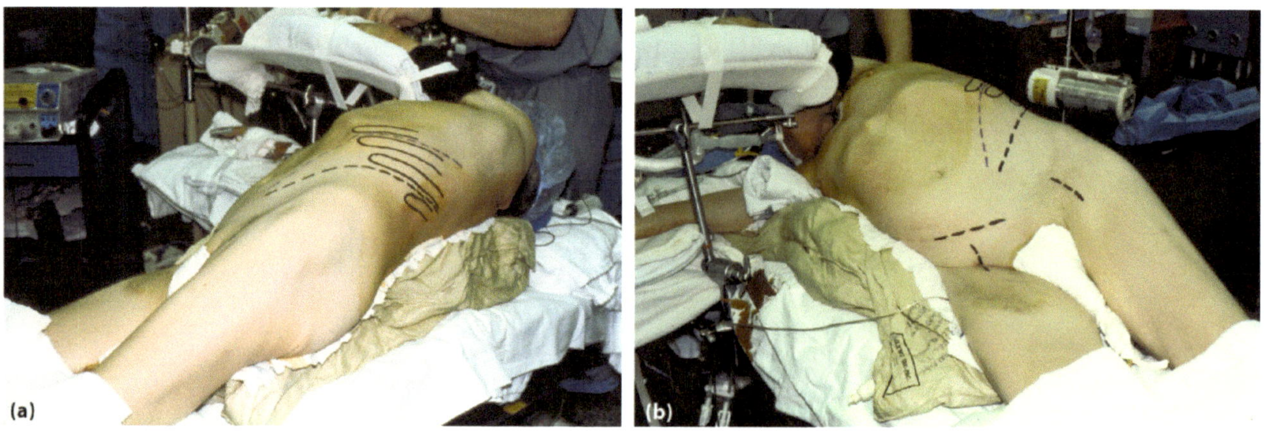

Figure 28.9 Patient positioning for left flank retroperitoneal approach: (a) view from the left (surgeon's) side of the table showing the vacuum "beanbag." The chest is at 70° to the table while the hips are rotated posteriorly. The lower-most incision in the 11th intercostal space (ICS) is typically used for infrarenal AAAs while the upper incision in the ninth ICS is most useful for extent IV TAAAs. The 10th ICS incision (not shown) is most commonly used for pararenal AAAs; (b) view from the right side of the table demonstrating bilateral vertical groin incisions and right lower quadrant counter incision sometimes used to expose right external iliac artery extraperitoneally.

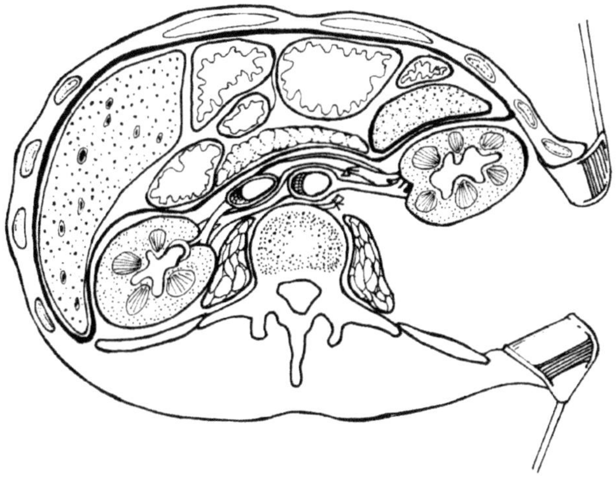

Figure 28.10 Cross-sectional view demonstrating the standard dissection plane posterior to the left kidney used with left flank retroperitoneal exposure. Ties on the divided ends of the lumbar branch of the left renal vein.

dividing overlying lymphatics and periaortic fat; an ultrasonic scalpel is helpful for this step as dissection is carried distally toward the bifurcation (Figure 28.11).

Following definition of the neck of the aneurysm, index finger dissection anterior and posterior to the aorta establishes a plane for placement of a cross-clamp; circumferential dissection is unnecessary as long as the clamp arms can pass beyond its far wall. The vena cava is not immediately adjacent to the aorta at this level so caval injury is not a concern. When SR control is necessary, aortic dissection proceeds cephalad toward the left diaphragmatic crus, identified as a firm tendinous band crossing the aorta just proximal to the origin of the left renal artery. The crural fibers are divided 2–3 cm along the axis of the aorta and the underlying aortic wall exposed. The origin of the left RA is cleared off and dissection anterior and posterior to the aorta creates a plane for clamp placement. There is frequently a pair of lumbar arteries at this level that can be inadvertently injured. For SC control, the crural fibers are divided an additional 5 cm and the fascia investing the aorta incised to allow fingertip passage anterior and posterior to the aorta. SC control is, in fact, easier to obtain via this approach than SR control because of the relative absence of retroperitoneal fat and lymphatics at this level. When anticipating the need for SC control preoperatively, access can be improved by a tenth interspace incision.

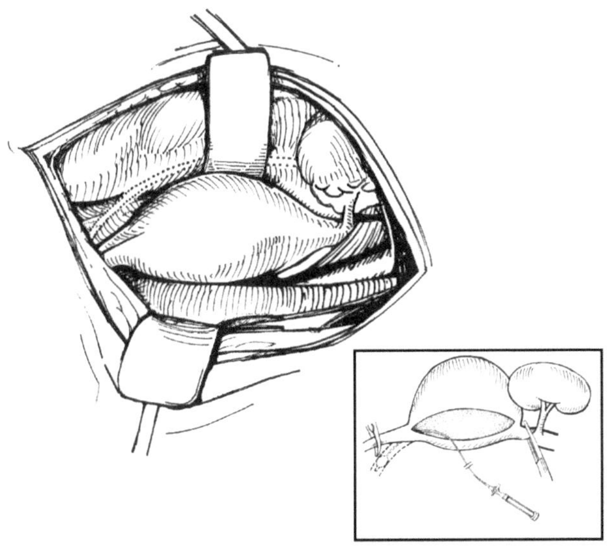

Figure 28.11 Left flank retroperitoneal exposure of infrarenal aorta from crus to aortic bifurcation with an infrarenal clamp in place. The dotted line is the course of the left ureter. Inset: a balloon occlusion catheter controlling the right common iliac artery in a patient with a large infrarenal (IR) AAA. The figure also demonstrates the ease of clamping the IR neck of a large AAA from this approach as opposed to a transperitoneal, midline approach.

After obtaining proximal control, the peritoneal sac is stripped out of the left iliac fossa to expose the iliac arteries. Care should be taken to mobilize the left ureter along with the peritoneal sac. The left common iliac artery can be readily visualized and controlled along most of its length, but only the proximal-most right common iliac can be exposed from this approach, particularly in the presence of a large aortic aneurysm. Division of the IMA (if this can be done safely) and further mobilization of the peritoneal sac to the patient's right can be helpful. A useful alternative is obtaining endoluminal control of the right iliac with a balloon occlusion catheter or a small Foley catheter inserted into the proximal artery after opening the aneurysm (Figure 28.11). More distal right iliac exposure is also facilitated by bringing the flank incision all the way to the midline, although even in this circumstance, exposure beyond the iliac bifurcation is not possible. If femoral anastomoses are necessary, groin incisions can be performed after the table has been rotated to the left as far as possible. In this circumstance, the location of the femoral arteries should be marked out preoperatively *after* the patient has been positioned as the required incisions will be shifted to the patient's left compared with supine exposure. In obese patients, the right groin may be obscured by an overhanging panniculus that may require significant retraction for exposure.

It is important to note that the right RA is relatively inaccessible with this approach. Endarterectomy of a short, discrete ostial lesion is possible as is bypass to the very proximal right RA, though this latter maneuver can be quite challenging. The left RA is accessible along its entire course.

After appropriate exposure, aneurysm repair with this approach is identical to TP, midline repair. Following hemostasis, the aneurysm sac is closed around the graft, but there is no need for re-peritonealization. Wound closure is facilitated by flattening the table out of the jackknife position (if used). Any incision made in the left diaphragm is oversewn during wound closure and pleural air evacuated through a temporary 16 Fr red-rubber catheter following lung insufflation. The ribs are re-approximated with looped #1 PDS on a blunt needle. The three muscle layers of the abdominal wall are closed separately with running 0 or 2-0 PDS suture.

Besides the limited exposure of the right iliac and right renal, disadvantages of this approach are the longer time required for positioning and wound opening/closure and the inability to fully explore the entire abdomen, a circumstance of less importance in an era of near-universal preoperative CT scanning. Advantages include reduced evaporative fluid losses, reduced ileus, reduced incisional pain, and reduced long-term complications related to adhesions and abdominal wall hernias. Given the complex nature of most open IR AAA repairs being performed today, left flank RP exposure is frequently the approach of choice.

TRICKS AND TRAPS

- Midline, transperitoneal, inframesocolic exposure is still the open repair approach chosen by most vascular surgeons.
- For suprarenal clamping from a TP approach, the left renal vein should be retracted following full mobilization (after ligating and dividing its adrenal, gonadal, and lumbar branches) rather than ligated and divided.
- Circumferential mobilization of the proximal aortic neck is unnecessary.
- Avoid circumferential mobilization of the proximal-most right common iliac artery to minimize the risk of venous injury.
- Avoid injury to the parasympathetic nerves around the origin of the IMA and crossing over the left common iliac origin.
- Create a sewing ring proximally by "T-ing off" the aortotomy laterally and leaving the posterior third of the aortic wall intact.
- Avoid PTFE grafts for AAA repair because of the risk of perigraft seromas.
- Preserve flow to at least one hypogastric artery to avoid pelvic ischemic complications.
- Avoid femoral exposure/anastomoses, if possible, to reduce infection risk.
- A left flank extraperitoneal approach is useful for more complex open aortic repairs and is associated with several advantages.
- The distal right common iliac and right renal arteries are relatively inaccessible with the flank approach. Ligation/division of the inferior mesenteric artery (if safe) improves right iliac exposure.

QUESTIONS

1. Pick the true statement:
   a. Femoral exposure/anastomoses add no risk to open AAA repair
   b. Tube graft AAA reconstructions do not affect sexual function
   c. Hypogastric revascularization is unimportant
   d. Circumferential mobilization of the right common iliac artery can be hazardous

   Answer: d

2. The best graft material for AAA repair is:
   a. Dacron
   b. PTFE
   c. Cryopreserved allograft
   d. Neoaortoiliac system (NAIS) constructed from femoral veins

   Answer: a

3. Resection and grafting are favored over intraluminal repair of AAA:
   a. Because it is faster and associated with less blood loss
   b. Because it is easier to control lumbar arteries from the outside of the AAA sac
   c. With mycotic AAA
   d. Because it is associated with less damage to surrounding structures

   Answer: c

4. Disadvantages of the left flank retroperitoneal approach include:
   a. Increased risk of incisional hernia
   b. Intraperitoneal adhesions
   c. Need to ligate the lumbar branch of the left renal vein
   d. Poor exposure of right renal artery and distal right iliac artery system

   Answer: d

REFERENCES

1. van Schaik J, Witt D, Albers L, Wever J, Elzevier H, Hamming J. Pilot study on feasibility and outcome of a nerve-preserving aortoiliac exposure technique. *Ann Vasc Surg*. 2024;98:388–397.

2. Kadakol AK, Karam JL, Lin JL, Nypaver TJ, Weaver MR, Reddy DJ, Haddad GK, West CA, Shepard AD. Perigraft seroma after open abdominal aortic aneurysm repair: frequency, risk factors and management. *J Vasc Surg*. 2011;54:637–643.
3. Indrakusuma R, Jalalzadeh H, van der Meij JE, Balm R, Koelemay MJW. Prophylactic mesh reinforcement versus sutured closure to prevent incisional hernias after open abdominal aortic aneurysm repair via midline laparotomy: a systematic review and meta-analysis. *Eur J Vasc Endovasc Surg*. 2018; 56:120–128.
4. Shepard AD, Reddy DJ, Evans JR, Elliott JP, Smith RF, Ernst CB. Left flank retroperitoneal exposure: a technical aid to complex aortic reconstruction. *J. Vasc. Surg*. 14:283–291, 1991.

29

Open ruptured abdominal aortic aneurysm repair

SACHINDER S. HANS

INTRODUCTION

Many patients with a ruptured abdominal aortic aneurysm (RAAA) present with sudden onset of back pain and/or flank pain with associated diaphoresis secondary to low blood pressure (BP). Because of severe pain, BP may be temporarily elevated, which is detrimental to continued bleeding. Pain may be in the periumbilical area and rarely in the inguinal area, masquerading as an incarcerated inguinal hernia. The location of pain depends on the site of rupture. Most ruptures occur in the left posterolateral wall of the aneurysm, and patients may remain hemodynamically stable for a few hours because of contained hematoma in the retroperitoneal space. On the other hand, anterior rupture is frequently associated with free rupture into the peritoneal cavity, with severe shock secondary to massive blood loss. Rarely, an AAA may develop a "chronic" contained rupture because bleeding from an opening in the posterior wall of the aneurysm sac is sealed by the anterior spinal ligament and other retroperitoneal structures.

Early transportation to an emergency department, prompt diagnosis (ultrasound/computed tomography angiography [CTA]) and resuscitation, preferably in the operating room, use of permissive hypotension (maintaining systolic BP between 80 and 100 mmHg), and immediate operation with proximal control of the aorta have a significant impact on the outcome of patients with a RAAA [1–6]. In most patients, there is time to obtain an emergency CTA of the abdomen and pelvis with less than 1 mm cuts. This not only confirms the diagnosis but allows evaluation for the mode of definitive treatment—endovascular aneurysm repair (EVAR) versus open repair—based on imaging-defined anatomic criteria. Although EVAR is currently the treatment of choice for a RAAA, some patients do not have suitable anatomy for an EVAR; therefore, open surgical repair is the only option. In patients with free rupture and/or profound hemodynamic instability, obtaining a CTA may not be possible and immediate transfer to the operating room for proximal aortic control is the best option.

OPERATIVE TECHNIQUE

By what means and how quickly proximal control of the aorta is obtained are critical in determining the outcome of patients with a RAAA. If the patient's condition suggests free rupture in the form of persistent hypotension, requiring large-volume fluid resuscitation, and increasing abdominal distention, obtaining rapid proximal control is of paramount importance. The patient is prepped from the nipple line to mid-thigh. To avoid cardiovascular collapse, close communication with the anesthesia team is critical because anesthetic induction/intubation should be withheld until the surgeon is ready to make the incision. Induction of general anesthesia relieves pain, relaxes the abdominal wall musculature, and completely releases sympathetic tone, all protective mechanisms that serve to maintain BP in a patient with a RAAA. A rapid transfusion protocol with blood products in the room, cell saver (autologous blood recovery system), and body warmers should be utilized. In most patients, a midline transabdominal incision from the xiphoid process to the symphysis pubis is performed. In selected patients with ileostomy/urinary stoma, or in patients with contained hematoma from a leaking suprarenal/paravisceral aneurysm, a left flank incision through the tenth intercostal space is preferable. This incision is extended toward the lateral border of the rectus abdominis muscle between the symphysis pubis and the umbilicus.

DOI: 10.1201/9781003452096-29

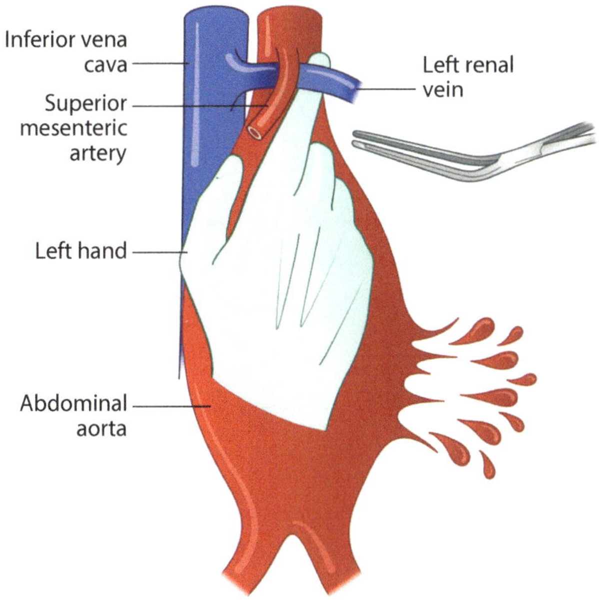

Figure 29.1 Mobilization of the pararenal aorta with the right index finger under the left renal vein.

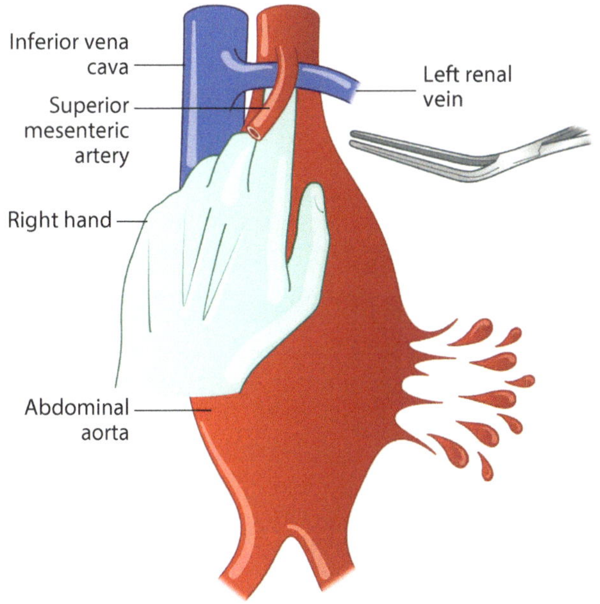

Figure 29.2 Mobilization of the pararenal aorta with left index finger under the left renal vein.

Proximal control

Proximal aortic control is best achieved at the supraceliac level (near the diaphragm) in patients with extensive retroperitoneal hematoma and shock. In some patients with a small-to-moderate retroperitoneal hematoma, blunt finger dissection of the infrarenal neck can be performed after mobilizing the ligament of Treitz. The left renal vein (LRV) is mobilized and retracted upward, and a vascular clamp is applied to the aorta just below the renal arteries (Figure 29.1).

Exposure of the supraceliac aorta

The left lobe of the liver is retracted toward the right following division of the left triangular ligament. Dissection is done through the gastrohepatic omentum. The esophagus with a nasogastric tube is retracted to the left; the author finds that encircling the esophagus with a Penrose drain can be helpful. Deep blades of a surgical retraction system (e.g., the Bookwalter III Retractor System, Symmetry Surgical, Antioch, TN, USA; or the Thompson retractor, Thompson Surgical Instruments, Traverse City, MI, USA) are inserted to expose the right crus of the diaphragm. The muscular fibers of the crus are separated with the help of long Metzenbaum scissors, and a 5–6 cm vertical opening is made. The index and middle fingers of the right hand are introduced through the opening, and the fascia surrounding the lower thoracic aorta is divided. With the help of the index and middle fingers of the right hand passed on either side of the aorta through the opening in the right crus, a long aortic clamp is guided into place with the left hand to clamp the lower thoracic aorta (Figures 29.2–29.4).

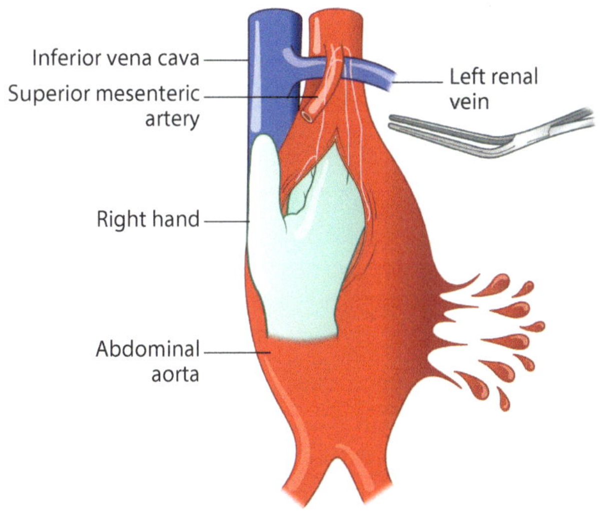

Figure 29.3 Insertion of right index and middle fingers into the neck of an abdominal aortic aneurysm to obtain proximal control.

In some patients with a RAAA, left medial visceral rotation (by mobilizing the spleen, tail of the pancreas, and colonic splenic flexure) is necessary to obtain adequate proximal aortic exposure. The peritoneal reflections of the colon and spleen are divided, and the viscera and left kidney are mobilized medially. With this maneuver, exposure of the suprarenal aorta is obtained and the left crus of the diaphragm is partially divided. Following control of the aorta at the supraceliac level, the clamp can then be moved distally to just below the renal arteries to reduce the visceral/renal ischemic time provided the aneurysm is not pararenal.

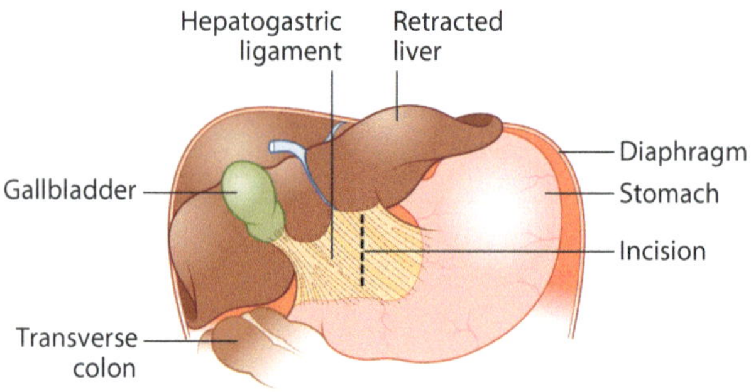

Figure 29.4 Transcrural supraceliac aortic control begins by making an incision in the gastrohepatic omentum.

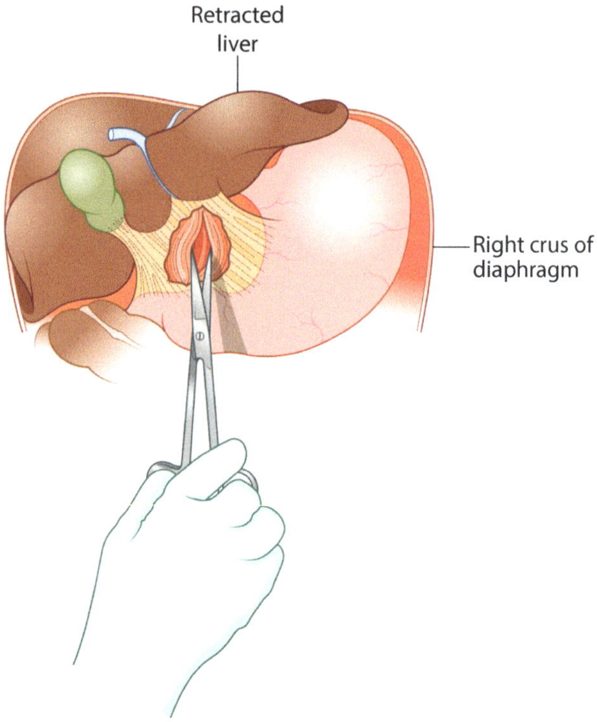

Figure 29.5 Scissors splitting the muscular fibers of the diaphragmatic crura to expose the supraceliac aorta.

Balloon occlusion control

An alternative technique for proximal control involves the insertion of a 28 cm long 12-Fr sheath into the femoral artery under local anesthesia to allow passage of a large-diameter occlusion balloon (e.g., 28–32 mm Z-MED™; B. Braun Interventional Systems Inc., Bethlehem, PA, USA), which can be inflated in the distal thoracic aorta to gain proximal control. Manual pressure by an assistant to keep the 12-Fr sheath in place is usually necessary because of the tendency of the sheath to slip out. Aortography to determine the suitability of EVAR can be undertaken after proximal balloon aortic occlusion is obtained (see Chapter 10). If the patient is not a suitable candidate for EVAR, open repair is commenced. A left thoracotomy for

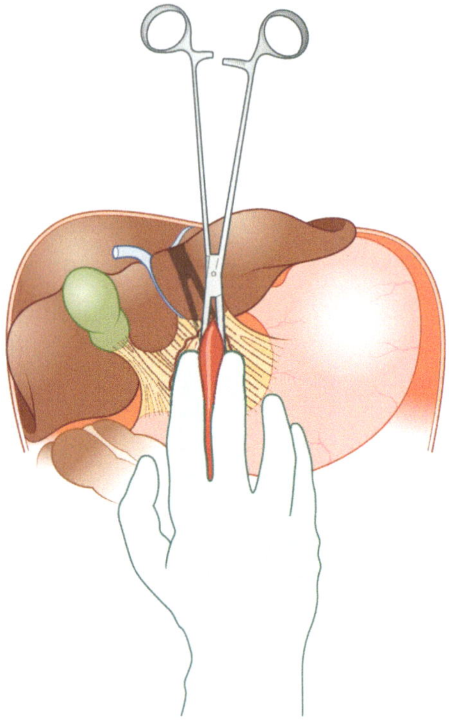

Figure 29.6 Transcrural application of proximal aortic clamp to supraceliac aorta.

proximal control of the thoracic aorta for RAAA repair is rarely necessary. In patients with acceptable hemodynamic stability, proximal control at the supraceliac level, as previously described, is usually preferred.

After obtaining proximal control, it is best to have the anesthesia team continue aggressive fluid and blood product resuscitation, even if the BP has improved. Without adequate resuscitation, any further blood loss can result in acute decompensation resulting in cardiac arrest. A decision should be made at this point whether to administer heparin. In patients with relatively stable BP and a small-to-moderate retroperitoneal hematoma, intravenous heparin (75 IU/kg) is administered by the anesthesia team with serial monitoring of activated clotting times. In patients with shock and very large retroperitoneal hematomas, intravenous heparin is administered after the proximal anastomosis is completed. The dose of heparin used (50 IU/kg) is smaller than for elective open AAA repair.

Following proximal aortic control, distal exposure is obtained. Both common iliac arteries can be controlled if they are not aneurysmal; otherwise, the origin of the external and hypogastric arteries need to be clamped separately. The author does not recommend circumferential mobilization of the aortic neck and iliac arteries nor passage of vessel loops or tapes because these maneuvers can result in injury to adjacent venous structures (e.g., the LRV, its lumbar branch, or the iliac veins). Iatrogenic major venous injury results in significant morbidity and mortality. It is better to perform anterior and lateral dissection of the aortic neck and the iliac arteries and place vascular clamps on the aortic neck and iliac arteries after compression between the index and middle fingers. The inferior mesenteric artery (IMA) is dissected and controlled with a silastic vessel loop close to its origin from the aorta. Alternatively, the IMA can be evaluated from inside the aneurysm sac. In patients with a small retroperitoneal hematoma, following proximal aortic control, the operation should flow in a careful and deliberative manner similar to elective open AAA repair.

After ensuring adequate volume resuscitation and proximal and distal control, the anterior wall of the aneurysm sac is opened to the right of the IMA origin with electrocautery and scissors and intraluminal thrombus is removed. Lumbar arteries are carefully controlled by figure-of-eight 2-0 silk sutures. Because of heavy calcified plaque, local endarterectomy of the origin of the lumbar arteries may be necessary to achieve hemostasis. The infrarenal/juxtarenal aorta is prepared for proximal anastomosis by dividing the aorta wall. A transverse incision distal to the origins of the renal arteries is made and joins the longitudinal aortotomy incision in a "T"-shaped manner. After lateral division of the aortic neck, the posterior wall of the aortic neck is divided a few millimeters longer than the anterior wall. Sometimes, the posterior wall of the aortic neck is not divided and is used as a double layer for proximal anastomosis. In most patients with a RAAA, an aorto-bi-iliac Dacron graft (18 × 9 mm or 20 × 10 mm) is required. If the aortic bifurcation is of suitable quality, a straight tube graft may be appropriate. A tube graft can decrease operative time, fluid requirements, and postoperative ileus. In rare cases, taking the graft to the femoral level(s) is necessary.

The proximal anastomosis of the main body of the Dacron graft to the aortic neck is first completed using a running 3-0 or 4-0 polypropylene suture (Ethicon US, LLC, Somerville, NJ, USA). In some patients with a dilated, friable aortic neck, a two-layer proximal anastomosis is performed [7]. The use of BioGlue® surgical adhesive (CryoLife Inc., Kennesaw, GA, USA) or FLOSEAL hemostatic matrix (Baxter International Inc., Deerfield, IL, USA) following completion of proximal anastomosis may help with hemostasis.

In preparation for distal anastomoses, posterior circumferential dissection of the de-compressed iliac arteries can now be undertaken. Graft limb-to-iliac artery anastomoses are done with a 4-0 cardiovascular polypropylene suture followed by retrograde and antegrade flushing prior to securing the suture line. With poor back-bleeding from one or both iliac arteries, consideration should be given to the distal passage of a moderate-diameter (5-Fr) Fogarty balloon catheter before completing the anastomosis, particularly if the patient was not heparinized before clamping. Following completion of the anastomosis, flow is gradually restored to the lower extremities to prevent declamping shock, which can be particularly severe in patients with a RAAA. Declamping shock results from redistribution of the blood volume below the clamp with falling cardiac pre-load and release of vasodilators from the re-perfused lower extremities. Volume loading and correction of metabolic acidosis should be aggressively undertaken by the anesthesia team with the monitoring of blood gases, electrolytes, and cardiac output. After restoration of flow to one iliac artery, there can be significant retrograde bleeding from missed lumbar arteries that should be promptly controlled with figure-of-eight 2-0 silk sutures. Distal pulses/Doppler signals should be carefully checked at this point and consideration given to further interventions (e.g., passage of Fogarty balloon embolectomy catheters) if distal flow is absent.

Once adequate distal flow has been documented, all efforts should be directed to obtaining hemostasis. This is best accomplished with protamine sulfate reversal of heparin (if given) and administration of clotting factors as necessary. Once hemostasis has been achieved, the retroperitoneum is closed, carefully separating the duodenum and small bowel from any contact with the prosthetic graft by suturing the remaining right lateral wall of the AAA to the descending mesocolon; the aneurysm sac is closed around the prosthetic graft. In the pelvic portion, the small bowel mesentery is sutured to the mesentery of the pelvic colon. The abdomen is closed with a single layer of No. 1 Maxon™ running monofilament absorbable suture (Medtronic, Minneapolis, MN, USA). If there is significant tension secondary to bowel edema or hematoma, open abdomen negative pressure therapy (AbThera™ 3M, Saint Paul, MN, USA) is used followed by delayed closure of the abdomen.

COMPLICATIONS

Bleeding

After open repair of a RAAA, postoperative bleeding may occur and is usually caused by coagulopathy associated with shock, hypothermia, and large-volume fluid resuscitation. We have found point-of-care thromboelastography extremely valuable in rapidly assessing hemostatic derangements and guiding appropriate component-specific correction. In institutions where this modality is not available, consider proactive component transfusion. For patients with a large retroperitoneal hematoma and associated shock, proactive transfusion encompassing two pooled buffy-coat platelet concentrates immediately and again 30 minutes before aortic unclamping together with fresh frozen plasma administered in a 1:1 ratio to the amount of red blood cells, should be instituted [8]. In a significant number of patients, coagulopathy is dilutional and can be corrected by administering appropriate blood products like fresh frozen plasma, cryoprecipitate, and in some instances, factor VII. However, disseminated intravascular coagulation is a very serious complication of RAAA repair and is associated with very high mortality.

Acute lower extremity ischemia

This is usually the result of in situ thrombosis of the distal vascular bed because of hypotension and inadequate anticoagulation. Occasionally, it may be the result of embolic occlusion of mural thrombus from the aneurysm sac. Significant lower extremity ischemia is a serious complication and should be investigated and treated before leaving the operating room. If a femoral pulse is absent, the iliac anastomosis should be checked; if the patient has good pulse distal to the anastomosis, the femoral artery should be opened via a groin incision and Fogarty balloon catheters passed proximally and distally. If femoral pulses are palpable but no posterior tibial or dorsalis pedis flow is demonstrated by Doppler, the feet should be warmed; if distal flow is not re-established soon, a No. 3 or 4 Fogarty embolectomy catheter is passed distally. If the patient is unstable and in shock, further interventions to improve lower extremity arterial flow should be postponed.

Colon ischemia

Colon ischemia is another very serious complication of RAAA repair and should be suspected in any patient with postoperative diarrhea, particularly if bloody. Flexible sigmoidoscopy should be performed as soon as the diagnosis is entertained. If colon ischemia is confined to the mucosa, improvement with general supportive care (intravenous antibiotics directed against gut flora, nothing by mouth, and total parenteral nutrition) is expected. However, if there is concern for full-thickness necrosis, the patient should be returned urgently to the OR for colectomy with colostomy. In these patients, mortality is very high. At the time of RAAA repair, the IMA should be ligated close to its origin to preserve collateral flow. Should the sigmoid colon appear to be ischemic, and if there is a large, liquefied hematoma involving the sigmoid mesocolon, consideration should be given to draining the hematoma to relieve compression of the branches of the IMA. If colon ischemia does not improve, then consideration should be given to reimplanting the origin of the IMA into the Dacron graft using a Carrel patch, though IMA reimplantation is rarely necessary.

Abdominal compartment syndrome

Abdominal compartment syndrome is a well-recognized complication of RAAA repair and occurs secondary to massive fluid resuscitation and prolonged aortic clamping on top of a large retroperitoneal hematoma. Using intraabdominal pressure (IAP) measurements from an indwelling Foley catheter, 50% of patients had an IAP >20 mmHg after open repair of RAAAs; of those, approximately 20% developed multiple organ dysfunction or failure [9]. Medical therapy includes neuromuscular blockade, positive end-expiratory pressure, albumin, and furosemide. In the presence of elevated IAP, peak airway pressures >30 cm H_20, and persistent oliguria, patients should undergo a decompressive celiotomy. The abdomen should be left open and care taken to prevent a small bowel fistula with proper coverage of the exposed intestines. Vacuum-assisted temporary abdominal closure (AbThera™ Advance Open Abdomen Dressing by 3M Medical) speeds resolution of swelling and is followed by delayed primary fascial closure.

Other complications

Cardiac arrhythmias, myocardial infarction, respiratory failure, acute renal failure, prolonged ileus, acute pancreatitis, and hepatic failure may all occur following RAAA repair; consultation with appropriate specialists may be helpful. Multiorgan failure following open repair of RAAAs is associated with high morbidity and mortality.

TRICKS AND TRAPS

1. Permissive hypotension in a patient with a RAAA (systolic BP 80–100 mmHg) reduces ongoing bleeding and is associated with improved outcomes.
2. Emergent high-quality, thin-section CTA of the abdomen and pelvis helps decide between endovascular and open repair of a RAAA. Whenever possible, endovascular repair is preferred because of documented better outcomes.
3. Resuscitation of unstable patients with RAAA should be done in hybrid OR and not in the ER.
4. Rapid supraceliac control is preferred in patients with a large retroperitoneal hematoma and/or severe hypotension.
5. Heparin should be administered to only those patients who are hemodynamically stable with a small retroperitoneal hematoma.
6. Tube graft, if feasible, is preferred to aorto-biiliac graft. Aortofemoral graft reconstruction should be avoided unless necessary.
7. Administration of packed red blood cells and fresh frozen plasma in 1:1:1 ratio along with the administration of platelets in patients with massive blood loss may help prevent coagulopathy.
8. In patients with significant edema of the viscera, delayed abdominal closure should be considered with application of the AbThera™ negative pressure wound system at the time of repair.
9. In patients with persistent metabolic acidosis in the post-op period, colon ischemia should be suspected.

QUESTIONS

1. Intraabdominal pressure greater than 20 mmHg, using a Foley catheter in the urinary bladder, following repair of ruptured AAA occurs in what percentage of patients?
   a. <20%
   b. 20–35%
   c. >35% but <50%
   d. >50%

   Answer: d

2. Following completion of distal anastomosis(es) during open repair for a RAAA, the patient has diffused oozing from exposed surfaces. Lab data: hemoglobin 9.2 g, hematocrit 26, platelets 84,000, INR 1.8, fibrin split products normal. Most common cause of this abnormality:
   a. Disseminated intravascular coagulopathy
   b. Secondary fibrinolysis
   c. Dilutional coagulopathy
   d. Mismatched blood

   Answer: c

3. Multisystem organ failure occurs in 1–3% of patients undergoing open repair of RAAA and is associated with a mortality rate of:
   a. 20%
   b. >20% but <40%
   c. 40–49%
   d. 50–70%

   Answer: d

4. A 72-year-old female presented to the ER with profound hypotension secondary to a RAAA. The patient should undergo:
   a. Balloon occlusion of the lower thoracic aorta via femoral artery access in ER
   b. Balloon occlusion of the lower thoracic aorta via brachial artery access in OR
   c. Supraceliac aortic control in OR
   d. Retrograde passage of large Foley catheter balloon from the opened aorta neck during laparotomy

   Answer: c

REFERENCES

1. Robinson WP, Schanzer A, Li Y, et al. Derivation and validation of a practical risk score for prediction of mortality after open repair of ruptured abdominal aortic aneurysms in a US regional cohort and comparison to existing scoring systems. *J Vasc Surg*. 2013 Feb;57(2):354–61.
2. Wang LJ, Locham S, Al-Nouri O, et al. Endovascular repair of ruptured abdominal aortic aneurysm is superior to open repair: propensity-matched analysis in the vascular quality initiative. *J Vasc Surg*. 2020 Aug;72(2):498–507.
3. Hans SS, Huang RR. Results of 101 ruptured abdominal aortic aneurysm repairs from a single surgical practice. *Arch Surg*. 2003 Aug;138(8):898–901.
4. Noel AA, Gloviczki P, Cherry KJ Jr, Bower TC, et al. Ruptured abdominal aortic aneurysms: the excessive mortality rate of conventional repair. *J Vasc Surg*. 2001 Jul;34(1):41–6.
5. Eslami MH, Messina LM. Ruptured AAA: open surgical management. *Semin Vasc Surg*. 2010 Dec;23(4):200–5.
6. Cho JS, Kim JY, Rhee RY, et al. Contemporary results of open repair of ruptured abdominal aortoiliac aneurysms: effect of surgeon volume on mortality. *J Vasc Surg*. 2008 Jul;48(1):10–17; discussion 17–8.
7. Hans SS, Robb HJ. A two-layer "telescoping" proximal anastomosis for repair of juxtarenal abdominal aortic aneurysms. *Am Surg*. 1997 Sep;63(9):839–41.
8. Phillips AR, Tran L, Foust JE, Liang NL. Systematic review of plasma/packed red blood cell ratio on survival in ruptured abdominal aortic aneurysms. *J Vasc Surg*. 2021 Apr;73(4):1438–1444.
9. Björck M. Management of the tense abdomen or difficult abdominal closure after operation for ruptured abdominal aortic aneurysms. *Semin Vasc Surg*. 2012 Mar;25(1):35–8.

30

Proximal abdominal aortic aneurysm repair

ALEXANDER D. SHEPARD

INTRODUCTION

The proximal abdominal aorta is defined as the aorta running from the aortic hiatus to the renal arteries. Aneurysms of this segment present unique challenges in management compared with those of the infrarenal (IR) aorta. Operative exposure is more extensive and unfamiliar, leading to longer procedure times and increased risk of injury to adjacent organs (e.g., spleen, pancreas). Proximal aortic clamping leads to obligatory periods of renal/visceral ischemia and increased cardiac stress compared with IR aortic clamping. Finally, aortic reconstruction techniques are more complicated than the end-to-end anastomoses of IR repair.

Assessment of cardiac, pulmonary, and renal function is essential to risk stratification. A high-quality (thin-cut) computed tomographic angiogram (CTA) is critical in preoperative evaluation; it allows one to plan the approach, determine a logical clamping/unclamping sequence, and devise an expeditious reconstruction. Careful preoperative planning is the key to good outcomes with this operation. Intraoperative monitoring with arterial line, central line, and Foley catheter is routine, supplemented by transesophageal echocardiography as needed.

OPERATIVE APPROACH

A standard transperitoneal (TP), inframesocolic exposure is suitable only for juxtarenal (JR) abdominal aortic aneurysms (AAA). Exposure of more proximal AAA can be done through a midline incision using medial visceral rotation (MVR) or through a left flank (LF) approach (thoraco-retroperitoneal or thoracoabdominal). The author greatly prefers the latter. With MVR, the abdomen is opened in the standard fashion with a long midline incision, and the peritoneal reflection lateral to the left colon and spleen is incised from the sigmoid colon cephalad to the aortic hiatus. A retrorenal plane is developed and the spleen, pancreas, and left kidney are retracted medially to expose the entire abdominal aorta from hiatus to bifurcation. If required, right renal artery (RA) and distal right iliac access can be obtained through standard TP exposure techniques. The major disadvantages of this approach are lack of access to the distal descending thoracic aorta, a high incidence of splenic injury (~20%), and complications of excessive visceral retraction (e.g., bowel ischemia and pancreatitis) [1].

For these and other reasons, we have favored a LF approach through a ninth or tenth intercostal space incision—ninth for paravisceral, extent IV thoracoabdominal aneurysms (TAAA) and tenth for pararenal AAAs. Positioning of the patient in a modified left thoracotomy position is key (Figure 28.9 in Chapter 28). When grafting to the bifurcation, the author leaves the patient in an almost pure lateral position, rotating the hips posteriorly only when iliac/femoral exposure is required. The incision is begun at the level of the umbilicus at the lateral margin of the left rectus sheath and carried obliquely into the appropriate intercostal space entering the left chest. More proximal aortic exposure can be gained by taking the incision further posteriorly (as far as the paraspinous muscles if necessary) while more distal exposure is facilitated by extending the incision to the midline. The diaphragm is divided circumferentially, beginning at the costal margin approximately 2 cm from its lateral attachments, to avoid injury to phrenic nerve branches. As much diaphragm is divided as necessary (usually no more than 50%) to avoid tearing it during subsequent rib retraction. We have avoided radial division of the diaphragm since a 2001 review of our experience revealed that this was the single most important factor associated with post-op respiratory failure following this operation [2].

A standard mechanical retraction system (e.g., Omni Tract or Thompson) provides good exposure. As described previously in Chapter 28, a retroperitoneal plane posterior to the left kidney is developed and the kidney and the peritoneal sac/visceral contents are retracted

DOI: 10.1201/9781003452096-30

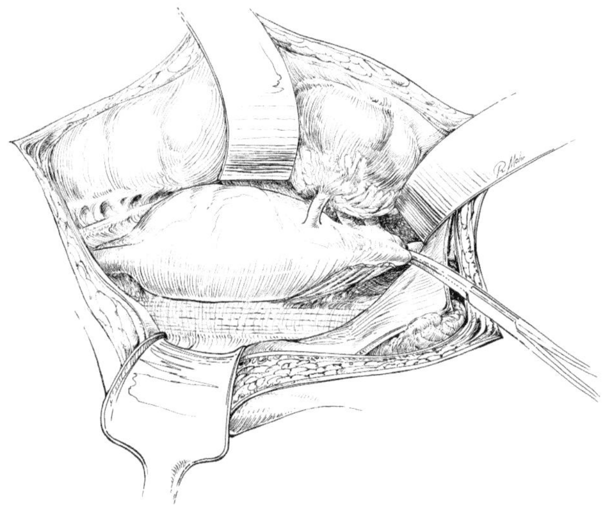

Figure 30.1 Exposure of a proximal AAA through a left flank retroperitoneal approach after left crus division.

to the patient's right. The lumbar branch of the left renal vein is carefully sought as it crosses over the aorta and divided, providing a guide to the location of the left RA. The left diaphragmatic crus is divided along the long axis of the aorta; this maneuver is facilitated by the operator inserting his/her left index finger under the crus (on top of the aorta) and dividing the muscle with electrocautery (Figure 30.1). This step is critical for exposing the supraceliac (SC) aorta and the celiac and superior mesenteric artery (SMA) origins. The left RA usually originates from the aorta just below the lowermost edge of the crus. For JR AAAs, it is unnecessary to dissect out more than the left RA and potentially the SC aorta depending on the planned clamp level. For suprarenal (SR) AAAs, control of the SMA and sometimes the celiac is beneficial, while for paravisceral AAAs, control of all three vessels is helpful. Lymphoareolar tissue overlying the PAA is divided with an ultrasonic scalpel.

Control of SC aorta is relatively simple to obtain through this approach; investing fascia is divided and the operator's index finger is passed just anterior and posterior to the aorta to allow passage of the blades of a cross-clamp. There is no need to circumferentially control the aorta at this level. Care should be taken when developing the posterior plane to avoid injuring any intervening segmental arteries. Supramesenteric (SM) aortic control is more tedious to obtain because of the presence of a vascularized lymphatic plexus lying on the anterior surface of the aorta between the celiac and SMA. Suprarenal control is easier than SM because of the absence of any tissue adherent to the aorta at this level. Once proximal aortic control has been obtained, the origins of the left RA, SMA, and celiac axis are dissected out as necessary. Though slightly more time-consuming, control of the celiac and SMA is associated with less blood loss than simply allowing these vessels to back bleed with a supraceliac aortic clamp on. Extraluminal control is also less cumbersome than intraluminal control with balloon occlusion catheters.

The IR component of the AAA is next exposed by dividing overlying tissues. Care should be taken to identify the left ureter and ensure that it is retracted with the peritoneal sac out of harm's way. Iliac control is obtained as previously described in Chapter 28. Lumbar arteries that can be preserved at either the proximal or distal anastomosis are controlled while those originating from the aneurysm sac and accessible are ligated to reduce blood loss after opening the aneurysm.

Aortic clamp site

Choosing an appropriate proximal clamp level is one of the most important determinants of operative success with PAAA repair. Anatomy and aortic disease dictate clamp level, which is chosen based on a careful review of the preoperative CTA. The more proximally the aorta is clamped, the greater the cardiac strain and the higher the visceral ischemia burden; in general, therefore, the most distal feasible clamp site is preferred. It is also important not to clamp diseased aorta with the consequent risk of renal/visceral and lower extremity atheroembolism. With SR clamping, the relationship between the RAs and SMA needs to be carefully assessed; when the SMA originates too close to the RAs, SR clamping may not be possible without risking injury to one of these vessels. One must also guard against injuring the unseen origin of the right RA when it arises more proximally off the aorta than the left RA.

When more proximal aortic clamping is required, we have favored SC over SM because the SC aorta is reliably the least diseased segment of abdominal aorta and because it is fast and easy to perform from an LF approach. Control at the SM level has the advantages of less cardiac stress and maintenance of visceral perfusion through the celiac; this exposure, however, is more tedious than SC and can be associated with significant SMA back bleeding if the SMA is not concomitantly controlled. Prior to proximal aortic clamping, we always consider preliminary IR clamping, if the aorta at this level is not too aneurysmal or diseased; this maneuver allows control of any back bleeding lumbar vessels and the IMA without wasting valuable visceral/renal ischemia time.

PROTECTION AGAINST VITAL ORGAN ISCHEMIA

With proximal aortic clamping comes obligatory renal ± visceral and occasional spinal cord ischemia (SCI). Acute kidney injury (AKI) is one of the most commonly reported complications of these repairs [3]. Minimizing clamp time is obviously critical. Prior to clamping, it is important to optimize hemodynamics; mannitol (25 gm) is administered 15–20 min prior to anticipated clamping. Selecting an appropriate clamp site reduces the risk of embolizing debris into the RAs. When utilizing a LF approach, the right RA is particularly vulnerable to this complication because of its dependent position; inflation of a small balloon occlusion catheter in the origin of this vessel can block the passage of such debris. When prolonged (>30 min) renal ischemia times are anticipated or patients have pre-existing chronic kidney disease, we routinely use cold renal perfusion to reduce renal metabolic demands; 250 ml of 4°C Ringers lactate (containing heparin 1000 units/L, methylprednisolone 500 mg /L, sodium bicarbonate 15 mL of 8.4%/L, 25% mannitol 12.5 mL/L) is infused into each kidney followed by 50 ml q 15 minutes for the duration of clamping. Infusion is accomplished through balloon-tipped Pruitt perfusion catheters (9 Fr) for large RAs or 4–5 Fr Fogarty irrigating balloon catheters for smaller or diseased RAs. Several papers have demonstrated the value of this technique in the prevention of AKI [3,4]. Although unproven, the author has utilized a similar approach for visceral protection by infusing the SMA (400 ml initially followed by 75 ml q 15 min) during SC clamping. Using this technique, we have noted less coagulopathy and fewer hemodynamic changes with unclamping. Recent research has suggested superiority of a 4°C histidine-tryptophan-ketoglutarate renal perfusion solution (Custodiol) compared with Ringer's lactate, but trials have been limited [5].

Spinal cord ischemia is uncommon with PAAA repair, but frequent enough that protective steps should be taken in higher-risk situations—defined in our experience as all extent IV TAAAs and whenever SC clamp times are anticipated to exceed 30 min. A lumbar drain is placed preoperatively, and cerebrospinal fluid is drained to maintain an intrathecal pressure ≤10 cm H_2O. Other adjuncts include moderate passive hypothermia (allowing the patient to cool to 34°C) and avoidance of high-dose vasodilators during cross-clamp.

AORTIC RECONSTRUCTION

Prior to aortic clamping, we routinely heparinize, believing that microvascular thrombosis is a major determinant of multisystem organ failure when it occurs. Careful communication with the anesthesia team is necessary during clamping and blood should always be immediately available when opening the aneurysm sac.

Construction of the proximal aortic anastomosis differs from IR repairs because of the need to maintain flow to the renal/visceral arteries. Repair of JR AAA (defined as aneurysms with no IR neck suitable for clamping and anastomosis) is the simplest. Although we perform most of these AAA repairs through the LF, they can also be done through a TP approach after full mobilization of the left renal vein (Figure 28.3 in Chapter 28). This maneuver allows full visualization of the JR aorta for both clamping and proximal anastomosis. The ostia of the two RAs are frequently incorporated into the anastomotic suture line (Figure 30.2).

Reconstruction of more proximal AAAs is more complicated and usually requires a beveled end-to-end anastomosis incorporating the renal and visceral artery origins. How this is performed depends on the relationship of the RAs to the aorta. If both RAs originate anteriorly with most of the aneurysmal wall extending posteriorly, a posterior bevel is possible. With this reconstruction, the aorta is trimmed to leave the two RAs, the SMA, and if necessary, the celiac on an anterior tongue of aorta while the graft is cut to leave a corresponding posterior bevel (Figure 30.3). Unfortunately, local anatomy is usually not amenable to this type of reconstruction.

More commonly, the proximal reconstruction is a laterally based, beveled anastomosis, which is used when the RAs are separated by a significant amount of aneurysmal aortic wall. This technique incorporates the right RA,

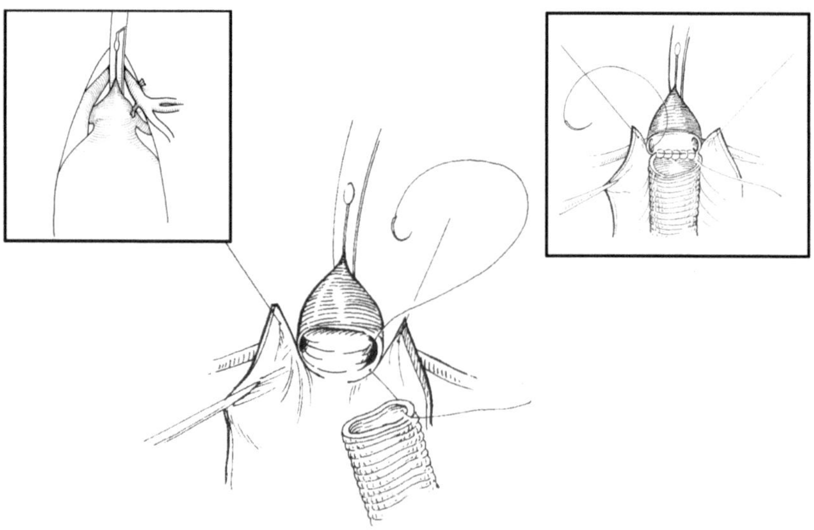

Figure 30.2 Construction of proximal aortic anastomosis during JR AAA repair demonstrating incorporation of RA ostia into the suture line.

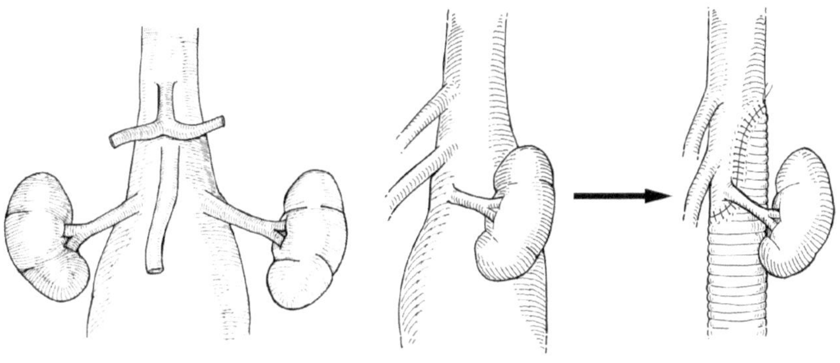

Figure 30.3 Proximal aortic reconstruction utilizing a posterior beveled anastomosis, leaving celiac, SMA, and both RAs on an anterior tongue of aorta. This reconstruction is only appropriate when RAs arise close to each other anteriorly.

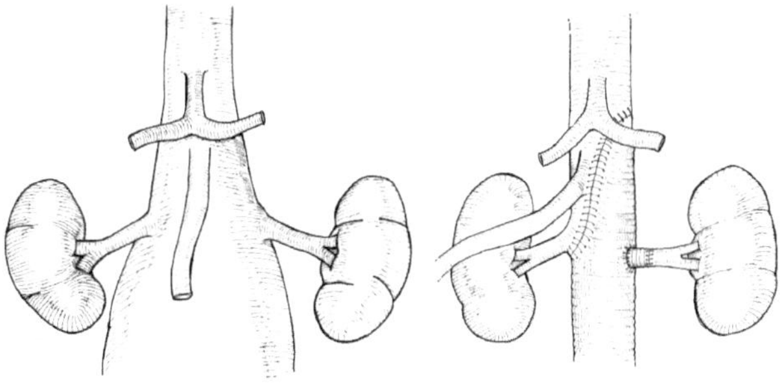

Figure 30.4 Proximal aortic reconstruction utilizing a lateral beveled anastomosis, incorporating celiac, SMA, and right RA on a tongue of aorta with either bypass to or reimplantation of the left RA. This is the most commonly performed proximal reconstruction and is utilized when there is significant aortic wall between the two RAs.

SMA, and celiac (as necessary) on a tongue of aorta, while the left RA is either reimplanted into the graft or more frequently bypassed with a small caliber sidearm graft previously sewn on to the aortic graft (Figure 30.4). When using a renal graft, it is imperative to carefully rotate/trim the aortic graft so that the sidearm is appropriately positioned; we have found the two o'clock position (SMA at 12 o'clock) to be the most satisfactory position to prevent subsequent sidearm kinking. The graft to aortic anastomosis is performed by the inclusion technique, taking the first suture bites at the level of the dependent right RA and then carrying the suture line up the posterior wall of the aorta, taking double-thickness bites until the transected edge of the aorta is encountered (Figure 30.5a). Single-thickness aortic wall stitches bring the suture line up to the level of the SMA or celiac, and then down the transected anterior wall. The anastomosis is completed by bringing the other suture along the anterior aortic wall (double-thickness transitioning to single-thickness bites) to the level of the first suture line (Figure 30.5b). When performing a beveled anastomosis of any type, it is important to leave as little aortic wall behind as possible to reduce the risk of future aortic wall degeneration and recurrent aneurysm formation. Following appropriate flushing maneuvers, the right RA perfusion catheter is removed, and the suture line is secured, allowing

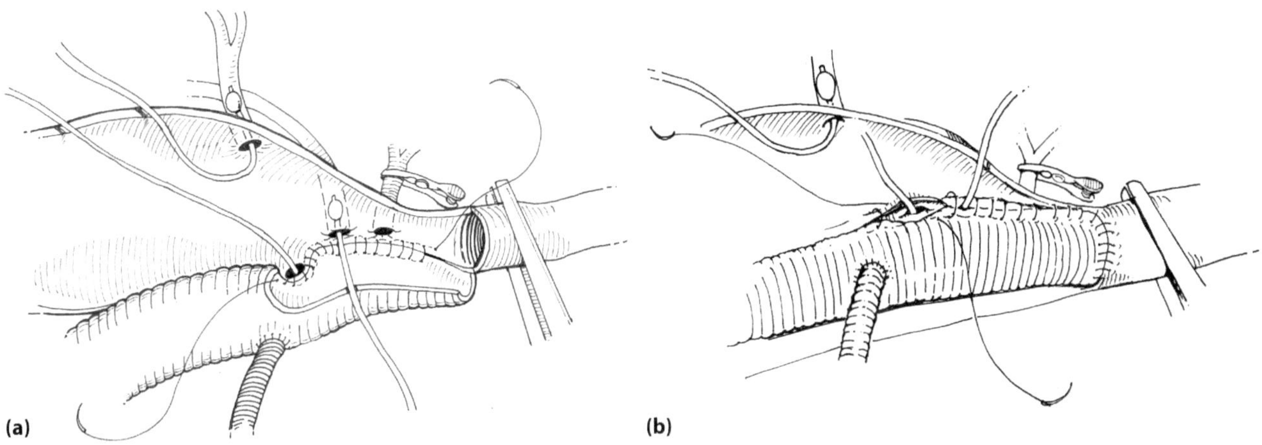

(a) (b)

Figure 30.5 Lateral beveled proximal anastomosis: (a) demonstrating placement of perfusion catheters in SMA and both RAs with construction of aortic suture line along the posterior wall; bulldog clamp on celiac artery; (b) completion of anterior wall suture line.

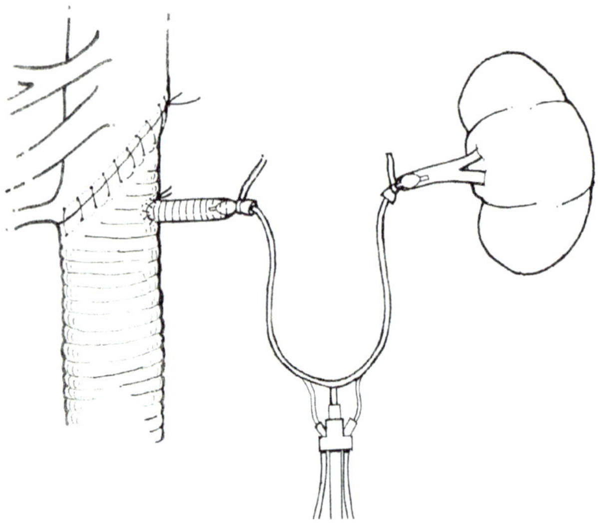

Figure 30.6 Pruitt carotid shunt between sidearm graft and left renal artery allowing left kidney perfusion during construction of distal aortic/iliac anastomosis.

sequential restoration of flow to the right RA, the celiac, and finally the SMA.

A decision is made at this point whether to proceed next with revascularization of the left kidney *or* the lower extremities. We usually proceed with the distal anastomosis first to restore hypogastric flow and reduce SCI risk. In addition, doing the distal anastomosis after the left RA increases the risk that the renal revascularization could be disrupted during distal aortic/iliac manipulation. Continued cold perfusion of the left kidney can be carried out during the distal anastomosis, or alternatively, the left kidney can be shunted using a Pruitt carotid shunt with one end placed in the renal sidearm and the other in the left renal artery (Figure 30.6). Once the distal anastomosis (or if to the iliacs, the right iliac anastomosis) has been completed, attention is directed to the left RA. It is imperative that this anastomosis be performed under tension since there is invariably redundancy in the graft/artery that can lead to kinking when the left kidney is returned to its normal anatomic location. Reimplantation of the left RA along with a cuff of aorta usually avoids this problem but requires placement of a partially occluding clamp on the graft, frequently at the level of the visceral/right RA patch that can disrupt this fresh suture line. If distal flow has been restored prior to this reconstruction, we usually check for pedal Doppler flow and, if adequate, reverse the heparin anticoagulation before completing the left RA bypass.

Sometimes, the aneurysm extends well above the origin of the celiac, mandating an end-to-end anastomosis between the graft and the aorta with reimplantation of the celiac, SMA, and right RA as a separate inclusion patch (Figure 30.7). In addition, in patients with the origins of the celiac, SMA, and right RA widely spaced apart, an inclusion patch with all three artery origins is simply not possible without leaving significant amounts of abnormal aortic wall behind. In this situation and in patients with

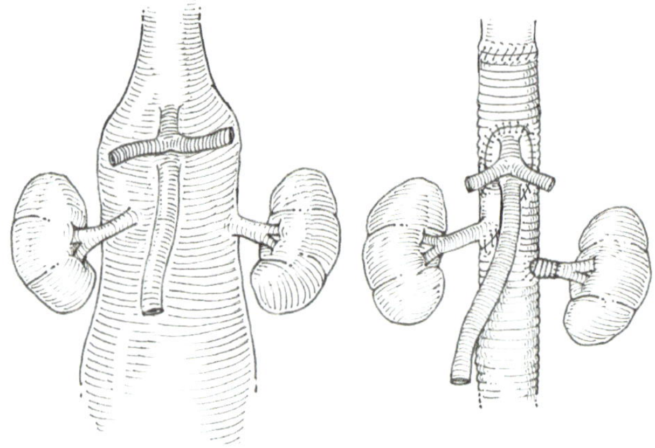

Figure 30.7 Extent IV TAAA showing end-to-end proximal aortic anastomosis with reimplantation of celiac, SMA, and right RA as a single patch and bypass of left RA.

documented connective tissue abnormalities, we have utilized a graft with prefabricated sidearms for reconstruction (Vascutek® Coselli Thoracoabdominal Graft) (Figure 30.8). The use of this graft requires significant attention to detail to ensure that the graft limbs line up with their respective branches. When using this graft, we perform the proximal aortic anastomosis followed by the right RA graft anastomosis, which is the key graft limb to line up appropriately. Once the right kidney is perfused, flow is restored to the SMA and left RA through shunts or perfusion catheters placed into the graft limbs. This technique reduces renal/visceral ischemia time while giving priority to the restoration of hypogastric flow and reduction in SCI. After the distal anastomosis is done, the SMA and celiac grafts are performed, saving the left RA for last. Doing the left renal graft prior to the viscerals constrains exposure and risks disruption of this bypass during visceral reconstruction. In

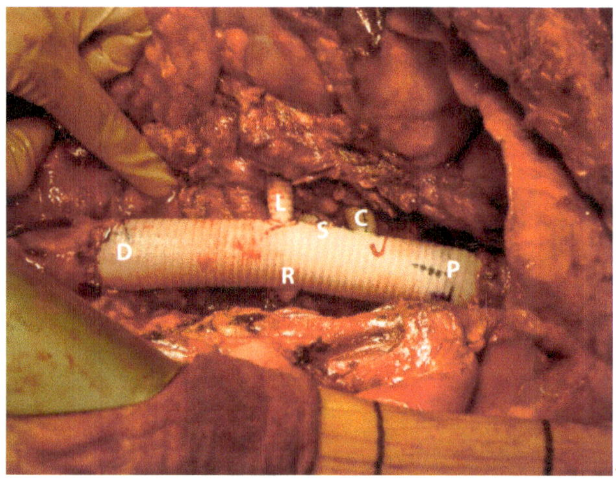

Figure 30.8 Branched (Coselli) graft reconstruction of an extent IV TAAA. Proximal aortic anastomosis to the right of the photo, distal aortic anastomosis to the left of the photo. P, proximal graft; C, celiac limb; S, SMA; L, left RA; R, right RA; D, distal graft.

most situations, the Coselli graft limbs are cut very short (no more than 15–30 mm) to avoid kinking.

Following completion of all anastomoses and assurance of good Doppler flow in all reconstructed vascular territories, heparin anticoagulation is reversed, and the hemostatic profile is corrected as necessary. The left chest is drained with a small (19 Fr) postero-basal pleural tube, the diaphragm closed with 0 or 2-0 polypropylene, the ribs re-approximated with looped #1 PDS, and the wound closed in layers with 0 PDS. Postoperatively, a spinal cord protection protocol is maintained for at least 24 hours in patients with a lumbar drain.

The key to this operation is reducing blood loss, which can be minimized by avoiding venous injuries, ligating lumbar arteries prior to opening the sac, and reducing the coagulopathy associated with gut/liver ischemia/reperfusion by cold SMA perfusion and expeditious visceral revascularization [6]. Cold renal perfusion reduces the risk of AKI. In experienced hands. the mortality and morbidity of open PAAA repair approaches that of IR AAA repair and remains the standard approach for managing these complex AAAs.

TRICKS AND TRAPS

1. A high-quality (thin-cut) computed tomographic angiogram (CTA) is critical in preoperative evaluation; it allows one to plan the approach, determine a logical clamping/unclamping sequence, and to devise an expeditious reconstruction.
2. A left flank thoraco-retroperitoneal approach through the tenth or ninth intercostal space is ideal for exposing most proximal AAAs.
3. Circumferential (as opposed to radial) division of the diaphragm reduces postoperative pulmonary dysfunction by avoiding injury to branches of the phrenic nerve.
4. The lumbar branch of the left renal vein crosses over the aorta just below the origin of the left renal artery. If very large, the CTA should be checked for the presence of a retroaortic left renal vein.
5. Longitudinal division of the left diaphragmatic crus is necessary to expose the supraceliac aorta.
6. Choosing a proximal aortic clamp site is based on careful review of pre-op CTA; in general, the most distal feasible clamp site is preferred.
7. Cold renal perfusion is a valuable adjunct to reduce postop acute kidney injury and is utilized when renal ischemia times >30 minutes are anticipated or in the presence of pre-existing chronic kidney disease.
8. Most proximal anastomoses are performed in beveled fashion to the aorta, leaving as little native aortic wall behind as possible.
9. Placing a short sidearm graft on the aortic graft for left renal revascularization allows shunting of the left kidney with a Pruitt carotid shunt after completion of the proximal aortic anastomosis so that the distal aortic/iliac anastomosis can be performed first.
10. The key to this operation is reducing blood loss, which can be minimized by avoiding venous injuries and reducing the coagulopathy associated with gut/liver ischemia/reperfusion by cold SMA perfusion and expeditious visceral revascularization.

QUESTIONS

1. Pick the true statement:
    a. A high-quality, thin-cut CTA is a critical preoperative planning test.
    b. Renal and visceral ischemic complications are rare with PAAA repair
    c. A standard midline transperitoneal approach is adequate for most PAAA repairs
    d. Proximal AAA repair is no more challenging than standard infrarenal AAA repair

    Answer: a

2. Pick the true statement re: left flank thoraco-retroperitoneal exposure for PAAA repair:
    a. The optimal patient position is hips flat with the chest rotated 30° to the table
    b. The aorta is best approached anterior to the left kidney
    c. Exposure of the right RA and distal right iliac system can be limited
    d. It does not matter if the diaphragm is divided radially or peripherally

    Answer: c

3. Pick the best statement re: proximal aortic clamping:
    a. There is no significant difference between the various clamp sites (SR vs. SM vs. SC)
    b. SR clamping can be associated with coagulopathy
    c. The best clamp site should be determined by the intraoperative appearance of the aorta
    d. The clamp level should be determined by the configuration of the aneurysm and the presence of aortic luminal disease

    Answer: d

4. During PAAA repair, cold renal perfusion:
    a. Should always be utilized
    b. Is associated with a reduction in the incidence of acute kidney injury
    c. Prevents the coagulopathy associated with visceral ischemia
    d. Works by increasing renal metabolic demands

    Answer: b

REFERENCES

1. Reilly LM, Ramos TK, Murray SP, Cheng SWK, Stoney RJ. Optimal exposure of the proximal abdominal aorta: a critical appraisal of transabdominal medial visceral rotation. *J Vasc Surg* 1994;19:375–390.
2. Anagnostopolous PV, Shepard AD, Pipinos II, Nypaver TJ, Cho JS, Reddy DJ. Factors affecting outcome in proximal abdominal aortic aneurysm repair. *Ann Vasc Surg* 2001;15:511–519.
3. Kabbani LS, West CA, Viau D, Nypaver TJ, Weaver MW, Barth C, Lin JC, Shepard AD. Survival after repair of pararenal and paravisceral abdominal aortic aneurysms. *J Vasc Surg* 2014;59:1488–1494.
4. Koksoy C, LeMaire SA, Curling PE, Raskin SA, Schmittling ZC, Conklin LD, Coselli JS. Renal perfusion during thoracoabdominal aortic operations: cold crystalloid is superior to normothermic blood. *Ann Thorac Surg* 2002;73:730–738.
5. Kahlberg A, Tshomba Y, Baccellieri D, Bertoglio L, Rinaldi E, Ardita V, Colombo E, Moscato U, Melissano G, Chiesa R. Renal perfusion with histidine-tryptophan-ketoglutarate compared with Ringer's solution in patients undergoing thoracoabdominal aortic open repair. *J Thor Cardiovasc Surg* 2023;165:569–579.
6. Anagnostopoulos PV, Shepard AD, Pipinos II, Raman SBK, Chaudhry PA, Mishima T, Morita H, Suzuki G. Hemostatic alterations associated with supraceliac aortic cross-clamping. *J Vasc Surg* 2001;35:100–108.

31

Thoracoabdominal aortic aneurysm repair

SAMIA D. ELLIAS AND MARK F. CONRAD

INTRODUCTION

Thoracoabdominal aortic aneurysms (TAAAs) constitute about 10% of aortic aneurysms and have shown an increased incidence with enhanced imaging. Modern surgical management, pioneered by E. Stanley Crawford, involves reconstructing the aneurysmal aorta with a Dacron graft with direct anastomoses of critical vital organ arteries, albeit posing a risk of ischemia to these structures. Despite evolving approaches, open repair of TAAAs still carries a 5–10% risk of perioperative complications, including renal, respiratory, and spinal cord ischemia (SCI).

CLASSIFICATION AND NATURAL HISTORY

Anatomy

The Crawford classification scheme has been used to delineate the extent of a TAAA and is useful in defining the associated risks of repair as well as the operative approach (Figure 31.1).

Natural history

TAAA risk factors include hypertension, atherosclerosis, smoking, and chronic obstructive pulmonary disease (COPD); 70% are degenerative aneurysms, with atherosclerosis contributing to medial degeneration. Hereditary factors (Marfan's, Ehlers–Danlos) account for 15–20% of cases. In patients with intact degenerative TAAAs, repair is reasonable when the diameter exceeds 6 cm; experienced surgeons can consider repair at >5.5 cm. Repair is recommended for patients with features indicating an increased rupture risk, even when the diameter is <5.5 cm (e.g., rapid growth [>0.5 cm/year], symptomatic aneurysm). Aortic event rates and five-year survival significantly change when TAAA diameters exceed 6.0 cm, with a risk of adverse events ranging from 9.3% to 19% [1]. Mortality at this diameter is two to four times higher than the median operative mortality of an open TAAA repair. A fixed diameter may be insufficient; body surface area (BSA), especially in women and shorter individuals, may be considered. More precise calculations, incorporating BSA, can yield the aortic size index (ASI), with its predictive role under investigation.

DIAGNOSTIC IMAGING

Accurate radiographic evaluation is crucial for operative planning. Computed tomography angiography (CTA) is preferred for evaluating aneurysm extent, visceral vessel patency, renal artery origin, distal repair extent, iliac vessels, and potential pelvic occlusive disease. CTA provides details on the aorta proximal to cross-clamp, renal artery topography, and iliofemoral access vessels. Some advocate preoperative imaging for the artery of Adamkiewicz to reduce SCI risk. Now magnetic resonance angiography can assess flow dynamics, aortic wall stress, and 4D MRI for TAAA evaluation.

PATIENT SELECTION AND PREOPERATIVE EVALUATION

Patients with aortic disease undergo preoperative investigations based on surgery urgency. TAAA repair candidates, typically with degenerative aneurysms, share features of diffuse atherosclerosis. Concurrent coronary artery disease is assessed via coronary catheterization or CTA. Considering the commonality of hypertension, smoking history, and COPD, pulmonary function testing with one-lung ventilation planning is considered. Renovascular disease and renal insufficiency coexist, impacting long-term renal function. Preoperative azotemia (serum creatinine >2.5 cm/dL) is a relative contraindication unless potential for renal function salvage exists.

DOI: 10.1201/9781003452096-31

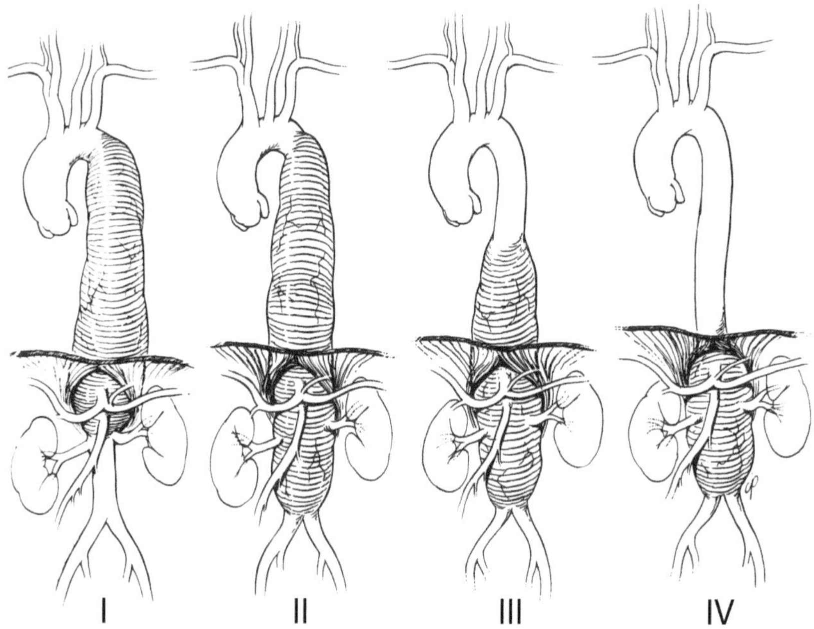

Figure 31.1 Crawford classification for TAAAs. Type I: distal to left subclavian artery to diaphragm above the celiac artery. Type II: extends beyond the celiac artery, often to aortic bifurcation. Type III: mid-descending thoracic aorta to aortic bifurcation. Type IV: the celiac artery to aortic bifurcation. Type V (not shown): distal descending thoracic aorta, including celiac and superior mesenteric origins but excluding renal arteries.

Abnormal preoperative serum creatinine correlates with perioperative mortality.

SURGICAL TREATMENT

Treatment options

AHA/ACC guidelines now suggest endovascular repair with fenestrated or branched grafts in patients with intact degenerative TAAA and suitable anatomy. These grafts, with fenestrations and branches, allow continued perfusion of aortic side branches during repair. The latest device is a multi-branched endograft, applicable in 88% of TAAA patients. The Zenith t-Branch system is the first commercialized off-the-shelf multi-branched endograft. However, anatomical suitability, peripheral access, and aortic lumen size are crucial considerations for this approach. Common combinations include two or three fenestrations for renal arteries and SMA, and one or two directional branches for CA and SMA [2].

The hybrid approach, combining visceral artery debranching with endovascular TAAA exclusion, is resource-efficient for extent I, II, and III patients, avoiding thoracotomy. It is non-inferior to open surgery for extent IV and pararenal aneurysms, eliminating aortic cross-clamping risks. However, its role in preventing SCI is controversial (0 to 30% paraplegia). While not a substitute for open repair, the hybrid approach remains an alternative for high-risk patients with prior aortic surgery, multiple comorbidities, and contraindications for aortic clamping and cardiopulmonary bypass (CPB) [3].

TECHNICAL COMPONENTS

Operative exposure

Operative success relies on exposure of the left posterolateral aspect of the TAA. The patient is positioned in the right lateral decubitus position. A CSF drainage catheter is inserted before positioning. We utilize motor evoked potential (MEP) monitoring for additional protection against SCI. Thoracic incision is determined by the proximal extent of the aneurysm. Typically, at the fifth or sixth intercostal space, with posterior division of the sixth or seventh rib providing adequate exposure and incision kept lateral along the edge of the rectus.

Abdominal aorta exposure is achieved by entering the plane posterior to the spleen, left kidney, and colon. Abdominal contents are reflected to the right, preserving the left ureter under laparotomy pads (Figure 31.2). Retroperitoneal tissues overlying the aorta are transected, and the lumbar branch of the renal vein is identified and divided. The left renal artery (LRA), topographically close to this vein, is identified and dissected toward its origin on the aorta, serving as the starting point for dividing retroperitoneal tissues over the aorta inferiorly and the median arcuate ligament and diaphragmatic crura superiorly. Circumferential division through the muscular portion of the diaphragm, leaving a few centimeters attached laterally, preserves phrenic innervation. The use of a large Penrose drain passed through the divided aortic hiatus facilitates retraction and is used liberally by the author.

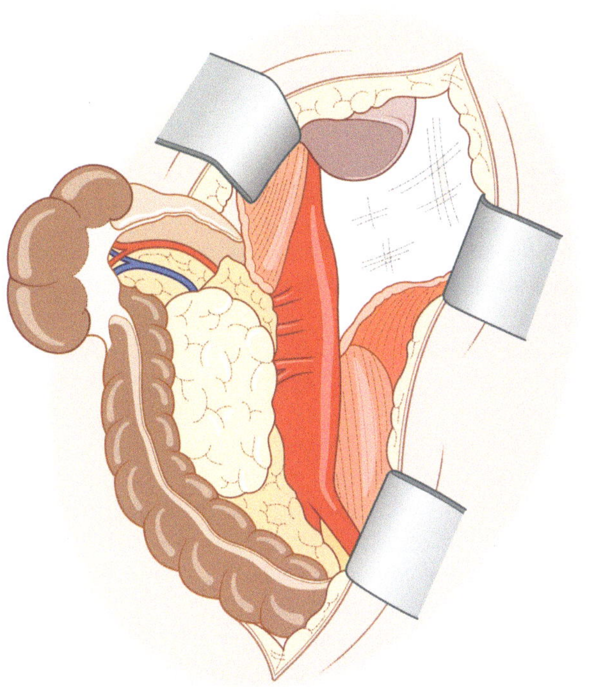

Figure 31.2 Exposure of the left chest and abdomen through a thoracoabdominal incision with the left kidney, spleen, pancreas, and left colon reflected medially. This approach exposes the entire left posterolateral aspect of the thoracoabdominal aorta.

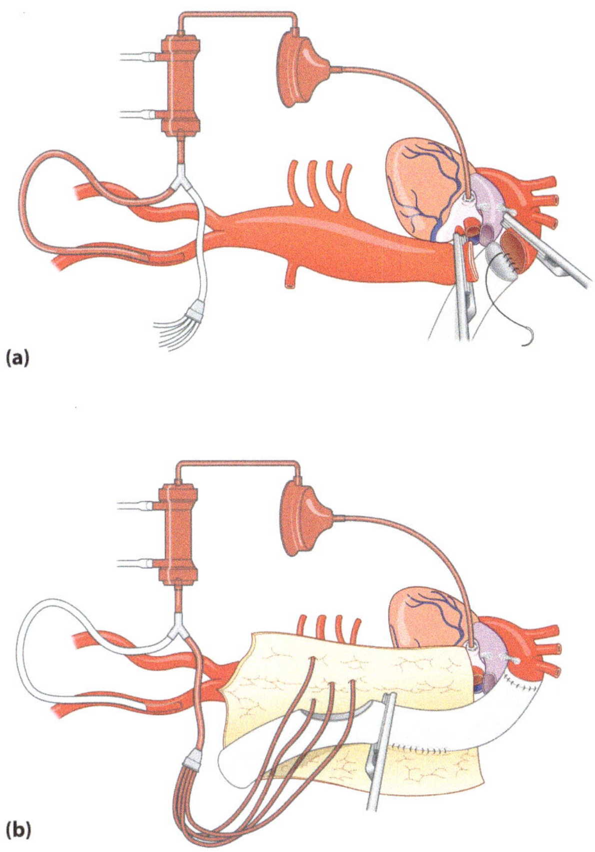

Figure 31.3 Operative conduct of TAAA repair involves (a) initial distal aortic perfusion (via left heart bypass) with the heparin-impregnated Biomedicus 560 Centrifugal Pump (Medtronic, Minneapolis, MN, USA) using the femoral artery, and (b) subsequent maintenance of perfusion by multiple catheters as reconstruction proceeds distally.

Dissection of left pleural space

After left lung deflation, the mediastinal pleura over the aneurysm and proximal aorta is divided. For type I–II aneurysms, proximal aortic control near the left subclavian artery (LSA) origin is necessary. The left vagus nerve is mobilized by dividing it distal to the left recurrent nerve origin, preserving the latter. If more proximal control is required, the ligamentum arteriosum beneath the aortic arch is divided, carefully avoiding the left main pulmonary artery. The aorta is encircled with a vessel tape on either side of the LSA, depending on the aneurysm's proximal extent. Blunt dissection is used on the posterior aspect of the aorta to clear sufficient normal aorta for clamp application while maintaining an adequate length for a precise proximal anastomosis. External control of the LSA is preferred, but intraluminal balloon control can be used if necessary. The left inferior pulmonary vein (IPV) is isolated for atrial femoral bypass, placing a 4-0 polypropylene purse-string suture for the venous cannula, which needs not be larger than 19 Fr.

Atriofemoral bypass

The author extensively employs atriofemoral bypass with a centripetal, motorized pump and low systemic heparin doses for extent I–III TAAAs, aligning with the spinal cord collateral network concept and emphasizing pelvic/hypogastric perfusion (Figure 31.3). The left heart bypass circuit's return line has a Y-connector for pump return to the distal aortic cannula and two 9-Fr Pruitt® balloon-tipped perfusion catheters to maintain continuous mesenteric perfusion during construction of the proximal aortic anastomosis. Another system with two 9-Fr Pruitt catheters is set up for 4°C cold solution delivery to the renal arteries. Suturing an 8-mm graft to the femoral artery prevents leg ischemia, and potential myoglobinuria [4].

Clamping sequence and proximal anastomosis

The aortic prosthesis is prepared by attaching a 6-mm polytetrafluoroethylene (PTFE) sidearm graft for LRA reconstruction; Dacron is preferred, but PTFE is used for mycotic aneurysms due to decreased infection susceptibility. Atriofemoral bypass is initiated with left IPV cannulation and arterial return via the left common femoral artery, maintaining distal mean perfusion pressures of 60–70 mmHg; any deterioration in MEPs should prompt an increase in stimulus intensity or an increase in distal perfusion pressures. A sudden drop in MEP amplitude (within two to ten minutes) or a sustained progressive drop (within ten to 40 minutes) of >75% from baseline is considered significant. Efforts are made to place the first sequential clamp to allow retrograde perfusion of the lower intercostals and renal/viscerals via the femoral cannula of the atriofemoral bypass circuit.

Prepare the proximal neck by opting for circumferential aortic control to allow for complete aortic division to avoid proximal suture line injury to the underlying esophagus and the potential for a late erosion/fistula. Position the proximal clamp chosen considering the left subclavian artery (LSA) and the presence of atheromatous debris and aortic dissection. Sequentially clamp the distal aorta from T6, progressing distally. Open the proximal descending thoracic aorta upon clamping, removing all thrombus. Swiftly oversew back-bleeding proximal intercostal vessel orifices (T4–T8). Use 3-0 polypropylene for a typical proximal anastomosis, 4-0 polypropylene for a fragile aortic wall, and for a calcified aorta, consider 2-0 polypropylene. Initiate the suture line at the posterior wall, reinforcing it with felt pledgets continuing anteriorly. Place the proximal clamp just distal to the graft anastomosis and move the distal clamp to the end of the descending aorta. Further open the remaining thoracic aorta and evaluate T9–L1 intercostal vessels for potential reimplantation based on MEP signals, controlling back-bleeding with balloon occlusion catheters. Unless significant MEP changes occur, defer intercostal reconstruction.

Renal/visceral artery reconstruction

Reposition the distal clamp below to the infrarenal aorta and open the visceral aorta. Identify and control the orifices of the celiac, superior mesenteric, and left and right renal arteries using bulldog clamps for the SMA and celiac arteries. Gently cannulate the renal arteries with 6-Fr Pruitt perfusion catheters under direct vision. Conduct orificial endarterectomy if significant occlusive lesions are present in the right renal artery (RRA) and SMA. In cases requiring aortic endarterectomy, ensure adequate dissection of the SMA and celiac artery for potential countertraction from the external side, if needed—this is not feasible with the RRA, requiring sharp excision under direct vision for the endarterectomy plane conclusion.

The author employs a single inclusion patch covering the origins of the celiac artery, SMA, and RRA. Tension is applied to the aortic graft, and an elliptical side island is excised, spiraling posteriorly toward the RRA origin. The posterior anastomosis is completed under tension using single stitches passing through both the aorta and Dacron graft. The 6-Fr perfusion catheter is exchanged for a 12-Fr catheter to temporarily stent the RRA origin. A balloon-expandable stent secures RRA flow, placed under direct vision after the proximal suture line passes the artery orifice to ensure that no narrowing has occurred. The anterior suture line, emphasizing stitches near the SMA and celiac artery origins, is finalized. Before completion, back-bleeding and patency of the celiac artery, SMA, and RRA are verified. A single flush of the proximal aortic cross-clamp ensures no clot or debris accumulation in the graft. When the origins of the visceral and right renal artery are at some distance from each other, individual buttons of each ostium can be re-implanted in the graft using running 4-0 polypropylene (Figure 31.4).

LRA reconstruction utilizes a 6-mm PTFE sidearm graft for direct end-to-end anastomosis. This approach is flexible for managing occlusive lesions, multiple renal

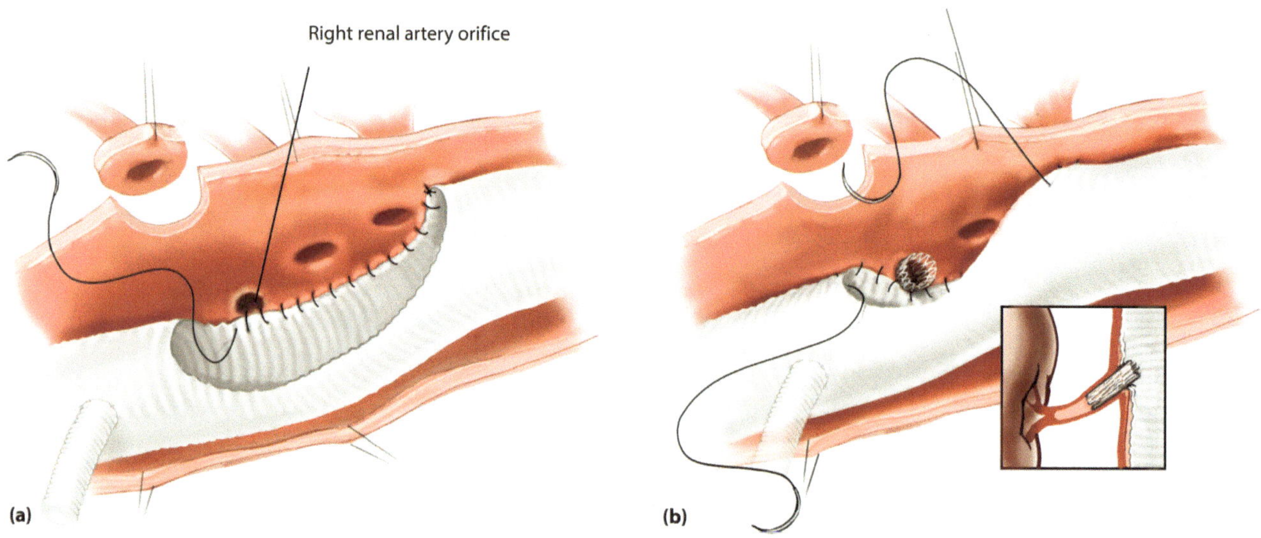

Figure 31.4 (a) Creation of visceral patch inclusion anastomosis of the celiac axis, SMA, and RRA with a 6-mm polytetrafluoroethylene sidearm bypass for left renal artery reconstruction; (b) deployment of a balloon-expandable stent into the RRA orifice to either treat occlusive lesions or prevent encroachment by the suture line.

arteries, and other complexities. Proper orientation of the sidearm graft is crucial to prevent kinking when returning the LRA to its anatomical position.

In patients with connective tissue disorder and under 60 years, or those with ostial separation exceeding 3 cm, a premanufactured side-branched thoracoabdominal aortic graft (STAG) is employed. Separate bypasses to each vessel start with the celiac and superior mesenteric arteries and conclude with the left renal artery [5]. To enhance spinal perfusion, prioritize performing the distal anastomosis before visceral and renal reconstruction to restore pulsatile flow to the pelvis.

Reconstruction of intercostal vessels

If MEP remains stable, occlusion balloons are removed, and vessels are oversewn with silk suture. Reconstruction, if needed, is achieved through an inclusion button anastomosis. Intercostal arteries near proximal or distal aortic anastomoses can be reconstructed with a long, beveled suture line. Additional revascularization methods include attaching short sidearm grafts to the main aortic graft or, in specific cases, implantation to the main aortic graft with Carrel patches containing intercostal vessels (Figure 31.5).

Distal anastomosis

The author prioritizes tube reconstructions to the aortic bifurcation, unless gross aneurysmal disease is present in the common iliacs. Extending reconstruction to the iliac or femoral arteries is a last resort. After restoring flow to the lower extremities, intraoperative checks include pulse recordings and Doppler signals in various arteries.

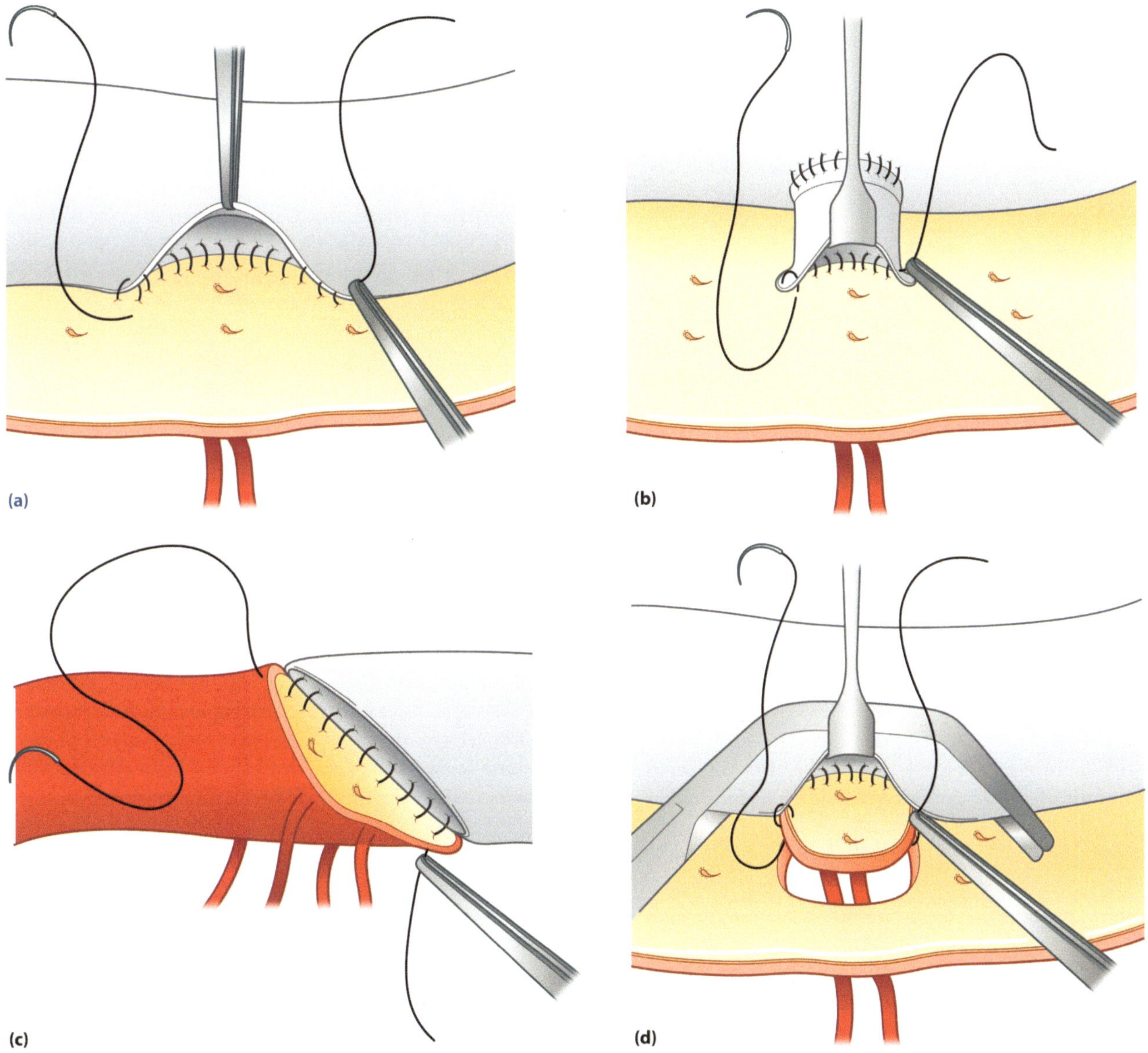

Figure 31.5 Methods of managing critical intercostal arteries: (a) inclusion button anastomosis; (b) separate sidearm graft; (c) beveled anastomosis preservation; (d) Carrel patch mobilization and direct reimplantation into the graft.

Hemostasis is typically sufficient after the distal anastomosis, with platelet and fresh frozen plasma (FFP) infusions increased as a precaution and minimal heparin use is crucial. Careful inspection of the aneurysm sac is done to detect potential sources of postoperative hemorrhage. The redundant sac is sutured over the aortic prosthesis, and renal artery reconstructions are verified before closure. The left kidney, when returned to its normal anatomic location, usually provides ample coverage with perinephric fat. A single pleural tube and a suction drain may be placed.

Postoperative care

Postoperatively, patients are closely monitored in the ICU to minimize hemodynamic shifts, reducing the risk of renal failure and SCI. Aggressive fluid administration is utilized in the first 24 hours to maintain a mean arterial pressure (MAP) of 80 to 90 mm Hg. Oxygen delivery is prioritized in early recovery, and if stable overnight, extubation may occur the next morning. Hematocrit is monitored for bleeding, coagulation disorders are promptly corrected, and intravascular volume is supported with FFP infusions for the initial 12 hours. CSF drainage continues for 48 hours postoperatively, followed by a 24-hour observation period. Gentle diuresis is considered 48 to 72 hours after the operation.

RESULTS OF TREATMENT AND COMPLICATIONS

Operative mortality

Operative mortality for TAAA repair is 8–16%, but in the author's experience, it is 4.4% for elective TAAA repaired with atriofemoral bypass. Higher comorbidities elevate operative risk, with preoperative coronary artery disease, COPD, and renal insufficiency linked to increased mortality. The extent of TAAA significantly affects the risk of SCI.

Renal failure

To minimize renal injury, renal ischemic times should be minimized. Other protective measures include cold renal perfusion, avoidance of intraoperative hypotension, and addressing renal stenotic lesions. Cold renal perfusion with crystalloid or blood is recommended, while furosemide, mannitol, or dopamine solely for renal protection is discouraged. In open TAAA surgery, cold renal fluid is directly instilled into the renal arteries before visceral reconstruction to help prevent renal ischemia-reperfusion injury. Various techniques are employed for renal artery reimplantation as discussed earlier. Dialysis is reserved for specific indications, with continuous venovenous hemodialysis preferred when needed.

Respiratory complications

Patients with TAAAs, often elderly with COPD and a smoking history, are at a high risk for postoperative pulmonary dysfunction. Approximately 40% experience respiratory complications, exacerbated by left hemidiaphragm paralysis and chest wall incision pain. A diaphragm-sparing technique is applied when possible. For failed extubation, early tracheostomy is preferred. In a recent study, 27% required prolonged ventilation, 15% needed at least one reintubation, and 11% required early tracheostomy [6]. Strategies to reduce complications include optimizing preoperative pulmonary function, meticulous intraoperative management, avoiding excessive blood administration, early extubation, and liberal use of early tracheostomy.

Spinal cord ischemia

The author identified greater extent of open TAAA repair as an independent predictor of SCI: 17% in type I versus 8% in type II [3]. The incidence of SCI has declined with staged aortic repair, distal perfusion, neuromonitoring, and cerebrospinal fluid drainage. Distal aortic perfusion with left atrial femoral bypass, coupled with MEP monitoring, is the principal strategy we employ for cord protection in type I–III TAAAs, based on studies suggesting collateral support mainly originating from the pelvis (i.e., hypogastric arteries). MEP monitoring provides objective criteria for selective intercostal reconstruction. The clinical spectrum ranges from complete flaccid paraplegia to varying degrees of paraparesis. Incomplete deficits suggest reasonable functional recovery and survival, but an SCI Deficit Scale score of I (flaccid paralysis) indicates a poor prognosis.

Late outcomes

Late survival post-TAAA repair aligns with elective AAA repair patients. Approximately 10% experience late aortic events, but graft-related complications are rare. Complications include occlusion of visceral vessel reconstructions, graft infections, and inclusion patch aneurysms. Most late aortic events stem from native aneurysmal disease in non-contiguous aortic segments. Improved perioperative outcomes have shifted the focus to long-term follow-up, revealing that most operative survivors return to preoperative independent living status.

TRICKS AND TRAPS

- Repair is recommended when the diameter exceeds 6 cm; experienced surgeons can consider repair at >5.5 cm. Consider repair <5.5 cm with features indicating an increased rupture risk.
- Endovascular repair is a viable option with parallel fenestrated and branched stent-grafts.
- Cerebrospinal fluid drainage is employed routinely for all TAAA repairs.

- Motor evoked potential monitoring is used for most extent I–III TAAAs.
- The left renal artery serves as the starting point for dividing retroperitoneal tissues over the aorta.
- Circumferential division through the muscular portion of the diaphragm, leaving a few centimeters laterally, preserves phrenic innervation and reduces postoperative pulmonary dysfunction.
- Extensive employment of atriofemoral bypass for extent I–III TAAAs, aligning with the spinal cord collateral network concept and emphasizing pelvic/hypogastric vessel perfusion is recommended to reduce the risk of spinal cord ischemia.
- Employ cold renal perfusion to reduce post-ischemic renal dysfunction.
- With young patients, those with connective tissue disorders, and those in whom the origins of the visceral/renal arteries are widely separated, consider the use of a pre-constructed branched graft.
- Reconstruct the left renal artery with a previously attached 6 mm sidearm graft taking care to align the graft properly to avoid kinking when the left kidney is returned to its normal anatomic position.
- Evaluate T9–L1 intercostal vessels for potential reimplantation based on MEP signals; unless significant MEP changes, defer intercostal reconstruction.
- To enhance spinal perfusion, prioritize performing the distal anastomosis before visceral and renal reconstruction with branched grafts to restore pulsatile flow to the pelvis.
- Inspection of the aneurysm sac detects potential sources of postoperative hemorrhage. Postoperatively recommend ICU care, with an aggressive hydration MAP goal of 80–90 mm Hg and FFP infusions for the initial 12 hours.

QUESTIONS

1. All of the following have been demonstrated to reduce the risk of spinal cord ischemia risk in TAAA except:
   a. Utilization of atriofemoral bypass
   b. Drainage of cerebrospinal fluid
   c. Maintaining mean arterial pressure at >80–90 mm Hg
   d. Cold perfusion of intercostal arteries
   e. Monitoring motor evoked potentials

   Answer: d

2. Branched graft reconstruction of TAAAs should be considered in all of the following situations except:
   a. Young patients
   b. Older patients
   c. Patients with connective tissue disorders
   d. Aneurysms where the ostia of the visceral and renal arteries are more than 3 cm apart
   e. Long segment visceral stenosis not amenable to endarterectomy

   Answer: b

3. Which of the following adjuncts does not reduce the risk of renal failure following TAAA repair?
   a. Cold renal perfusion
   b. Cold blood renal perfusion
   c. Normothermic renal perfusion
   d. Minimizing renal clamp time
   e. Furosemide

   Answer: e

4. The most common postoperative complication following TAAA repair is:
   a. Spinal cord ischemia
   b. Renal failure
   c. Myocardial infarction
   d. Respiratory failure
   e. Stress ulceration with bleeding

   Answer: d

REFERENCES

1. Isselbacher EM, Preventza O, Black III JH, et al. ACC/AHA guideline for the diagnosis and management of aortic disease: a report of the American Heart Association/American College of Cardiology Joint Committee on Clinical Practice Guidelines | *Circulation*. 2024 Mar 20.
2. Tenorio ER, Dias-Neto MF, Lima GBB, et al. Endovascular repair for thoracoabdominal aortic aneurysms: current status and future challenges. *Ann Cardiothorac Surg*. 2021 Nov;10(6):744–67.
3. Conrad MF, Crawford RS, Davison JK, et al. Thoracoabdominal aneurysm repair: a 20-year perspective. *Ann Thorac Surg*. 2007 Feb 1;83(2):S856–61.
4. Ouzounian M, LeMaire SA, Weldon S, et al. Open repair of thoracoabdominal aortic aneurysm: step-by-step. *Oper Tech Thorac Cardiovasc Surg*. 2018 Mar 1;23(1):2–20.
5. Tanaka A, Smith HN, Safi HJ, et al. Open treatments for thoracoabdominal aortic aneurysm repair. *Methodist DeBakey Cardiovasc J*. 2023;19(2):49–58.
6. Etz CD, Luozzo GD, Bello R, Luehr M, et al. Pulmonary complications after descending thoracic and thoracoabdominal aortic aneurysm repair: predictors, prevention, and treatment. *Ann Thorac Surg*. 2007 Feb 1;83(2):S870–6.

32

Surgical repair of inflammatory aortic aneurysms

CHARLES A. WEST JR. AND JOHN L. CRAWFORD

INTRODUCTION

Inflammatory aortic aneurysms are uncommon vascular lesions ranging in frequency from 3% to 10% of surgically repaired abdominal aortic aneurysms (AAAs). They represent unique additional challenges to the vascular surgeon, compared with those seen during open repair of routine degenerative AAAs. The likelihood of these technical difficulties increases as the extent of the aneurysm and size of the inflammatory mass increase.

Inflammatory aortic aneurysms (IAAAs) occur at a younger age, have a stronger familial tendency, and occur more predominantly in men compared with noninflammatory aneurysms. These patients are almost uniformly smokers. The majority are symptomatic at presentation with abdominal or back pain, weight loss, and elevated erythrocyte sedimentation rate and c reactive protein as common clinical and laboratory findings. Also, distinct from diffuse atherosclerotic aortic aneurysms, IAAAs may present with ureteral obstruction, hydronephrosis, and renal dysfunction secondary to periaortic fibrosis. These aneurysms, if untreated, may result in rupture, a fatal complication, that most commonly occurs on the posterior aortic wall. The diagnosis is made preoperatively with 90% sensitivity using computed tomography angiography or magnetic resonance angiography. Inflammatory aortic aneurysms are usually isolated to the infrarenal segment of the abdominal aorta. A characteristic inflammatory cuff of periaortitis and perianeurysmal fibrosis encasing the aneurysm wall, which enhances with contrast, is the classic radiographic feature (Figure 32.1). At surgical exploration, the presence of a pearly white, glistening aortic wall with dense adhesions of retroperitoneal structures to its surface is the *sine qua non* of the inflammatory aortic aneurysm (Figure 32.2). The aortic wall is

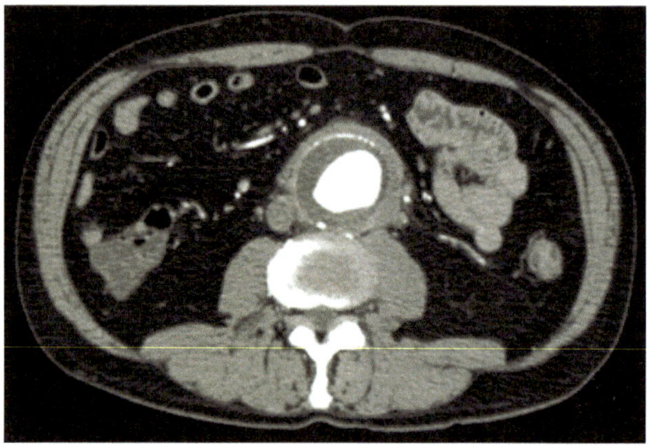

Figure 32.1 Computed tomography angiography axial image of an inflammatory abdominal aortic aneurysm with classic thickened and fibrotic aneurysm wall.

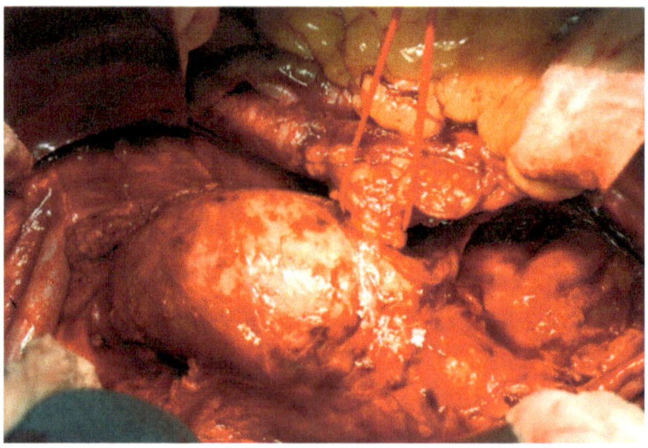

Figure 32.2 Intraoperative image of an inflammatory abdominal aortic aneurysm with its characteristic pearly white, glistening appearance.

DOI: 10.1201/9781003452096-32

three to four times thicker and more rigid than degenerative aneurysms, and the inflammatory process is limited to the anterior and lateral aortic wall. These features increase the incidence of injury to both vascular and visceral retroperitoneal structures during aneurysm repair as neighboring structures (duodenum, inferior vena cava, and ureters) are frequently encased and/or adherent to the aneurysm wall.

Endovascular aneurysm repair (EVAR) has been used in the treatment of inflammatory aortic aneurysms with success and some studies have demonstrated regression of periaortic fibrosis and the inflammatory response. Results from EVAR for treating uncomplicated IAAAs appear similar to those for noninflammatory AAAs. Compared with open repair, EVAR offers slight advantages of reduced morbidity and mortality. However, controversy exists as to whether treatment with EVAR offers an equivalent resolution of the inflammatory response involving the diseased aorta compared with treatment from open repair surgery. Open surgical repair has demonstrated a greater degree in the reduction of periaortic inflammation and fibrosis and many reports document complete resolution of aortic wall thickening and fibrosis. When comparing relief of ureteral obstruction in those with complicated presentations, open surgery has shown superior results.

We believe that the use of open aortic surgical techniques for the repair of inflammatory aortic aneurysms are still important and necessary for optimum patient outcomes, although endovascular repair is also a useful technique.

OPERATIVE MANAGEMENT

Exposures

The abdominal aorta can be approached from two sectors, anteriorly or laterally. The anterior, via a midline celiotomy using a xipho-pubic incision, affords specific advantages in treating aneurysmal and occlusive disease. The lateral approach can be from a thoracoabdominal incision involving two body cavities or a direct left lateral approach from a flank incision with the patient turned in a 90-degree position. The anterior approach offers the advantage of ease and facility in addressing the aorta and its branches from the renal artery level to beyond the femoral bifurcation in those with juxtarenal or infrarenal aortic aneurysms. Operating room preparation is simpler and easily reproducible for emergent procedures.

ANTERIOR EXPOSURE

Infracolic aortic exposure

The patient is placed in a supine position with both arms tucked and protected. The skin is sterilized from just above the nipple level to the knees. Fluorescent ureteral stents are placed before the skin incision to prevent injury in the event of ureteral adhesion to the inflammatory aneurysm. A midline incision that extends from the xiphoid process to just above the pubis creates the space required to safely expose the proximal aorta at the renal and mesenteric level down to the iliac bifurcations. For added exposure, the xiphoid process may be resected and the skin incision carried further cephalad. An Omni-Tract Wishbone Retractor System (Integra LifeSciences Corporation, Plainsboro, NJ, USA) is placed to provide the required upward and lateral retraction. As the exposure is created, shallow blades are transitioned to longer blades for retraction of the posterior peritoneal tissues, the abdominal wall, and the lower chest wall. The retractor system must be properly placed to achieve lateral and superior retraction of the upper abdominal cavity. The retractor's central lock hinge is positioned in the midsternal region with the wishbone arms spread wide several centimeters lateral to the midaxillary line. The hinge lock mechanism and arms are elevated 15–20 cm above the horizontal surface of the chest and abdomen. The wishbone arms are kept parallel and slightly abducted. This allows the force vector generated by the retractors to be at a 45-degree angle from the horizontal plane of the anterior abdominal wall directed upward and outward.

After the abdomen has been opened, the nasogastric tube placement has been confirmed, and the abdomen has been explored, the falciform ligament is taken down between heavy ties. This is followed by division of the triangular ligament toward the dome of the diaphragm. The right side of the transverse colon is tucked above the liver. The mid-transverse colon and splenic flexure are lifted above and over the stomach and placed under the diaphragm with dry laparotomy pads. A longitudinal posterior peritoneal incision is made over the aneurysm from the base of the pancreas directed toward the right side of the aorta and biased toward the right iliac artery. The small intestinal contents are wrapped in saline moist cloth towels, kept within the abdominal cavity when possible, and retracted to the right with use of a slotted malleable or Fence Omni blade.

In the setting of an inflammatory aneurysm, the duodenum is generally adherent to the anterior right lateral aneurysm wall. This segment should be left undisturbed until the proximal dissection is complete. The ligament of Treitz is mobilized completely before completing the full length of the posterior retroperitoneal incision. The duodenum adherent to the aneurysm is allowed to escape the enclosed towel; the remaining duodenum and small bowel are held.

At this juncture, the inferior mesenteric vein is divided between heavy ties. The long retractor blades are advanced deeper and the posterior peritoneal structures are hooked by the blades and retracted to the right and left.

The upper abdominal wall and lower rib cage are spread widely apart. Proximally, a transverse posterior peritoneal incision is made at the base of the pancreas in the avascular plane, perpendicular to the longitudinal incision over the aneurysm. This incision is carried laterally above the left renal vein (LRV) and toward the inferior vena cava (IVC) on the right side. A Harrington blade is placed in the midline over the central mesenteric root for proximal gentle retraction of the body of the pancreas.

Deep to the pancreas, the LRV is either dissected in a comprehensive manner or divided. If the renal vein is densely adherent to the aneurysm, it is transected and closed with monofilament sutures or a vascular stapler near the IVC and just to the left of the aorta, preserving the critical branches. Preserving the branches of the LRV during this process is important for kidney viability, and the decision should be made early to avoid undesirable bleeding. The branches are taken down sequentially between 3-0 silk ties to include the adrenal vein, accessory renal branches, and the lumbar-renal vein. A renal vein retractor may be placed anterior to the pararenal aorta to retract the vein superiorly by several centimeters.

At this point, both renal arteries are dissected out sharply and encircled with silastic vessel loops. The diaphragmatic crura on either side of the aorta in the space above the renal arteries are visible. These are divided posteriorly down to the spine. These maneuvers release the aorta anteriorly and permit safe clamping of the suprarenal aorta after gentle circumferential digital exploration to ensure complete tissue clearance. The superior mesenteric artery can be dissected out sharply, excising lymphatic tissue if needed, and looped for a supramesenteric aortic clamp position, if necessary. This is the maximum proximal limit of aortic exposure with the infracolic approach.

The inferior abdominal wall retraction is expanded by dividing the inferior mesenteric artery and placing a deep retractor blade lateral to the left side of the midportion of the aneurysm, sweeping the posterior peritoneal structures laterally, including the mesentery of the sigmoid colon. The iliac arteries are sharply dissected out, as needed, down to the iliac artery bifurcations.

LATERAL APPROACHES

Thoracoabdominal and flank exposures

A thoracoabdominal or flank approach may be adopted to avoid structures that adhere to the inflammatory aneurysm, such as the duodenum and LRV. The thoracoabdominal approach involves a two body cavity exposure with the patient turned 60 degrees at the chest and 45 degrees at the hip, with an "S" incision through the eighth intercostal space from a left side up position. The dissection can be retroperitoneal or the parietal peritoneum can be opened, followed by an extended left medial visceral rotation. The author's preference is to open the abdomen and chest and divide the diaphragm circumferentially toward the hiatus, before embarking on the medial visceral rotation (MVR).

Generally, complete diaphragm division is not required. Once retractors are placed, the MVR begins by taking down the white line of Toldt from the left lower quadrant extending superiorly and medially. The kidney is brought anteriorly, to avoid the adherent LRV, and the crura on the left are divided. The mesenteric vessels are exposed with sharp dissection after dividing the crura and releasing the medial arcuate ligament. Location of the proximal clamp is established, and iliac vessel control is obtained via sharp dissection with Cooley vascular scissors (Becton, Dickinson and Company, Franklin Lakes, NJ, USA). The iliolumbar vein is divided, and care is taken to avoid injury to the left ureter.

The lateral flank approach is described in Chapter 34 and performed from a 90-degree right lateral decubitus position. The incision begins at the lower costal margin and is transversely oriented toward the umbilicus. The dissection is kept in a true retroperitoneal plane. The 12th rib is often removed and the diaphragm is partially incised. This approach avoids the anatomic hazards encountered anteriorly. One disadvantage is the extreme posterior displacement of the right iliofemoral vessels, but this may be favored based on surgeon preference and experience.

Reconstruction

The reconstructive phases are like traditional methods of open degenerative aortic aneurysm repair. After systemic heparin administration (100 IU/kg), an activated clotting time of >250 seconds is achieved before aortic clamping. Curved, heavy iliac clamps are placed first, followed by a curved aortic clamp placed suprarenal for the juxtarenal repair. The renal arteries are clamped with coarctation clamps. The aneurysm is opened, the thrombus is removed, lumbar bleeding is controlled, and a graft is sewn end-to-end in a standard fashion. A bifurcated graft is preferred, and this is sewn end-to-end to the appropriate iliofemoral vessels in a sequential manner (Figure 32.3). After unclamping is completed and hemostasis

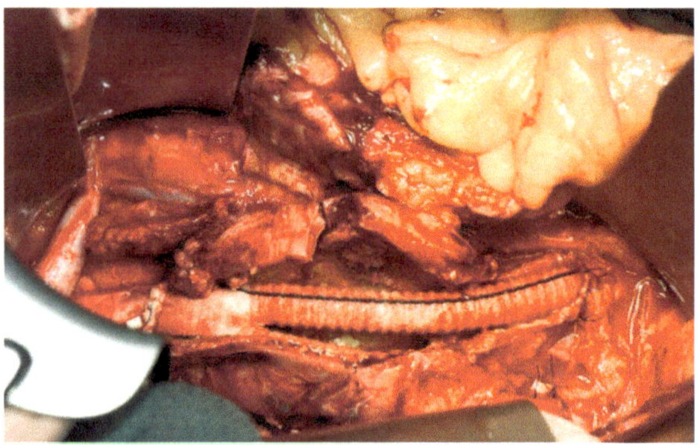

Figure 32.3 Intraoperative image of a completed aortobiiliac bypass graft. Note the markedly thickened anterior aneurysm wall.

is achieved, enough of the inflammatory aneurysm sac is resected to allow for graft coverage by the remaining aneurysm wall. The posterior peritoneum is closed, followed by abdominal wall closure.

CONCLUSION

Open aortic reconstruction for complex aneurysms is becoming an infrequently applied skill set in contemporary vascular surgery. As a result, familiarity and facility with the technical steps and open surgical skills required to safely repair these aneurysms are still important for vascular surgeons in the modern era of endovascular surgery. Tertiary high-volume vascular centers where skilled teams are available to offer comprehensive care may be the best directed care for these patients.

TRICKS AND TRAPS

Open surgical repair indications

- We believe open surgical treatment of IAAAs is indicated for good-risk patients who present with ureteral obstruction or who have severe symptoms associated with periaortic inflammation.
- Hostile aortic necks that are short and angulated and/or diseased aorto-iliac artery anatomy unsuitable for endograft placement are generally recommended for open repair.

Endovascular aortic aneurysm repair

- We believe good-risk patients with IAAAs who have minimal inflammatory symptoms and that are anatomically suitable for an endovascular stent graft should be considered for EVAR as first-line therapy.
- High-risk surgical patients with symptomatic IAAAs, including ureteral obstruction, should undergo EVAR.
- We recommend employing EVAR for all ruptured aneurysms that are deemed anatomically suitable.

Technical tips

The primary key to the operation is wide exposure. This permits the surgeon to reliably control the aorta and its surrounding structures, preventing injury to vascular and visceral structures.

Before the initial incision is made, the placement of ureteral stents is used in all cases.

Early division of the LRV in the setting of anterior aortic wall adherence prevents undesired bleeding and provides better exposure.

We employ a two vascular attending team approach to expedite all complex aortic reconstructions. This significantly decreases operative times, reduces complications, and improves patient outcomes.

QUESTIONS

1. The preoperative diagnosis of inflammatory abdominal aortic aneurysm is best made by:
   a. Abdominal aortic ultrasound
   b. Catheter-based aortography
   c. CTA
   d. PET scan

   Answer: c

2. During exposure of inflammatory AAA using the transperitoneal approach, the following veins should not be sacrificed:
   a. Inferior mesenteric vein
   b. Left renal vein lateral to adrenal/gonadal vein
   c. Left renal vein medial to adrenal/gonadal vein
   d. Posterior lumbar vein forming a renal collar vein

   Answer: b

3. Periaortic inflammatory fibrosis in inflammatory AAA extends from:
   a. Supraceliac aorta to the iliac artery bifurcation
   b. The renal artery to the iliac artery bifurcation
   c. Inferior mesenteric artery to the mid-external iliac artery
   d. Distal abdominal aorta to the femoral arteries

   Answer: b

REFERENCES

Crawford JL, Stowe CL, Safi HJ, et al. Inflammatory aneurysms of the aorta. *J Vasc Surg.* 1985;2:113–24.

Goldstone J, Malone JM, Moore WS. Inflammatory aneurysms of the abdominal aorta. *Surgery.* 1978;83:425–30.

Hill J, Charlesworth D. Inflammatory abdominal aortic aneurysms: a report of thirty-seven cases. *Ann Vasc Surg.* 1988;2:352–57.

Kakkos SK, Papazoglou KO, Tsolakis IA, Lampropoulos G, Papadoulas SI, Antoniadis PN. Open versus endovascular repair of inflammatory abdominal aortic aneurysms: a comparative study and meta-analysis of the literature. *Vasc Endovascular Surg.* 2015 Jul-Aug;49(5–6):110–8. doi: 10.1177/1538574415602780.

Maeda H, Umezawa H, Hattori T, Nakamura T, Umeda T, Kobayashi H, Kawachi H, Iida A, Shiono M. Early and late outcomes of inflammatory abdominal aortic aneurysms: comparison with the outcomes after open surgical and endovascular aneurysm repair in literature reviews. *Int Angiol.* 2013 Feb;32(1):67–73.

Paravastu SC, Ghosh J, Murray D, Farquharson FG, Serracino-Inglott F, Walker MG. A systematic review of open versus endovascular repair of inflammatory abdominal aortic aneurysms. *Eur J Vasc Endovasc Surg*. 2009 Sep;38(3):291–7. doi: 10.1016/j.ejvs.2009.05.005. Epub 2009 Jun 21.

Pennell RC, Hollier LH, Lie JT, et al. Inflammatory abdominal aortic aneurysms: a thirty-year review. *J Vasc Surg*. 1985;2:859–69.

Rasmussen TE, Hallett JW Jr. Inflammatory aortic aneurysms. A clinical review with new perspectives in pathogenesis. *Ann Surg*. 1997;225:155–64.

Stone WM, Fankhauser GT, Bower TC, Oderich GS, Oldenburg WA, Kalra M, Naidu S, Money SR. Comparison of open and endovascular repair of inflammatory aortic aneurysms. *J Vasc Surg*. 2012 Oct;56(4):951–5; discussion 955–6. doi: 10.1016/j.jvs.2012.03.253. Epub 2012 Jun 15.

Tang T, Boyle JR, Dixon AK, et al. Inflammatory abdominal aortic aneurysms. *Eur J Vasc Endovasc Surg*. 2005;29:353–62.

van Bommel EF, van der Veer SJ, Hendriksz TR, Bleumink GS. Persistent chronic peri-aortitis ('inflammatory aneurysm') after abdominal aortic aneurysm repair: systematic review of the literature. *Vasc Med*. 2008 Nov;13(4):293–303. doi: 10.1177/1358863X08091147.

Walker DI, Bloor K, Williams G, et al. Inflammatory aneurysms of the abdominal aorta. *Br J Surg*. 1972;59:609–14.

33

Open thoracic aortic aneurysm repair

KYLE G. MILETIC

INTRODUCTION

While the exact prevalence of descending thoracic aneurysms is unknown due to underreporting, various autopsy studies have shown a prevalence of asymptomatic aneurysmal disease as high as 670 per 100,000 [1] or ten cases per 100,000 person-years [2]. Additionally, both the prevalence of aneurysmal disease and the number of operations for the same has increased substantially over the past 30 years [3]. Cystic medial degeneration (often associated with arteriosclerosis) is the most frequent pathology that leads to aneurysmal degeneration. Genetically mediated aortopathies, such as Marfan and Loeys–Dietz syndromes, are also quite common, and there is increasing recognition of a wide variety of genetic disorders associated with aortopathy. Currently, commercially available assays can test for well over 25 different genetic mutations that are associated with an increased risk for aortopathy.

Most patients with thoracic aortic aneurysms are asymptomatic. Increasing use of computed tomography, such as for lung cancer screening, has resulted in increased detection and detection at smaller sizes. When symptoms do develop, they often do so much later in the course of the disease when the aorta is large enough to impinge on adjacent structures. This includes dysphagia and stridor from esophageal and tracheal compression, dyspnea from compression of the lung, and hoarseness from stretching of the recurrent laryngeal nerve.

In patients with known or suspected aneurysmal disease, computed tomographic angiography (CTA) is the gold standard for diagnosis. CTA is vital in determining aneurysm extent, size, and other incidental findings, such as mural thrombus and location of intercostal vessels that are relevant for operative planning.

The decision to offer repair—whether open or endovascular—is primarily based on size. The 2022 ACC/AHA guidelines [4] for management of aortic disease recommend repair at a diameter of ≥5.5 cm in patients without identifiable risk factors for aortopathy. In patients with risk factors for rupture (such as genetic aortopathy, growth of >0.5 cm/y, symptomatic aneurysm, saccular or infectious aneurysm, or female sex), repair may be considered at a smaller diameter.

The choice between thoracic aortic endovascular repair (TEVAR) or open repair can be challenging. No randomized controlled trials comparing TEVAR with open repair exist. Analysis of Medicare claims data has shown improved perioperative mortality with TEVAR, although open repair was associated with a reduced late hazard of death and reintervention [5]. Thus, the guidelines recommend TEVAR for most patients but with consideration of open repair in low-risk patients with a life expectancy of at least ten years, as well as patients with anatomy unfavorable for TEVAR.

OPERATIVE TECHNIQUE

After complete preoperative workup including echocardiogram, cardiac catheterization, and high-quality CTA of the chest, abdomen, and pelvis, open intervention can be undertaken. Anesthetic considerations include cerebrospinal fluid (CSF) drainage and epidural catheters placed prior to induction. It is our practice to drain 50 mL of CSF from the time the spinal drain is placed until aortic cross-clamping. Standard general anesthesia with a double lumen endotracheal tube is routinely used for lung isolation. A right-sided femoral 9 French central venous catheter for large volume fluid infusion as well as femoral arterial lines are utilized. A right-sided radial arterial line and a left-sided Swan-Ganz catheter are placed as well. If repair with extracorporeal mechanical support is anticipated, we have moved to percutaneous cannulation of the femoral artery and vein on the left. Owing to difficulty with percutaneous access once the patient is in the lateral decubitus position, we obtain access to both the femoral artery and vein with the patient supine. The artery is preclosed with two Perclose Proglide™ devices (Abbott Cardiovascular) and 8 French sheaths are left in

DOI: 10.1201/9781003452096-33

both the artery and vein. These are sterilely prepped into the operative field after positioning.

The patient is then positioned in the right lateral decubitus position. A left posterolateral thoracotomy is performed. We typically use the preoperative CT scan to guide selection of intercostal space. Often, the fourth intercostal space is adequate for proximal repairs and the sixth for mid to distal repairs. In aneurysms going to the diaphragmatic hiatus, eighth intercostal space exposure may be necessary. For patients with very extensive aneurysms, a single skin incision centered over the sixth intercostal space with mobilization of the extrathoracic musculature and two thoracotomies— in the fourth and eighth intercostal spaces—may be considered, although this is associated with significant postoperative pain. Once the chest is entered, the left lung is deflated, and the aorta is mobilized away from the pleura.

At this point, the proximal neck of the aneurysm is identified and the decision regarding necessity of deep hypothermic circulatory arrest (DHCA) is made. It has become our practice to, if anatomically favorable, place a short TEVAR just distal to the left subclavian artery. The open graft is thus sewn to the distal end of the TEVAR stent, thus obviating the need for DHCA. In many cases, however, open repair is performed due to lack of anatomic features suitable for TEVAR. Thus, the neck of the aneurysm is examined and the decision regarding DHCA is made. If there is enough healthy aorta to clamp distal to the left subclavian artery, then partial cardiopulmonary bypass (CPB) is utilized. If DHCA is undertaken, full bypass is initiated, and cooling is commenced.

In patients who do not need DHCA, it has been our practice to use partial CPB without a reservoir. This allows lower ACT goals (250–300 seconds) and reduces postoperative coagulopathy. The cardiotomy suction is still used, but the blood collected is returned to a rapid transfuser and whole, heparinized blood is reinfused into the patient. Avoiding the use of cell saver allows for salvage of platelets and various clotting factors. Intravenous tranexamic acid is used routinely as well.

In patients who do not need DHCA, once partial CPB is initiated, the patient is slightly cooled to 34°C for spinal cord protection. Approximately ten minutes prior to aortic cross-clamp, we instill 30 mg of preservative-free papaverine into the spinal drain catheter as an adjunct for spinal cord protection. This is allowed to dwell for five minutes with the patient in the Trendelenburg position and then the CSF is drained to maintain an intrathecal pressure of $\leq$10 cmH_2O for the remainder of the procedure, with a maximum of 120 mL CSF drained for the duration of the case.

Aortic cross-clamps are then applied proximally and distally to the aneurysm, ensuring sufficient neck of normal aorta is available to sew. Once the clamps are in place, the perfusionist adjusts the partial bypass flows to target a lower body mean arterial pressure of 80–90 mmHg. The aorta is then opened proximally and transected to ensure complete separation from the underlying esophagus. Care must be taken to identify and preserve the recurrent laryngeal nerve in its typical course on the anterior surface of the aorta in zone 2 of the arch (Figure 33.1). A previously sized Dacron graft is then brought into the field and prepared. The proximal anastomosis is typically constructed with running 4-0 polypropylene suture usually reinforced with a thin strip of bovine pericardium (Figure 33.2). In exceptionally fragile aortas (particularly those with prior aortic dissection), a strip of PTFE felt may be used to reinforce the anastomosis. The graft is then clamped and the proximal cross-clamp is removed. The proximal anastomosis is checked for hemostasis and the fully distended graft is then tailored to appropriate length. The distal anastomosis proceeds in a similar fashion to the proximal anastomosis (Figure 33.3). Based on CTA and direct visualization, there are often several intercostal vessels posteriorly that may be

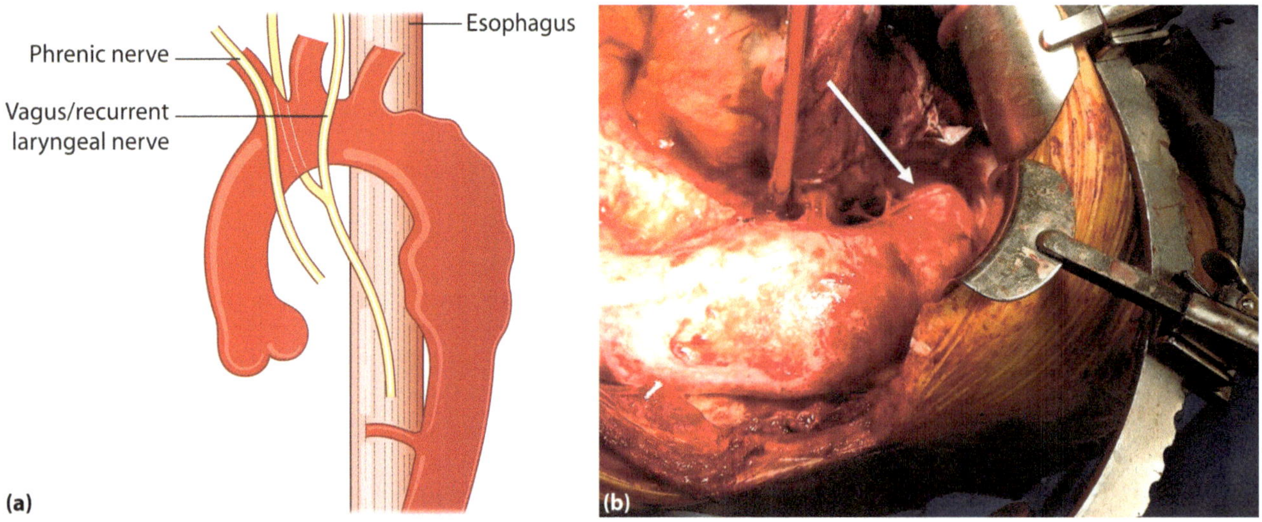

Figure 33.1 (a) Anatomic position of the phrenic, vagus, and left recurrent laryngeal nerves; (b) intraoperative photograph of pre-repair thoracic aortic aneurysm showing exposed recurrent laryngeal nerve (white arrow).

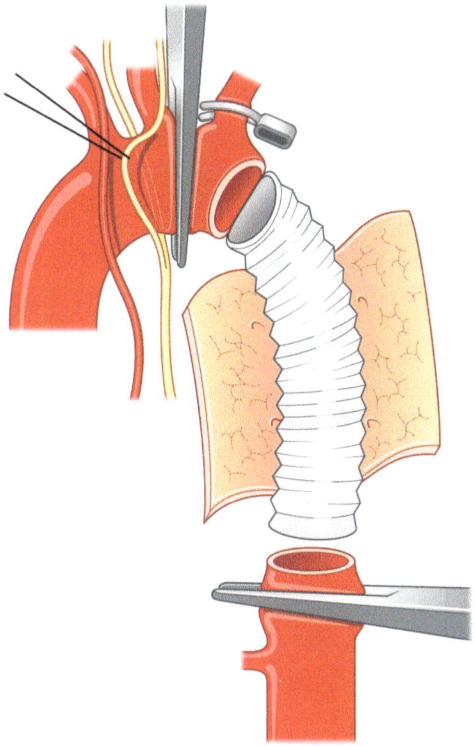

Figure 33.2 Construction of the proximal anastomosis.

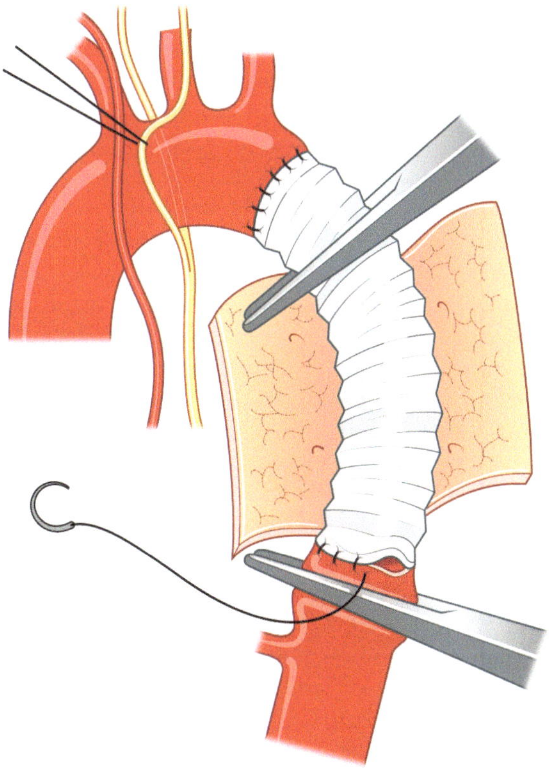

Figure 33.3 Construction of the distal anastomosis.

saved by beveling the aorta and incorporating them into an oblique anastomotic suture line with the graft, with particular attention paid to intercostals below the sixth intercostal space, as these are most likely to contribute to spinal cord perfusion.

If large intercostal vessels are unable to be incorporated into an oblique aortic anastomosis, an island of native aortic tissue incorporating the ostia of these vessels is fashioned and a segment of the graft opposite the island is excised. The island is then anastomosed to the posterior aspect of the graft utilizing 4-0 polypropylene suture. Alternatively, a short piece of 6 mm or 8 mm straight Dacron graft can be used as an interposition graft to anastomose intercostal arteries directly to the graft (Figure 33.4). This technique is particularly useful in the very fragile or aneurysmal aorta where there is concern regarding late development of a patch pseudoaneurysm.

In patients who require DHCA, full CPB is utilized after passing a venous cannula into the right atrium from the left groin as confirmed by transesophageal echocardiography. Prior to initiation of CPB, the arterial line of the bypass circuit is bifurcated into a Y configuration in preparation for upper and lower body perfusion. Once the patient is cannulated via the groin, bypass and systemic cooling are initiated to a nasopharyngeal temperature of 18°C. The heart will likely fibrillate during cooling and a left-sided vent may need to be placed via the left inferior pulmonary vein to prevent distension in the case of aortic insufficiency. Once the patient is fully cooled, the distal thoracic aorta is clamped at the T5 level to maintain lower body perfusion. Upper body blood flow thus ceases. The aorta is opened, and the proximal anastomosis thus proceeds in a similar fashion to the non-DHCA technique. However, a Dacron graft with a prefabricated 8- or 10-mm side branch is chosen. Once the proximal anastomosis is completed, the second limb of the arterial bypass line is attached to the side branch and both upper- and lower-body perfusion are reinitiated. The distal clamp is then moved caudally to normal aorta. The patient is rewarmed to normothermia while the distal anastomosis and intercostal reimplantation proceed.

Routine de-airing maneuvers are then performed. The patient is separated from CPB upon reaching normothermia. Hemostasis is assured. Banked blood products are usually required due to coagulopathy. Prior to closure, the graft is wrapped in the native aneurysmal aorta. If there is not sufficient tissue to completely wrap the aorta, a large sheet of bovine pericardium is used. Regardless, it is important to ensure that there is no exposed Dacron graft in the thoracic cavity to prevent erosion of the graft into the lung. Routine placement of chest tubes and closure then proceeds.

Postoperative management of these patients is relatively similar to standard postoperative cardiac and vascular surgical patients but with some important caveats. First, it

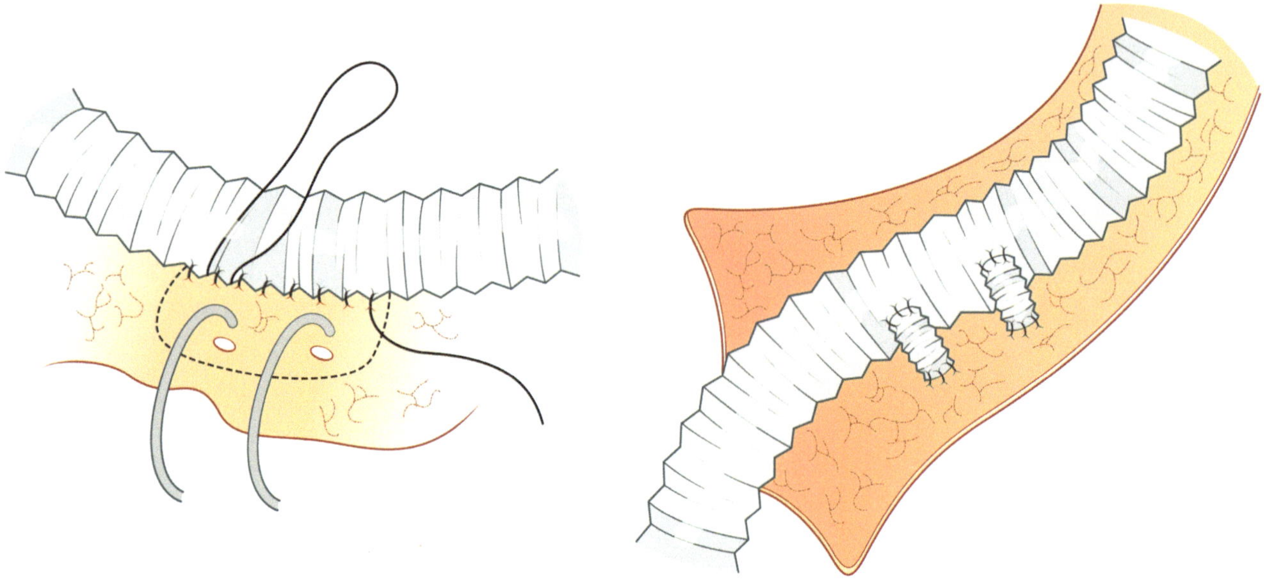

(a) (b)

Figure 33.4 Intercostal artery patch reimplantation techniques: (a) direct intercostal island implantation; (b) implantation using interposition grafts.

is our practice to maintain endotracheal intubation until at least the morning of the first postoperative day as these patients often have pulmonary and airway edema due to the substantial fluid shifts as well as direct trauma to the left lung from surgical manipulation. Second, CSF drainage to a pressure of 10 cmH_2O is continued for at least 36 hours postoperatively. After this, the drain is clamped for at least six hours prior to removal with close monitoring of lower extremity neurologic status.

COMPLICATIONS

The most feared complication following repair is spinal cord injury (SCI) manifesting as paraparesis or paraplegia. As discussed earlier, CSF drainage is of paramount importance in the prevention of SCI. Regardless of use of CSF drainage, risk of SCI increases linearly with duration of aortic clamping. Thus, ensuring optimal exposure and dissection of as much of the aorta as possible prior to clamping is helpful in reducing clamp times. Whenever possible, the proximal clamp should be placed beyond the left subclavian artery to allow for continuous spinal cord perfusion via the left vertebral artery. Distal clamping should be done as proximal as possible to preserve intercostal arteries, especially below the sixth intercostal space.

Reattachment of intercostal arteries can reduce the prevalence of postoperative neurologic deficit [6]. Though somewhat subjective, it has been our practice to reimplant intercostal arteries with sluggish back bleeding. Those with no back bleeding are likely chronically occluded and of no clinical consequence. Those with very vigorous, pulsatile back bleeding are likely very well collateralized and should be oversewn as early as possible in the repair to prevent a "steal" phenomenon. However, those with relatively sluggish bleeding are likely patent but not well collateralized, suggesting that they may provide an important source of blood to the spinal cord.

The patient who develops evidence of SCI postoperatively is treated as a surgical emergency. The first step in management is to raise the blood pressure to a mean arterial pressure of at least 90 mmHg. Urgent insertion of a CSF drain (if not already present) is then performed and the drain is set to maintain an intrathecal pressure of 0 cmH_2O. Often, this is enough for patients to regain neurologic function. CSF drain is then left in for at least 48 additional hours and the drain is slowly weaned.

Brain injury is an important additional complication for this patient population, particularly in patients in whom DHCA is required. There are two main types of neurologic injury: temporary dysfunction (manifesting as lethargy, agitation, and disorientation) and stroke. Temporary dysfunction is generally attributable more to hypoxic-ischemic injury and stroke to embolus. Like spinal cord injury, brain injury is linearly associated with duration of DHCA [7].

Lung injury is the most common complication following open repair, with prolonged (>48 hours) mechanical ventilation occurring in 20–30% of patients [8]. Risk factors for prolonged ventilatory support include age, division of the diaphragm, duration of aortic clamping, number of transfused blood products, and smoking [9].

Finally, renal dysfunction is not uncommon, although its incidence is lower in isolated descending thoracic aneurysm repair as opposed to thoracoabdominal repair. Rates of dialysis after thoracic aneurysm repair are as high as 5% [10]. The true rate of clinically significant renal dysfunction is likely much higher, but prevalence is difficult

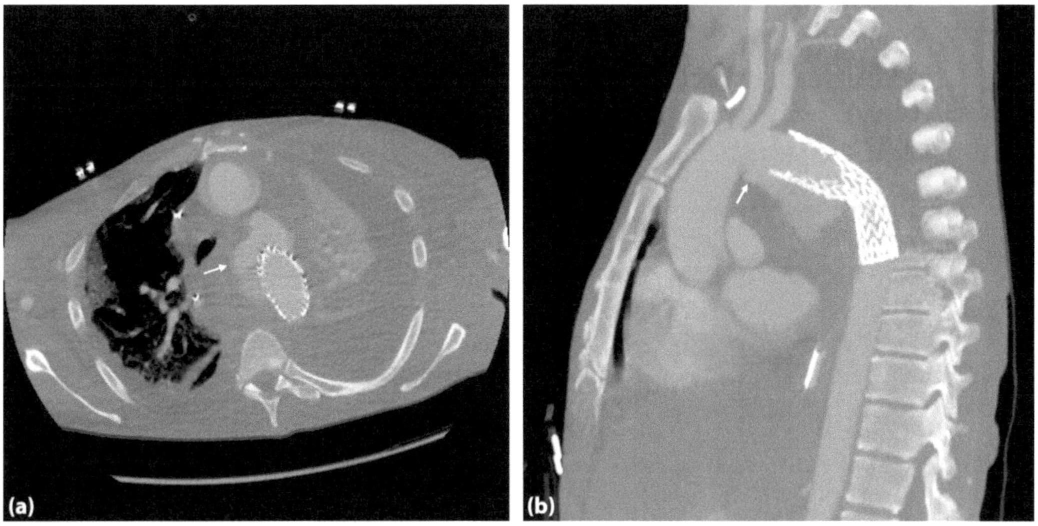

Figure 33.5 Computed tomographic angiogram showing large proximal aortic pseudoaneurysm with contained rupture causing compression of the left lung in the setting of an infected thoracic endograft: (a) axial view with tracheal shift to the right; (b) sagittal view. White arrows point to contrast extravasation from pseudoaneurysm.

to determine given the variability in definitions and reporting. Distal clamping alone without visceral perfusion via partial CPB is a risk factor for renal dysfunction.

SPECIAL SITUATIONS

The increasing adoption of TEVAR (and its usefulness in avoiding DHCA in patients with proximal descending aneurysms) means that in many cases, a stent graft may already be present in a patient undergoing subsequent open repair. This scenario can present a technical challenge as the TEVAR stent may be quite large (40 mm or greater) and the distal, normal aorta quite small (often as small as 20 mm). This makes graft choice difficult, as a large graft will make the distal anastomosis challenging and a small graft will be very difficult to sew to a large, rigid stent graft. In this case, we have used a Gelweave™ Siena aortic arch graft (Terumo Aortic). The elephant trunk portion of the Siena graft is removed, and the Siena collar is used to construct the proximal anastomosis to the oversized stent graft (with felt reinforcement). The smaller main body of the graft is then used for the distal anastomosis. This allows for essentially unlimited taper of the large stent to small, normal aorta. In the case of a thoracoabdominal repair, the Siena cuff can be anastomosed to a Gelweave™ Coselli thoracoabdominal graft on the back table prior to implantation. When using this technique, careful measurement of the distance between the proximal anastomosis and visceral vessels is necessary to avoid kinking or stretching of the graft.

Infectious (mycotic) aneurysms or pseudoaneurysms present an additional challenge. These aneurysms have a very high probability of rupture regardless of size. Therefore, urgent operation should be considered without delay for control with antibiotic therapy. Other than the profoundly unstable patient who would not tolerate open operation, TEVAR should be avoided as much as possible given the high risk of seeding the endograft. Surgical repair proceeds similarly to a standard open operation. However, care must be taken to ensure complete excision of the infected segment of aorta to obtain source control and prevent rupture. Both rifampin-soaked Dacron grafts as well as cryopreserved allografts are reasonable options for reconstruction with similar early results [11].

The infected aortic graft or TEVAR endograft presents a formidable technical challenge with high morbidity and mortality (Figure 33.5). Following the surgical principles of wide debridement and removal of all infected tissue (including suture lines) are of paramount importance. If a new graft is to be used, pedicled flaps of muscle or omentum may be used to cover the graft. The infected TEVAR with subclavian involvement is particularly challenging as a septic patient will likely not tolerate the DHCA that is required to completely remove all infected tissue. In this case, we have managed this patient in a multiple-step process. First, open arch debranching with carotid-subclavian bypass (or complete arch debranching, depending on the extent of infection) is performed. Next, extra-anatomic bypass (ascending to descending thoracic aortic bypass tunneled behind the inferior vena cava) utilizing a rifampin-soaked Dacron graft is performed via median sternotomy. Finally, posterolateral thoracotomy with excision of the stent graft and all infected tissues followed by ligation of the involved portion of thoracic aorta proceeds. This is a complex and morbid undertaking, but it allows complete excision of infected tissue without the added risk of CPB and DHCA.

TRICKS AND TRAPS

- Careful preoperative review of the CT angiogram is of vital importance in choosing the interspace used for thoracic access to ensure optimal exposure.
- As much dissection and mobilization of the aorta should be done prior to initiation of CPB and aortic clamping to both limit bleeding and the risk of spinal cord injury.
- If possible, maintaining flow to the left subclavian artery and flow in the aorta below T6 will help to reduce the risk of spinal cord injury.
- If anatomically favorable, a short TEVAR graft placed at the level of the left subclavian artery can allow for the avoidance of hypothermic circulatory arrest.
- When choosing to reimplant intercostal arteries, particular attention should be paid to those below the sixth intercostal space as they are more likely to be involved in critical spinal cord perfusion.
- The placement of a transesophageal echocardiogram probe into the stomach is very helpful in marking the esophagus to avoid injury.
- In patients with large and tortuous aneurysmal disease, entry to the right pleural space is often inevitable—an empiric right-sided chest tube should be placed after turning the patient supine at the conclusion of the operation.

QUESTIONS

1. Which of the following is the principal advantage of open thoracic aneurysm repair over endovascular stent grafting?
   a. Reduced risk of spinal cord ischemia
   b. Reduced late hazard of death
   c. Reduced perioperative mortality
   d. Reduced risk of perioperative renal failure

   Answer: b

2. Regardless of absolute size, what rate of aneurysmal growth would prompt surgical intervention?
   a. 1 mm/year
   b. 3 mm/year
   c. 5 mm/year
   d. 1 cm/year

   Answer: c

3. Utilization of deep hypothermic circulatory arrest results in an increased risk of all of the following EXCEPT:
   a. Stroke
   b. Renal failure
   c. Coagulopathy
   d. Respiratory failure

   Answer: d

4. Which of the following techniques of intercostal artery reattachment should be avoided due to the high incidence of early thrombosis?
   a. Direct intercostal artery reattachment to the graft
   b. Reattachment with an island of surrounding aortic tissue
   c. Interposition graft to the intercostal artery
   d. Beveling of proximal or distal anastomosis to incorporate the intercostals in a suture line

   Answer: a

REFERENCES

1. Svensjö S, Bengtsson H, Bergqvist D. Thoracic and thoracoabdominal aortic aneurysm and dissection: an investigation based on autopsy. *The British Journal of Surgery*. 1996;83(1):68–71. doi:10.1002/bjs.1800830122.
2. Clouse WD, Hallett JW, Schaff HV, Gayari MM, Ilstrup DM, Melton LJ. Improved prognosis of thoracic aortic aneurysms: a population-based study. *JAMA*. 1998;280(22):1926–1929. doi:10.1001/jama.280.22.1926.
3. Olsson C, Thelin S, Ståhle E, Ekbom A, Granath F. Thoracic aortic aneurysm and dissection: increasing prevalence and improved outcomes reported in a nationwide population-based study of more than 14,000 cases from 1987 to 2002. *Circulation*. 2006;114(24):2611–2618. doi:10.1161/CIRCULATIONAHA.106.630400.
4. Isselbacher EM, Preventza O, Hamilton Black J, et al. 2022 ACC/AHA guideline for the diagnosis and management of aortic disease: a report of the American Heart Association/American College of Cardiology Joint Committee on clinical practice guidelines. *Circulation*. 2022;146(24):e334–e482. doi:10.1161/CIR.0000000000001106
5. Chiu P, Goldstone AB, Schaffer JM, et al. Endovascular versus open repair of intact descending thoracic aortic aneurysms. *Journal of the American College of Cardiology*. 2019;73(6):643–651. doi:10.1016/j.jacc.2018.10.086
6. Cheung AT, Pochettino A, McGarvey ML, et al. Strategies to manage paraplegia risk after endovascular stent repair of descending thoracic aortic aneurysms. *The Annals of Thoracic Surgery*. 2005;80(4):1280–1288; discussion 1288–1289. doi:10.1016/j.athoracsur.2005.04.027
7. Coselli JS, Crawford ES, Beall AC, Mizrahi EM, Hess KR, Patel VM. Determination of brain temperatures for safe circulatory arrest during cardiovascular operation. *The Annals of Thoracic Surgery*. 1988;45(6):638–642. doi:10.1016/s0003-4975(10)64766-2

8. Kulik A, Castner CF, Kouchoukos NT. Outcomes after thoracoabdominal aortic aneurysm repair with hypothermic circulatory arrest. *The Journal of Thoracic and Cardiovascular Surgery*. 2011;141(4):953–960. doi:10.1016/j.jtcvs.2010.06.010
9. Engle J, Safi HJ, Miller CC, et al. The impact of diaphragm management on prolonged ventilator support after thoracoabdominal aortic repair. *Journal of Vascular Surgery*. 1999;29(1):150–156. doi:10.1016/s0741-5214(99)70356-3
10. Coselli JS, LeMaire SA, Preventza O, et al. Outcomes of 3309 thoracoabdominal aortic aneurysm repairs. *The Journal of Thoracic and Cardiovascular Surgery*. 2016;151(5):1323–1337. doi:10.1016/j.jtcvs.2015.12.050
11. Tabiei A, Cifuentes S, Kalra M, et al. Cryopreserved arterial allografts versus rifampin-soaked Dacron for the treatment of infected aortic and iliac aneurysms. *Annals of Vascular Surgery*. 2023;97:49–58. doi:10.1016/j.avsg.2023.04.015

34

Endovascular aortic stent graft explantation

TIMOTHY J. NYPAVER AND LOAY S. KABBANI

INTRODUCTION

With improvement in endovascular techniques and continued refinements/modifications of stent grafts, along with the technical experience accumulated over the past two decades, endovascular aneurysm repair (EVAR) has become the primary means of infrarenal abdominal aortic aneurysm (AAA) repair in greater than 85% of patients. In patients with shorter aortic necks (<15 mm) as well as those with challenging anatomic configurations (iliac tortuosity, aortic neck angulation, small diameter access vessels), EVAR is now often possible. Fenestrated EVAR now provides a means for repairing juxtarenal AAAs as well. The practice of physician-modified endografts (PMEGs) has expanded endovascular repair to more proximal anatomic levels with four-vessel (celiac, superior mesenteric artery, and renal) fenestrations most frequently performed. While the initial morbidity and mortality of EVAR are lower compared with open AAA repair, EVAR patients require lifelong radiographic surveillance to identify endoleaks, graft migration, limb thrombosis, and sac expansion. Thirty percent of EVAR patients develop endoleaks, with 30% of these patients requiring some type of intervention. Fortunately, the majority of endoleaks can be successfully treated with endovascular techniques, whether through embolization of a feeding vessel (type II endoleak), placement of a proximal or distal extension stent graft (type I endoleak), or a bridging stent graft (type III endoleak). However, these endovascular "rescue" techniques may also fail, leading to continued sac expansion or even rupture. Graft infections and recurrent graft limb thrombosis (in which endovascular techniques are no longer possible or indicated) are additional situations where aortic stent explantation and concomitant open aortic reconstruction may be required. Aortic stent graft explantation is a complex procedure requiring unique and specialized techniques for a successful outcome.

INDICATIONS FOR EVAR EXPLANT

The incidence of late open conversion after EVAR should be less than 5% (range, 0–9%) [1–3]. In one recent series, the conversion rate was 1.5% [1]. The main indications for graft explantation include endoleak (with or without graft migration), graft infection, or refractory graft occlusion. Sac enlargement secondary to endoleaks can occur in up to 40% of EVARs. While the majority of these endoleaks can be repaired endovascularly, some persist despite multiple attempts at endovascular rescue, and such patients may require conversion with EVAR explantation and open aortic reconstruction. Graft infection, while less frequent after EVAR than open repair, is a major life- and limb-threatening complication that typically requires stent graft explantation. When performed with concomitant in-situ aortic graft reconstruction as is the current guideline, a replacement conduit relatively resistant to infection is required. This step requires experience with the use of cryopreserved allografts or rifampin-soaked Dacron grafts. Many of the operative considerations are similar to the management of infected aortic grafts placed via an open approach. Graft thrombosis is the least common indication for EVAR explant; graft thrombosis is usually confined to a graft limb and can be successfully managed with endovascular techniques or an extra-anatomical bypass. In situations where such techniques are not feasible or have repetitively failed, conversion to an open repair may be the only option.

Type Ia endoleaks account for the majority of endoleaks that require explant [1–4]. Type Ia endoleaks and graft migration are noted to occur more commonly with EVARs placed outside the indications for use (IFU) as detailed by the endograft manufacturer. Short, heavily calcified necks, severe aortic neck angulation (>60 degrees), and diseased distal iliac seal zones are common underlying factors associated with EVAR failure. In one study, 56% of patients requiring graft explants had EVARs performed outside the recommended IFU criteria [1]. Additionally, it

DOI: 10.1201/9781003452096-34

has been noted that larger aortic neck diameters of 30 mm to 32 mm, despite meeting IFU criteria, can predispose to type Ia endoleaks [2].

Type II endoleaks occur in 14–30% of all EVARs. Most type II endoleaks do not cause sac expansion. Patients with persistent type II endoleak associated sac expansion, despite endovascular attempts to control or eliminate the endoleak, may require an open procedure, ranging from ligation of feeding vessels to graft explantation and replacement. In patients with sac expansion thought to be secondary to a type II endoleak, one should always be concerned about the possibility of an occult type I endoleak. Additionally, type II endoleaks causing sac enlargement can predispose to the development of a type I endoleak. One needs to take this into consideration when selecting the appropriate treatment of an enlarging aneurysm sac presumed to be secondary to a type II endoleak. Lastly, there is the real possibility, after direct ligation or internal suturing of feeding vessels (repair of type II endoleak), of developing new type II endoleaks or even a new type I endoleak.

Type V endoleaks are a unique concern with sac expansion despite the absence of an identifiable endoleak with imaging studies (computed tomographic angiography, catheter angiography, or ultrasound-based duplex imaging). As no precise endoleak is identified and therefore cannot be targeted for treatment, aortic stent graft explantation is often necessary in the setting of continued sac expansion. It is presumed that many type V endoleaks are unrecognized type I endoleaks. An additional option for type V endoleaks, prior to graft explanation, is "relining" the endograft with a new stent graft. Following a relining procedure, the patient must be monitored frequently (every four to six months) to ensure sac stabilization or regression.

ANATOMY

The proximal aortic seal zone for the majority of EVARs is infrarenal, with the exception being for fenestrated/branched EVARs that are performed for pararenal aneurysms. Most EVAR devices have suprarenal fixation adding a further layer of complexity to EVAR explants. Exposure of the infrarenal aorta is mandatory to accomplish the repair and suture the replacement aortic graft to the native aortic neck. Periaortic inflammatory changes invariably occur post-EVAR, making exposure of the infrarenal neck and iliacs more challenging than in de novo open repair. In addition, the infrarenal neck loses some integrity following EVAR, making infrarenal clamping hazardous. More proximal aortic control is frequently necessary. It is the authors' experience that one should be prepared to accomplish the proximal repair with suprarenal or supraceliac clamping following graft explantation.

OPERATIVE TREATMENT

With aortic stent graft explantation, there are several variables that impact the conduct of the operation including indication(s) for explantation, type of endograft utilized, replacement graft planned, operative approach (transabdominal vs. left flank retroperitoneal), aortic clamp level (suprarenal or supraceliac or infrarenal), and extent to which the endograft is explanted (partial vs. complete).

We prefer a transperitoneal transabdominal approach when infrarenal clamping is possible. This is often the case when proximal endograft graft has migrated distally and a suitable infrarenal neck is still available for clamp placement. When suprarenal or supraceliac control is required (as is the case in most patients) or when patients have had extensive prior abdominal operations, a left flank retroperitoneal approach is preferred.

Clamp level will be dictated by the anatomic findings as noted on preoperative imaging. Factors that influence clamp position are the relationship of the renal and visceral vessels to the endograft and the superior extent of the suprarenal fixation component. In one series, supraceliac clamping was utilized in 25% of patients [3]. However, exposure of the supraceliac aorta is time well spent as paravisceral aortic dissection is often difficult. Inflammation in the proximal neck, secondary to the graft and in particular penetration by endo-hooks, can make pararenal dissection difficult, rendering the placement of a suprarenal clamp problematic.

The steps for supraceliac aortic exposure (transperitoneal, transabdominal) are well described. In brief, the left lobe of the liver is retracted toward the right following division of the left triangular ligament; the peritoneal reflection over the gastroesophageal junction is divided; the gastrohepatic ligament is opened through a longitudinal incision; deep blades of a self-retaining retractor are applied; and finally, an opening is made through the overlying crus. With careful blunt finger dissection, the anterior surface of the aorta is exposed and the fascia surrounding the aorta divided. The aorta is then dissected toward the spine on each side, enough to allow aortic clamp placement. Circumferential dissection of the aorta is unnecessary and may be potentially risky.

Suprarenal clamping remains technically feasible in patients without an inflammatory response and in whom an adequate distance between the renal ostia and the superior mesenteric artery exists.

The aortic neck and the proximal extent of the endograft are exposed via an inframesocolic approach, with the fourth portion of the duodenum mobilized after dividing the ligament of Treitz. The transverse colon, stomach, and greater omentum are retracted superiorly with the small bowel retracted to the right and sigmoid colon retracted down and to the left. The left renal vein is encountered and carefully exposed to allow cephalad retraction. It may be necessary to ligate and divide its lumbar, gonadal, and adrenal branches, keeping in mind that if the renal vein is to be divided, these vessels should be preserved. Mobilization is facilitated by the placement of a Penrose drain around the renal vein, allowing both superior and inferior retraction and further aortic exposure.

The extent of endograft excision often depends on the pre-existing device seal, presence (or absence) of suprarenal fixation struts, and whether underlying graft infection is suspected. Suprarenal stents and barb fixation can make complete excision especially challenging. Technical aids to facilitate this maneuver are detailed below.

Graft replacement

With complete graft excision in the absence of infection, one performs standard aorto-bi-iliac or aorto-bifemoral reconstruction with a bifurcated woven polyester (Dacron) graft. With partial graft preservation (detailed below), a bifurcated graft is used with anastomosis to the previous endograft main body proximally *or* to the endograft limbs distally. Construction of these distal graft-to-endograft anastomoses can be challenging, and whenever possible, the surgeon should incorporate suture bites on the anastomosis into the EVAR graft material *and* the surrounding native vessel wall. Care must be taken to avoid detaching the loose pseudo-intima (i.e., compacted fibrin layer) lining the stent graft limbs. In the presence of an established or highly suspected graft infection, all prosthetic graft material should be completely excised. For infection, the authors follow the most recent guidelines and favor in-situ reconstruction with an infection-resistant graft—cryopreserved aortic allograft if available, if not, a rifampin-soaked Dacron graft is utilized.

Retroperitoneal approach

The retroperitoneal approach is favored by the authors when suprarenal or supraceliac exposure will be required to gain proximal control. Advantages include complete single field exposure of the paravisceral aorta to allow for selection of the proximal clamp site. This approach may be problematic if distal right iliac artery exposure is anticipated. Exposure is accomplished through a left flank incision in the tenth or ninth intercostal space extending to the lateral rectus sheath with division of the musculature of the abdominal wall and entry into the retroperitoneal space. Mobilization of the peritoneal sac and intraperitoneal contents to the midline ensues, maintaining the psoas muscle on the posterior aspect of the exposure and then developing a plane posterior to the left kidney. The dissection continues superiorly to the level of the left diaphragmatic crus, which is then divided, allowing exposure of the supraceliac aorta. The crus can be divided slowly with Bovie cauterization with a right-angle clamp protecting the underlying aorta. Suprarenal or supraceliac exposure can then ensue with the intention of clamping the aorta above the most superior hooks of the suprarenal attachment stent.

Intraoperative challenges: Proximal

In the absence of infection, it is common and preferred to suture the proximal anastomosis to the fabric of a well-incorporated endograft, while incorporating native aortic tissue into the suture line (Figure 34.1). When complete excision of the EVAR graft and suprarenal stent is required (as in aneurysmal degeneration of the pararenal aorta), several strategies are available to facilitate complete excision of these suprarenal struts. One method is to circumferentially release the barbs from the polyester-covered main body with a wire cutter. Another method involves use of a 20 mL syringe as a large-caliber sheath to encircle and collapse the suprarenal component (effective only with the Cook Zenith Endograft). Some authors have described using iced saline on the nitinol elements to help collapse the metal to its pre-deployment state to facilitate removal. If these techniques are unsuccessful, we do not hesitate to leave the bare stent segments in situ even in an infected setting, assuming all the prosthetic graft material has been excised.

It is important to note that wall penetration by the barbs of a suprarenal fixation device can make complete removal of such an endograft very difficult. A reliable set

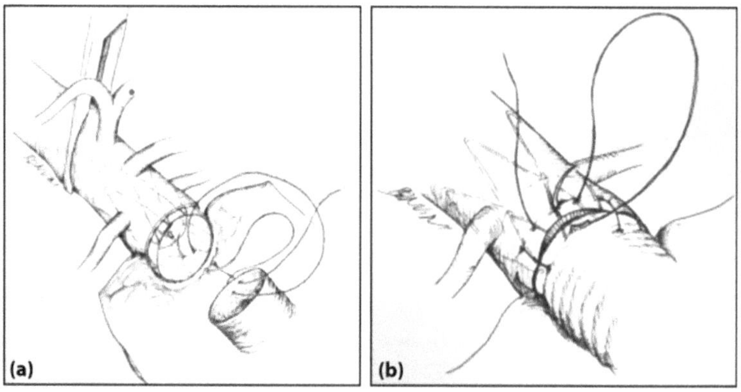

Figure 34.1 (a) Initiation of end-to-end anastomosis between Dacron prosthetic graft and transected endograft combined with partially divided aortic neck using a "parachute" technique. (b) Completion of this anastomosis again taking suture bites through both the native aortic wall and the endograft.

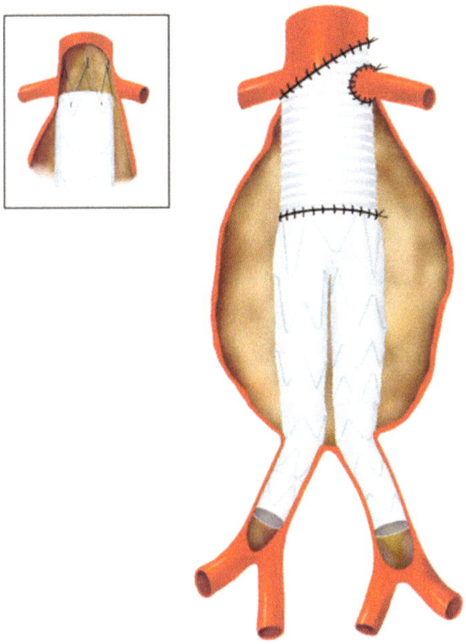

Figure 34.2 Beveled proximal anastomosis between prosthetic graft and aorta incorporating the right renal artery ± the superior mesenteric artery; the left renal artery is re-implanted into the graft. Distally, the prosthetic graft is sewn to the distal endograft that remains in situ.

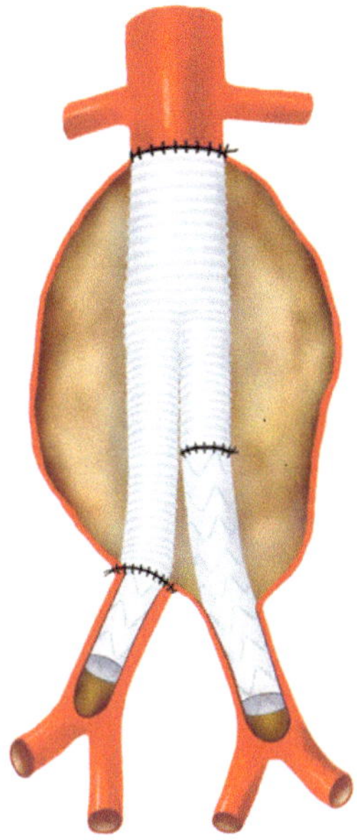

Figure 34.3 Proximal prosthetic graft anastomosed to infrarenal aorta. Distally, the iliac limbs are sewn to the distal limbs of the endograft (left in situ). The right limb anastomosis incorporates the right iliac artery wall.

of wire cutters and sturdy needle holders can be indispensable. Removal of the suprarenal component can tear the aorta, injure the origins of the adjacent renal and/or visceral arteries, and require prolonged suprarenal clamping, all of which contribute to adverse outcomes. Complete excision of the endograft may necessitate extension of the aortotomy to above the level of the renal orifices. When this is required, we perform a beveled anastomosis to incorporate the superior mesenteric and right renal arteries and then either bypass or reimplant the left renal artery reimplantation or bypass. (Figure 34.2) A retroperitoneal approach simplifies this maneuver with much easier exposure to allow the construction of a beveled proximal anastomosis.

Intraoperative challenges: Distal

Given the extensive peri-aortic/arterial inflammation in the pelvis associated with a prior EVAR, obtaining distal iliac control can be challenging. Several techniques are available to obtain distal control. If the distal endograft limbs are well incorporated and without issue and the plan is to leave them in situ, then they can simply be clamped after opening the aneurysm sac. Fogarty clamps are best to avoid damage to the metallic struts and the fragile pseudointima lining these grafts can sometimes "fold up" with potential problems. The transected iliac limbs of the stent graft are then used as distal anastomotic sites for the new prosthetic bifurcation graft (Figure 34.3). This technique is particularly useful in patients with ruptured aneurysms where time and blood loss are of the essence. If feasible, it is preferred that the native iliac artery wall and graft limb are incorporated together into a single distal suture line. Passing the stitches through the graft fabric and the vessel wall provides better hemostasis. Frequently, it is simply easier to just sew to the endograft limb proximal to the aortic bifurcation. Selecting a small caliber segment of endograft makes for a better size match to the prosthetic graft. When sewing to an endograft limb alone, one must be cognizant of how thin-walled its polyester fabric is compared with a standard graft and the fact that it can be easily torn. We recommend using a small caliber needle when performing this anastomosis. Reinforcement with felt or bovine pericardium is occasionally necessary.

In the presence of infection (or a type 1b endoleak), it is necessary to remove the iliac endograft limbs. In this situation, distal control can be obtained by passing large balloon occlusion catheters into the native iliac arteries through the transected endograft limbs. Transfemoral balloon occlusion of both iliac limbs is an alternative option. In the presence of a type 1b endoleak or infection, the distal endograft limbs can usually be removed with firm traction, taking care not to dislodge the occluding balloon catheter.

A less common situation occurs with a type 1b endoleak in which it is determined that the proximal attachment site is intact and the problem leading to the sac expansion is related to distal seal, either unilaterally or bilaterally. Most type Ib endoleaks can be managed via extension of the iliac limbs into the distal common iliac or further down into the external iliac. The hypogastric

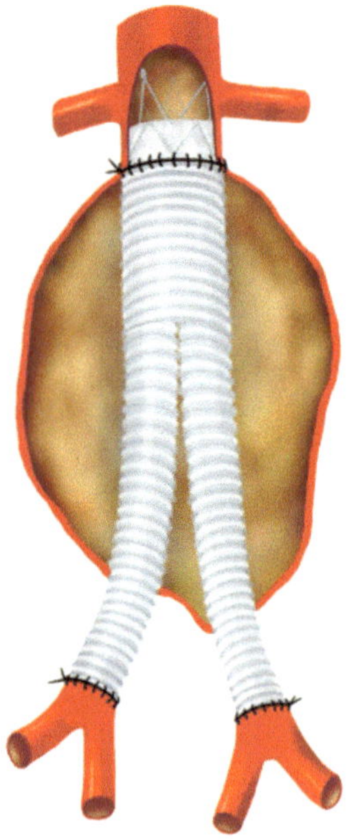

Figure 34.4 Incorporated proximal endograft anastomosed to the main body of a new aorto-bi-iliac prosthetic graft. Proximal suture line incorporates both the aortic wall and the transected endograft wall.

artery in this situation can be embolized or if preservation is desired, an iliac branch device can be deployed. Rarely, in the emergent open repair setting of a rupture AAA with a prior endograft (and once it is determined that the source of the rupture is a distal type Ib), the proximal endograft can be left in place with the new graft sutured to the prior endograft and extended to the native iliac vessel beyond the prior seals zones of the endograft (Figure 34.4). Iliac artery exposure for anastomosis can be quite challenging in these cases and great care should be taken in the required dissection. As with any re-do aortic surgery, selective placement of ureteral catheters preoperatively can be quite helpful.

OUTCOMES

This is an extensive operation with a significant physiologic insult to the patient. Bleeding from the proximal anastomosis can result from inadequate incorporation of healthy native aortic tissue into the anastomosis. If graft infection is the indication for explant, recurrent infection remains a risk but should be minimized by performing wide debridement and utilizing an omental wrap. Similarly, bleeding from distal anastomosis can occur secondary to failure to incorporate healthy iliac vessel into the distal anastomosis. Iliac artery degeneration progressing to iliac rupture after complete endograft removal from the iliac arteries can occur. This may be related to disruption of iliac artery wall integrity while excising the iliac limbs.

EVAR explant has significant morbidity and mortality with a complication rate of 27–60% [4, 5]. Major complications include renal dysfunction, respiratory failure, and cardiac complications inclusive of myocardial infarction. Due to concern of the potential for significant blood loss, we recommend using cell saver in non-infected cases.

Outcomes for EVAR explantation/conversion are dependent on the indication for excision and repair with mortality rates of 40% reported in the setting of post-EVAR ruptured AAAs and somewhat less for infections [4, 5]. However, when EVAR explants are performed electively in the absence of infection, mortality rates should be approximately 5–6% [5, 6]. Patients with EVAR failures not amenable to endovascular salvage need evaluation for EVAR explantation to avoid an urgent/emergent operation. Referral to a high-volume aortic center is recommended. Postoperative imaging surveillance is of paramount importance, particularly for those patients who have had partial graft explantation.

TRICKS AND TRAPS

1. Aortic stent graft explantation is required in the setting of a prior EVAR complicated by significant endoleak-induced sac expansion, aortic rupture, graft infection, and recurrent graft thrombosis.
2. This is a complex procedure with worse outcomes compared with standard open AAA repair.
3. Suprarenal or supraceliac proximal control is frequently required and the retroperitoneal approach is favored when it is anticipated that infrarenal clamping is not feasible.
4. Transperitoneal exposure and infrarenal clamping are sometimes suitable when stent graft migration has occurred with a preserved infrarenal neck.
5. One of the technical challenges of aortic endograft explantation is management of the suprarenal fixation apparatus if present. The operating surgeon must have in his arsenal several different and tailored methods for complete or partial excision of the suprarenal fixation stent to allow the secure construction of a proximal anastomosis.
6. Endograft infection requires complete graft excision and ideally in-situ replacement with an infection-resistant conduit.
7. Partial graft excision and reconstruction can be judiciously employed in instances of sac expansion secondary to endoleak without evidence of infection.

QUESTIONS

1. The indication for endograft explant with the highest perioperative mortality is related to:
   a. Persistent type 2 endoleak despite prior embolization
   b. Recurrent graft limb thrombosis
   c. Type 3 endoleaks
   d. Graft infection

   Answer: d

2. Which of the following is associated with an increased incidence of type I endoleak post-procedurally?
   a. Aortic neck diameter of 34 mm
   b. Aortic neck angulation less than 60 degrees
   c. Type 2 endoleaks without sac expansion
   d. Smaller aneurysms

   Answer: a

3. Select the best option for a patient with a lumbar artery type 2 endoleak without evidence of sac expansion:
   a. Trans-arterial trans-hypogastric embolization
   b. Exploratory laparotomy with opening of aneurysm and over-sewing of patent lumbar orifices
   c. Repeat CTA in six months
   d. Relining of the endograft

   Answer: c

4. Which of the following endoleaks can be best managed by endovascular techniques as opposed to an open procedure?
   a. Type 5 endoleak with sac growth and prior relining procedure
   b. Type Ib endoleak with aneurysm expansion and direct flow into the aneurysm sac
   c. Type 2 endoleak without sac expansion
   d. Type 1 endoleak with suspected graft infection

   Answer: b

REFERENCES

1. Kansal V, Nagpal S, Jetty P. Editor's choice – late open surgical conversion after endovascular abdominal aortic aneurysm repair. *Eur J Vasc Endovasc Surg.*, 2018. 55(2): p. 163–169.
2. McFarland G, Tran K, Whitt VD, Sgroi M, Chandra V, Well MW, et al. Infrarenal endovascular aneurysm repair with large device (34- to 36-mm) diameters is associated with higher risk of proximal fixation failure. *J Vasc Surg.*, 2019. 69(2): p. 385–393.
3. Dubois L, Harlock J, Gill HL, Chen JC, Rheaume P, Jetty P, Boyd A, et al. A Canadian multicenter experience describing outcomes after endovascular abdominal aortic aneurysm repair stent graft explantation. *J Vasc Surg.*, 2021. 74(3): p. 720–728. e1.
4. Arnaoutakis DJ, Sharma G, Blackwood S, Shah SK, Menard M, Ozaki CK, Belkin M. Strategies and outcomes for aortic endograft explantation. *J Vasc Surg*, 2019. 69(1): p. 80–85.
5. Lyden SP, et al., Technical considerations for late removal of aortic endografts. *J Vasc Surg.*, 2002. 36(4): p. 674–678.
6. Lopez Espada C, Behrendt CA, Mani K, D'Oria M, Lattman T, Khashram M. VASCUNExplant collaborator group. Editor's choice – the VASCUNExplanT project: an international study assessing open surgical conversion of failed non-infected endovascular aortic aneurysm repair. *Eur J Vasc Endovasc Surg.* 2023 Nov;66(5):653–660.

35

Primary and secondary aortoenteric fistula

TIMOTHY J. NYPAVER

INTRODUCTION

An aortoenteric fistula (AEF), whether primary or secondary, represents one of the most challenging and dreaded of vascular surgical complications. Primary AEFs are relatively rare and represent a direct communication between the native aorta and the overlying bowel. Secondary AEFs are related to a prior aortic reconstruction and are more common, occurring in 0.5–1.2% of all aortic reconstructions [1–3]. The patient with an AEF of either type may have significant hemodynamic compromise with active or recent gastrointestinal (GI) bleeding. In addition, increasing experience suggests that both primary and secondary AEFs can occur after endovascular abdominal aortic aneurysm (AAA) repair. While logic dictates that AEFs after endograft placement should be classified as secondary, there may be instances in which a pressurized aneurysm sac from an ongoing endoleak ruptures into an adjacent bowel segment [4, 5]. Since it would have no direct communication with the endograft, it is reasonable to consider these as primary AEFs.

Important prioritizing considerations for the vascular surgeon faced with a suspected AEF include: (1) whether the patient is hemodynamically stable, or whether there is an active, life-threatening hemorrhage; (2) the overall risk to the patient for cardiopulmonary complications and their ability to undergo a difficult major operation; (3) the indication for the prior aortic reconstruction; (4) the location of the distal anastomoses (distal aorta, iliac, or femoral arteries); and (5) based on the computed tomography (CT) findings, whether there is enough aortic neck to allow a new proximal anastomosis below the renal arteries. The hemodynamic status of the patient and whether there is active hemorrhage determine the rapidity of transit to the operating room and the algorithm for operative management (Figure 35.1).

SECONDARY AEF

Secondary AEFs occur because of communication between a previously placed aortic graft or endograft and the bowel, typically located at the third and fourth portions of the duodenum. The patient most often presents two to three years after placement of the aortic graft, with manifestations of GI bleeding. Manifestations of infection are present in up to 50% of patients and include fever and leukocytosis [1–3]. Patients often present with a "herald" bleed, which allows for timely diagnostic evaluation in any patient with previous aortic reconstruction. Massive hemorrhage, without antecedent bleeding, is unusual and accounts for <5% of presentations [1–3]. The communication between the GI tract and the graft material can either involve the anastomosis (true AEF) or the graft body or limb (prosthetic-enteric erosion) [2]. The source of bleeding for the true AEF is from the aorta itself, while the prosthetic-enteric erosion typically bleeds from the edge of the bowel wall. One-fourth of patients present with manifestations of infection and sepsis alone without evidence of GI bleed [1–3, 6].

The stable patient should undergo esophagogastroduodenoscopy (EGD) with attention paid to the third and fourth portions of the duodenum, looking for ulceration. While visualization of graft material on EGD is pathognomonic, this is rarely seen and not required to make the diagnosis. CT angiography (CTA) may be of benefit by demonstrating perigraft fluid, bowel wall thickening and inflammation, periprosthetic air, or proximal anastomotic pseudoaneurysm formation, and provides important anatomic information that has an impact on the operative approach (Figure 35.2). While there are often indirect findings of AEF on CTA, one rarely makes a definitive diagnosis; the treating surgeon must maintain a high index of suspicion and proceed with operative repair even though the diagnosis may be in question.

DOI: 10.1201/9781003452096-35

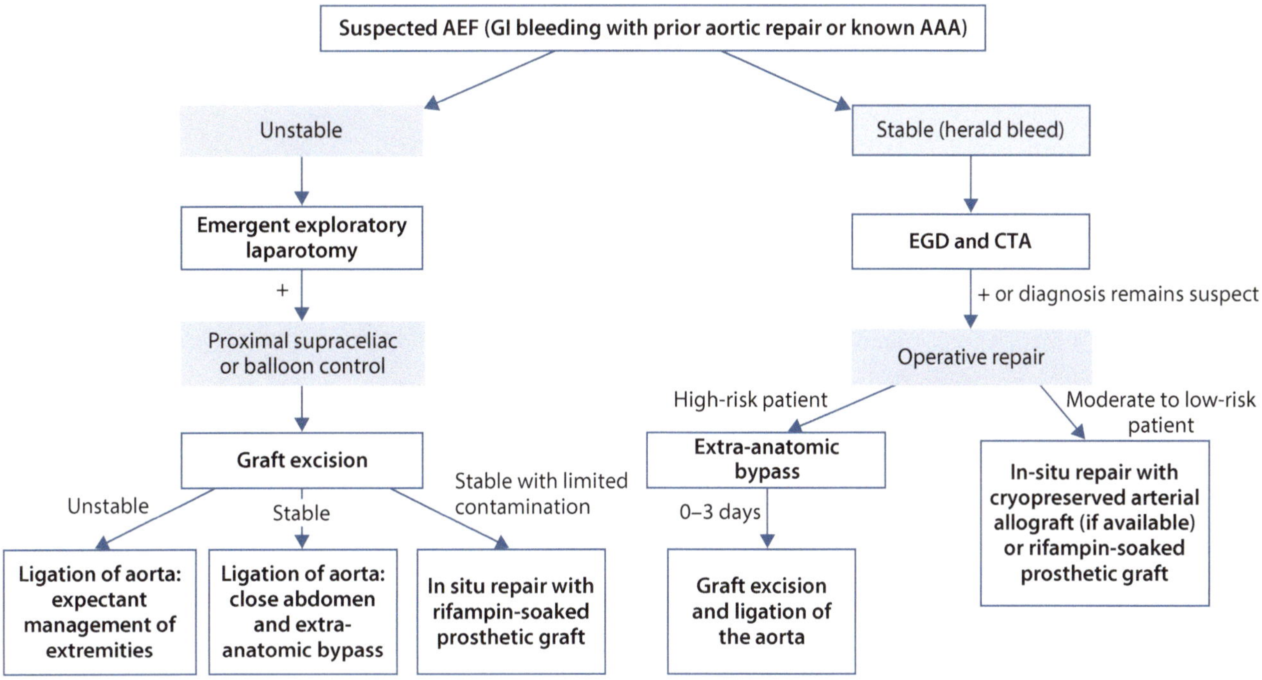

Figure 35.1 Management algorithm for the patient with suspected aortoenteric fistula. AAA, abdominal aortic aneurysm; AEF, aortoenteric fistula; CTA, computed tomography angiography; EGD, esophagogastroduodenoscopy; GI, gastrointestinal.

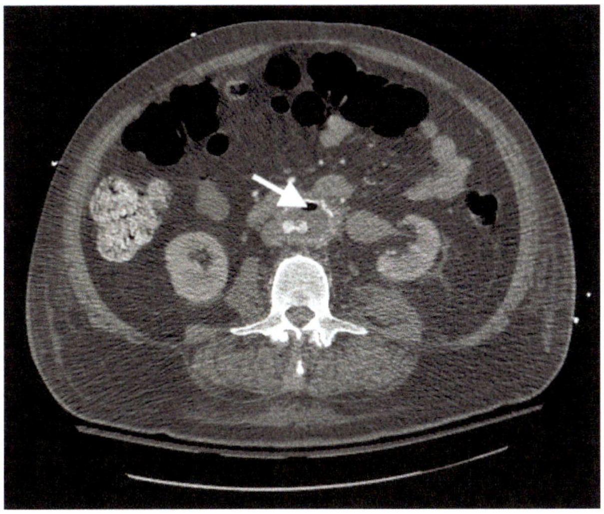

Figure 35.2 Computed tomography angiography of a patient with secondary aortoenteric fistula. There is gas accumulation within the aneurysm sac in proximity to the bifurcated graft (white arrow pointing to air within the aneurysm sac).

In the hemodynamically stable patient, once the diagnosis is either confirmed or highly suspected, the operating surgeon must decide between two radically different approaches: (1) staged or sequential extra-anatomic bypass (clean planes) followed by aortic graft excision (infected); or (2) aortic graft excision with in-line aortic graft replacement with one of the following conduits: femoral vein (venous autograft), cryopreserved arterial allograft, or a new prosthetic graft with antimicrobial impregnation, typically with rifampin. Over the past decade, there has been a progressive adoption of the in-line (or in-situ) treatment for aortic graft infections, inclusive of aortoenteric fistula. For all in-line graft replacement options, extensive debridement of the aortic wall and any inflammatory tissue, along with omental coverage, is essential. The author's preference is graft excision with in-line replacement with cryopreserved arterial allografts. If the cryopreserved allograft is not readily available, then rifampin-impregnated Dacron grafts are utilized. Staged extra-anatomic bypass and graft excision are reserved for patients who, because of their comorbidities, are unlikely to tolerate direct excision and in-line replacement (Figure 35.1). Generally, the author has not used the neoaortoiliac system (venous autograft) in the management of AEF. In addition, the author has not utilized a bovine pericardial tube in the management of AEFs, however, does recognize that it may have utility in aortic graft infection reconstruction [7]. The patient should receive broad-spectrum antibiotics because most cultures from AEFs yield polymicrobial organisms. The following describes the author's operative management in the patient with hemodynamic stability, with a good-to-moderate operative risk in whom at least 3 mm of aortic neck is present between the renal arteries and the graft.

The patient is positioned supine and prepped from the neck to the knees. The author prefers a long midline incision with control at the supraceliac aorta. This is accomplished via mobilization of the left lobe of the liver, retraction of the gastroesophageal junction to the left, and separating out the crura of the diaphragm to expose the aorta. This area is almost always free of prior adhesions. Distal control is obtained either at the level of the iliac vessels or distal graft anastomoses. This latter maneuver may require bilateral femoral artery exposure before making the abdominal incision. Any omentum encountered is preserved for later use. Finally, exposure of the graft and AEF, including a segment of aorta below the renal arteries, is undertaken. The new in-line graft should be prepared and ready for use before any exposure of the AEF. If bleeding is encountered around the AEF, supraceliac and distal clamps are quickly applied. The dissection continues expeditiously with the goal of exposing a segment of the infrarenal aorta. Proximal control is moved from the supraceliac to the infrarenal location as soon as possible to minimize visceral/renal ischemic time. Often, it is necessary to place the clamp between renal or suprarenal levels to allow visualization of viable noninvolved aorta to accomplish an anastomosis. If suprarenal control is difficult, the supraceliac clamp is left in place while the proximal anastomosis is accomplished.

Before clamp placement, the patient is given an appropriate heparin dose and intravenous mannitol 25–50 g. If the proximal clamp is positioned suprarenal or supraceliac, the author limits the initial debridement to the proximal perirenal aorta and proceeds with the anastomosis to limit renal and mesenteric ischemia time. The opening in the bowel is encountered and covered with wet laparotomy pads with the intention of repairing this later. The anastomosis is accomplished in a typical fashion with 3-0 polypropylene suture in a circumferential fashion. The anastomosis is checked, and if hemostatic, large Fogarty clamps with soft inserts are applied to the graft. With release of the suprarenal clamp, renal perfusion is restored. Debridement of any periaortic inflammation or infection is completed, including removal of any remaining graft material. The time spent excising any grossly infected or inflammatory tissue is a critically important component of in-line replacement therapy and should not be accomplished in haste. Complete excision of the pre-existing graft is mandatory. Following this, the anastomoses are performed to each uninvolved iliac artery, preferably beyond the prior graft anastomoses (Figure 35.3). The duodenal defect is debrided and closed primarily. If the duodenal defect is large, a segmental resection with end-to-end anastomosis is performed.

If the infected graft extends down to the femoral arteries, groin incisions are accomplished first with exposure of the femoral arteries and graft. The native arteries are exposed proximally and distally to the site of the prior anastomosis. A two-team approach, each working on one groin, is beneficial. Access to the tunnels is maintained with an umbilical tape; laparotomy pads can be passed through the tunnels, accomplishing some minor debridement while maintaining access. Because of the significant retroperitoneal adhesions that are typically encountered, the creation of a new tunnel is difficult, with a significant risk of iliac

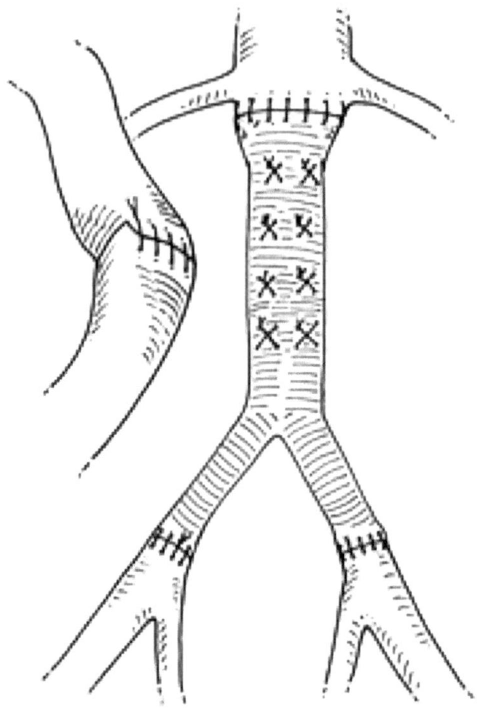

Figure 35.3 Depiction of the cryopreserved arterial allograft as an in-line repair. Note the anteriorly placed lumbar orifices that have been oversewn.

vein injury. At the time of the initial graft debridement, the author has found it helpful to divide the graft limb just above the anastomosis so that the common femoral-profunda femoris-superficial femoral artery circuit is maintained, limiting distal ischemia. Once the surgeon is ready to do the distal anastomosis of the new conduit, the arteries are clamped, any remaining graft material is completely excised, and the distal anastomosis is performed. In most instances, when doing the groin reconstruction, the author attempts to preserve retrograde flow. The author has used rotation of the sartorius muscle to provide coverage of the groin anastomoses. The skin of the groin wound is left open with the application of a vacuum-assisted closure dressing. Intra-abdominally, a segment of the omentum is mobilized on a vascular pedicle and wrapped around the newly placed prosthesis or graft (Figure 35.4).

PRIMARY AEF

Primary AEFs most frequently involve rupture of an infrarenal or pararenal AAA directly into the third or fourth portion of the duodenum, although other areas of the bowel may be involved. In the setting of GI bleeding and a known AAA, CTA may reveal the presence of extraluminal gas in the periaortic area in close approximation to a segment of bowel. The most common symptom is GI bleeding, with hemorrhage the most likely cause of death. The diagnosis is rarely made preoperatively and delays in diagnosis can lead to a disastrous outcome. Once suspected or diagnosed, the patient should

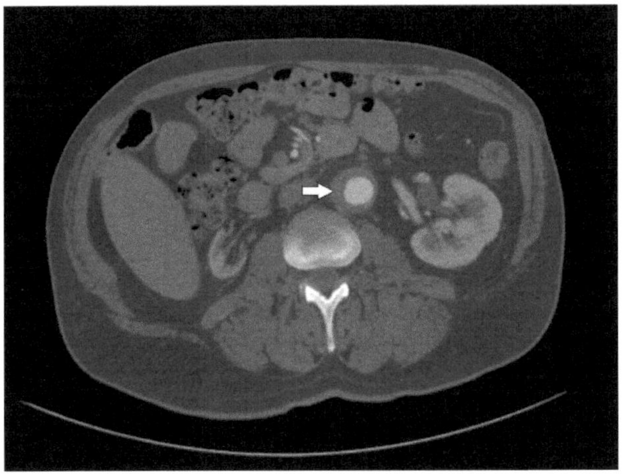

Figure 35.4 Computed tomography angiography of patient status post-excision of infected aortic graft secondary to an aortoenteric fistula, repaired via an in-line rifampin-impregnated Dacron graft with an omental wrap. The white arrow indicates the omental wrap positioned around the prosthetic graft.

be taken emergently to the operating room. The repair proceeds much like that of an open repair of a ruptured AAA with the following caveats: (1) temporary proximal supraceliac control is obtained; (2) the proximal clamp is transitioned to the infrarenal aortic level as soon as possible; (3) debridement of any inflammatory tissue is performed; and (4) a two-layered closure of the bowel defect is undertaken. Throughout the operation, one attempts to minimize bowel contamination. As a primary AEF typically does not indicate long-standing infection, in-line replacement with a rifampin-impregnated Dacron graft is selected as the method of repair and revascularization. Endovascular repair can be accomplished as a bridge to definitive therapy in patients with hemodynamic instability and massive GI bleeding, or in extremely high-risk patients, as a method of palliative repair [8].

OTHER CONSIDERATIONS

Very limited to nonexistent aortic neck on CT scan

In this situation, if performed electively, the author has selectively used medial visceral rotation of the spleen and tail of the pancreas to allow for exposure of the pararenal aorta. While this is beneficial for performance of the proximal anastomosis, it carries significant risk, including splenic capsular injury, bleeding, pancreatic injury, and longer operative time and dissection, further complicating what is already a difficult operation.

The high-risk patient

If the patient's medical comorbidities make them high-risk for a prolonged operation, consideration is given to extra-anatomic bypass followed by graft excision. It should be noted the author favors graft excision with in-line replacement with either a cryopreserved allograft or a rifampin-impregnated Dacron graft, and that extra-anatomic bypass, as a means of restoring lower extremity perfusion, is now rarely employed. Regardless, extra-anatomic bypass remains in the armamentarium of surgical treatment options and is a valuable technique in selected high-risk patients. This approach minimizes the extent of the open abdominal portion of the operation and reduces ischemia-reperfusion injury associated with prolonged pelvic and lower extremity clamp time. When prior aortic reconstruction is confined to the abdomen, extra-anatomic reconstruction is performed with a standard axillobifemoral bypass graft placement (Figure 35.5). Within zero to three days of this operation, the patient undergoes excision of the infected graft and any inflammatory tissue, repair of the bowel defect, and closure of the aortic stump. Proximal supraceliac control and distal vessel control are necessary before dissection around the AEF. Distal control is necessary because there is excellent retrograde perfusion supplied by the recently placed extra-anatomic bypass. All graft material is excised. The aortic stump is oversewn in a standard two-layered closure with 2-0 or 3-0 polypropylene suture, with a row of interrupted mattress sutures and an over-and-over stitch

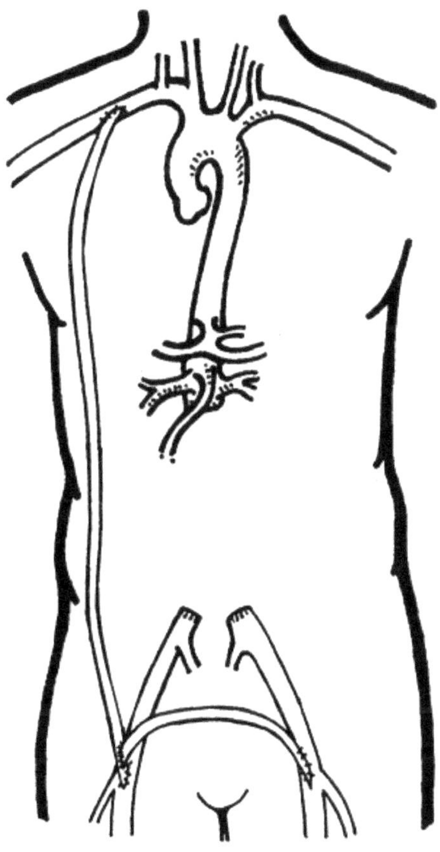

Figure 35.5 Depiction of the extra-anatomic reconstruction used in the repair of an aortoenteric fistula in which the original graft is completely intra-abdominal.

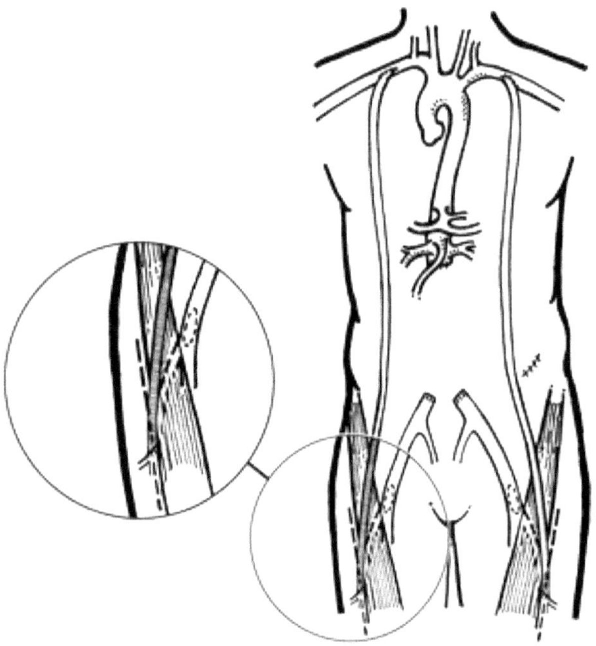

Figure 35.6 Depiction of the most common type of extra-anatomic reconstruction used in the repair of an aortoenteric fistula in which the original graft extends down to the femoral arteries. Note the lateral location of the incision used to expose the mid-to-distal profunda femoris artery.

for the second layer. Any other foreign material (pledgeted suture) is avoided. When the original graft extends down to the femoral arteries, the extra-anatomic reconstruction by necessity becomes more elaborate. The author favors performance of bilateral axilloprofunda bypass graft placement with de novo incisions made lateral to the sartorius muscle to dissect out the mid-to-distal profunda femoral artery that serves as the site for the clean distal anastomosis and outflow (Figure 35.6).

In this high-risk patient population, endovascular therapies are also attractive alternatives. If the high-risk patient is an endovascular candidate anatomically, then consideration could be given to the application of endovascular graft placement as a definitive treatment option. However, this is to be applied to a relatively small subset of patients, as endovascular repair alone has been associated with higher rates of recurrence, sepsis, and AEF-related death [9, 10].

Hemodynamic instability

In the hemodynamically unstable patient, the decision is made to move directly to the operating room or hybrid operating room suite (Figure 35.1). The author has used emergent percutaneous access in instances of aortic pathology and bleeding with proximal balloon control of the hemorrhage. With ultrasound guidance, femoral access can easily be obtained, even in the setting of prior aortofemoral bypass. Once wire access is obtained to the suprarenal level, a larger-diameter sheath (>10 Fr) can be advanced into the aorta and a CODA® Balloon Catheter (Cook Medical Inc., Bloomington, IN, USA) is inflated for proximal control. This has the potential to be lifesaving and allows some stabilization of the patient before operative management. If endovascular repair were an option anatomically, then the author would proceed with it as a bridge to stability. One important caveat would be to avoid suprarenal fixation endografts as this complicates subsequent open repair. If endovascular options are limited or anatomically not possible, the patient would then undergo midline incision with proximal supraceliac aortic control as described previously. Once proximal control is obtained, the operative team would proceed with infrarenal exposure and, if the patient is critically ill, ligation of the aorta (two-layered closure). Further reconstruction of the extremities is pursued as the patient's condition allows. If there is limited contamination with minimal overall blood loss, one could consider proceeding with in-situ repair with an antibiotic impregnated graft.

Rifampin-impregnated Dacron graft

The most used method for antimicrobial impregnation of prosthetic grafts is soaking the graft in an antibiotic solution of rifampin (Figure 35.7). Prosthetic grafts form an ionic bond with rifampin primarily through the gelatin that is used in the sealant process. The antibiotic is released locally and gradually for up to five days.

Cryopreserved arterial allograft

When time allows, this is the author's preferred treatment method for in-line repair of AEF. First, the graft and appropriate sizes of the aortic allograft are determined. The graft is prepared as the operation ensues because there is a defined thawing process when preparing a cryopreserved allograft. The thawing process averages approximately 30–40 minutes. Slits to enlarge the circumference of the proximal portion of the graft may have to be made to accommodate the anastomosis because of size discrepancy. Rather than using a single opening in the allograft, incisions are made into the allograft at both the 3 o'clock and 9 o'clock positions for appropriate sizing. The graft is rotated so that the lumbar orifices are positioned anteriorly; each lumbar artery is oversewn with interrupted 4-0 polypropylene suture.

CONCLUSION

The management goals of AEF, whether primary or secondary, remain the control of hemorrhage and infection, maintenance or preservation of lower extremity perfusion, and the elimination of future morbidity or recurrence related to the repair procedure. With the approaches outlined in this chapter, morbidity and mortality can be reduced (mortality <20%), and a durable, infection-resistant, limb-saving reconstruction can be accomplished [6, 10]. The vascular surgeon, in addition to expeditiously

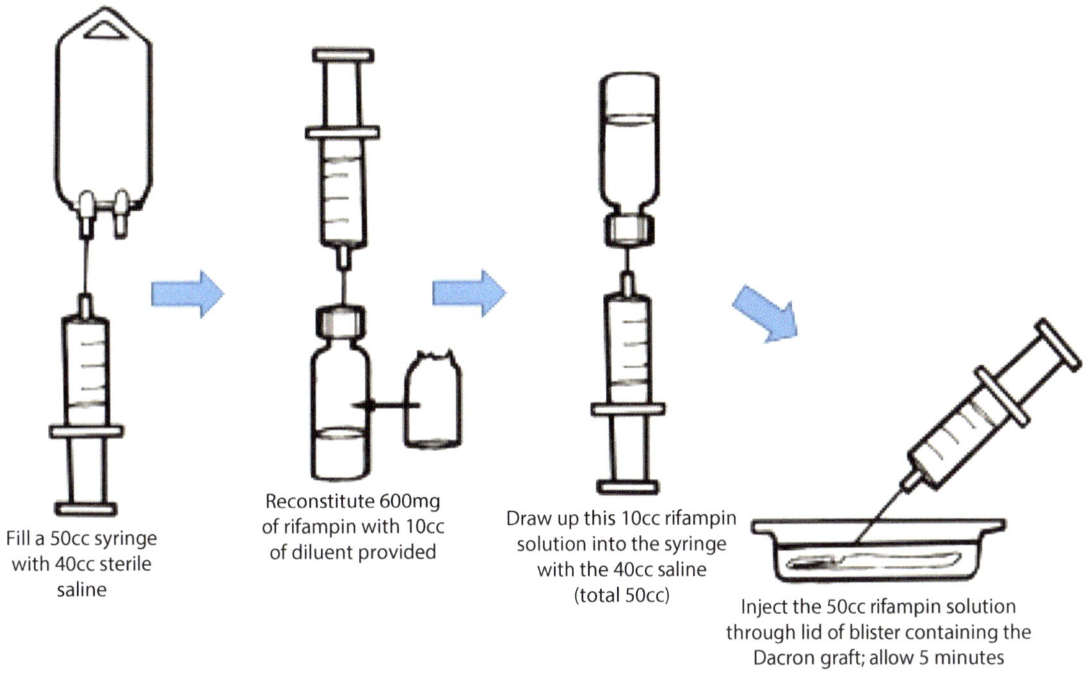

Figure 35.7 Sequence of the procedure for the preparation of a rifampin-impregnated Dacron graft to be used for in-line repair of an aortoenteric fistula.

arriving at the proper diagnosis, must be able to apply a variety of skills, techniques, and experience, including endovascular and complex redo abdominal open repair, to save the patient's life and maximize their long-term survival.

TRICKS AND TRAPS

1. Aortoenteric fistula, whether primary or secondary, represents one of the most challenging and dreaded of vascular surgical complications; an algorithmic expeditious diagnostic and therapeutic approach must be adopted if satisfactory outcomes are to be achieved.
2. Bleeding may be small initially (herald bleed) and the diagnosis may not be established until one is in the operating room.
3. Both primary and secondary AEFs can occur after endovascular aneurysm repair.
4. In-line aortic repair is favored in the hemodynamically good-risk stable patient with use of a cryopreserved arterial allograft (preferred if available) or a new rifampin-soaked Dacron prosthetic graft.
5. Primary AEFs can uniformly be repaired with an antibiotic impregnated in-situ prosthetic graft.
6. In-line graft repair, regardless of the conduit, requires extensive debridement of the aortic wall and any inflammatory tissue, closure of the duodenal defect, and omental coverage of the new graft.
7. Endovascular coverage or repair of the bleeding site, if possible, can be accomplished as a bridge to definitive therapy in patients with hemodynamic instability or significant GI bleeding, or in extremely high-risk patients as a method of palliative repair.

QUESTIONS

1. The most appropriate management of a primary aortoenteric fistula in a hemodynamically stable moderate-risk patient who presented with one episode of melena would be:
   a. In-line graft replacement with a neo-aortic venous autograft
   b. In-line graft replacement with a cryopreserved allograft
   c. In-line replacement with a rifampin-soaked Dacron graft
   d. Extra-anatomic bypass with aortic ligation postoperative day number two
   e. Bovine pericardial patch repair of the aortic defect

   Answer: c

2. Regarding the cryopreserved allograft, which of the following statements is true?
   a. The allograft will need to be replaced within five years of implantation
   b. The allograft does not require any prep time
   c. It is recommended that the allograft be sewn in with the oversewn lumbar arteries on the anterior surface
   d. Cryopreserved allograft can only be used if the distal anastomosis is confined to the iliac vessels
   e. As an allograft, it is rare to have any size mismatch

   Answer: c

3. An 80-year-old male with a prior open aneurysm repair (eight years ago) presents with a massive gastrointestinal bleed and hemodynamic instability. He undergoes open emergent exploratory laparotomy and is found to have a secondary aorto-enteric fistula. A proximal aortic clamp is placed supra-renally, however, the patient remains unstable. The most appropriate next step in management would be:
   a. Aortic ligation and expectant management of extremities
   b. In-situ repair with a Dacron prosthesis
   c. In-situ repair with a cryopreserved allograft
   d. Aortic ligation followed by bilateral ax-fem bypass
   e. Neo-aortic venous autograft repair

   Answer: a

4. The open management of a secondary aortoenteric fistula in a stable patient would typically include all the following except
   a. Debridement of the aortic wall
   b. A pedicled omental flap around the new graft
   c. In-situ graft replacement
   d. Duodenal resection with primary end-to-end anastomosis
   e. Excision of all primary prosthetic material

   Answer: d

REFERENCES

1. Elliot, J. P., Jr, Smith, R. F., & Szilagyi, D. E. Proceedings: aortoenteric and paraprosthetic-enteric fistulas. Problems of diagnosis and management. *Arch Surg.* 1974; 108: 479–490.
2. Bunt, T. J. Synthetic vascular infections. II. Graftenteric erosions and graft-enteric fistulas. *Surgery.* 1983; 94: 1–9.
3. Hallett, J. W., Jr, Marshall, D. M., Petterson, T. M., et al. Graft-related complications after abdominal aortic aneurysm repair: reassurance from a 36-year population-based experience. *J Vasc Surg.* 1997; 25: 277–286.
4. McPhee, J. T., Soybel, D. I., Oram, R. K., et al. Primary aortoenteric fistula following endovasular aortic repair due to type II endoleak. *J Vasc Surg.* 2011; 54: 1164–1166.
5. Fatima, J., Duncan, A. A., de Grandis, E., et al. Treatment strategies and outcomes in patients with infected aortic endografts. *J Vasc Surg.* 2013; 58: 371–379.
6. Kuestner, L. M., Reilly, L. M., Jicha, D. L., et al. Secondary aortoenteric fistula: contemporary outcome with use of extraanatomic bypass and infected graft excision. *J Vasc Surg.* 1995; 21: 184–195.
7. Weiss S, Mallorqui MH, Czerny M, et al. Physician made bovine pericardial tube graft in aortic infection: a European multicentre study. *Eur J Vasc Endovasc Surg.* 2024; 67: 997–1005.
8. Marone, E. M., Mascia, D., Kahlberg, A., et al. Emergent endovascular treatment of a bleeding recurrent aortoenteric fistula as a "bridge" to definitive surgical repair. *J Vasc Surg.* 2012; 55: 1160–1163.
9. Antoniou, G. A., Koutsias, S., Antoniou, S. A., et al. Outcome after endovascular stent graft repair of aortoenteric fistula: a systemic review. *J Vasc Surg.* 2009; 49: 782–789.
10. Kakkos, S. K., Bicknell, C. D., Tsolakis, I. A., et al. Editor's choice. Management of secondary aorto-enteric and other abdominal arterio-enteric fistulas: a review and pooled data analysis. *Eur J Vasc Endovasc Surg.* 2016;52:770–786.

36

Open repair of femoral and femoral anastomotic aneurysms

SEMERET T. MUNIE AND ALEXANDER D. SHEPARD

INTRODUCTION

Arterial aneurysms in the lower extremities are clinically important because of their potential to cause limb-threatening ischemia, from thrombosis or embolization of mural thrombus, or in rare circumstances, rupture. Intervention is preferred before aneurysms become symptomatic. Most true aneurysms of the lower extremities are degenerative in nature, while false aneurysms are related to anastomotic, traumatic, and mycotic etiologies. Common risk factors for aneurysm formation include male gender, older age, smoking, and hypertension. In rare cases, connective tissue abnormalities (e.g., Marfan's syndrome) can also lead to aneurysmal degeneration.

DEGENERATIVE FEMORAL ANEURYSMS

True femoral artery aneurysms (FAAs) are more common in the common femoral artery (CFA) (57%) than they are in the superficial femoral artery (SFA) (26%) or profunda femoris artery (PFA) (17%) [1]. Aneurysms confined to the CFA are classified as type I, while those involving the origin of the PFA are type II [2]. This classification scheme is important for determining reconstruction options.

The presentation of true FAAs can range from asymptomatic to severe lower extremity ischemia. Approximately 40% of patients are asymptomatic at the time of diagnosis, another 40% present with signs of lower extremity ischemia from embolization of mural thrombus or thrombosis, and 20% have local pain or notice a groin mass [3]. Rarely, very large FAAs can compress the femoral vein causing limb swelling while femoral nerve compression can result in femoral neuropraxia. The diagnosis is usually made on physical exam by palpation of a pulsatile groin mass. A variety of imaging modalities (ultrasonography, computed tomographic angiography [CTA], or magnetic resonance imaging [MRI]) can confirm the diagnosis. Catheter-based angiography has limited ability to assess the presence of an aneurysm as it only demonstrates the lumen of an artery and may miss the diagnosis in aneurysms lined with significant mural thrombus. Angiography can be helpful in evaluating the vascular anatomy of the lower extremity for operative planning, though in most situations high-quality thin-cut CTA will suffice.

Indications for treatment

Previous studies have shown that the diameter of the CFA increases with age, male sex, and larger body surface area. The normal size in men is approximately 1.0 cm and 0.8 cm in women [4]. In patients with asymptomatic disease, standard guidelines advise surgical repair for FAAs ≥2.5 cm in diameter or those containing a significant amount of mural thrombus. A recent study looking at 182 patients with degenerative FAAs raised the question as to whether current management guidelines are too aggressive for their natural history. This study found that acute complications rarely occurred in aneurysms <3.5 cm in diameter and recommended adjusting current criteria [5]. On the other hand, all symptomatic FAAs should be treated regardless of size to prevent life- and limb-threatening complications (i.e., thrombosis, embolization, local compression, and rupture).

Preoperative planning

Perioperative assessment of cardiovascular risk is essential in this patient population. Imaging of the aorta, iliac, superficial femoral, and popliteal arteries, usually with CTA, should also be performed to evaluate for presence of any concurrent aneurysms. Bilateral lower extremity perfusion should also be evaluated with segmental pressure testing.

DOI: 10.1201/9781003452096-36

Operative repair

The surgical treatment of FAAs usually involves open repair where the aneurysmal segment is replaced with an interposition graft. Synthetic vascular grafts such as polytetrafluroethylene (PTFE) or Dacron are usually preferred over vein grafts due to their reported better patency rates and closer size matches. General or regional (epidural) anesthesia is preferred in case operative time is prolonged.

A longitudinal groin incision is used to expose the aneurysm. Control of the CFA or external iliac artery proximally and of the SFA and PFA distally is obtained. Most degenerative aneurysms arise just below the origins of the inferior superficial epigastric and lateral iliac circumflex branches, making control at the external iliac level the norm. Efforts should be made to preserve these branches to avoid local groin wound ischemic complications. When controlling the external iliac at this level, it is usually necessary to divide a small portion of the inguinal ligament. In addition, care should be exercised in searching for (and dividing if necessary) the crossing iliac circumflex vein also known as "the vein of pain" to avoid later inadvertent injury. At the femoral bifurcation, one should always look for and control a posteriorly exiting arterial branch from the CFA or the proximal-most PFA. Failure to control this branch prior to opening the aneurysm can lead to troublesome back bleeding. If the aneurysm is very large or ruptured, a retroperitoneal approach through a short, transverse suprainguinal incision may be necessary to obtain proximal control of the external iliac artery. An alternative approach is the placement of a 5.5 Fr balloon occlusion catheter in the distal external iliac from the contralateral femoral or retrograde from a patent ipsilateral SFA. Following therapeutic heparinization, the inflow and outflow vessels are clamped and the aneurysm opened. Most aneurysms can be simply excised, though this is not necessary. Debulking the groin of all aneurysm wall can make the reconstruction easier. However, complete aneurysm excision also has the potential to disrupt more lymphatics, which can induce troublesome postoperative lymphedema of the involved extremity.

Type I aneurysms are generally reconstructed with a CFA-to-CFA interposition graft of either Dacron or PTFE (Figure 36.1a). Type II aneurysms can be repaired with an interposition graft to the PFA and re-implantation of the SFA or vice-versa (Figures 36.1b, 36.2, 36.3). If the SFA is chronically occluded with minimal clinical symptoms prior to surgery, then an interposition graft to the PFA alone is appropriate. Although an appealing reconstruction option, small caliber bifurcation grafts (12 mm × 6 mm or 14 mm × 7 mm) fare poorly in this position. For unclear reasons, such grafts are associated with unacceptably high rates of limb thrombosis, in our experience.

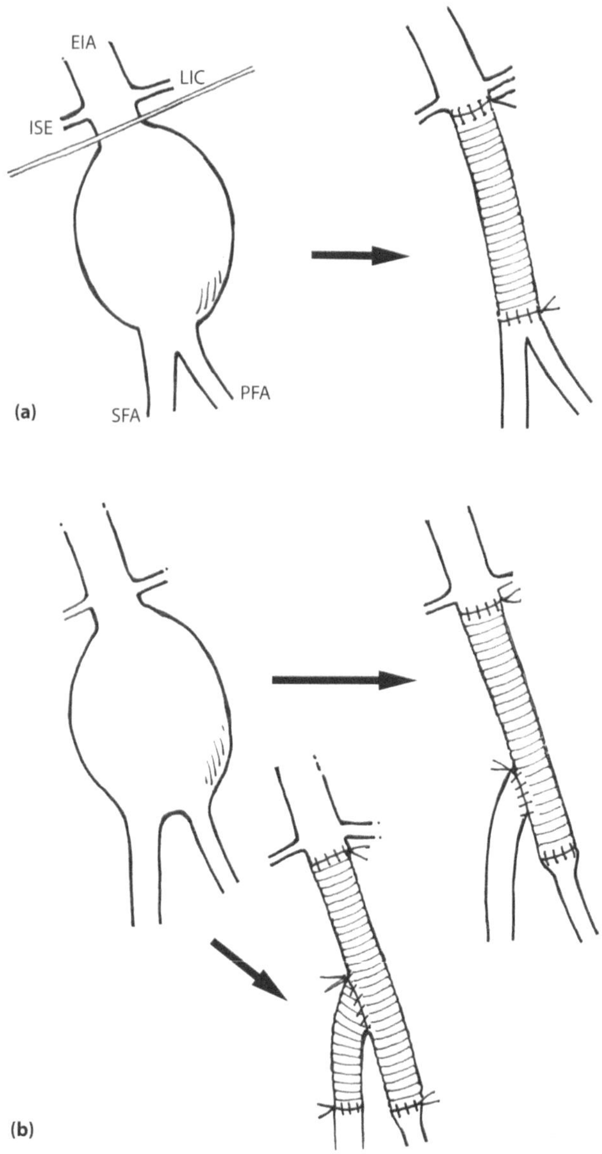

Figure 36.1 (a) Type I aneurysms are confined to CFA and can be repaired with a CFA-to-CFA interposition graft of either Dacron or PTFE; (b) type II aneurysms involve the bifurcation and can be repaired with an interposition graft to the PFA and re-implantation of the SFA or vice-versa, or with use of a second interposition graft.

Following a check for distal perfusion, anticoagulation reversal, and careful hemostasis, the wound is closed in layers. Meticulous wound closure is critical to avoid any postoperative wound breakdown, which could be catastrophic in the presence of a prosthetic graft.

FEMORAL ANASTOMOTIC ANEURYSMS

Anastomotic aneurysms have traditionally been described as resulting from a disrupted suture line between a graft

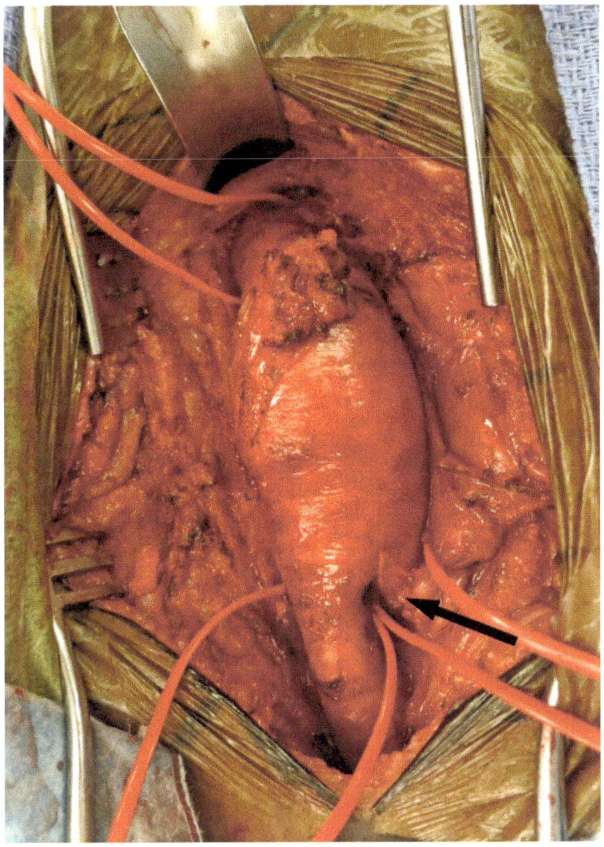

Figure 36.2 Intraoperative image of a type II femoral aneurysm with involvement of PFA origin. Red vessel loops are around CFA proximally and SFA and PFA distally. The black arrow points to PFA.

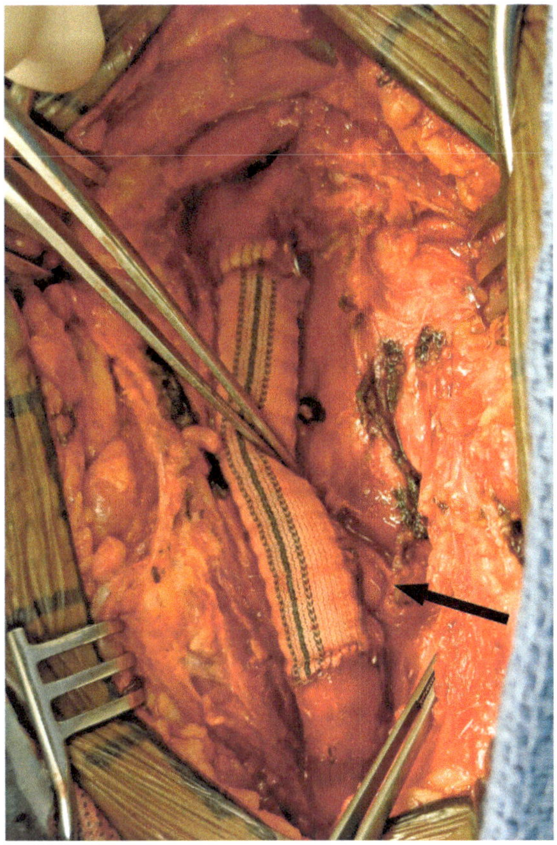

Figure 36.3 Post-aneurysm excision with end-to-end Dacron graft anastomosis to CFA proximally and SFA distally with re-implantation of PFA into the side of the graft (black arrow).

and the host artery. In the groin, this most commonly occurs at the femoral anastomosis of an aortofemoral bypass. Careful analysis, however, suggests that degeneration of the femoral artery wall is a more important contributory factor [6]. Complications are uncommon in femoral anastomotic aneurysms less than 2 cm in diameter. Larger aneurysms are associated with local complications and limb ischemia. Risk factors for the development of anastomotic aneurysms include chronic obstructive pulmonary disease, current smoking, and postoperative groin wound infection. The incidence is higher with prosthetic grafts than autogenous vein.

Clinical presentation

Anastomotic aneurysms typically present more than five years after the original bypass surgery. The diagnosis is suggested by the presence of a painless pulsatile mass in 60–70% of patients and symptoms of acute limb ischemia in another 20%. Less frequent presentations include a painful pulsatile mass and rupture. Patients may also present with a clinical picture suggestive of graft infection such as groin erythema, pain, fever and/or chills, or a draining sinus.

Diagnosis

Every patient with a suspected femoral artery anastomotic aneurysm should undergo CT angiography of the *entire* graft to evaluate for the presence of infection (i.e., gas, or fluid, around the graft) as well as to rule out any synchronous aneurysms (Figure 36.4).

Indications for treatment

In a patient who presents with history of femoral arterial anastomosis, a pulsatile groin mass and symptoms, repair is indicated. Symptoms can be pain from expansion/rupture, ischemia from thrombosis or embolization of mural clot, or venous obstruction/deep vein thrombosis from compression of the adjacent vein. Repair in asymptomatic patients depends on the size of the aneurysm (≥2.5–3 cm in diameter), the degree of associated mural thrombus, and documentation of rapid expansion.

Surgical repair

In the absence of any signs of infection, the pseudoaneurysm is ideally approached through the old groin incision that can be extended proximally or distally as needed. Occasionally, the old incision is so poorly situated that only a portion of it can be incorporated into the new incision. In rare circumstances, it is necessary to make an entirely new incision that should be vertically oriented to provide the most options for adequate exposure. Great care should be exercised in these situations because of the risk of healing complications from local wound ischemia. With very large aneurysms, proximal control can be obtained through a transverse suprainguinal incision or a balloon occlusion catheter passed from the arm into the distal graft limb or from a retrograde catheter passed from a patent SFA. Due to the re-operative nature of these cases, dense scar tissue is the rule and is best managed with sharp scalpel dissection, rather than scissors. These patients are at increased risk for postoperative lymphatic complications, hence care should be taken to ligate any suspected lymphatic channels. It is important to avoid entry into the plane between the adventitia and media of the artery, which can often seem like an "easy" dissection plane. Such an "exarterectomy" will result in a vessel wall too weak to hold stitches at the time of vascular reconstruction.

Just as with true FAAs, an attempt at control of inflow and outflow vessels should be made before opening anastomotic aneurysms. Dense scar tissue can make it challenging. Occasionally, it is easier to obtain intraluminal control with balloon occlusion catheters. Important principles to follow while performing anastomotic aneurysm repair are good vascular control, excision of the aneurysm with debridement of proximal and distal ends of vessels back to normal arterial wall, use of an appropriately sized interposition graft, anastomotic sutures placed in healthy tissue, and creation of a tension-free anastomosis. A variety of reconstruction techniques are available. Primary repair is almost never anatomically possible, and even if it is, should be avoided because such a reconstruction never addresses the root cause of the aneurysm and is, therefore, associated with an unacceptably high recurrence rate. The most frequent scenario involves an end-to-side anastomosis between a prosthetic aortofemoral graft limb and the CFA. When the proximal CFA and SFA are occluded, an interposition graft between the graft limb and the PFA is straightforward (Figure 36.5a). When the CFA is patent with significant retrograde flow into the pelvis, a decision has to be made as to whether to preserve this vessel in the reconstruction. If so, then it may be necessary to place an interposition graft between the CFA and PFA with a second interposition graft between the graft limb and this new graft (Figure 36.5b). Maintaining flow in a patent SFA is another scenario that may require re-implantation of the PFA or SFA into an interposition graft or even a second interposition graft (Figure 36.5c).

If graft infection is suspected preoperatively, removal of the infected graft and revascularization through noninfected tissue planes is indicated. The approach to this problem is beyond the scope of this chapter and is covered in more detail in the chapter on graft infections. The one exception to this rule is a prosthetic graft infection with *staphylococcus epidermidis*. This low virulence organism has been frequently cultured from uninfected appearing femoral anastomotic aneurysms resulting from prior aortofemoral bypass and has been implicated as the causative factor. Identification of this organism from surgical specimens is difficult and requires special attention by the microbiology lab to release the bacteria from its protective biofilm, but when it is found, consideration should be given to lifelong suppressive antibiotics.

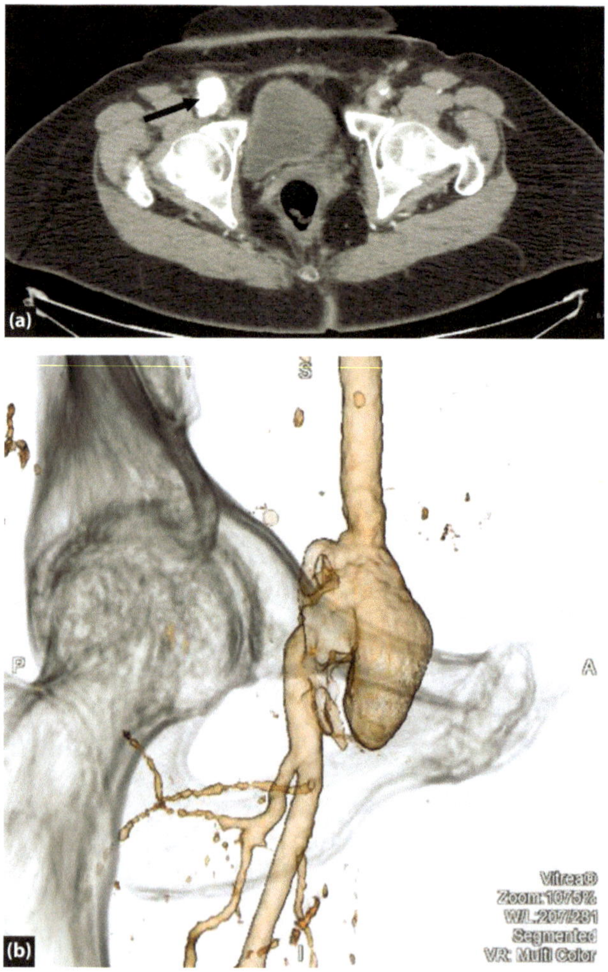

Figure 36.4 Right femoral anastomotic aneurysm (black arrow) in a 58-year-old patient five years s/p aortobifemoral bypass: (a) axial CTA image with the black arrow pointing to the aneurysm, note that left femoral artery is occluded following a prior attempted revision; (b) three-dimensional CTA image of aneurysm documenting occlusion of right SFA and outflow through the PFA.

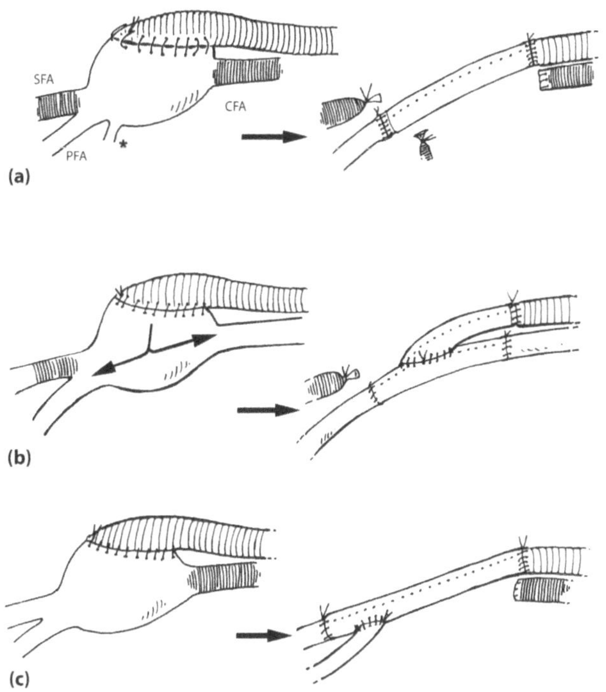

Figure 36.5 (a) When both the SFA and proximal CFA are occluded, an interposition graft between the aortofemoral graft limb and the PFA can be performed; (b) when the CFA is patent with significant retrograde flow into the pelvis, preservation of retrograde flow requires placement of an interposition graft between the CFA and PFA with a second interposition graft between the graft limb and this new graft; (c) when both the SFA and PFA are patent, distal reconstruction can be performed to the SFA with re-implantation of the PFA or vice-versa.

Postoperative care

Postoperative complications after true femoral and anastomotic FAA repair are similar and include hemorrhage, lymphatic leak, wound infection, graft infection, graft occlusion, major limb amputation, and recurrent femoral anastomotic aneurysm. Given its re-do nature, anastomotic aneurysm repair is associated with a higher incidence of local wound complications, which highlights the need for meticulous operative technique.

In general, femoral artery aneurysms can be repaired with good success. The literature reports mortality rates of less than 5%, which can be higher in emergency settings. As with all arterial reconstructions, the key to good outcomes is thorough preparation of the patient, thoughtful preoperative planning, and good operative technique.

TRICKS AND TRAPS

- FAAs are best exposed through a longitudinal groin incision.
- Proximal control is usually gained at the distal external iliac level just above the inferior superficial epigastric and lateral iliac circumflex branches.
- Complete aneurysm resection is usually easiest, taking care not to injure the femoral vein or nerve.
- Reconstruction with as short a segment of prosthetic graft as possible is best, with re-implantation of the profunda (or SFA) into the side of the graft.
- While tempting, reconstruction with a small caliber (14 × 7 mm or 12 × 6 mm) bifurcation graft should be avoided because of a higher thrombosis rate.
- Anastomotic FAAs can be quite challenging secondary to associated scarring, which is best dealt with using sharp scalpel dissection.
- Avoid groin lymphatic complications, particularly with anastomotic FAAs.
- Meticulous wound closure is critical given the presence of a prosthetic graft.

QUESTIONS

1. The most common presentation of a femoral artery aneurysm (FAA) is?
   a. Painful pulsatile groin mass
   b. Femoral neuropraxia from femoral nerve compression
   c. Lower extremity ischemic symptoms
   d. Asymptomatic

   Answer: d

2. All of the following are indications for FAA repair except?
   a. Diameter >2.5 cm
   b. Common femoral DVT from aneurysm compression
   c. Pregnancy
   d. Distal thromboembolism from mural thrombus

   Answer: c

3. Pick the true statement:
   a. The preferred graft material for repair of a FAA is the greater saphenous vein
   b. Bifurcated prosthetic grafts are a good operative option for the repair of FAAs
   c. With large FAA, it is sometimes best to achieve proximal control through a midline celiotomy
   d. Low virulence staph epidermidis is a rare cause of anastomotic FAAs

   Answer: d

4. All of the following are causes of a FAA, except?
   a. Degenerative changes
   b. Anastomosis from prior grafting
   c. Trauma
   d. Fibromuscular dysplasia

   Answer: d

5. Pick the true statement. Wound complications after FAA repair:
   a. Are minimized with anastomotic FAAs if the prior incision is used
   b. Are rarely associated with lymphatic complications
   c. Can be avoided by the routine use of transverse incisions
   d. Are of no great concern

   Answer: a

REFERENCES

1. Sapienza P, et al. Femoral artery aneurysms: long-term follow-up and results of surgical treatment. *Cardiovasc Surg.* 1996;4:181–184.
2. Graham LM, Zelenock GB, Whitehouse WM Jr, et al. Clinical significance of arteriosclerotic femoral artery aneurysms. *Arch Surg.* 1980;115:502–507.
3. Shepard AD, Jacobson GM. Anastomotic aneurysms. In: Towne JB, Hollier LH (Eds.), *Complications in vascular surgery.* New York: Marcel Dekker; 2004:139–153.
4. Sandgren T, et al. Arterial dimensions in the lower extremities of patients with abdominal aortic aneurysms: no indications of a generalized dilating diathesis. *J Vasc Surg.* 2001;34:1079–1084.
5. Lawrence PF, Harlander-Locke MP, et al. The current management of isolated degenerative femoral artery aneurysms is too aggressive for their natural history. *J Vasc Surg.* 2014;59:343–349.
6. Szilagyi DE, Smith RF, Elliott JP, Hageman JH, Dall'Olmo CA. Anastomotic aneurysms after vascular reconstruction: problems of incidence, etiology, and treatment. *Surgery.* 1975;78:800–816.

37

Iliofemoral endarterectomy and bypass

YASAMAN KAVOUSI

INTRODUCTION

Endarterectomy remains the gold standard treatment for occlusive disease of the common femoral artery (CFA) and femoral bifurcation with low 30-day mortality (<2%) and excellent five-year and ten-year patency rates (>90%) [1]. The severity of atherosclerotic disease in the CFA will determine one's candidacy for percutaneous interventions. Plaque in the CFA/femoral bifurcation with >40–50% stenosis of the CFA on pre-operative imaging studies and appropriate symptoms should be treated with open femoral endarterectomy and patch angioplasty with simultaneous aorto-iliac or infrainguinal stenting as needed. This hybrid approach represents an alternative to a purely open approach (e.g., aortofemoral or femoral-distal bypass). It is associated with less morbidity and shorter length of hospitalization [2]. In select patients, isolated CFA endarterectomy has been shown to be a safe and effective method in treating chronic limb-threatening ischemia [3].

Due to mechanical and anatomic reasons, endoluminal treatment of CFA disease remains controversial. There is no evidence to suggest that an endoluminal approach has comparable results to the open technique. Femoral endarterectomy should, therefore, maintain a prominent place in the armamentarium of every vascular surgeon.

OPERATIVE TECHNIQUE

The patient is placed supine on the operating room table. In most cases, surgery is performed under general anesthesia. However, it can also be performed under spinal or local anesthesia with monitored conscious sedation. A Foley catheter is placed. The arms are tucked to facilitate intra-operative angiography. Bilateral groins and lower abdomen are prepped and draped when there is associated iliac disease that will be addressed at the time of endarterectomy. If a concomitant intervention for infrainguinal disease is to be performed, then the groin and ipsilateral lower extremity should be prepared. Bony landmarks including the anterior superior iliac spine and the pubic tubercle are marked on the skin. A line is drawn connecting the two landmarks to mark the inguinal ligament. We routinely use ultrasound to mark the CFA bifurcation even when there is a femoral pulse. Such localization allows precise incision placement and avoids blind dissection of the CFA with the potential for creating false dissection planes risking wound complications.

An 8–10 cm vertical incision is made over the CFA and extended as necessary for adequate exposure. A transverse incision just distal to the inguinal ligament can also be utilized in cases of very focal disease that does not require endarterectomy of the deep and superficial femoral arteries (SFA). Transverse incisions have been reported to have a lower rate of post-operative wound complications, particularly in the obese. The incision is deepened through the subcutaneous tissues with the use of electrocautery or ultrasonic dissector. We have found the ultrasonic device is helpful in reducing the risk of lymphatic complications. If the ultrasonic device is not available, lymphatic channels are identified and ligated with 3-0 sutures.

Palpation of a calcified tubular artery is helpful to maintain proper orientation. The inguinal ligament serves as a landmark for the junction of the CFA with the external iliac artery (EIA). Exposure is best accomplished with large self-retaining Weitlaner, or in more obese patients, Adson Cerebellar retractors. Once the femoral sheath is encountered, electrocautery is used sparingly and with caution. Dissection at this point is done sharply with Metzenbaum scissors. However, a #15 blade scalpel is preferred in cases of "re-do" groins to facilitate dissection of the artery from the surrounding scar tissue. Dissection is kept close to the artery to avoid injury to the surrounding structures and minimize bleeding. Obtaining proximal control of the artery should be prioritized, particularly in cases of hostile groins. A right-angle clamp is used to dissect the artery circumferentially. The dissection should be performed around a plaque-free or less diseased area of the artery, where it can be safely clamped. Care should

DOI: 10.1201/9781003452096-37

be taken not to injure the back wall of the artery during this step. The inguinal ligament can be partially divided to gain access to the distal EIA just beneath the ligament. The use of a small table-mounted retractor system (e.g., Omni-Tract) is ideal for retraction of the inguinal ligament and exposure of this vessel. Care should be taken to identify the iliac circumflex vein or "vein of sorrow" that crosses anterior to the CFA at this level. It should be ligated and divided. The superficial inferior epigastric artery and the lateral iliac circumflex arteries should be identified and encircled (the author's preference is to use 3-0 silk suture to keep the surgical field less crowded). These two branches mark the junction between the EIA and the CFA and the EIA immediately proximal to them is frequently disease-free and a good clamp site. Once the artery is mobilized, it is doubly encircled with a silastic vessel loop.

After proximal control, attention is turned to identification of the femoral bifurcation, which is marked by an abrupt caliber change in the artery. The profunda femoris artery (PFA) is usually oriented posterolaterally and courses deep (Figure 37.1a). In addition, there is usually a large posterior branch of the distal CFA or proximal PFA that should always be sought and controlled prior to making an arteriotomy. The PFA typically gives rise to three main branches, namely the lateral circumflex femoral artery, the medial circumflex femoral artery, and the perforating branches. The lateral and medial circumflex

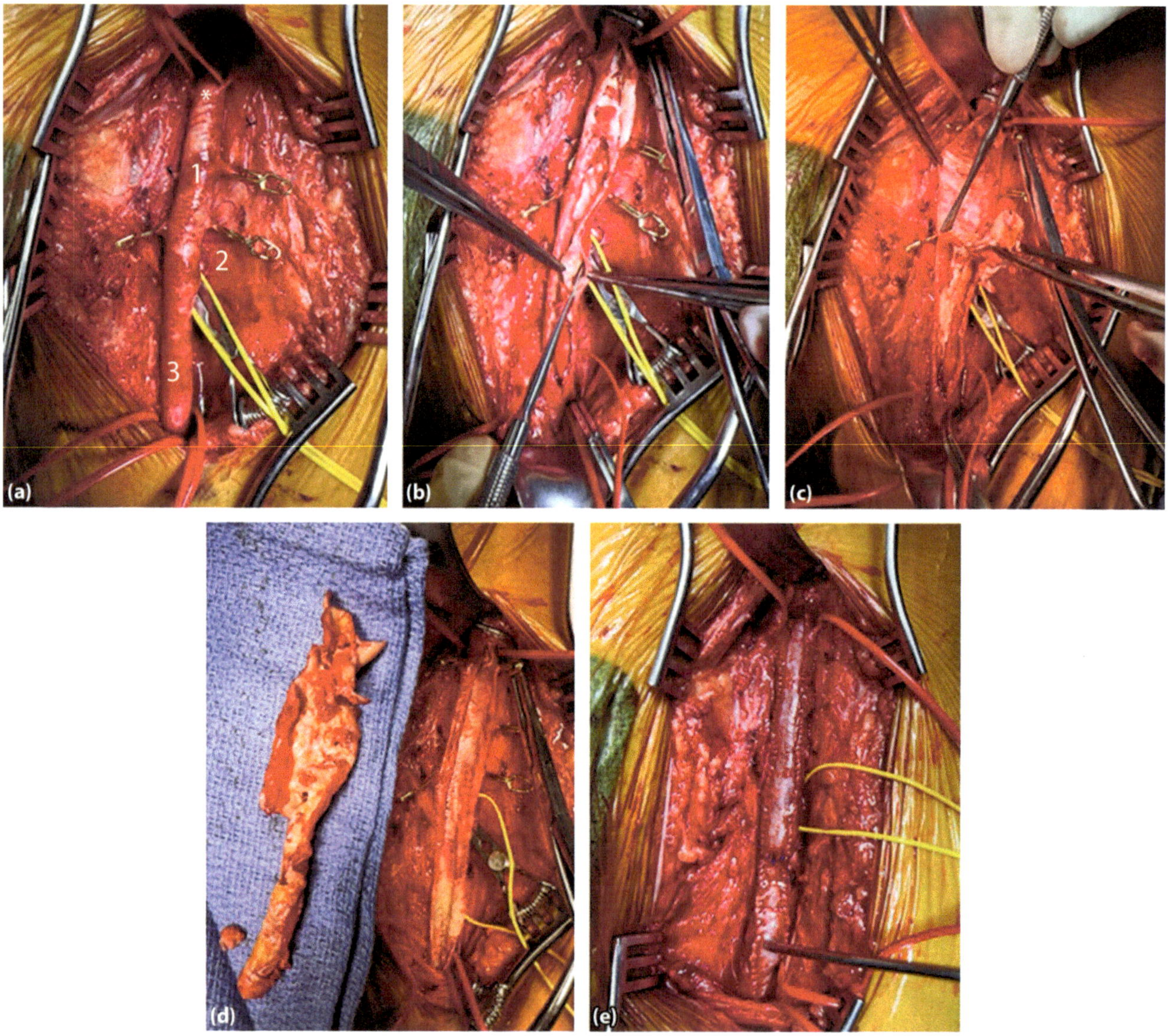

Figure 37.1 (a) Open exposure of the left common (1), deep (2), and superficial femoral (3) arteries. (*) Red vessel loop around distal-most external iliac artery just above the lateral iliac circumflex and superficial inferior epigastric arterial branches; (b) initiation of endarterectomy cleavage plane laterally at the level of deep femoral artery takeoff; (c) endarterectomy being carried distally along the medial edge of common femoral; (d) completed endarterectomy of common and superficial femoral arteries along with the origin of the deep femoral artery with excised plaque next to arteries; (e) completed bovine pericardial patch closure. Note: length of arteriotomy such that two separate patches were required for closure.

femoral arteries can also originate directly from the CFA (14% and 20% of the time). Exposure of the PFA beyond its origin usually requires ligation and division of at least one large crossing deep femoral vein that passes under the SFA and crosses over the PFA 3–5 cm from its origin. If large, this vein should be suture-ligated to prevent tie dislodgment during later manipulation with troublesome bleeding. The main PFA and its branches are encircled with vessel loops. Past the femoral bifurcation, the CFA continues as the SFA (3), which is dissected free in the same fashion and encircled with a vessel loop (Figure 37.1a).

Careful study of the pre-operative CTA is important in cases where profundaplasty is indicated for limb salvage. This review should include information regarding the extent of the endarterectomy, presence of a viable endarterectomy endpoint, and the number and location of branches in reference to vessel origin. If a longer length of PFA exposure is required, the incision should be extended along the course of the PFA and medial to the medial border of the sartorius muscle for ease of exposure.

Once all major arteries are isolated, the patient is systemically heparinized with an ACT goal of >250 seconds, which is maintained throughout the period of clamping. The CFA is clamped with a small right-angled Cooley clamp. Padded vascular clamps such as a Fogarty hydragrip can be used for heavily calcified distal EIA or proximal CFA. The PFA is clamped with a small Gregory profunda clamp. In some instances, and particularly with small PFA, gentle traction on the vessel loop may be enough control. SFA is clamped with an angled DeBakey clamp.

In cases of isolated CFA occlusive disease, once distal and proximal control is obtained, a relatively soft spot is identified on the anterior wall of the artery. Using a #11 scalpel, a small arteriotomy is created with the blade directed upward, taking care to avoid back wall injury and ensuring entry into the arterial lumen. The arteriotomy is extended cephalad and caudal using Potts scissors and should remain in the midline anteriorly. Distally, the arteriotomy is carried to the level of normal artery in the SFA. In cases of SFA occlusion, where the PFA is the only outflow artery, the arteriotomy is carried into the PFA until normal.

Using a Freer elevator, a plane is developed between the atheromatous plaque and the deeper media (Figure 37.1b). The depth of this endarterectomy plane depends on the depth of the plaque, and in some cases, the resulting wall is quite thin and should be handled carefully to avoid tearing. Very rarely, with full-thickness calcific plaque, it may be necessary to resect the CFA and replace it with a prosthetic graft. Once the plane is developed medially and laterally, the plaque is divided sharply in the middle (Figure 37.1c). The atheromatous plaque is now elevated distally, and the same plane is developed to a relatively disease-free zone. The same is done proximally. These zones may not be completely normal but it is of utmost importance to avoid overzealous endarterectomy at the end points. The goal is to achieve a smooth tapering of the plaque at both ends, but particularly distally. Leaving a slight shelf (<20% narrowing) of plaque proximally is acceptable. Residual debris and medial fibers are removed with fine forceps (Figure 37.1d). Heparinized saline on an olive-tip needle is used to identify these small and translucent fibers. If there is any concern, the distal end point can be tacked down with 6-0 or 7-0 Prolene sutures to prevent an intimal flap, which can then result in antegrade dissection of the artery and possible thrombosis. The artery is closed with a patch to prevent narrowing. Bovine pericardium is our patch material of choice (Figure 37.1e). Vein is appropriate in a contaminated field. It is important not to size the patch too large to reduce the risk of late aneurysm formation. The closure begins at either apex with a 6-0 Prolene suture, and is carried down on either side to be tied at the midway point. After appropriate venting, the suture line is completed and the clamps are serially released, starting with the PFA, then the CFA, and lastly the SFA.

Isolated profundaplasty

The PFA is arguably the most important artery of the lower extremity. Due to its rich collateral network, it can serve as a perfusion bridge between the abdominal and pelvic inflow arteries and the distal SFA-popliteal circulation. In severe infrainguinal occlusive disease, the profunda circulation is frequently spared and remains patent beyond the femoral circumflex artery. When present, atherosclerotic disease is often limited to the orifice and proximal portion of the artery. The origin of the PFA is variable. Pre-operative CTA can help define the anatomy and location of PFA.

Orifical disease can be treated with eversion endarterectomy as described in the previous section. As for more distal PFA disease, exposure is obtained through the same incision as above following the course of PFA laterally. One of the challenging aspects of distal PFA exposure is the presence of crossing veins, which should be carefully dissected and divided. Up to 10–15 cm of the artery can be exposed using this approach (Figure 37.2). Great care should be taken to preserve all small branches; we have found small Yasargil clips to be quite helpful in controlling them. Endarterectomy of the PFA is done in the same fashion as that of the CFA. It is of utmost importance to secure a good endarterectomy endpoint. Chasing the plaque further distally is not always possible. Utilization of 7-0 Prolene tacking sutures on the PFA endarterectomy endpoint can help ensure its patency.

Concomitant iliac and infrainguinal occlusive disease

Concomitant iliac and SFA-popliteal occlusive disease is frequently seen with CFA disease and can be treated with a hybrid approach. When treating external iliac lesions, the

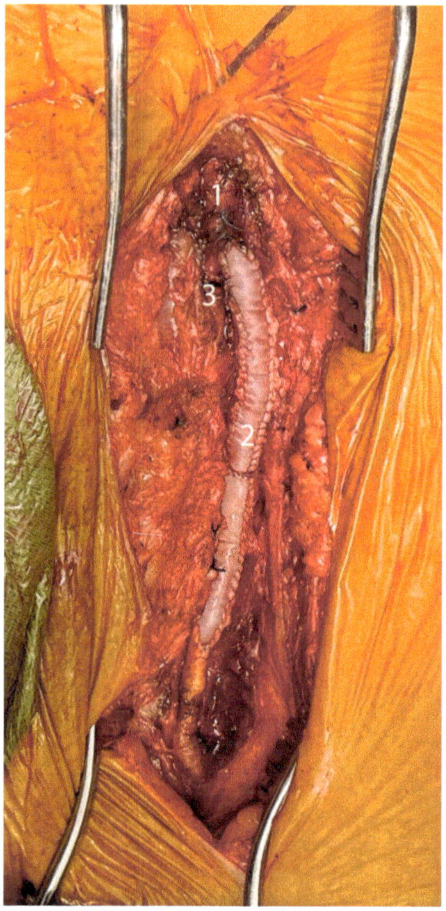

Figure 37.2 (1) Left common femoral artery; (2) isolated, extensive profunda femoris endarterectomy with bovine pericardial patch angioplasty; (3) chronically occluded superficial femoral artery.

proximal portion of the femoral patch is brought onto the distal EIA. This allows for an iliac stent (or stent graft) to extend into the proximal patch, ensuring a healthy distal landing zone. After completion of patch closure, the patch is punctured as far distally as possible under direct vision and a micropuncture sheath is inserted. Angiography is performed through the sheath to define the anatomy. The sheath is then upsized to the appropriate size depending on the size of the intended stent/stent graft. The iliac artery lesion is crossed using a hydrophilic wire and a supporting catheter. If the wire cannot be passed in a retrograde fashion, a percutaneous approach from the contralateral femoral artery, or the brachial artery, can be used to traverse the iliac lesion. The guidewire can then be brought out through the bovine patch, creating through-and-through access. Balloon-expandable or self-expandable stents/stent grafts can be placed proximally but a self-expanding stent is best to be placed into the proximal-most portion of the patch because of its flexibility that allows for clamping if needed. Sizing of the stent/stent graft is done based on pre-operative CT angiography with 5–10% oversizing.

An alternative method is to access the CFA artery prior to endarterectomy and perform iliac artery stenting first. This can be done in cases of CFA disease, where the lumen of the artery can still be accessed. Self-expanding stents should be used to stent the EIA, as they can be safely clamped during the endarterectomy portion. Alternatively, balloon occlusion can be done for proximal vascular control using an over-the-wire 5Fr balloon thrombectomy catheter with balloon inflation in the distal EIA. Once the endarterectomy has been completed and the proximal portion of the patch is sewn onto the artery, the balloon can be removed, leaving the wire in place, for subsequent stent placement, and the proximal patched artery can be clamped instead. Near completion of the patch closure, the end of the wire is brought out from the middle of the patch after puncturing it with a 19G needle. This allows for sheath insertion once the patch angioplasty is completed.

For concomitant infrainguinal interventions, the endarterectomy and subsequent patch should be carried into the SFA for a few centimeters. Prior to or following completion of the patch closure, a wire can be passed distally in preparation for intervention. In most cases, a self-expanding stent is positioned across the SFA endpoint into the patched portion. The proximal and distal patch endpoints are marked with clips for future radiographic identification.

Adjunctive techniques

Remote endarterectomy is defined as an en-bloc plaque removal of a long-segment plaque in the EIA. This is achieved by creating a cleavage between the plaque and the deep media/adventitia layer. A ring stripper that matches the diameter of the occlusive plaque is placed over the freed end of the transected plaque and advanced proximally into the EIA under fluoroscopy. The plaque is transected proximally using a MollRing Cutter™ (Vascular Architects, Inc., San Jose, CA, USA). The atheromatous plaque is then removed in one piece (Figure 37.3). The endarterectomized artery can either be stented or left alone. The proximal transection zone should always be stented. This technique can be achieved with good technical success and long-term patency [4].

ILIOFEMORAL BYPASS

Endoluminal revascularization is not always possible with chronically occluded EIA. In this situation, a prosthetic bypass from a relatively non-diseased common iliac artery can be considered. The donor iliac can be exposed through a modified lower quadrant "transplant" incision. The retroperitoneal space is entered laterally, and the peritoneal sac is retracted medially, along with the ureter to expose the psoas muscle. The EIA is identified and traced proximally to the common and internal iliac arteries. Exposure of the femoral artery is done as described

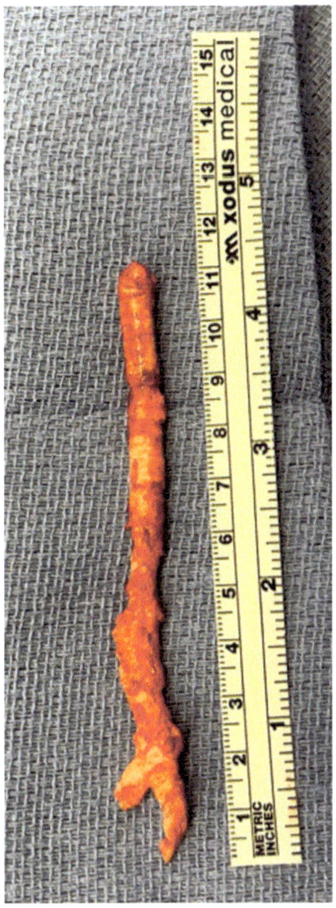

Figure 37.3 Remote endarterectomy with en-bloc external iliac–common femoral plaque removal. The bifurcated plaque at the bottom represents plaque removed from the origins of superficial femoral and profunda femoris arteries.

previously. A tunnel is created anterior to the EIA and CFA. The tunnel should pass posterior to the ureter. An umbilical tape is then passed through the tunnel. A 7- or 8-mm Dacron or polytetrafluoroethylene (PTFE) graft is used as the bypass conduit. Once the patient is fully heparinized, the common iliac or iliac bifurcation is clamped proximally and distally, and a longitudinal arteriotomy is made in a disease-free segment. An end-to-side anastomosis is performed with 5-0 Prolene after appropriately beveling the graft. Distally, an end-to-side anastomosis is performed to a disease-free segment of CFA, which frequently requires a local endarterectomy when diseased (Figure 37.4).

COMPLICATIONS

Even though femoral endarterectomy is a highly effective revascularization technique, performed via a single incision, it remains an invasive procedure with consequent morbidity, particularly in frail patients. Wound complications are the "Achilles' heel" of this procedure, and can occur in up to 10% of the cases, and include infection, hematoma, seroma, and lymph leak. The 30-day mortality is <2%. Careful monitoring of the incision is imperative

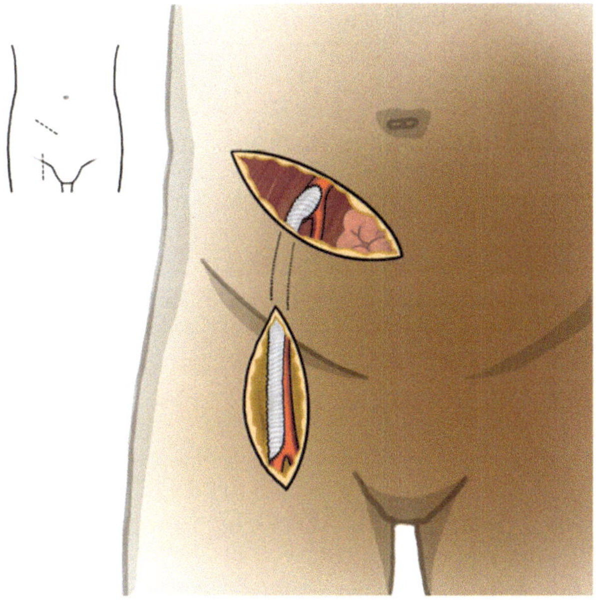

Figure 37.4 Right iliac artery to femoral artery prosthetic bypass from common iliac bifurcation proximally to femoral artery bifurcation distally.

for early identification of surgical site complications and early intervention as needed.

TRICKS AND TRAPS

1. Partial division versus lateral mobilization of the inguinal ligament can allow for more proximal CFA/distal EIA exposure.
2. Correction of proximal PFA disease is imperative for a durable outcome, particularly with concomitant severe SFA disease/occlusion.
3. Except for large-diameter CFAs with focal disease, patch closure of the arteriotomy should be mandatory. In cases of concurrent PFA occlusive disease, endarterectomy to the point of a normal PFA lumen is not always possible and the endarterectomy can be ended in partially diseased artery. Tacking sutures can be used to secure the endpoint.
4. In combined femoral endarterectomy with stenting of the EIA, the stent/endoprosthesis should be placed into the patch, preferably above the groin flexion point.
5. In combined femoral endarterectomy with stenting of the proximal-most SFA, the endarterectomy and patch should be carried down on to the SFA and the proximal-most SFA stent landed in this patch.
6. Self-expanding stents are favored over balloon-expandable stents in these two locations given their increased flexibility.
7. With combined iliac disease, iliac stenting can be performed either prior to or following femoral endarterectomy.

QUESTIONS

1. A 70-year-old man with insulin-dependent diabetes and current smoking presents to your clinic with bilateral leg pain. His symptoms are worse on the right side and are present at rest. His right femoral pulse is not palpable. He has a 1+ femoral pulse on the left side. He has dependent rubor of his right foot on exam. His ABIs are 0.3 on the right and 0.8 on the left. Arterial duplex study reveals no flow in the right common femoral artery and reduced velocities in the proximal deep femoral artery. What is the next step in management?
   a. Observation
   b. Initiation of cilostazol and smoking cessation
   c. CTA abdomen/pelvis with run off
   d. Bilateral lower extremity arteriogram via right groin access
   e. Right common femoral endarterectomy

   Answer: c

2. A 69-year-old man with hypertension and well-controlled diabetes presents with lifestyle-limiting claudication of his left lower extremity. The patient is fully risk stratified. CTA with run off is obtained, which reveals a high-grade stenosis of the external iliac artery, as well as near total occlusion of the common femoral artery. Profunda femoris artery is patent. What is the best next step in the management of this patient?
   a. Supervised walking program and initiation of cilostazol
   b. Common and external iliac artery angioplasty and stenting
   c. Common iliac to profunda bypass
   d. Common femoral artery endarterectomy
   e. Common femoral artery endarterectomy with stenting of the common and external iliac arteries

   Answer: e

3. A 59-year-old woman with history of prior tobacco use, insulin-dependent diabetes, and hypertension presents with left lower extremity pain. She reports that it has been worsening in severity and is now present at rest. She also reports nocturnal pain. On exam, she had a weak right femoral pulse. She did not have a left femoral pulse. Her ABIs are 0.35 on the left side and 0.7 on the right side. CTA with run off reveals near total occlusion of the left common femoral artery and high-grade stenosis of the proximal profunda femoris. Her superficial femoral artery is occluded with reconstitution of the popliteal artery via profunda femoris collaterals. Iliac arteries are patent bilaterally. She is evaluated in the pre-optimization clinic and deemed to be an appropriate risk surgical candidate. What is the best next step in the management of this patient?
   a. Left common femoral endarterectomy with bovine pericardial patch angioplasty
   b. Left common femoral endarterectomy with left superficial femoral artery stenting
   c. Left common femoral endarterectomy and left deep femoral artery eversion endarterectomy with bovine pericardial patch angioplasty
   d. Left external iliac to popliteal artery bypass
   e. Left external iliac to deep femoral artery bypass

   Answer: c

4. A 65-year-old man with previous history of left below-knee amputation in the setting of mid-foot osteomyelitis presents with pain in his below-knee stump four years post-op. On exam, the skin over the distal stump feels cool to touch. He reports pain at rest that wakes him up at night. He does not have a left femoral pulse. CTA with run off reveals patent left iliac system but near occlusion of the common femoral artery and occlusion of the proximal deep femoral artery. He has been ambulatory with his prosthetic leg. What is the next best step in the management of this patient?
   a. Observation and pain control
   b. Initiation of cilostazol
   c. An above-knee amputation
   d. Revision of the below-knee amputation
   e. Left common femoral endarterectomy and left deep femoral artery eversion endarterectomy with bovine pericardial patch angioplasty

   Answer: e

REFERENCES

1. Boufi M, Ejargue M, Gaye M, Boyer L, Alimi Y, Loundou AD. Systematic review and meta-analysis of endovascular versus open repair for common femoral artery atherosclerosis treatment. *J Vasc Surg*. 2021 Apr;73(4):1445–1455. doi: 10.1016/j.jvs.2020.10.026. Epub 2020 Oct 22. PMID: 33098944.
2. Piazza M, Ricotta JJ, Bower TC, Kalra M, Duncan AA, Cha S, Gloviczki P. Iliac artery stenting combined with open femoral endarterectomy is as effective as open surgical reconstruction for severe iliac and common femoral occlusive disease. *J Vasc Surg*. 2011 Aug;54(2):402–411. doi: 10.1016/j.jvs.2011.01.027. Epub 2011 Apr 30. PMID: 21531527.
3. Chaney M, Joshi G, Cataneo Serrato JL, Rashid M, Jacobs A, Jacobs CE, White JV, Schwartz LB, El Khoury R. The natural history of isolated common femoral endarterectomy for chronic

limb-threatening ischemia. *J Vasc Surg*. 2024 May 31:S0741-5214(24)01229-1. doi: 10.1016/j.jvs.2024.05.050. Epub ahead of print. PMID: 38823529.

4. Bekken JA, de Boer SW, van der Sluijs R, Jongsma H, de Vries JPM, Fioole B. Remote iliac artery endarterectomy: a case series and systematic review. *J Endovasc Ther*. 2018 Feb;25(1):140–149. doi: 10.1177/1526602817749620. PMID: 29338645.

38

Aortofemoral bypass

HASSAN CHAMSEDDINE AND ALEXANDER D. SHEPARD

INTRODUCTION

Primary operative therapy for aortoiliac occlusive disease (AIOD) has shifted from open bypass to endoluminal techniques with aortofemoral bypass (AFB) being reserved for patients with the most advanced disease. This group often presents with significant inflammatory changes associated with prior in-dwelling stents and femoral artery punctures, which can significantly complicate the arterial dissection and graft tunneling during AFB. These challenges are compounded by the infrequent performance of AFB today due to the success of endoluminal procedures.

Indications for AFB mirror those of any peripheral artery disease procedure: lifestyle-limiting claudication and chronic limb-threatening ischemia. AFB patients typically exhibit severe multilevel involvement, often featuring TASC D disease in the aortoiliac segment with heavily calcified arteries and aortoiliac hypoplasia. Juxtarenal aortic occlusion is another circumstance necessitating AFB. Simultaneous occlusive plaque in the femoral arteries is the rule and concomitant femoral endarterectomy is frequently necessary.

Like any open aortic reconstruction, preoperative assessment of the patient's cardiac, pulmonary, and renal function is necessary. Preoperative imaging options include angiography, or more commonly, a thin-cut, high-quality computed tomographic angiogram (CTA) of the abdomen/pelvis and bilateral lower extremities (LE). Imaging allows for a comprehensive evaluation of the disease and anatomy, with emphasis placed on key factors such as the degree of aortoiliac calcification, concurrent renal/visceral artery occlusive disease (with particular attention to the patency of the inferior mesenteric artery [IMA]), presence of juxtarenal aortic plaque, and any vascular anomalies (e.g., accessory renal arteries, retroaortic left renal vein [LRV]). Imaging plays a pivotal role in effective procedure planning, determining the clamp site, and identifying the need for concomitant proximal or distal endarterectomy(ies). Anesthetic monitoring typically involves an arterial line and a central line, except for high-risk patients, where transesophageal 2D echocardiography can be beneficial. The use of a Foley catheter is routine.

Operative steps

AFB is usually performed through a midline celiotomy with a transperitoneal (TP), infra-mesocolic approach to the aorta. The patient is positioned supine with the right arm tucked at the side to facilitate anchoring a mechanical retraction system (e.g., Thompson or Omni Tract) to the table. Controversy exists regarding whether to expose the femoral arteries or open the abdomen first. Our preference is to start in the groins, thus ensuring a shorter peritoneal cavity exposure time, minimizing evaporative fluid losses, and reducing hypothermia risk.

Groin exposure

Pre-incision ultrasound is utilized to determine the level of the femoral bifurcations, allowing for precise groin incision placement. In patients with absent femoral pulses, this minimizes dissection in false planes, reducing the risk of wound complications. Groin exposure is best performed through a longitudinal incision. Transverse incisions are rarely used due to their restricted exposure but may be helpful in obese patients with limited femoral artery disease to reduce wound complications. When performed in patients with multiple prior endoluminal procedures, dissection of the femoral vessels can pose significant challenges. The scarring in such patients often requires sharp scalpel dissection with a #15 blade. We have found an ultrasonic scalpel to help reduce lymph leaks in virgin groins and reserve ties only for lymph nodes and large crossing vessels. In cases of heavily scarred and re-do groin procedures, identification and dissection of a diseased superficial femoral artery (SFA), which can

DOI: 10.1201/9781003452096-38

be palpated as a firm cord just below the femoral bifurcation, is useful. Once identified, dissection proceeds proximally to the common femoral artery (CFA). After achieving circumferential control of these arteries, the profunda femoris artery (PFA) is dissected out last, with careful attention to the presence of a posterior branch of the distal-most CFA which originates at the level of the bifurcation. Failure to control this branch before making a femoral arteriotomy can lead to problematic back bleeding.

The extent of femoral dissection is contingent on the degree of disease, but even with a normal CFA, at least 5 cm of mobilized artery is needed to provide a site for a femoral anastomosis. With a diseased SFA, occlusive plaque within the origin of the PFA is typical and must be addressed to ensure an optimal outcome; failure to correct such disease compromises outflow and jeopardizes long-term patency. If this can be corrected with an eversion endarterectomy of the PFA, then only 1–2 cm of this artery needs to be mobilized. However, it is common for bifurcation disease to extend further distally, necessitating more extensive exposure. Achieving distal PFA exposure usually requires the division of at least one, and often two, crossing veins; if large, these should be suture ligated to prevent subsequent tie dislodgment during manipulation.

After completing the groin dissections, the distal portion of the retroperitoneal (RP) tunnels in the abdomen is initiated for subsequent passage of the graft limbs. A small portion of the inguinal ligament is divided when creating these tunnels. This maneuver not only reveals the distal-most external iliac artery (EIA) but also prevents postoperative graft limb compression by the undivided ligament. During this exposure, a large crossing vein (lateral iliac circumflex vein) is invariably visualized on the anterior surface of the distal EIA. Commonly known as the "vein of pain," this venous branch should be divided between ligatures to avoid injury during graft tunneling. The operator's index finger, with the fingernail down, is then passed along the surface of the EIA proximally to start the RP tunnel for the graft limb.

Abdominal exposure

Most surgeons prefer a midline celiotomy with a TP, infra-mesocolic approach to the infrarenal (IR) aorta. While a transverse incision may be helpful for patients with severe pulmonary disease because of less incisional pain, it sacrifices thoraco-epigastric collaterals, often an important source of LE perfusion in AIOD patients. Alternatively, a left flank RP approach can be used (see later in the chapter).

In the TP approach, the abdomen is opened from xiphoid to midway between the umbilicus and symphysis pubis. A table-mounted mechanical retraction system (i.e., Thompson or Omni Tract) provides excellent exposure without the need for a second assistant. The transverse colon and greater omentum are retracted cephalad, while the small bowel is packed into the right abdomen. Packing the bowel, as opposed to retracting it out of the abdomen, reduces bowel edema. Division of the ligament of Treitz enhances small bowel mobility and allows duodenal mobilization off the aortic neck (Figure 38.1). The posterior retroperitoneum overlying the aorta is incised longitudinally from the reflected duodenum to below the IMA. Cephalad dissection reveals the LRV, demarcating the proximal extent of exposure (Figure 38.2). From the lower border of the LRV to just below the IMA, an ultrasonic scalpel is used to clear the anterior surface of the aorta of overlying RP fat. The inferior mesenteric vein (running obliquely and more superficially) can be ligated/divided as necessary, and lymphatics along the LRV are ligated as encountered to avoid chyle leaks.

The aorta immediately distal to the LRV is suitable for proximal anastomosis in most patients. While the aorta at this level can be controlled circumferentially, we usually mobilize just enough to allow placement of a vertically oriented cross-clamp to avoid injury to posterior lumbar arteries. Distal circumferential control of the aorta is achieved just below the IMA, with special attention to preserving the hypogastric plexus and parasympathetic nerves. These structures course anterior to the aorta and travel caudally over the origin of the left common iliac

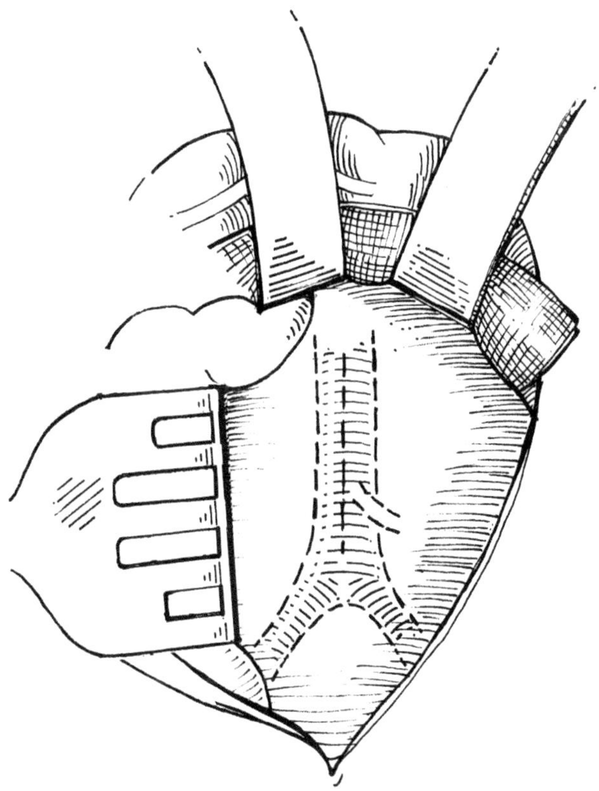

Figure 38.1 Midline, transperitoneal, infra-mesocolic approach to the IR aorta with the transverse colon reflected superiorly and the small bowel packed to the right.

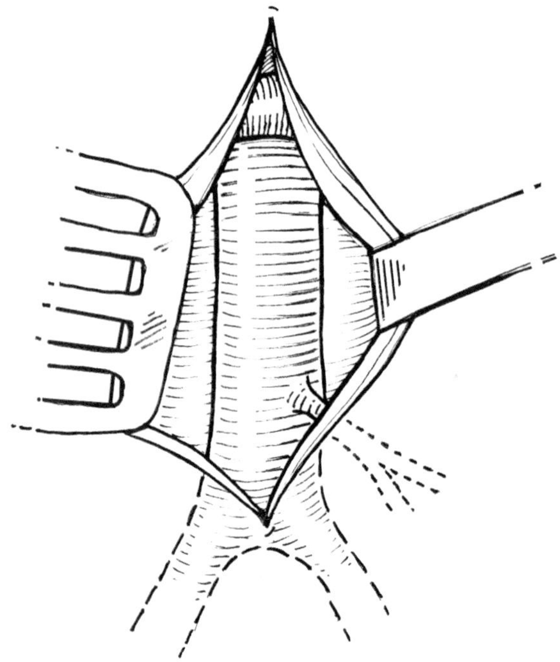

Figure 38.2 Retroperitoneal incision to expose the IR aorta from the LRV to just above the bifurcation.

artery, and their injury can lead to erectile dysfunction in men. RP tunnels from the exposed aorta to the groins are then completed with blunt index finger dissection (again fingernail down) *under* the ureters (Figure 38.3). Tunneling a graft limb anterior to the ureter poses a risk of ureteral entrapment from scarring between the limb and underlying iliac artery, potentially leading to post-operative ureteral obstruction. To demarcate these tunnels, a long aortic clamp is passed from the groin into the aortic RP space, and silastic tubing or umbilical tape is pulled through.

Reconstruction

We perform end-to-end proximal anastomoses almost universally for AFB. After heparinization to a therapeutic ACT (>250 seconds), the IR aorta is clamped just below the renal arteries after clamping the IMA, if patent. Subsequently, a TA-30 stapler (with 2.5 mm staples) is passed around the aorta and fired—just above the IMA if occluded *or* below the IMA if patent. After transection, the aorta is clamped 4–5 cm distal to the proximal cross-clamp to prevent back bleeding from intervening lumbars and the aorta is transected at the proposed proximal anastomotic site. It is important to place the proximal anastomosis close to the renal arteries to minimize the risk of future graft compromise from progression of atherosclerotic disease in this residual aortic stump. A segment of aorta is then resected to just above or below the IMA with care taken to leave a small piece of aortic wall attached to the IMA, if patent. Excision of this aortic segment creates a "trough" for the main graft shaft to lie in and facilitates graft coverage at the end of the case. Back-bleeding lumbar arteries are suture ligated as encountered.

An appropriately sized bifurcated prosthetic graft, typically 16 × 8 mm for men and 14 × 7 mm for women, is selected. Factors that are believed to enhance long-term patency include using a polytetrafluoroethylene (PTFE) graft and maintaining a short main shaft of the graft (a length of 3–4 cm). The proximal aortic cuff is prepared by removing any adherent debris or thrombus, and an end-to-end anastomosis is performed with a running 3-0 or 4-0 polypropylene stitch using the parachute technique (Figure 38.4). After ensuring a hemostatic anastomosis, the main graft is clamped, and the limbs pulled into the groins through the RP tunnels.

Graft limb anastomoses are performed to the CFAs and in the presence of bifurcation disease extended distally through the origins of the PFAs. The CFA, SFA,

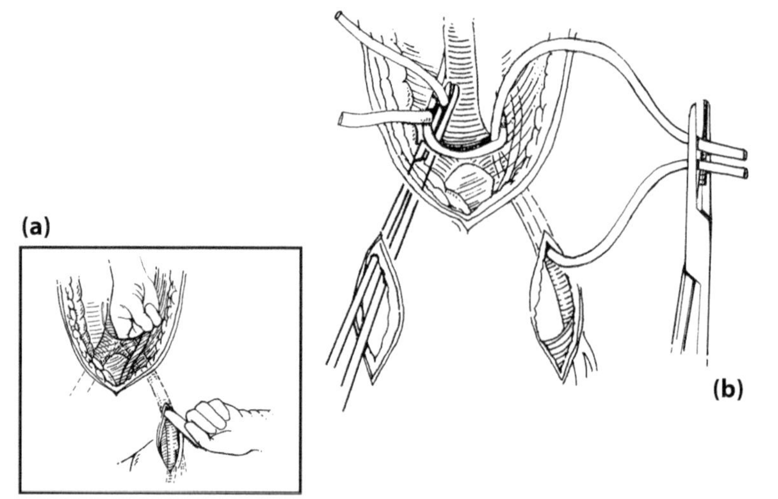

Figure 38.3 (a) Creation of retroperitoneal tunnel from the aorta to the left groin by blunt index finger dissection from above *and* below along the anterior surfaces of the iliac artery and *behind* the ureter; (b) tunnels from both groins below the ureters to the retroperitoneal space around the aorta marked by umbilical tapes.

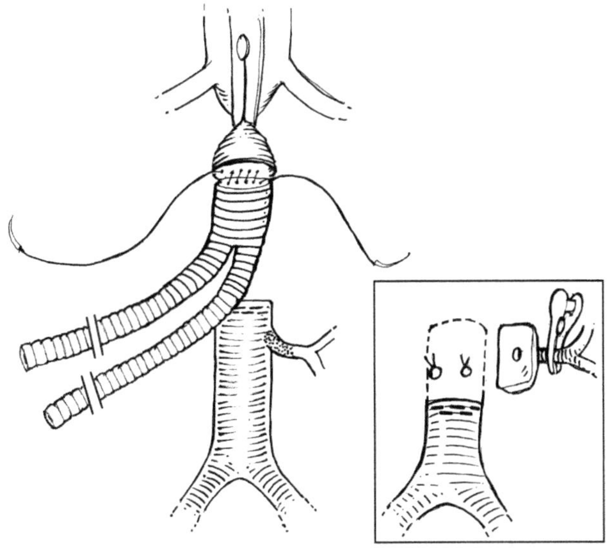

Figure 38.4 IR aorta clamped and divided with resection of a segment of aorta to the level of the IMA. The distal aorta is stapled closed (above the IMA if the IMA is occluded) and intervening lumbar arteries are ligated. A bifurcated aortic prosthesis is sewn end-to-end to the aorta using a "parachute" technique. Inset: if the IMA is patent, the aorta is stapled off below it after clamping the IMA, and the IMA and an aortic patch are preserved for possible re-implantation into the graft if back bleeding is poor.

and PFA are clamped, along with the posterior branch artery at the bifurcation. A 2.5–3 cm (longer if necessary) longitudinal arteriotomy is performed on the CFA and extended into the PFA or, less frequently, the SFA, as needed (Figure 38.5). Concomitant endarterectomy is frequently necessary to clear disease from the proximal PFA. Given this artery's role as the dominant outflow vessel in most patients with significant SFA disease, failure to do so can compromise long-term graft patency. Ostial disease in the PFA can sometimes be addressed with an eversion endarterectomy, but caution must be exercised to ensure that the vessel distal to the plaque is normal to avoid raising a distal flap that could lead to luminal narrowing/occlusion. Long arteriotomies necessitated by extensive endarterectomies can be patched by extending the graft hood several centimeters; however, in some situations, it is best to patch a long femoral arteriotomy with bovine pericardium and sew the graft limb into the patch (Figure 38.6).

After the distal anastomotic site is prepared, the proximal main shaft clamp is temporarily removed and the graft distended, pulled to length, trimmed, and appropriately beveled to fit the arteriotomy. An end-to-side anastomosis is then performed in "parachute" fashion, starting at the "heel" of the graft. Near completion of the anastomosis, the graft and arteries are "vented," the suture line is secured, and flow restored to the extremity, giving the anesthesia team adequate warning to prepare for any hemodynamic changes. Opening the CFA first, the graft limb second, the PFA third, and the SFA last reduces the risk that any intraluminal debris will embolize distally. Following completion of the other groin anastomosis, Doppler flow signals in the feet are checked to ensure patency of the reconstruction.

Back bleeding from a patent IMA is checked before reversing heparin anticoagulation. In the setting of AIOD, a patent IMA often provides collateral circulation to the lower extremities, so restoration of pulsatile flow to the femoral level is usually enough to ensure adequate IMA back bleeding, in which case, the IMA can be safely ligated. In the rare event of inadequate back bleeding, re-implantation of the IMA into the left limb of the graft is considered.

Protamine is administered to reverse anticoagulation, and after ensuring hemostasis, closure is affected. The retroperitoneum is closed over the graft in two layers before the groins are closed in three layers, followed by

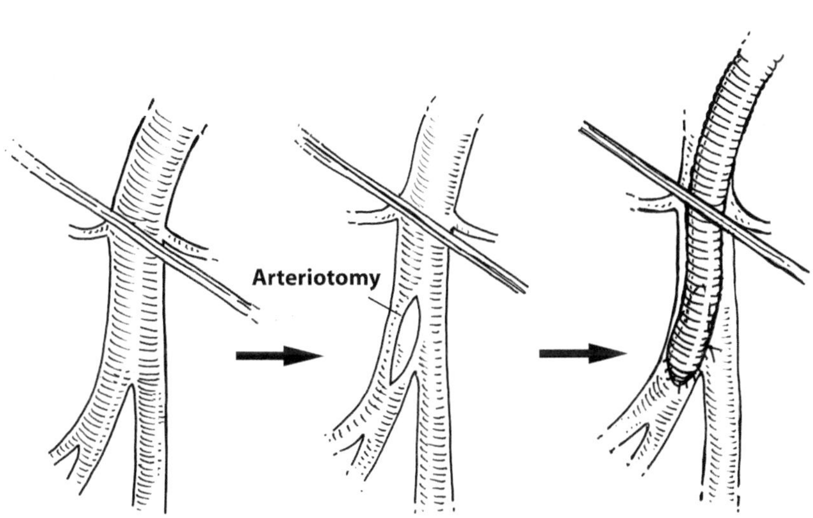

Figure 38.5 Right femoral artery exposed and opened across the profunda femoris origin in preparation for an end-to-side graft limb to femoral artery anastomosis.

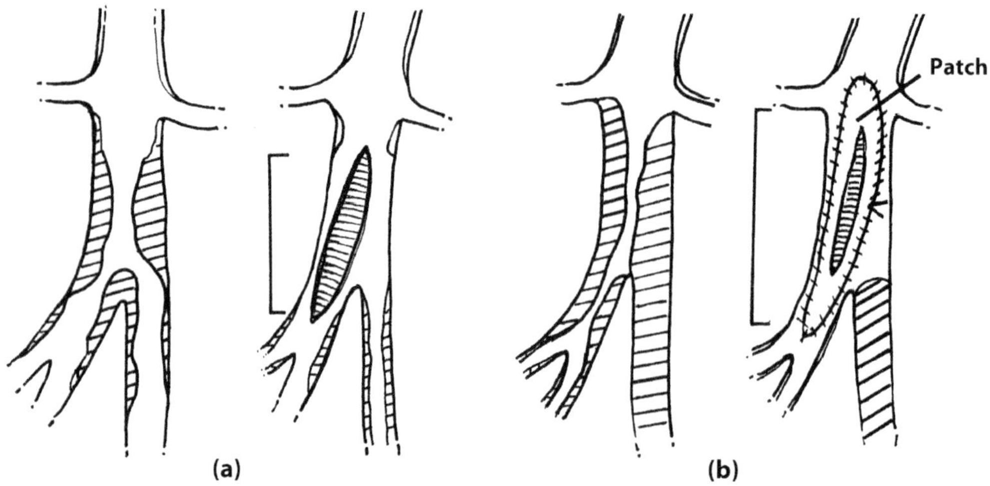

Figure 38.6 (a) Local endarterectomy of CFA and origin of PFA can be performed to clear occlusive plaque; (b) more extensive plaque requires long segment arteriotomy/endarterectomy and separate patching prior to graft limb anastomosis.

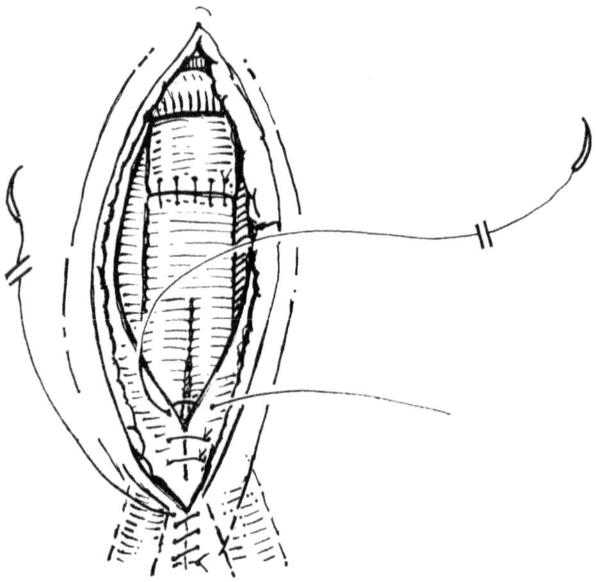

Figure 38.7 Retroperitoneal closure over the graft in two layers to avoid graft exposure to the bowel and the possibility of a graft-enteric erosion/fistula.

the abdominal wall (Figure 38.7). Negative pressure incisional wound dressings are routine for the groins.

Special circumstances

In situations when suprarenal (SR) aortic clamping is necessary, such as juxtarenal aortic occlusion, more proximal aortic exposure is required. In these cases, the LRV may be either mobilized or ligated/divided. Mobilization involves freeing up the vein from the inferior vena cava back toward the left kidney with the division of the three branches distal to the kidney (lumbar branch, gonadal, and adrenal veins) (Figure 38.8). If the LRV is to be divided, however, preserving these branches is vital for providing collateral venous outflow for the kidney. Following SR clamping, the IR aorta is transected, and the thrombotic plug is carefully removed. A sufficiently long aortic cuff should be left to allow placement of an IR

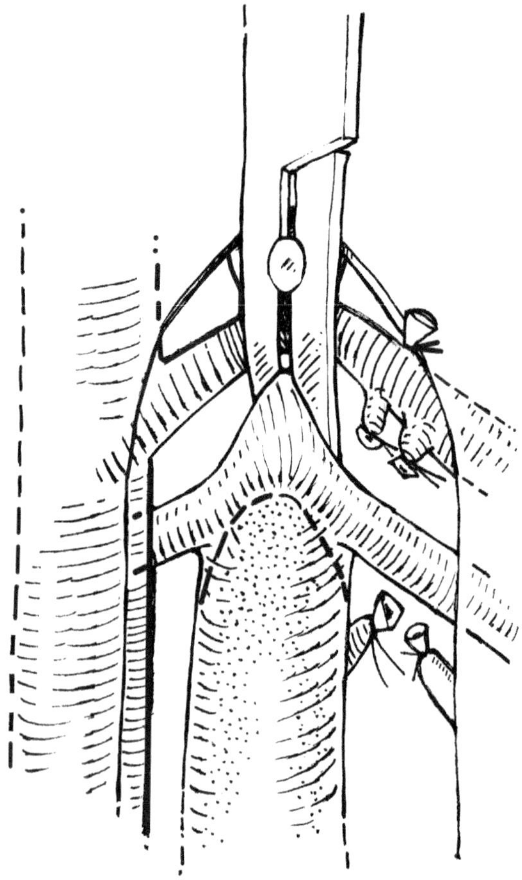

Figure 38.8 Following division of its adrenal, gonadal, and lumbar branches, the LRV is widely mobilized and retracted to allow placement of a SR aortic cross-clamp.

clamp once the occlusive plug is removed for quick restoration of renal flow.

A "porcelain aorta" (severe, circumferential calcification of the IR aorta) may also mandate temporary SR clamping to allow endarterectomy of a calcified plaque plug from the transected IR aorta. This maneuver creates an aortic cuff soft enough to accept stitches but must be performed meticulously to avoid full-thickness injury to the aortic wall. Sewing to such an endarterectomized aortic cuff is best performed with a 4-0 polypropylene on a small needle.

RETROPERITONEAL APPROACH TO THE AORTA

A left flank RP approach to the aorta is advantageous in certain circumstances. Proper positioning is key with the patient in a modified right lateral decubitus position—shoulders at 60–70° to the table and the hips rotated as far as possible posteriorly. The primary operator stands on the patient's left, rotating the table to the left for optimal groin exposure and all the way to the right for abdominal exposure. Marking the groin incisions when the patient is properly positioned is essential, as these incisions will be shifted to the patient's left compared to when they are supine. Right femoral exposure can be challenging in obese patients with an overhanging panniculus.

For IR aortic exposure, the flank incision begins at the level of the umbilicus and extends from the lateral margin of the left rectus into the 11th intercostal space for 8–10 cm. The flank and intercostal musculature are divided, and the RP space is entered at the tip of the 12th rib. The peritoneum is stripped away anteriorly as far as the rectus and an RP plane is developed behind the left kidney and ureter, which are reflected anteriorly. The peritoneal sac and viscera are retracted to the right, and the IR aorta and left iliac artery are exposed. Proximally, the lumbar branch of the LRV crosses over the aorta and serves as a reliable landmark to the origin of the LRA. This vein is ligated and divided to expose the IR aortic neck; a much larger-than-normal lumbar branch should prompt concern for a retroaortic LRV. To avoid ligating such an LRV, the aorta should be exposed anterior to the kidney. An ultrasonic scalpel is used to divide overlying periaortic fat and lymphatics along the left lateral wall of the aorta down to the bifurcation. The aorta just below the LRA is cleared off and index finger dissection anterior and posterior to the aorta creates planes for clamp placement. When SR control is required, the left diaphragmatic crus (a firm tendinous band crossing the aorta just proximal to the origin of the LRA) should be divided 2–3 cm along the axis of the aorta to expose and clear the origin of the LRA, allowing blunt finger dissection anterior and posterior to the aorta. After achieving proximal control, the IMA is identified and preserved if patent; if not, it is ligated and divided to improve exposure for the right RP tunnel. While the tunnel to the left groin is easily made from this approach, the right side is more challenging and demands care to avoid inadvertent entry into the peritoneal cavity.

After completing the vascular reconstruction and achieving hemostasis, any incision made in the left diaphragm is closed with 3-0 polypropylene and pleural air is evacuated through a temporary 16 Fr red-rubber catheter with lung insufflation. Ribs are re-approximated with looped #1 PDS, while the muscle layers of the abdominal and chest walls are closed separately with running 0 or 2-0 PDS suture.

Though more time-consuming than a standard midline TP approach, an RP approach has several advantages: a reduction in evaporative fluid losses/ileus, less incisional pain making it better for those with significant pulmonary dysfunction, better exposure for SR clamping, and avoidance of adhesions from multiple prior celiotomies.

RE-DO AORTOFEMORAL BYPASS

Re-do AFB is significantly complicated by scarring, which greatly impedes exposure and tunnel creation. Ureteral stents, inserted preoperatively, can assist in identifying and subsequently avoiding injury to the ureters. While a RP approach can aid proximal exposure, especially when SR clamping is necessary, re-do groin exposure is much more challenging. Creating a new tunnel to the right groin is undeniably the most difficult aspect of this approach and requires careful execution to avoid a right ureteral injury or inadvertent entry into the abdomen. In situations where this cannot be safely accomplished, an aorto-uni-femoral bypass to the left femoral artery followed by a femoral-femoral bypass to the right side may be considered. When severe scarring precludes IR aortic exposure, a descending thoracic aorta to femoral bypass serves as an acceptable alternative. Adopting a two-team approach to re-do groin dissections has proven beneficial. Sharp dissection with a #15 blade is preferred to avoid dulling multiple pairs of scissors, and debulking thrombosed graft segments helps create space for the new graft. This operation is highly challenging and should be reserved for reasonable-risk patients operated on by only the most experienced surgeons.

Though less frequently performed in the endovascular era, AFB remains a highly effective operation for AIOD with excellent long-term patency. Commonly encountered complications, including groin lymphatic leaks, venous injury, and ischemic colitis, can be avoided by thorough preoperative planning and careful operative technique.

TRICKS AND TRAPS

- Groin dissection prior to opening the abdomen decreases the time of peritoneal cavity contents exposure, minimizing evaporative fluid losses and hypothermia risk.

- Circumferential control of the SFA and CFA precedes dissection of the PFA.
- Control of the posterior branch of the distal-most CFA, at the level of the bifurcation, is essential before femoral arteriotomy.
- Dividing a portion of the inguinal ligament during RP tunnel creation helps visualize the distal-most EIA and prevents postoperative graft limb compression.
- RP tunnels to the groins should pass posterior to the ureters.
- A midline, TP, infra-mesocolic approach to the IR aorta is preferred by most vascular surgeons.
- The proximal anastomosis is best performed in an end-to-end fashion close to the renal arteries with a short main shaft to enhance graft patency.
- Correcting significant occlusive disease in the PFA improves long-term graft patency.
- For SR clamping from a TP approach, the LRV can be divided *or* mobilized and retracted. If divided, it is important to preserve its adrenal, gonadal, and lumbar branches.
- A left flank RP approach is increasingly useful for complex open aortic repairs, offering several advantages.
- The distal right common iliac artery and right renal artery are inaccessible with the left flank approach. Ligation/division of the IMA (if safe) improves right iliac exposure.

QUESTIONS

1. Circumstances that may necessitate aortofemoral bypass over endovascular therapy include:
   a. Prior aortoiliac interventions
   b. TASC D disease in the aortoiliac segment
   c. Concomitant significant occlusive disease in the femoral arteries
   d. All of the above

   Answer: d

2. During the creation of the distal portion of the retroperitoneal tunnels into the abdomen, it is essential to divide a small portion of the inguinal ligament to:
   a. Reveal the distal-most external iliac artery
   b. Prevent postoperative graft limb compression
   c. Prevent inadvertent ureteral injury
   d. a and b

   Answer: d

3. If the inferior mesenteric artery does not back bleed well after completing the femoral anastomoses and restoring flow, one should consider:
   a. Performing additional distal endarterectomies on the femoral arteries
   b. Administering heparin to maintain anticoagulation
   c. Re-implanting the IMA to the left limb of the graft
   d. Ligating and dividing the IMA

   Answer: c

4. Which of the following is not an advantage of utilizing a left flank retroperitoneal approach to the aorta?
   a. Improved exposure for suprarenal clamping
   b. Enhanced exposure for the right retroperitoneal tunnel
   c. Reduced postoperative incisional pain
   d. Reduced evaporative fluid losses

   Answer: b

SUPPLEMENTAL READING

1. Chiu KWH, Davies PG, Nightingale AW, Bradbury AW, Adam DJ. Review of direct anatomical open surgical management of atherosclerotic aorto-iliac occlusive disease. *Eur J Vasc Endovasc Surg.* 2010;39(4):460–471.
2. Kakkos SK, Haurani MJ, Shepard AD, Nypaver TJ, Reddy DJ, Weaver MR, Lin JC, Haddad GK. Patterns and outcomes of aortofemoral bypass grafting in the era of endovascular interventions. *Eur J Vasc Endovasc Surg.* 2011;42:658–666.
3. Sharma G, Scully RE, Shah SK, Madenci AL, Arnaoutakis DJ, Menard MT, Ozaki CK, Belkin M. Thirty-year trends in aortofemoral bypass for aortoiliac occlusive disease. J Vasc Surg. 2018;68(6):1796–1804.e2.
4. Shepard AD, Tollefson DFJ, Reddy DJ, Evans JR, Elliott JP, Smith RF, Ernst CB. Left flank retroperitoneal exposure: a technical aid to complex aortic reconstruction. *J Vasc Surg.* 1991;14(3):283–291.
5. Szilagyi DE, Elliott JP, Smith RF, Reddy DJ, McPharlin M. A thirty-year survey of the reconstructive surgical treatment of aortoiliac occlusive disease. *J Vasc Surg.* 1986;3(3):421–436.

39

Renal aneurysm repair

ABDUL KADER NATOUR AND ALEXANDER D. SHEPARD

INTRODUCTION

Renal artery aneurysms (RAAs) are rare entities occurring in approximately 0.1% of the population, with a peak incidence between the ages of 40 and 60 years. They most commonly arise secondary to congenital degenerative defects or fibrodysplasia with atherosclerotic changes as a secondary phenomenon. The overwhelming majority are asymptomatic and discovered incidentally on imaging studies. About 75% of these aneurysms are saccular and most commonly arise at the main renal artery bifurcation; 10% are bilateral [1, 2]. Rupture is the most dangerous presentation of RAA, carrying significant morbidity and mortality, and patients at risk for rupture should be repaired electively. The major risk factors for rupture are size and pregnancy. Traditionally, a 2 cm diameter was the cutoff for repair; however, current SVS guidelines recommend watchful waiting until the size is >3 cm [3, 4]. In addition, repair is indicated in patients of childbearing potential since pregnancy is associated with high maternal and fetal mortality. Symptoms of hypertension can result from fibromuscular dysplasia (FMD) aneurysms with associated stenosis and rarely from distal embolization of mural thrombus causing segmental renal hypoperfusion and vasoconstriction.

Thin-cut, high-quality computed tomographic angiogram (CTA) of the abdomen is performed preoperatively. Careful review of this study with three-dimensional (3D) reconstruction is crucial in planning operative repair as it defines the anatomy of RAA and associated arterial branches (Figure 39.1).

OPERATIVE STEPS

The patient is placed on the table in a supine position with the contralateral arm tucked to the side, which creates enough space to anchor a mechanical retraction system such as the Omni Tract or Thompson to the table. A firm foam pad is placed under the ipsilateral flank to elevate the affected kidney. A modified transverse supraumbilical ("frown") incision is best suited for these procedures, though some surgeons prefer a standard midline laparotomy to expose the involved kidney. The lower chest, abdomen, and both groins are prepped and draped. When

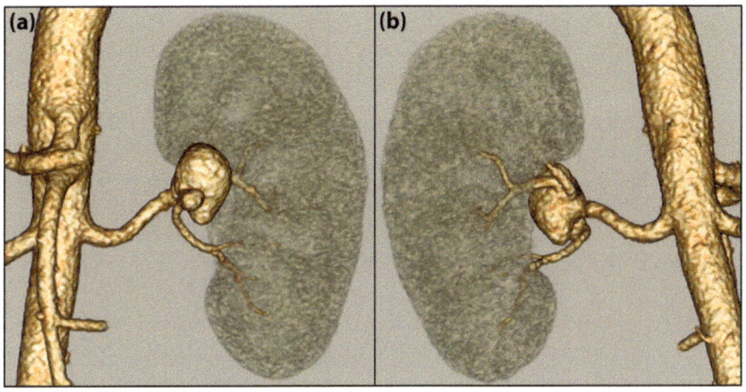

Figure 39.1 Three-dimensional CTA reconstruction of a left RA aneurysm: (a) anterior view demonstrating a lower pole segmental branch originating anteriorly; (b) posterior view showing mid-renal and upper pole segmental arteries arising in close proximity to each other from the posterior surface of the aneurysm.

DOI: 10.1201/9781003452096-39

treating unilateral disease, an upper transverse abdominal incision from the contralateral anterior axillary line to the ipsilateral posterior axillary line crossing the midline 3 cm to 5 cm above the umbilicus is made or extending to both flanks if treating bilateral disease (unusual). The incision is carried through the rectus abdominis and oblique muscles, which are divided in the direction of their fibers.

Right renal artery exposure

The small intestines are wrapped in moist pads and retracted to the left. The lateral peritoneal reflection from the cecum to the hepatic flexure is incised, and blunt dissection is used to fully mobilize the hepatic flexure, right colon, and mesentery toward the midline. The duodenum is similarly mobilized by dividing retroperitoneal attachments to the level of the hepatoduodenal ligament, which permits medial reflection of the duodenum and pancreas (Kocher maneuver), exposing the aorta, inferior vena cava (IVC), and renal vessels (Figure 39.2). The right renal vein (RV) is dissected free from its junction with the IVC to the renal pelvis and looped with a Penrose drain. Small tributaries of the right RV may require sacrifice to allow its complete mobilization and retraction off the underlying right renal artery (RA), which is usually situated posterior to it.

Dissection of the right RA is carried out in a proximal-to-distal fashion relative to the aneurysm and is carried all the way to its aortic origin. It is usually necessary to divide small branches of the IVC including lumbar veins when exposing the proximal-most right RA under the IVC. Larger tributaries should be carefully suture-ligated to avoid inadvertent tie dislodgement and problematic bleeding during IVC retraction medially off the proximal RA. After gaining control of the proximal RA, branches distal to the aneurysm are identified and controlled with small caliber elastic loops. This usually requires some dissection of the aneurysm itself, which should be minimized as large aneurysms are thin-walled and can be easily torn. Careful review of preoperative imaging will ensure that no branches are inadvertently missed. The aneurysm itself is subsequently mobilized once both inflow and outflow vessels have been controlled. Posterior branches may not be fully controlled until after aneurysm resection.

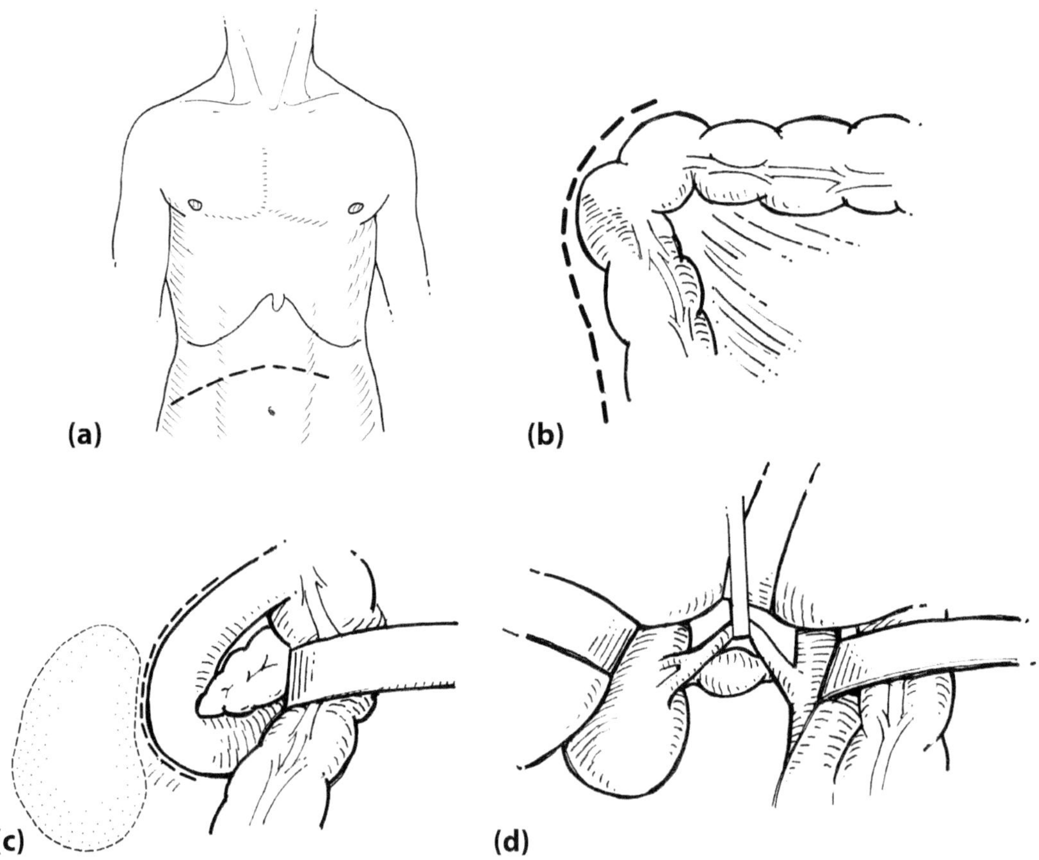

Figure 39.2 Exposure of the right RA using limited right medial visceral rotation: (a) upper abdominal, transverse incision extending from the right anterior axillary line to the left midclavicular line; (b) incision in peritoneal reflection to mobilize hepatic flexure/part of ascending colon marked by dashed line; (c) the duodenum is mobilized off the right kidney (Kocher maneuver); (d) right RA aneurysm exposed by retracting right RV cephalad after wide mobilization.

Left renal artery exposure

Exposure of the left RA follows a similar retroperitoneal dissection as performed on the right but with a partial left medial visceral rotation. The small intestines are retracted to the right. The lateral peritoneal attachments of the left colon from the level of the sigmoid colon to the splenic flexure are incised (Figure 39.3). A combination of blunt and sharp dissection, taking care not to injure the mesocolon medially, is used to develop a retroperitoneal plane anterior to the left kidney with the splenic flexure of the colon, spleen, and pancreatic tail retracted medially. This plane is more difficult to develop than a retro-renal plane. This approach provides much better exposure of the left RA, which often lies directly beneath the upper border of the left RV than from the midline through the mesocolon. The left RV is encircled with a Penrose drain and mobilized by ligating the adrenal, gonadal, and lumbar branches. This helps expose mid and distal left RA aneurysms. For aneurysms arising posteriorly off the left RA, a retro-renal approach with elevation of the left kidney can be helpful. This approach avoids the need for RV mobilization but often results in significant stretch of the left RA that can complicate subsequent repair. A left flank oblique incision in the tenth intercostal space is helpful if such an approach is chosen. Dissection of the left RA follows the same steps as the ones described on the right.

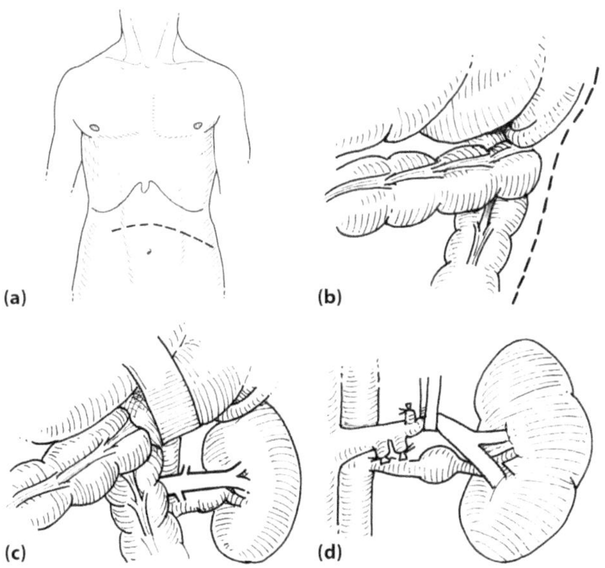

Figure 39.3 Exposure of the left RA using limited left medial visceral rotation: (a) upper abdominal, transverse incision extending from right midclavicular line to left anterior axillary line; (b) the dotted line is the incision in peritoneal reflection used to mobilize splenic flexure and the descending colon along with the spleen; (c) left kidney and left renal vasculature – the left RV is anterior to the left RA exposed by retracting the left colon and spleen medially; (d) left RV mobilized by dividing its lumbar, gonadal, and adrenal branches, and retracted cephalad to expose RA aneurysm.

After obtaining proximal and distal control and mobilization of the aneurysm, the patient is systemically heparinized to achieve an activated clotting time of ≥250 seconds. We routinely administer 25 g of mannitol 20 minutes prior to clamping to induce osmotic diuresis, though recent studies have questioned mannitol's renal protective effect. Regardless, we ensure that the patient is volume-loaded with a good urine output prior to clamping. When the RA clamp time is expected to be more than 30 minutes *or* in the presence of baseline significant kidney disease, we strongly encourage the utilization of renal cooling strategies. Our preferred approach is cold renal perfusion using an iced Ringers lactate solution (4°C containing heparin, mannitol, and methylprednisolone). Following proximal RA clamping, the distal RA is infused with 300 cc of this solution over 5–6 minutes. With larger aneurysms, a balloon-tipped irrigation catheter or a 16G angiocath can be placed directly into the aneurysm. Alternatively, a pediatric feeding tube can be used to perfuse individual branches after opening the aneurysm while taking great care not to injure them. After perfusion is complete, the distal arteries are occluded with microvascular clamps. We prefer to use Yasargil (cerebral aneurysm) microclips for the small caliber vessels. These low-profile clips reduce the clutter associated with larger clamps and provide a less-obstructed surgical field. Small conventional clamps are suitable for the main renal artery. Afterward, the aneurysm sac is resected, leaving a small rim of aneurysmal tissue attached to the ostia of the involved arteries. Care must be taken to preserve all sizeable branches including those originating from the posterior surface of the aneurysm. Subsequent reconstruction might be difficult, if not impossible, if these vessels are inadvertently trimmed too short.

RECONSTRUCTION TECHNIQUES

In situ reconstruction techniques available for RAA repair include aneurysmorrhaphy (defined as excising only the aneurysmal portion of a saccular RA aneurysm) with primary angioplastic closure or patch angioplasty, and the more commonly performed aneurysm resection with either bypass (aorto-renal or splanchnic-renal) or interposition vein grafting. When chosen appropriately in accordance with the patient's RA and aneurysm anatomy, studies have shown that there is little to no difference in short- or long-term outcomes between these different types of reconstruction.

Generally, the most suited for aneurysms involving the main RA are aorto-renal bypass or interposition grafting (Figure 39.4). For patients with saccular aneurysms, resection with primary closure is most commonly performed, or vein patch angioplasty if there are concerns the artery will be narrowed. When using primary closure, it is important to leave a small (1–2 mm) rim of aneurysmal wall attached to the artery to minimize the risk of luminal narrowing with vessel closure. The use of interrupted

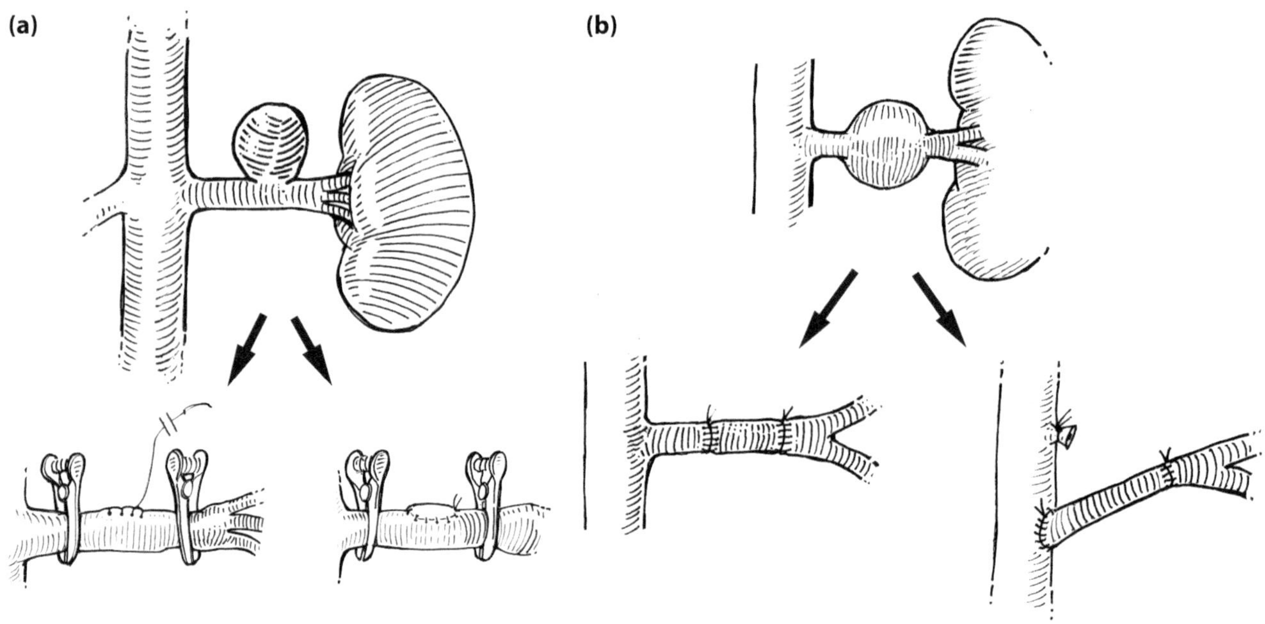

Figure 39.4 Repair techniques for aneurysms of the main RA: (a) saccular aneurysms can be primarily repaired with lateral aneurysmorrhaphy or patch closure; (b) full circumference aneurysms require interposition grafting or aortorenal bypass.

stitches as opposed to a running suture may also be helpful in avoiding luminal narrowing. In the setting of RAA associated with FMD, aorto-renal bypass may reduce the risk of future complications from retaining potentially diseased artery wall. Aorto-renal and extra-anatomic bypasses from the hepatic or splenic arteries may also be suited for aneurysms involving the main RA.

Aneurysms involving branch points (most commonly at the main RA bifurcation) are more frequent than main RA aneurysms and require more complex repairs. As with main RAAs, saccular aneurysms are best treated with aneurysmorrhaphy with or without patching. However, salvage of all branches frequently requires resection and grafting with or without branch reimplantation (Figure 39.5). A common orifice for reimplantation or bypass can be created in cases where separate branches arise in close proximity to each other after aneurysm excision. In most reconstructive cases, saphenous vein grafts are the preferred conduits over prosthetic grafts. However, in young patients with large caliber main renal arteries, a prosthetic graft is probably adequate as it avoids the very long-term risk of vein graft aneurysmal degeneration. An alternative when small branches of the main renal artery are involved is to use the hypogastric artery as a branched autologous graft. This technique is usually reserved for very young patients. Regardless of the method used, meticulous technique with loupe magnification and fine (6-0 or 7-0) polypropylene suture is mandatory. For very small branches, interrupted sutures as opposed to running may be more appropriate to avoid "purse-stringing" the anastomosis. At the completion of the reconstruction, technical adequacy is confirmed with intraoperative duplex scanning, and any significant defect is fixed immediately.

OTHER MODALITIES

Aneurysm plication. Plication of small (<1 cm in diameter) branch aneurysms is recommended when encountered during operations for larger, clinically significant aneurysms. The redundant arterial wall is oversewn with a running 6-0 or 7-0 polypropylene suture. Aneurysms involving very distal branches supplying limited parenchyma can be sacrificed with little to no consequences and are best addressed with endovascular techniques.

Ex vivo repair with auto-transplantation. This approach may be helpful if multiple or distal complex branch vessels are involved, if the cause of the renal artery aneurysm is dissection resulting in vessel friability, or if renal ischemia is expected to be >45 minutes. A complete description of this approach is beyond the scope of this chapter.

Nephrectomy. Nephrectomy is the best approach in patients with uncontrollable rupture of a RAA. It may also be appropriate for non-reconstructible aneurysms or aneurysms in the presence of a nonfunctioning, atrophic kidney.

ENDOVASCULAR REPAIR

Endovascular stent-graft exclusion using covered stents can be performed for main RAAs with adequate proximal and

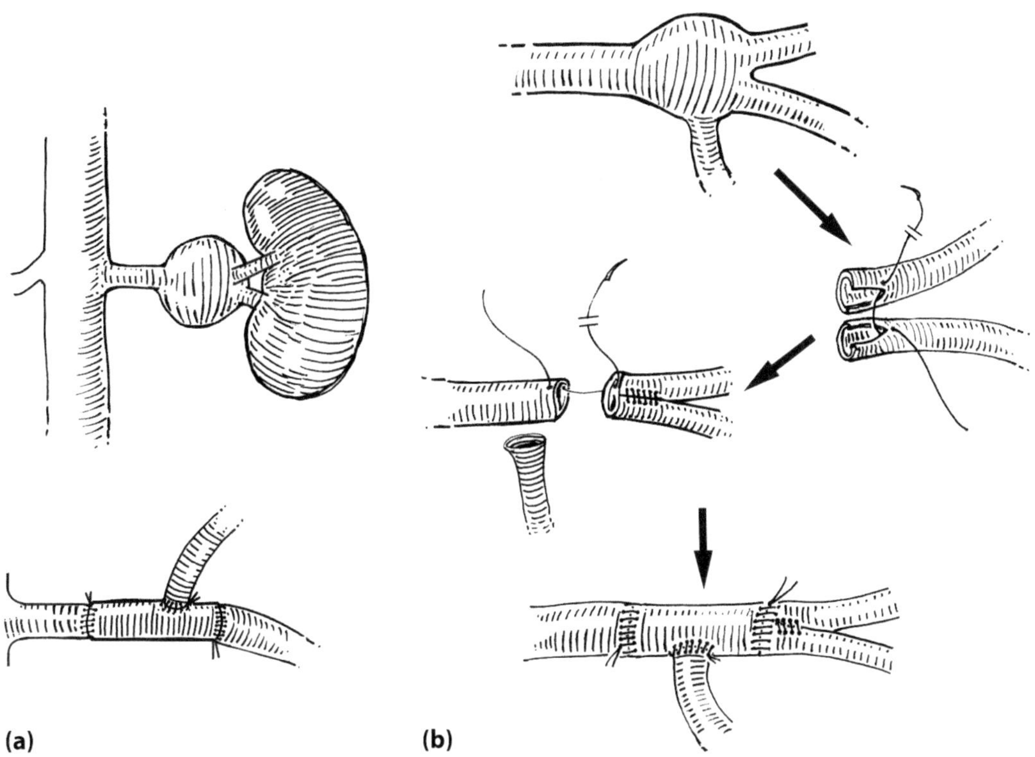

(a) (b)

Figure 39.5 Repair techniques for aneurysms involving RA bifurcation or branch arteries: (a) vein interposition graft to the larger RA branch with reimplantation of the smaller branch; (b) two large branches sewn together to create a common outflow for an interposition vein graft on which a third branch is reimplanted.

distal seal zones, particularly in patients with poor operative risk. Long-term data on patency of such reconstructions is lacking. However, inferring from contemporary experience with small caliber stent grafts in the performance of branched endograft repair of thoracoabdominal aneurysms, patency of these grafts is probably reasonable though probably inferior to an open reconstruction. Embolization techniques can be used for distal intraparenchymal aneurysms where there is a low risk for significant loss of renal mass. The risk of inducing renovascular hypertension from the small segments of ischemic parenchyma must be weighed against the risk of the aneurysm. Narrow-based saccular aneurysms, regardless of their location, can be treated with coil embolization using techniques like those utilized for cerebral artery aneurysms. Detachable coils are preferred in these scenarios to minimize the risk of coil malpositioning or distal embolization. In cases of wide-mouthed saccular aneurysms, stent-assisted coiling as with intracerebral aneurysms is helpful. A jailing technique is utilized where the stent is placed across the neck of the aneurysm after the sac has been microcatheterized. Coils are subsequently deployed through the microcatheter to induce aneurysm sac thrombosis [5].

POSTOPERATIVE CARE

Patients with prolonged renal ischemia may experience a significant diuresis during the immediate postoperative period which requires careful attention to intravenous fluids' administration and close monitoring of electrolytes, particularly potassium and magnesium levels. Acute thrombosis of the reconstructed renal artery may be heralded by a sudden drop in urine output. Occlusions of smaller branches are usually well-tolerated, though a significant volume of renal parenchymal ischemia can cause renovascular hypertension. A thin-cut surveillance CTA is obtained prior to discharge to ensure a technically adequate repair. An antiplatelet agent plus a statin are maintained for at least six months. Outpatient follow-up includes a renal duplex every six months for the first two years, plus regular checks of blood pressure and renal function. Any concerns should be addressed with a CTA or a catheter-directed arteriogram. Renal artery dissection after endovascular repair may occur and should be addressed prior to leaving the OR suite.

OUTCOMES

Renal artery aneurysm repair is an uncommonly performed operation that can be quite challenging. Open repairs should only be performed in reasonable-risk patients by experienced surgeons in centers of excellence. Under these circumstances, open renal artery reconstructions have durable outcomes with excellent long-term patency (95%) and freedom from recurrence. Up to 75% of patients have reported improvement in hypertension. Short- and mid-term outcomes of endovascular repair demonstrate a low risk of rupture and improved hypertension and renal function, though long-term patency rates are poorly documented.

TRICKS AND TRAPS

- A modified transverse supraumbilical ("frown") incision provides excellent operative exposure.
- Wide mobilization of the overlying renal vein is usually necessary for adequate RA exposure.
- Dissection of the RA is carried out in a proximal-to-distal fashion relative to the aneurysm.
- Dissection of the aneurysm itself should be minimized until adequate proximal control has been achieved as large aneurysms are thin-walled and easily torn.
- When anticipating RA clamp times >30 minutes, consider utilizing renal cooling strategies.
- Preserve and reconstruct all sizeable arterial branches.
- A common orifice for bypass can be created in cases where separate branches arise near each other after aneurysm excision.
- For small branches, consider interrupted sutures to avoid "purse-stringing" the anastomosis.
- Utilize intraoperative duplex for quality control, repairing any significant defects immediately.

QUESTIONS

1. The most common cause of a renal artery aneurysm (RAA) is?
   a. Fibromuscular dysplasia
   b. Atherosclerosis
   c. Pregnancy-related hormonal changes
   d. Degenerative changes in the arterial wall that may have a congenital basis

   Answer: d

2. The most common location for a RAA is?
   a. Ostium
   b. Proximal 1/3
   c. Middle 1/3
   d. At distal branch points

   Answer: d

3. Pick the true statement:
   a. The diagnostic modality of choice for a RAA is MRI because it avoids the use of radiocontrast media
   b. A high-quality thin-cut CTA is the best method to plan the operative repair of a RAA
   c. Duplex ultrasound scanning is only helpful as a preoperative test
   d. Completion angiography is highly recommended following repair of a RAA

   Answer: b

4. Endovascular RAA repair is a reasonable option in all of these situations except:
   a. An elderly, frail patient
   b. A localized aneurysm of the main RA with 1.5 cm proximal and distal landing zones
   c. A large aneurysm of the distal RA involving multiple branches
   d. A distal intraparenchymal aneurysm of a small branch artery

   Answer: c

5. All the following statements are false except:
   a. Wide mobilization of the renal vein should be avoided during RAA repair because of the risk of bleeding
   b. A midline, infra-mesocolic approach is the best exposure for most RAAs
   c. The greater saphenous vein is the best conduit if interposition grafting is necessary for RAA repair
   d. Preservation of all branches is unnecessary—only the major outflow artery from a RAA needs be reconstructed

   Answer: c

REFERENCES

1. Henke PK, Cardneau JD, Welling TH, et al. Renal artery aneurysms: a 35-year experience with 252 aneurysms in 168 patients. *Ann Surg*. 2001;234:454–62.
2. Klausner JQ, Lawrence PF, Harlander-Locke M, et al. The contemporary management of renal artery aneurysms. *J Vasc Surg*. 2015;61978–84. doi10.1016/j.jvs.2014.10.107.
3. Coleman DM, Stanley JC. Renal artery aneurysms. *J Vasc Surg*. 2015;62(3):779–85. doi:10.1016/j.jvs.2015.05.034.
4. Chaer RA, Abularrage CJ, Coleman DM, et al. The Society for Vascular Surgery clinical practice guidelines on the management of visceral aneurysms. *J Vasc Surg*. 2020;72(1S):3S–39S. doi:10.1016/j.jvs.2020.01.039.
5. Wang Y, Song S, Zhou G, et al. Strategy of endovascular treatment for renal artery aneurysms. *Clin Radiol*. 2018:73:414–19. doi.org/10.1016/j.crad.2017.11.009.

40

Infrainguinal bypass for lower extremity arterial occlusive disease

JAMAL JAWAD HOBALLAH, HASSAN CHAMSEDDINE, AND MARWAN BAHMAD

INTRODUCTION

Despite the advances in endovascular technology, infrainguinal bypass (IIB) continues to play a pivotal role in the management of patients with chronic limb-threatening ischemia. This chapter will focus on the technical aspects of conducting IIB. Simply put, the outcome of an IIB depends on planning, procedural execution, and strategic follow-up.

PLANNING

In planning an IIB, the surgeon needs to identify a dependable inflow artery, select the most appropriate outflow vessel, and connect these two with the best available conduit.

Preoperative evaluation of the inflow and outflow vessels

The selection of appropriate inflow and outflow vessels is dependent on a good-quality preoperative imaging study. A digital subtraction angiography (DSA) or a thin-cut computed tomography angiography (CTA) that includes the foot vessels is ideal for providing the needed information. In patients with renal dysfunction, a CO_2 angiogram can provide the needed information. Rarely, an on-table pre-reconstruction angiogram may be needed to further confirm the target artery. Preoperative duplex evaluation of the target vessel may complement the selection made by DSA or CTA by locating the segment least affected by calcification and guiding the selection of the distal anastomosis site. It is our practice to routinely interrogate the distal tibial arteries and pedal vessels preoperatively with duplex. The availability of a single-segment venous conduit can also influence the selection of the inflow and outflow vessels. A single-segment vein shorter than what is ideally needed can push for the selection of a more distal inflow source or a more proximal outflow vessel.

Inflow vessels

The most distal disease-free inflow source proximal to the occlusive pathology is chosen to allow for a shorter bypass. The common femoral artery (CFA) is frequently selected as it is usually less involved with the occlusive pathology, is easily accessible, and allows for a generous non-hampered anastomosis. In the presence of concomitant iliac artery stenosis, an intraoperative iliac angioplasty and stenting can be performed.

In cases of prior surgery in the groin (e.g., aorto-bifemoral bypass), avoiding re-exposure of the CFA is desired and a more distal inflow vessel (e.g., the profunda femoris artery) may be chosen. The superficial femoral artery (SFA) can also be used as an inflow vessel if it is relatively free of disease [1], typically proximal to the adductor canal where it is easily accessible. If the length of available vein is limited and in the presence of significant SFA disease, balloon angioplasty/stenting of the SFA can be performed and the popliteal artery can then be used as the inflow source [2]. The infrageniculate popliteal artery can be selected as it is usually disease-free and will provide a shorter bypass to the tibial or pedal vessels, especially in the presence of a limited vein conduit.

Outflow vessels

The larger and most accessible outflow vessel that provides non-obstructed pulsatile flow to the ischemic area in the foot is the most desired site for the distal anastomosis. If possible, it is logical to select the target vessel that supplies the angiosome or woundosome of the foot when tissue loss is present.

DOI: 10.1201/9781003452096-40

If both the anterior and posterior tibial arteries are potential targets, the posterior tibial artery (PTA) is usually preferred due to easier exposure and tunneling. In diabetic patients, it is not uncommon to find that the only revascularization option to the foot is through the peroneal artery, which contributes to pedal flow indirectly through its terminal branches [3]. The pedal vessels can also be used as targets for the distal anastomosis if a more suitable tibial artery is not available [4,5].

Preoperative conduit evaluation

A key step in the construction of an IIB is the evaluation of available vein conduits by a venous duplex examination. Saphenous veins with diameters smaller than 3 mm have been associated with lower patency rates [6]. If the ipsilateral great saphenous vein (GSV) is not available, autogenous conduit options include the contralateral GSV, the short saphenous vein, and arm veins. Prosthetic conduits are typically used as a last resource as they are associated with poorer outcomes.

Bypass configuration

The decision to perform a reversed, non-reversed/translocated, or in-situ vein bypass is based on the surgeon's preference, experience, and the GSV diameter. If the vein has a good diameter (≥3.5 mm), all three configurations are comparable [7,8]. If the vein has a uniform diameter throughout its length, the reversed configuration is attractive as it avoids dealing with the valves and the associated risks. However, if the vein has a large diameter at the saphenofemoral junction and a small diameter distally (~3 mm), a reversed bypass could result in a size mismatch between the vein and inflow and outflow arteries. In this case, a non-reversed/translocated or in-situ bypass may be preferred, using the larger end of the vein at the proximal anastomosis and the smaller end for the distal anastomosis. The disadvantage of not reversing the vein relates to the valves—valvulotomy can result in an incomplete cutting of a valve leaflet, missing the valve completely, or inadvertent vein wall injury. Another disadvantage of the in-situ bypass is the higher incidence of wound complications, which can jeopardize the subcutaneously located bypass [9]. In the reversed and non-reversed configurations, the bypass can be tunneled in a fresh location out of harm's way in the case of infection or wound breakdown.

Inflow and outflow procedures

In patients with combined inflow and outflow disease, the bypass procedure may be done simultaneously with the inflow procedure, often as a hybrid procedure involving CFA endarterectomy and iliac artery angioplasty/stenting. Most surgeons avoid combining *open* inflow procedures (e.g., aorto-bifemoral bypass) with distal bypasses due to increased complications.

EXECUTION

Infrainguinal bypasses can be performed under general or regional anesthesia with advantages and disadvantages of both.

VEIN HARVESTING

Harvesting of the GSV can be done using a single longitudinal incision or using multiple 5–10 cm incisions with 3 cm bridges of skin to avoid a very long skin incision with potential healing issues. The key principle is to harvest the vein in the least traumatic way without predisposing the incision to healing issues. Vein mapping by inking the skin overlying it preoperatively helps avoid creating unnecessary skin flaps and defines potential venous anomalies that could be present. Branches are ligated at least 1 mm from the vein wall to avoid a constricting adventitial waist or band at the site of the ligature. The vein is typically flushed with heparinized saline or heparinized cold blood.

When a single-segment vein that can connect the selected inflow and target vessels cannot be secured, a composite or spliced vein bypass can be performed. Very acceptable outcomes have been achieved with the all-autogenous composite vein bypasses, especially when coupled with an intensive postoperative surveillance protocol. Selected vein segments will depend on vein availability and the best configuration that prevents a size mismatch between the vein and the target outflow vessel. One technique is to use one segment in a reversed fashion with the second segment used in a non-reversed fashion after valvulotomy. A composite bypass may also be made of a prosthetic bypass joined to a vein segment, though such bypasses may not provide any patency advantage over a prosthetic bypass with an adjunctive distal anastomotic patch.

EXPOSURE OF THE INFLOW AND TARGET VESSELS

Most of the lower extremity target vessels are exposed through a medial approach except for the anterior tibial artery which is located on the lateral aspect of the leg. The peroneal artery can also be exposed laterally, typically requiring excision of a segment of the fibula.

Common femoral artery

The CFA and the proximal part of the SFA are exposed through a longitudinal incision placed over the femoral pulse. The artery is dissected sharply, and overlying lymphatics ligated and divided. When the CFA is very diseased, an endarterectomy may be necessary. Exposure of the external iliac artery at the level of the inferior epigastric vessels will typically identify a disease-free segment suitable for safe clamping. It is essential when performing a CFA endarterectomy to preserve flow to the profunda femoris artery (PFA). Tacking of the distal end point or extending the endarterectomy distally as needed into the PFA may be necessary. The arteriotomy can be closed preferentially using a patch or by including it in the proximal IIB anastomosis.

Profunda femoris artery

The PFA can be approached by extension of the initial longitudinal incision. Alternatively, and preferably in redo procedures, the PFA can be approached through a lateral approach, lateral to the sartorius muscle, which avoids previous groin scarring. Division of crossing veins is typically needed to provide adequate exposure.

Superficial femoral artery

The SFA can be reached through the same incision used for vein harvesting. After deepening the incision through the subcutaneous tissue until the sartorius muscle is identified, the overlying fascia is divided, and the SFA is identified deep to the sartorius muscle.

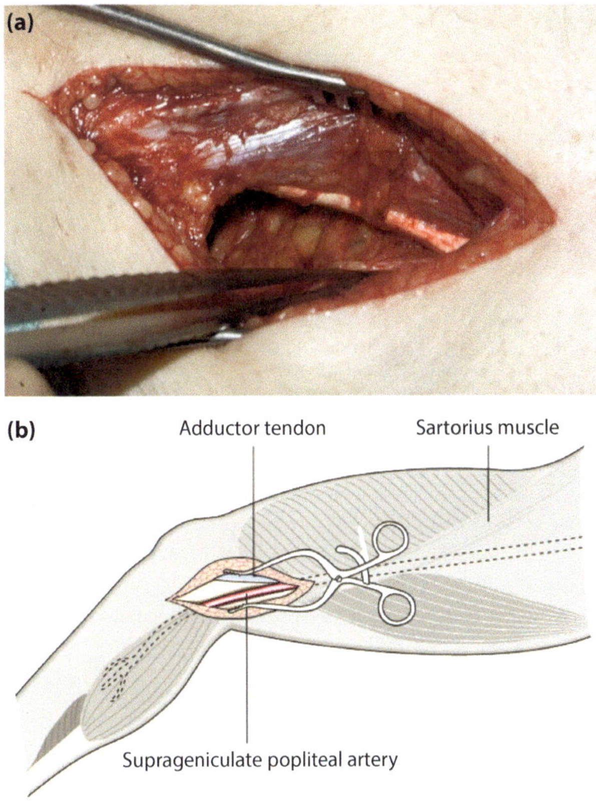

Figure 40.1 (a) Above-knee popliteal artery exposure showing the adductor tendon; (b) the abductor tendon is retracted superiorly and the sartorius muscle is retracted inferiorly.

Medial exposure of the popliteal artery

A rolled towel is placed underneath the proximal thigh and the knee is bent, which helps in exposing the popliteal vessels. The above-knee (AK) popliteal artery is exposed through a skin incision along the anterior border of the sartorius muscle from the level of the knee joint, extending 10–12 cm proximally, usually through the bed of the saphenous vein harvest site. The fascia of the popliteal space between the adductor tendon and the sartorius muscle is incised and a self-retaining retractor separates the two muscles apart. The popliteal artery can be palpated as a firm tubular structure just deep to the popliteal vein and encircled with a vessel loop to provide gentle traction (Figure 40.1). The dissection can be carried distally until a soft area suitable for anastomosis is identified, avoiding injury to the saphenous nerve as it exits from the adductor canal.

The below-knee (BK) popliteal artery is exposed via a longitudinal skin incision made from the level of the knee joint and extended distally for 10–12 cm, usually through the same incision used to harvest the below-knee GSV. Generally, the vein is mobilized out of harm's way and the superficial fascia is incised to enter the popliteal space with a sweeping motion of the index finger. The semimembranosus and semitendinosus tendons can be divided proximally to enhance exposure without functional consequence (Figure 40.2). The overlying popliteal vein is mobilized posteriorly, exposing the popliteal artery. Frequently, the popliteal artery is accompanied by two veins; care should be made to avoid injuring either when passing a right-angle clamp to encircle the artery with a silastic loop.

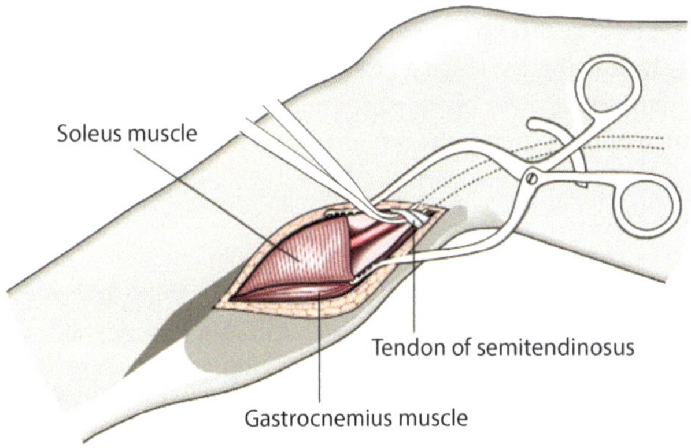

Figure 40.2 Exposure of the infrageniculate popliteal artery where division of semitendinosus and semimembranosus tendons will open up the popliteal space and facilitate exposure. The right-angle clamp is under the tendon of the semitendinosus.

The popliteal artery is then mobilized to identify a soft area for anastomosis. For subcutaneously tunneled grafts,

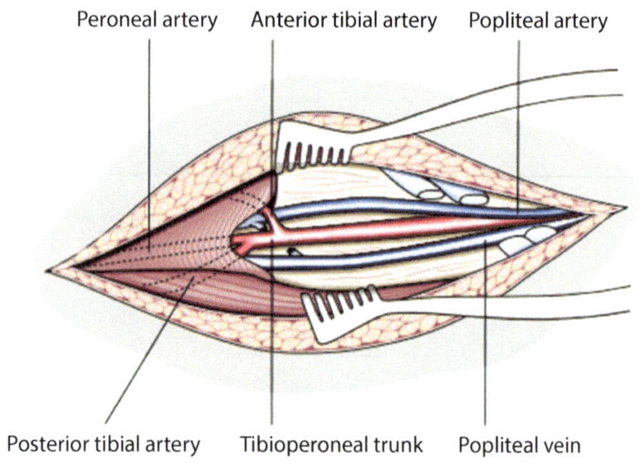

Figure 40.3 Division of the soleus muscle overlying the distal part of the infrageniculate popliteal artery allows exposure of the popliteal bifurcation and origin of the anterior tibial artery and the tibioperoneal trunk.

the most distal part of the popliteal artery allows a gentler curve of the vein graft to the anastomotic site.

Exposure of the popliteal trifurcation and the tibioperoneal trunk

The same incision used to expose the BK popliteal artery is extended distally. The soleus muscle covers the popliteal artery at the level of its trifurcation. The space between the popliteal artery and the soleus muscle is widened and a right-angle clamp is placed under the soleus muscle, which is divided by electrocautery exposing the underlying popliteal trifurcation. The first branch exposed is the anterior tibial artery (ATA). Ligation and division of the crossing anterior tibial vein and other veins allow exposure of the tibioperoneal trunk (Figure 40.3).

Posterior tibial artery

The posterior tibial artery is exposed through the same incision used to harvest the GSV. The deep fascia is incised, then the soleus muscle can be detached from its attachment to the tibia or by incising it longitudinally until the deep posterior compartment fascia is identified. This fascia is then incised, the posterior tibial neurovascular bundle is identified, and the accompanying veins separated from the artery by dividing the venae comitantes (Figure 40.4).

Plantar arteries

A 6–8 cm skin incision is performed between the medial malleolus and the calcaneus. After deepening the incision through the subcutaneous tissue, the flexor retinaculum is identified and incised, exposing the PTA and veins. The PTA is followed distally until it bifurcates into the medial and lateral plantar arteries (Figure 40.5). The lateral plantar artery can be further exposed by dividing the overlying muscles.

Peroneal artery

Medial exposure of the peroneal artery in the upper leg starts by exposing the posterior tibial neurovascular bundle, which can be retracted anteriorly along with the flexor digitorum longus muscle or posteriorly along with the flexor hallucis longus muscle (Figure 40.6). After exposing the posterior tibial vessels, the dissection is continued toward the fibula in the tissue plane (intermuscular septum) between the posterior tibialis muscle and the flexor hallucis longus muscle. Deep in the wound, a fascial layer will be identified and incised to expose one of the veins surrounding the peroneal artery. Further dissection and mobilization of this vein expose the peroneal artery. This usually requires division of a few small and delicate venae comitantes crossing over the peroneal artery. The exposure of the peroneal artery in the lower leg can be challenging in patients with heavy musculature and large-sized legs and a lateral approach may be preferred.

Anterior tibial artery

The ATA is exposed through a lateral approach via a longitudinal incision performed parallel to the tibia. The incision

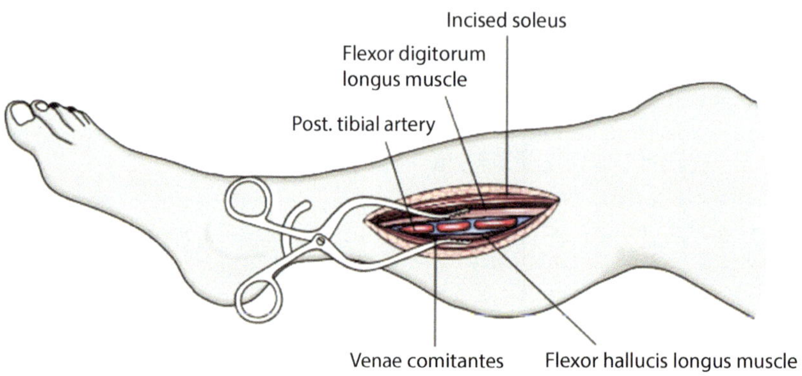

Figure 40.4 Exposure of the posterior tibial artery in the mid-leg.

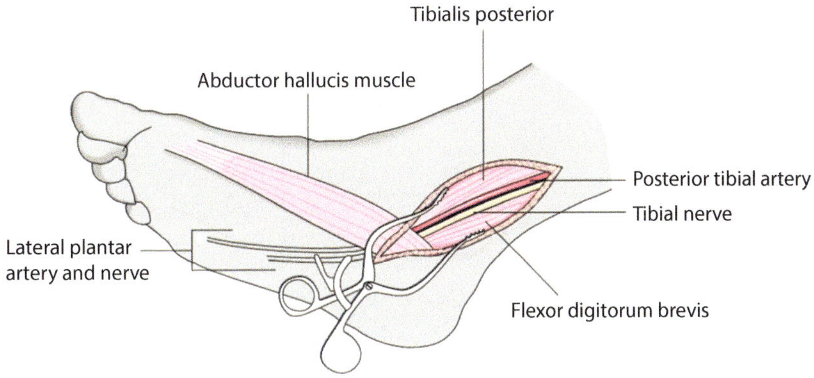

Figure 40.5 Exposure of the posterior tibial artery at the ankle and its bifurcation into the medial and lateral plantar arteries.

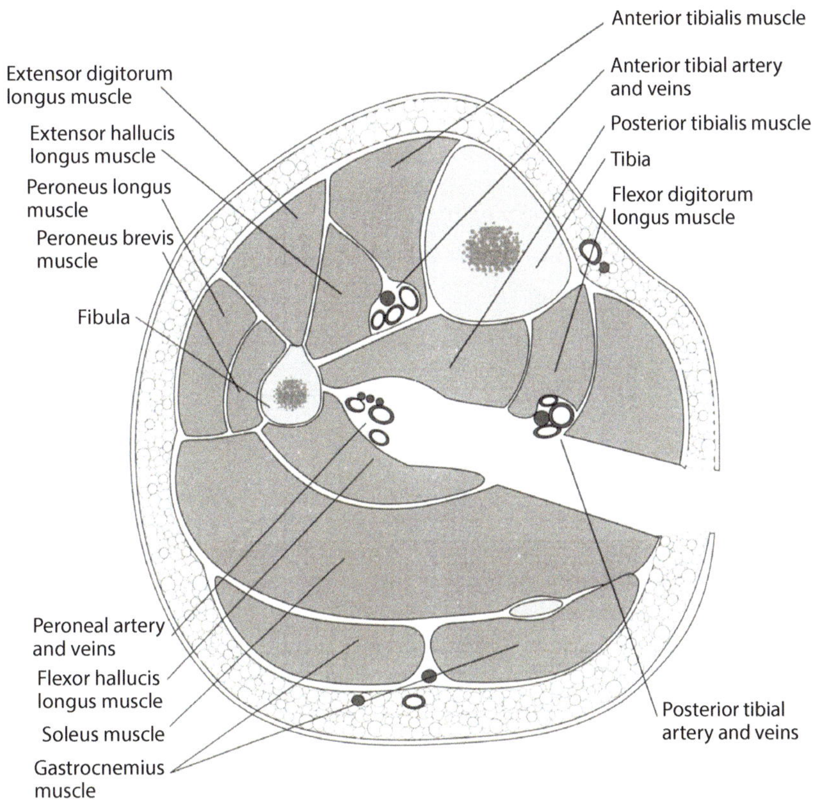

Figure 40.6 Medial exposure of the peroneal artery in the proximal leg.

starts 2 cm lateral to the tibial crest and extends for 10–12 cm. The skin incision is deepened through the subcutaneous tissue until the fascia is identified and incised longitudinally. The longitudinal cleft between the tibialis anterior muscle and the extensor hallucis muscle is entered. Gentle blunt dissection is carried out toward the interosseus membrane. A self-retaining retractor is placed deeper in the wound to enhance the exposure of the ATA and veins that will be seen at the deepest aspect of the incision.

In the lower leg, the ATA lies between the tendinous portions of the extensor muscles. A 10–12 cm incision is made parallel to the tibia and 2 cm inferior and lateral to it. The first tendon close to the tibia is the tibialis anterior muscle tendon. More distally, just above the ankle, the ATA is exposed by a short longitudinal incision with retraction of the extensor digitorum longus muscle laterally and the extensor hallucis longus muscle medially (Figure 40.7).

Dorsalis pedis artery

The dorsalis pedis artery is best exposed beyond the flexor retinaculum in the first metatarsal space (Figure 40.8). Mapping the dorsalis pedis artery preoperatively with duplex ultrasonography can guide the placement of the skin incision.

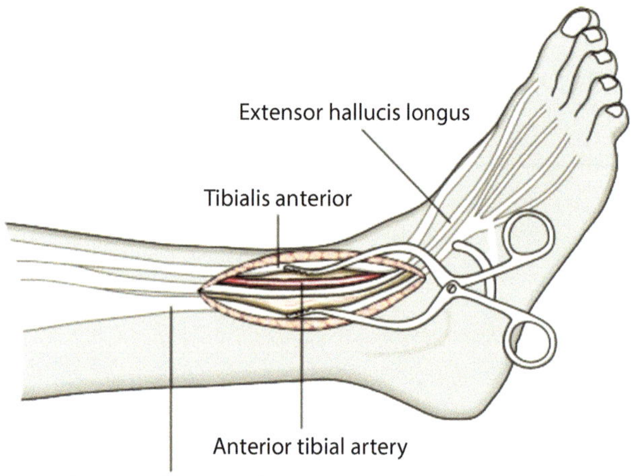

Figure 40.7 Exposure of the anterior tibial artery at the ankle.

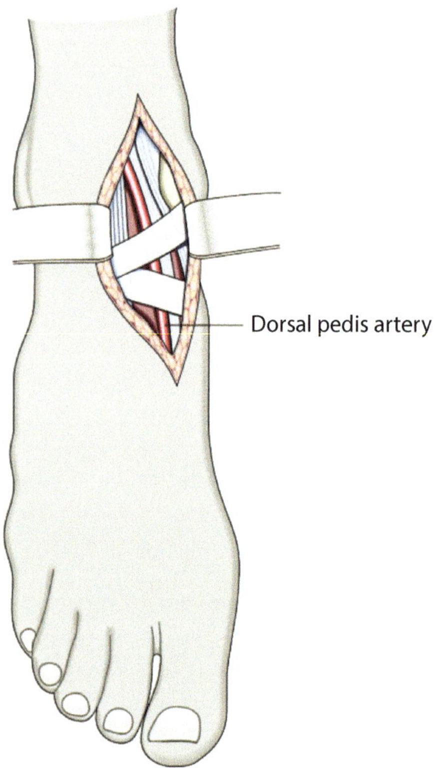

Figure 40.8 Exposure of the dorsalis pedis artery.

LATERAL APPROACH TO LOWER EXTREMITY VESSELS

Several of the lower extremity arteries that are usually exposed medially can also be reached through a lateral approach, a valuable technique in the presence of medial infection or scarring.

Lateral exposure of the profunda femoris and superficial femoral arteries

The PFA and SFA can be approached through an incision lateral to the sartorius muscle. Once the edge of the sartorius is reached, the sartorius muscle is retracted superiorly and medially. The SFA is located posterior to the sartorius muscle. The PFA can be more challenging to reach, and Doppler interrogation of the field can help identify its location.

Lateral exposure of the above-knee popliteal artery

In the presence of medial thigh infection, the suprageniculate popliteal artery can also be exposed through a lateral approach via a skin incision placed on the lateral aspect of the thigh and extending 10–12 cm proximally along the direction of the iliotibial tract, 1 cm posterior to and parallel to the iliotibial tract. It is deepened through the subcutaneous tissue until the deep fascia is identified and incised, opening the space between the iliotibial tract and the biceps femoris muscle, which then allows exposure of the AK popliteal artery (Figure 40.9). The distal SFA can be exposed by extending the incision more proximally and incising the adductor magnus muscle.

Lateral exposure of the below-knee popliteal artery

The popliteal artery can be reached by excising the proximal 7 cm of the fibula along with its head through a longitudinal incision starting proximal to the head of the fibula and extending distally for 10 cm. The incision is deepened through the subcutaneous tissue with care to identify the common peroneal nerve as it crosses over the neck of the fibula, which is then gently dissected, mobilized, and protected. The incision is deepened, exposing the fibular

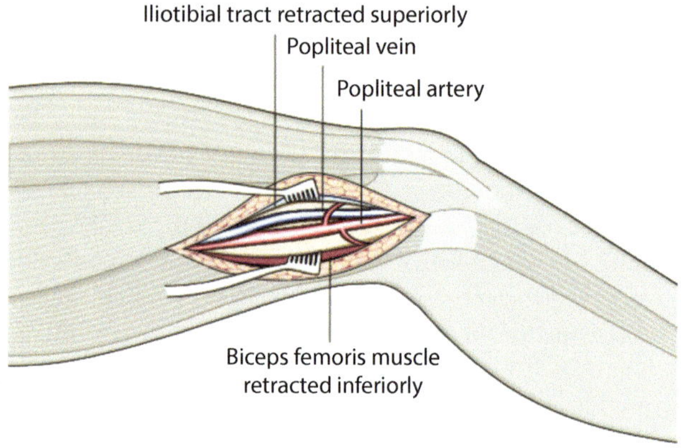

Figure 40.9 Lateral exposure of the suprageniculate popliteal artery

periosteum, which is stripped off the bone along with its muscular attachment. The fibula is then transected using a Micro-Sagittal saw 6–8 cm distal to its neck. The transected segment is held with a bone grasper and lifted gently, allowing for further release of all the posterior muscular attachments to the fibula and the attachment of the biceps femoris tendon. The proximal segment of the fibula is then removed, exposing the popliteal fossa. The tibial nerve is typically noted crossing the BK popliteal artery, which can then be palpated, dissected, and separated from the adjacent popliteal vein(s).

Lateral exposure of the peroneal artery

The peroneal artery can also be approached through a lateral approach, especially in redo procedures or when bypassing to its most distal segment. A 10 cm skin incision is performed along the length of the fibula over the selected segment of the peroneal artery and is deepened until the fibula is exposed. The muscular attachments to the fibula are released with electrocautery and the fibular periosteum stripped off ostium circumferentially. Care is taken to avoid injuring the peroneal vessels lying just deep to the fibula. A Micro-Sagittal saw can be used to divide the fibula at the desired levels, excising an 8–10 cm segment. The posterior periosteum is then incised, and the peroneal artery is identified deep to the excised fibular segment (Figure 40.10).

TUNNELING

Tunneling is an essential step in all bypasses to prevent graft compression, kinking, or twisting leading to bypass thrombosis.

For femoral to AK popliteal bypasses, the tunneling from the inguinal area to the AK popliteal space can be done subcutaneously, subfascially, or subsartorially, with the latter two being more common.

For BK popliteal artery bypasses, the same tunneling is done for the thigh segment, then the vein can be tunneled anatomically from the AK to the BK popliteal space between the heads of the gastrocnemius muscles (Figure 40.11). Subcutaneous tunneling is also possible but may require a steep curve between the AK and BK popliteal levels. This curve can be minimized by selecting an anastomotic site on the most distal part of the popliteal artery.

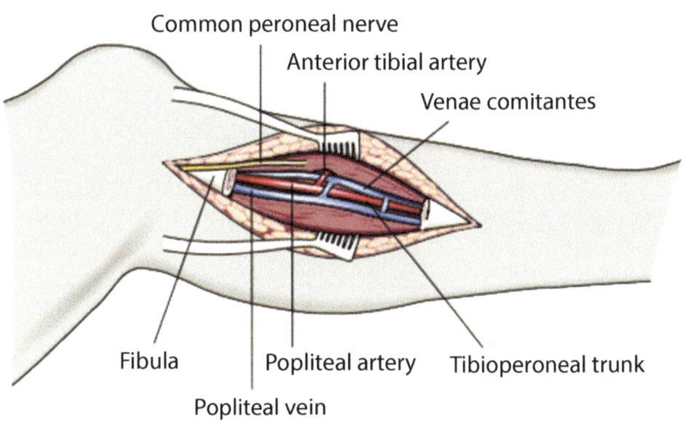

Figure 40.10 Lateral exposure of the peroneal artery.

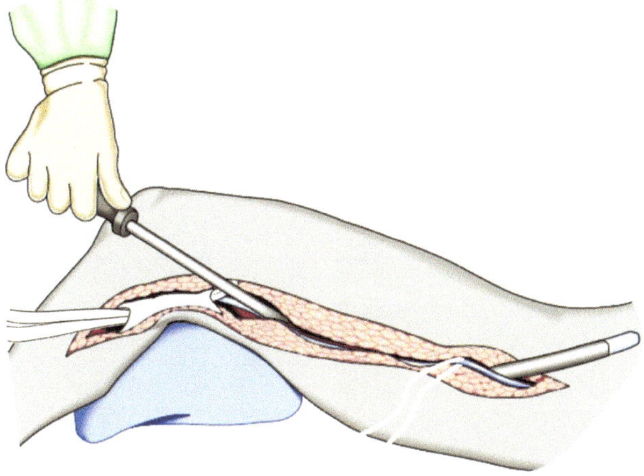

Figure 40.11 Tunneling to the below-knee popliteal artery using a large clamp across the popliteal space and a graft tunneler from the above-knee popliteal space to the groin.

Tunneling to the posterior tibial and peroneal arteries can be done entirely subcutaneously, or subcutaneously/subsartorially in the thigh, then anatomically at the knee and BK, and finally subfascially or subcutaneously below the knee.

For the ATA, the graft typically crosses from the medial to the lateral aspect of the leg. This can occur in the upper or mid-thigh and continued along the lateral aspect of the knee down to the ATA subcutaneously. Alternatively, it can cross subcutaneously from medial to lateral below the knee over the shin and the tibia and fibula, or deeply through the interosseous membrane, exiting into the anterior compartment of the leg and continuing to the target ATA (Figure 40.12).

ANTICOAGULATION

Once tunneling is performed, anticoagulation is carried out by the administration of intravenous heparin at 75 units/kilograms and followed up by checking the activated clotting time (ACT) to be maintained at >250 seconds.

CONSTRUCTION OF THE PROXIMAL ANASTOMOSIS

After administering intravenous heparin, atraumatic clamps are placed for proximal and distal control. The arteriotomy is performed in a soft part of the inflow vessel, occasionally requiring a localized endarterectomy. To avoid any narrowing at the proximal anastomosis, the GSV may be harvested with a cuff of the femoral vein for a wider anastomosis. Alternatively, the vein may be spatulated at a branch using a T-junction (Figure 40.13).

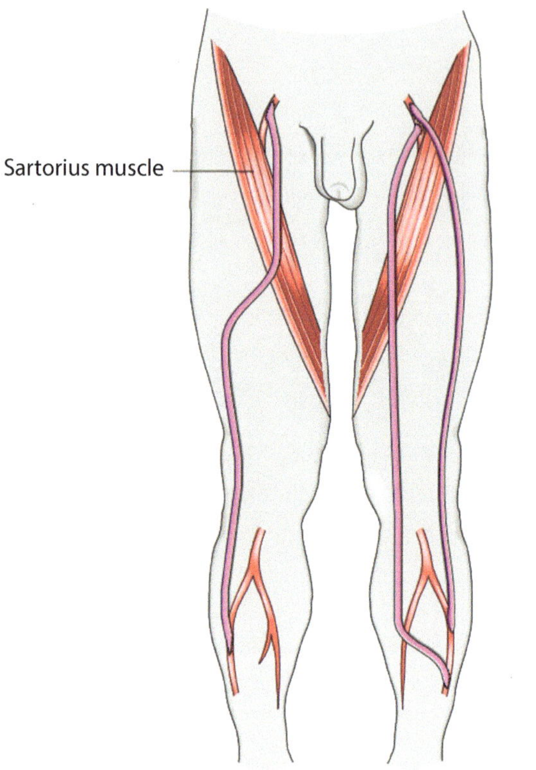

Figure 40.12 Various options for tunneling to the anterior tibial artery.

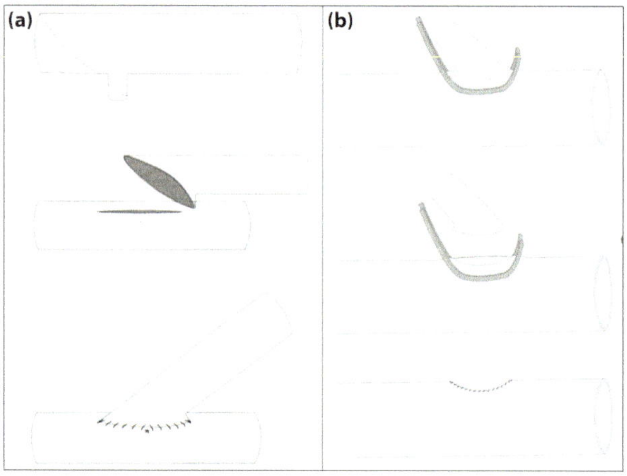

Figure 40.13 (a) Incorporating a T-junction branch in the proximal anastomosis; (b) incorporating a rim of the femoral vein in the proximal anastomosis.

If the wall is thickened or the vein diameter is small, the arteriotomy may be closed with a vein patch angioplasty and the proximal anastomosis constructed to the vein patch. If there is any concern of narrowing of the proximal anastomosis after its construction, a vein patch angioplasty of the proximal anastomosis is conducted. In the presence of significant disease at the origin of the PFA, the proximal portion of the PFA is exposed, the arteriotomy is carried out through its origin, and a vein patch angioplasty is performed to enhance flow into the PFA.

LYSING THE VALVES

In case of an in-situ or non-reversed, translocated bypass, disruption of the valves is required. For the non-reversed vein, this step should take place prior to passing it in the previously prepared tunnel. The Mill's valvulotome is a commonly used reusable valvulotome that is introduced through a side branch or through the distal end of the vein. The vein may be telescoped over the Mill's valvulotome. It is imperative during the valvulotomy to make sure that the tip of the Mill's valvulotome is not engaged in a side branch, which could then tear the vein.

PASSING THE VEIN IN THE TUNNEL

Once the vein is fully arterialized, the flow from the vein is checked in a cup and the vein checked for missed side branches that need to be oversewn to avoid bleeding in the tunnel. Care is taken to avoid twisting the vein while being passed in the tunnel. Additionally, ensuring that the tunnel does not "porpoise" from subcutaneous to subfascial planes and back again is crucial to avoid constriction by the fascia in that transition zone.

CONSTRUCTION OF THE DISTAL ANASTOMOSIS

Appropriate vascular control prior to creating the arteriotomy is essential to ensure excellent visualization in a bloodless field. Control of the tibial vessels should be done without any crushing injuries to the vessel. A sterile tourniquet can provide the least traumatic control to the vessels and is often preferred in diabetic patients (Figure 40.14). Alternatively, small atraumatic vascular bulldogs or clips (e.g., Yasargil clips, Heifetz clips) can be used, though they may induce spasm. Other options include

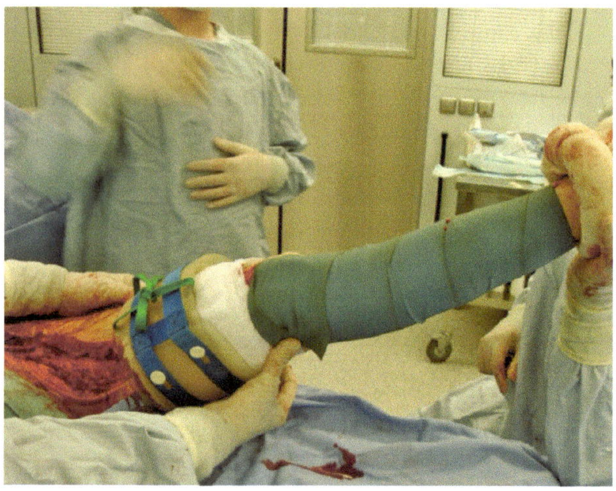

Figure 40.14 A sterile tourniquet is placed, and the leg is exsanguinated using an Esmarch bandage prior to inflating the tourniquet and constructing the distal anastomosis.

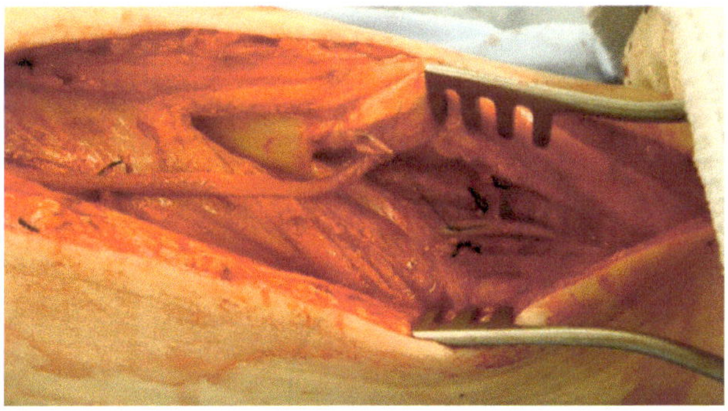

Figure 40.15 Constructing the distal anastomosis using a parachute technique.

internal flow occluder devices, or very rarely, small size 2 or 3 Fogarty catheters.

A 6-mm arteriotomy is performed and the anastomosis is carried out with a running 6-0 monofilament Prolene suture, ensuring there is excellent intima-to-intima apposition (Figure 40.15). Once completed, back bleeding from the target vessel along with forward bleeding from the bypass is performed. The anastomosis is flushed with heparinized saline solution and flow is resumed in the tibial artery. Prior to tying the knots, the flow in the bypass and in the target vessel distal to the anastomosis is checked by continuous wave sterile Doppler and should diminish when pinching the bypass and augment when resuming flow in the bypass.

Adjunctive techniques for the distal anastomosis with prosthetic bypasses

Although prosthetic bypasses to the above-knee popliteal artery have shown comparable patency rates to vein bypasses at two to three years [10], these bypasses are less frequently performed due to advances in endovascular technology. For below-knee target vessels, our preference continues to be composite vein bypasses over prosthetic bypasses. Prosthetic bypasses are only considered as a last resort prior to amputation if no venous conduit is available. Several adjunctive techniques can improve outcomes for prosthetic bypasses to the infrageniculate popliteal or tibial arteries. These include Linton patch, Miller cuff, Saint Mary's boot, Taylor Patch, and an adjunctive arteriovenous fistula, but are beyond the scope of this chapter.

COMPLETION ANGIOGRAM

An important step in bypass construction is the completion angiogram, performed by inserting a 20-gauge angiocath through a side branch or by direct puncture of the graft. This allows for evaluation of the flow in the bypass and detection of any issues that could lead to early failure or thrombosis.

WOUND CLOSURE

Wound closure is critical and should not be left to an unsupervised junior resident. It is very important to ensure that hemostasis is well-secured before closing the wound. The soft tissue over the anastomoses is closed in layers with gentle approximation of the tissues using interrupted or running suture of absorbable material such as Vicryl. Large figure-of-eight sutures that are tied too tightly can cause ischemic fat necrosis with subsequent wound dehiscence or infection. The skin may be closed with staples, subcuticular sutures, or simple nylon if good skin-to-skin apposition is achieved.

We do not reverse the heparin at the end of the case. Aspirin is resumed on the first postoperative day. If the wound is still oozing despite a meticulous attempt at hemostasis, a closed suction drain may be left in the popliteal space or the groin.

Management of concomitant foot wounds

Concomitant foot wounds are typically addressed two days postoperatively unless there is an active infection that needs to be promptly addressed.

POSTOPERATIVE FOLLOW-UP

A predischarge duplex scan of the bypass is conducted to provide a baseline evaluation. Duplex examination is repeated at one month postoperatively and at three months' intervals in the first postoperative year, and then every six months in the following year and yearly thereafter.

TRICKS AND TRAPS

- Preoperative imaging with digital subtraction angiography, high-quality thin-cut CT angiography, or MR angiography is crucial for the proper selection of inflow and outflow vessels.
- Opting for the most distal disease-free inflow source facilitates a shorter bypass. The common femoral artery is often chosen as it is usually less involved with occlusive pathology, is easily accessible, and allows for a generous non-constrained anastomosis.
- The popliteal artery can also serve as an inflow vessel even if endovascular techniques are used to treat proximal SFA disease.
- The outflow vessel that provides non-obstructed pulsatile flow to the ischemic area in the foot is the most desired site for the distal anastomosis.
- A single-segment great saphenous vein is the preferred conduit for infrainguinal bypass. Preoperative vein mapping is essential for effective case planning and conduit selection.

- In the absence of an adequate single-segment autologous vein, a composite all-autologous vein bypass can serve as an acceptable alternative. Composite prosthetic-vein bypasses may not provide much advantage over prosthetic bypasses with adjunctive patches at the distal anastomosis.
- The decision between reversed, non-reversed/translocated, or in-situ bypass depends on the surgeon's preference and experience and may be influenced by the anatomic dimensions of the great saphenous vein.
- When the CFA is very diseased, an endarterectomy prior to performing the proximal anastomosis may be necessary, making sure that proximal PFA disease is corrected. Adjunctive techniques including vein patch angioplasty may be needed.
- Atraumatic vascular control is essential for the construction of a flawless distal anastomosis in a bloodless field.
- A completion angiogram at the end of the case is important to detect imperfections or technical issues that could lead to early bypass graft failure.

QUESTIONS

1. A 72-year-old diabetic man presents with a non-healing ulcer over the right great toe of four weeks' duration. He was referred after a CT angiogram revealed extensive calcification in his tibial vessels, with poor visualization of the distal tibial and pedal vessels. Non-invasive testing reveals infra-popliteal tibial disease and a toe pressure of 20 mmHg. His creatinine level is 1.3mg/dl. What is the best next step?
   a. Obtain an MRA of the lower extremity
   b. Obtain a digital subtraction angiogram
   c. Great toe amputation
   d. Intraoperative exploration of the tibial and pedal vessels
   e. Below-knee amputation as no target vessels are visualized

   Answer: b

2. Digital subtraction angiography on the patient above revealed patent common femoral, superficial femoral, and popliteal arteries with totally occluded anterior tibial, posterior tibial, and peroneal vessels with reconstitution of the dorsalis pedis artery and an intact pedal arch in the foot. An endovascular approach was attempted and was unsuccessful. The patient has a 3.5 mm GSV in the thigh that becomes smaller than 2 mm below the knee. The best treatment option is:
   a. Common femoral to dorsalis pedis artery bypass using a reversed GSV
   b. Superficial femoral to dorsalis pedis artery in-situ bypass
   c. Infrageniculate popliteal to dorsalis pedis artery bypass
   d. Exploration of the dorsalis pedis artery and an attempted retrograde atherectomy of the tibial vessels
   e. PTFE bypass from the common femoral artery to the dorsalis pedis artery with an adjunctive Miller cuff at the distal anastomosis

   Answer: c

3. Assume the same patient had undergone prior varicose vein surgery and his saphenous veins had been treated by stripping on one side and radiofrequency ablation on the contralateral leg. Duplex evaluation revealed a patent cephalic vein measuring 3.5 mm from the mid-forearm to the deltopectoral groove. The best option would now be:
   a. PTFE bypass with adjunctive AV fistula
   b. PTFE bypass with Saint Mary's boot
   c. Cryopreserved vein bypass
   d. Cephalic vein bypass
   e. Reattempted endovascular approach

   Answer: d

4. A diabetic patient with left second toe wet gangrene and incompressible ankle vessels and a flatline toe waveform on non-invasive testing. After undergoing an open-toe amputation, CT angiography reveals a 60% left common iliac stenosis, diffuse calcific disease of the left common femoral artery including a 90% ostial stenosis of the profunda femoris, and a long segment occlusion of the SFA with reconstitution of the below-knee popliteal artery and patent tibial runoff to the foot. Duplex revealed a patent GSV measuring 4.0 mm from the ankle to the groin. The best option would be:
   a. Left common iliac stenting with close follow-up
   b. Left common femoral endarterectomy with GSV bypass to the posterior tibial artery
   c. Left common iliac stenting with left common femoral endarterectomy and GSV bypass to the below-knee popliteal artery
   d. GSV bypass from the left external iliac artery to the below-knee popliteal artery
   e. Aortofemoral bypass with concomitant GSV bypass from the left limb of the graft to the below-knee popliteal artery

   Answer: c

REFERENCES

1. Veith, F.J., et al., Superficial femoral and popliteal arteries as inflow sites for distal bypasses. *Surgery*, 1981. 90(6): p. 980–90.

2. Schneider, P.A., et al., Intraoperative superficial femoral artery balloon angioplasty and popliteal to distal bypass graft: an option for combined open and endovascular treatment of diabetic gangrene. *J Vasc Surg*, 2001. 33(5): p. 955–62.
3. Synn, A.Y., et al., Are there angiographic predictors of success for vein bypass to the peroneal artery? *Am J Surg*, 1992. 164(3): p. 276–80.
4. Pomposelli, F.B., et al., A decade of experience with dorsalis pedis artery bypass: analysis of outcome in more than 1000 cases. *J Vasc Surg*, 2003. 37(2): p. 307–15.
5. Hughes, K., et al., Bypass to plantar and tarsal arteries: an acceptable approach to limb salvage. *J Vasc Surg*, 2004. 40(6): p. 1149–57.
6. Wengerter, K.R., et al., Influence of vein size (diameter) on infrapopliteal reversed vein graft patency. *J Vasc Surg*, 1990. 11(4): p. 525–31.
7. Chang, H., et al., Non-reversed and reversed great saphenous vein graft configurations offer comparable early outcomes in patients undergoing infrainguinal bypass. *Eur J Vasc Endovasc Surg*, 2022. 63(6): p. 864–73.
8. Shah, D.M., et al., Long-term results of in situ saphenous vein bypass. Analysis of 2058 cases. *Ann Surg*, 1995. 222(4): p. 438–46; discussion 446–48.
9. Corson, J.D., et al., Technical aspects and results of the open in situ saphenous vein bypass technique. *Int Angiol*, 1993. 12(2): p. 162–67.
10. Klinkert, P., et al., Saphenous vein versus PTFE for above-knee femoropopliteal bypass. A review of the literature. *Eur J Vasc Endovasc Surg*, 2004. 27(4): p. 357–62.

41

Extra-anatomic reconstruction for aortoiliac occlusive disease

FARAH H.A. MOHAMMAD AND ALEXANDER D. SHEPARD

FEMOROFEMORAL BYPASS

This bypass is well tolerated even by high-risk patients as no aortic clamping is required. Factors to consider preoperatively include the confirmation of healthy inflow in the donor artery. The aorta and ipsilateral iliac artery should be patent with no significant occlusive disease. An easily palpable femoral pulse on physical exam is suggestive of good inflow, however, this must be confirmed with further testing. Imaging with computed tomography angiography (CTA) or conventional multiplanar angiography is ideal. Ultrasound can also be a good adjunct to evaluate the adequacy of inflow. The common femoral artery (CFA), superficial femoral artery (SFA), or profunda femoris artery (PFA) can be used as a recipient target for outflow. Additional endarterectomy may be required to optimize the outflow. Other factors to consider include previous operations, multiple prior arterial access for vascular, or cardiac interventions, as well as the body habitus.

Depending on the physiologic status of the patient, "fem-fem" bypass can sometimes be performed under local anesthesia with sedation if necessary, if the duration of these cases is short. General and regional anesthesia are also good options. If the patient is a good candidate for general anesthesia, then that is the anesthetic of choice in the author's practice. The patient is positioned supine on an OR table with extended or tucked arms depending on the operator's preference. The entire abdomen and both groins are prepped and draped sterilely. Pre-operative antibiotics are given. A pulseless CFA is expected on the recipient side. To avoid imprecise dissection, careful attention should be given to the bony landmarks. A line between the anterior superior iliac spine and pubic tubercle is drawn identifying the underlying inguinal ligament. The CFA lies approximately 2.5 cm lateral to the pubic tubercle. This location along with the level of the femoral bifurcation can be marked using ultrasound prior to prepping.

A vertical incision allows adequate exposure. The length depends on the extent of endarterectomy required. Once the incision is made with the scalpel, electrocautery or an ultrasonic scalpel can be used to deepen the incision through the subQ until the inguinal ligament is identified. The ligament can be mobilized by retracting it superiorly. The femoral artery can then be palpated as a pulsatile structure or a firm, rubbery to calcific tubular structure. For limited exposure, two Wheitlaner retractors can be used. For distal external iliac artery exposure, a Thompson (Thompson Surgical Instruments, Traverse City, MI, USA) or mini-Omni retractor (Omni-Tract Surgical Retractor Set) can be used. Lymphatics can be mobilized medially or laterally to avoid transection. Larger lymphatics should be ligated. The ultrasonic scalpel is helpful to avoid lymphatic leaks, which can be a potentially catastrophic complication of this procedure given the presence of a prosthetic graft and its usual superficial tunnel through the subcutaneous tissues. During exposure of the proximal PFA, a crossing deep femoral vein, if encountered, should be carefully ligated. Vessel loops can be used to encircle the CFA, PFA, and SFA. A tunneler can be used to create a gentle C-shaped suprapubic tunnel (Figure 41.1). This is created in the adipose layer along the anterior abdominal wall fascia. Some resistance is always met when crossing the midline. Great care should be taken when crossing a midline incisional scar. The curve of the tunnel should be smooth to avoid any kinking of the graft as it exits from the incision. The distal anastomotic sites should be carefully chosen to minimize problems with graft kinking and angulation. The common femoral artery immediately adjacent to the inguinal ligament should be avoided because of the tendency of grafts anastomosed to this segment to kink as the abdominal wall pannus "drops" when the patient stands (Figure 41.2). Graft angulation can also occur with hip flexion during sitting. For these reasons, we usually place the femoral

DOI: 10.1201/9781003452096-41

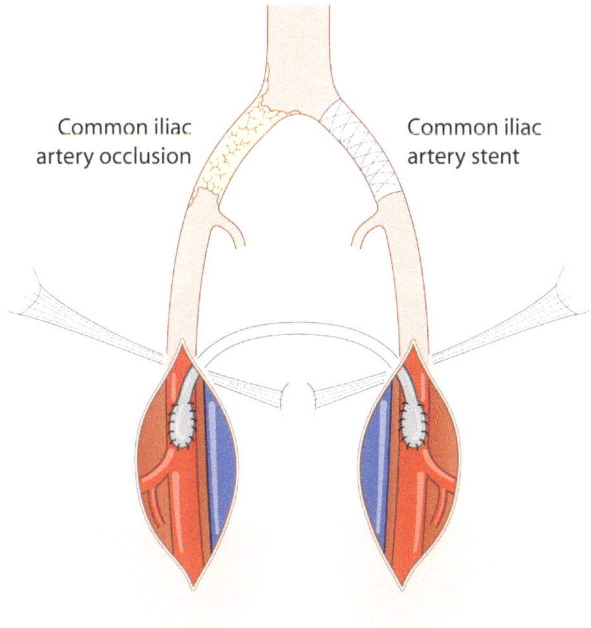

Figure 41.1 Typical femorofemoral bypass reconstruction with a C-shaped suprapubic tunnel. Inflow has been optimized with left common iliac stenting.

anastomosis(es) at the level of the femoral bifurcation(s), crossing over the origins of either the profunda femoris or SFA (Figure 41.3). Pre-peritoneal tunneling can be helpful in the case of previous surgery and excessive scarring. The prosthetic conduit should be at least 6–8 mm in size and both Dacron or ringed polytetrafluoroethylene (PTFE) can be used, although we prefer PTFE.

Vascular clamps versus vessel loops can be used for control. The author prefers the Satinsky DeBakey clamp for CFA, the angled DeBakey clamp for SFA, and a Gregory Profunda clamp for PFA. In the case of very calcific vessels, a No. 5 Fogarty balloon catheter can be used for proximal balloon occlusion. Patients should be heparinized before clamping but after the tunnel is created. The graft can then be passed through the tunnel. The inflow anastomosis is created first. An arteriotomy is made over the donor CFA with a #11 blade and extended with Potts scissors. If there is a need for extensive endarterectomy, then a bovine patch can be used prior to the graft anastomosis. It is critical that the disease at the origin of the profunda femoris is corrected to ensure adequate outflow. The graft is sewn after adequate spatulation. PTFE sutures can be used to decrease PTFE graft suture line bleeding. After graft pressurization, careful measurement, and appropriate trimming, the distal anastomosis is performed in a similar fashion. Adequate hemostasis is essential to avoid

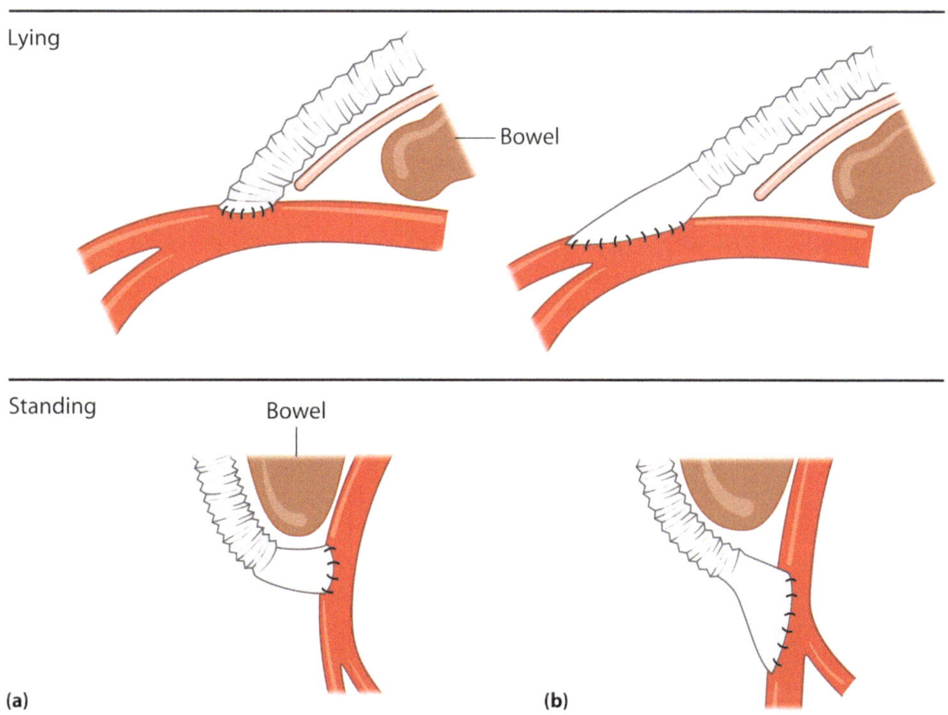

Figure 41.2 Femorofemoral graft showing avoidance of acute angulation at the inguinal ligament. (**a**) Kinking of the graft at the anastomosis when placed too close to the inguinal ligament. (**b**) Anastomosis placed further distal on the femoral artery to avoid kinking.

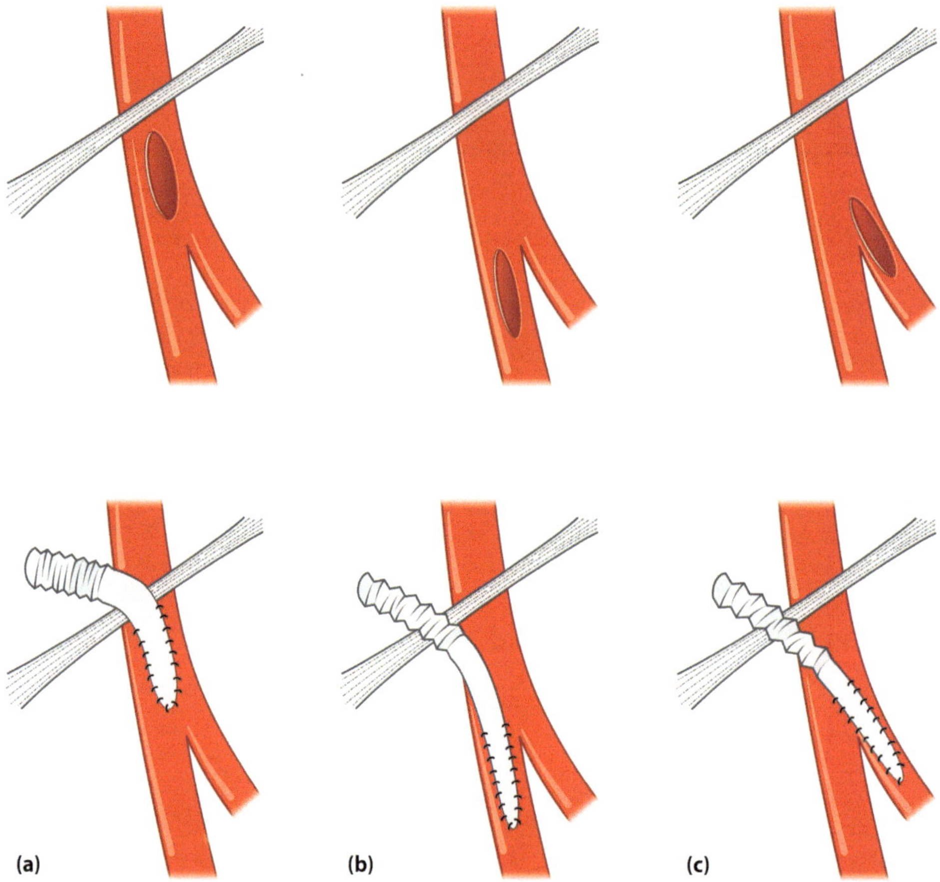

Figure 41.3 Construction of femorofemoral bypass anastomoses. (**a**) Arteriotomy on the proximal common femoral artery can lead to angulation. (**b**) More distal femoral arteriotomy, usually over bifurcations or onto either the superficial femoral artery or pro-funda femoris artery (PFA) can avoid this angulation. (**c**) Oblique arteriotomy onto the proximal PFA lessens the angle of curvature of the graft.

any hematomas. Hematomas can increase the risk of surgical site infection and thus graft thrombosis. Protamine can be given once pedal signals are confirmed. The incisions are then closed in layers with absorbable sutures. Skin can be closed with subcuticular sutures or staples. An incisional negative-pressure dressing is routine to reduce groin wound complications but is particularly important in redo exposures and in patients with high BMI.

AXILLO-(BI)FEMORAL BYPASS

The axillary artery can be used for inflow. The right axillary artery is usually preferred as the right subclavian artery (SA) is more reliably disease-free. In addition to physical exam, upper extremity segmental pressures, arterial duplex, or CTA can be used to rule out inflow stenosis to this artery.

The arm is positioned on a narrow arm board at the patient's side but prepped free to allow abduction during the case. The donor arm, shoulder, hemi-thorax, abdomen, and both groins are prepped and draped. If available, two teams can be utilized to perform this procedure more expeditiously. While one team performs the axillary dissection, the other can expose the femoral arteries.

A 7–8 cm incision is made a finger breadth below the clavicle toward the lateral two-thirds end of the clavicle. A muscle-splitting incision of the pectoralis major exposes the underlying clavipectoral fascia, which is incised. Underlying small venous tributaries are traced back to the axillary vein that lies just anterior and slightly caudal to the artery. Adequate exposure of the axillary artery requires the division of these small veins along with a branch or two of the artery (e.g., the thoracoacromial trunk). The first portion of the axillary artery (between the lower margin of the clavicle proximally and the medial edge of the pectoralis minor distally) is mobilized for a distance of 4–5 cm and controlled with vessel loops. Care should be taken to avoid injury to the brachial plexus, which tracks just above and behind the artery. Lateral exposure can be facilitated by dividing the medial portion of the head of the pectoralis minor, although the second portion of the axillary artery (the segment lying directly behind the pectoralis minor) should never be used to originate the graft because of the increased risk of anastomotic disruption with arm abduction when this segment is used. Posterior branches of the axillary artery in the region selected for anastomosis should usually be divided when encountered to avoid subsequent inadvertent injury and/or troublesome back bleeding during the performance of the anastomosis.

The femoral arteries can be exposed as described previously. The distal anastomotic sites should be carefully chosen to minimize problems with graft kinking and angulation as previously described for femoral-femoral bypass.

Using blunt digital dissection, a tunnel can be started either between the two pectoralis muscles or beneath the pectoralis minor depending on the type of proximal anastomosis chosen and continued with a tunneler in a gentle arc along the anterior axillary line, curving just medial to the ASIS into the ipsilateral groin. A counter incision can be made at the mid-point between the inferior costal margin and iliac crest as needed. An externally supported ringed PTFE graft is tunneled between the axillary and femoral incisions and subsequently through the femoral-to-femoral tunnel. A pre-constructed 8 mm graft with an already attached cross-femoral limb can be used versus sewing on the femoral limb separately (Figure 41.4). We prefer the modified proximal anastomosis technique wherein the graft runs parallel along the axillary artery with enough redundancy to prevent avulsion but just enough to avoid any kinking (Figure 41.5). After heparinization, the axillary artery is clamped proximally and distally. The arteriotomy is made on the antero-inferior surface of the artery. An end-to-side anastomosis is constructed with a 5-0 suture of choice. Femoral anastomoses are constructed similarly to the femoral-to-femoral bypass, again taking care to correct significant femoral level disease, particularly at the origin of the profunda femoris. Once good flow is confirmed, protamine can be given. Meticulous hemostasis should be achieved prior to closure. The axillary incision is closed in layers with absorbable sutures. Skin is then closed with subcuticular sutures.

POSTOPERATIVE MANAGEMENT

Medical management should include at a minimum an antiplatelet agent and statin therapy. The authors prefer an oral anticoagulant as well. Monitoring the groin incision to avoid any groin complication is the key. Routine surveillance with duplex US and ankle brachial pressure indices are performed at six weeks, three months, six months, and thereafter annually. Progressive disease in the outflow vessels is the most common cause of graft thrombosis. Anastomotic peak systolic velocities >300 cm/sec may need further investigation to rule out stenosis. With surveillance, a five-year patency for femorofemoral bypass of 50–60% can be achieved. Axillo-bifemoral bypass patency at five years can vary from 35–80%.

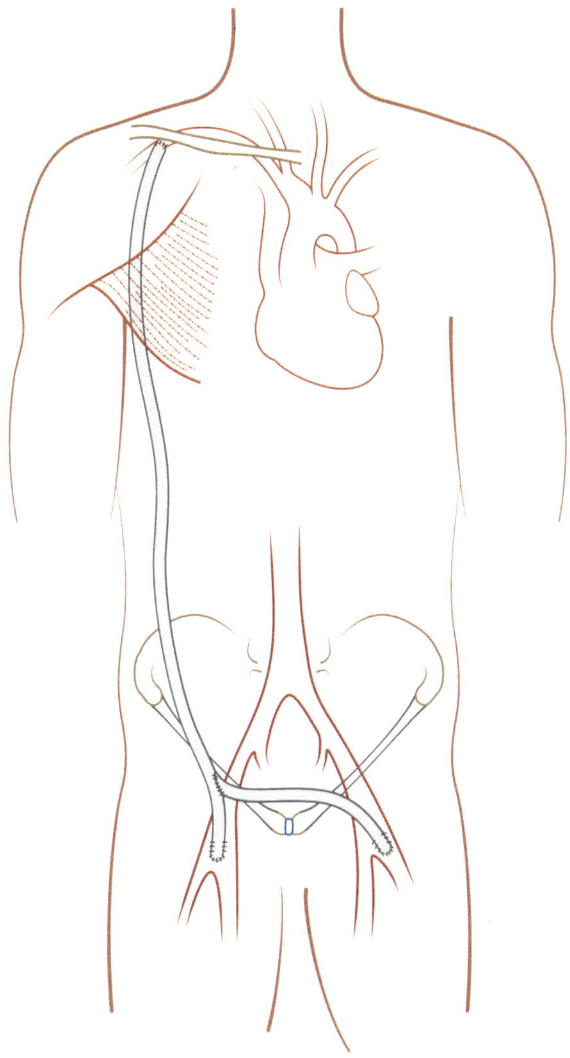

Figure 41.4 Axillobifemoral graft configuration.

COMPLICATIONS

Two rare but well-documented complications of axillofemoral grafting require mention. Disruption of the axillary anastomosis can occur following an episode of forceful abduction of the donor arm (e.g., as might occur during opening a garage door). To avoid this, place the proximal anastomosis as far medial as possible on the axillary artery and leave a slightly redundant segment of graft just beyond this anastomosis. The other unusual complication is perigraft seroma. While such seromas can occur following any placement of a prosthetic graft, they seem to be more frequent after axillo-femoral grafting. Although the cause is unknown, graft porosity produces a transudate of fluid surrounding the distal limb(s) of the graft which can extend up the flank. Patients complain of painless "lumps" in the groin(s). Management is conservative. Aspiration can be diagnostic and at least temporarily therapeutic; repetitive aspirations should be avoided, however, because of the risk of infection. In rare cases, graft replacement with a different type of graft material

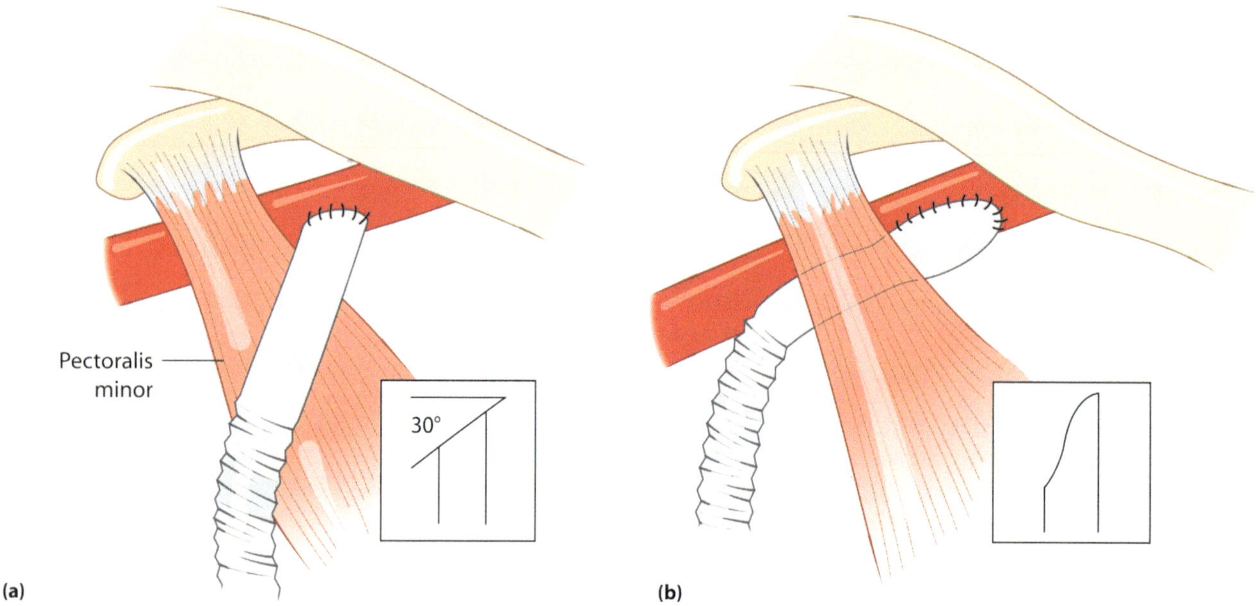

Figure 41.5 Axillary anastomosis construction technique. (**a**) Classic construction with graft cut at a 30-degree bevel and tunneled between the pectoralis muscles. (**b**) Modified technique favored by the authors with a more traditional, acutely angled graft bevel tunneled behind the pectoralis minor.

(e.g., exchanging PTFE for Dacron) through fresh tissue planes has been advocated.

TRICKS AND TRAPS

- Endovascular stenting can be used to optimize the inflow to the donor CFA if needed.
- Ultrasonography to mark the femoral bifurcations prior to making incision minimizes blind dissection and wound complications.
- A prior low midline celiotomy incision can make suprapubic tunneling difficult. Tunneling in the pre-peritoneal space is an alternative approach.
- Planning the arteriotomy is key to avoid acute angulation of the graft. If there is a need for extensive endarterectomy, sewing a patch prior to the graft may help with the lie and configuration of the graft.
- Groin wound complications are potentially catastrophic given the presence of a subcutaneously tunneled prosthetic graft.
- The right subclavian artery is more likely to be disease-free, thus making the right axillary artery more suitable as an inflow vessel for axillo-femoral grafting. Noninvasive testing should be performed to confirm the absence of hemodynamically significant disease in these donor arteries.
- The proximal anastomosis of an axillo-femoral bypass should be performed to the first portion of the axillary artery, which is relatively fixed.
- Pre-constructed axillo-bifemoral bypass grafts can be used to avoid graft-to-graft anastomoses.
- Adequate graft redundancy just distal to the axillary anastomosis is essential to avoid risk of avulsion of the graft with extreme arm abduction.

QUESTIONS

1. An 86-year-old male with COPD on 2L of home oxygen presents with symptoms of rest pain and critically low ABIs. Imaging shows infrarenal aortic and bilateral common iliac and proximal external iliac occlusions. What would be the best management?
   a. Aorto-bifemoral bypass
   b. Aorto-bi-iliac bypass
   c. Femoralfemoral bypass
   d. Axillo-bifemoral bypass

   Answer: d

2. Which artery is used as inflow for axillo-bifemoral bypass?
   a. First portion of the axillary artery
   b. Second portion of the axillary artery
   c. Third portion of the axillary artery
   d. Proximal-most brachial artery

   Answer: a

3. All of the following are recognized complications of axillo-femoral bypass except?
   a. Groin lymph leak
   b. Axillary anastomosis disruption after forceful abduction of the donor arm
   c. Perigraft fluid collection
   d. Aortic stump "blow-out"

   Answer: d

4. Extra-anatomic bypass is appropriate in all of these situations except:
   a. Mycotic aneurysm of the infrarenal aorta requiring aortic ligation
   b. CLTI in an elderly patient with extensive aortoiliac occlusive disease
   c. A 52-year-old postal worker with AIOD who experiences job-interfering bilateral calf claudication
   d. A 70-year-old male with juxtarenal aortic occlusion with severe short-distance claudication and history of aortoiliac radiation for lymphoma

   Answer: c

42

Thoracofemoral bypass graft for aortoiliac occlusive disease

ALI H. HAKIM, YUQIAN TIAN, AND IRAKLIS I. PIPINOS

INTRODUCTION

Thoracofemoral bypass for aortoiliac occlusive disease is a challenging procedure best suited for the subset of patients with aortoiliac disease who have either occlusion of a previous aortobifemoral bypass or a hostile abdomen due to prior surgery or other abdominal pathology.

INDICATIONS AND PREOPERATIVE PLANNING

Patients present with symptoms of severe aortoiliac occlusive disease including severe lifestyle-limiting claudication or critical limb-threatening ischemia. Diagnosis can usually be made with detailed history, physical examination, and non-invasive vascular studies. This procedure is ideal for low-risk patients with preserved lung function and a healthy thoracic aorta. Usually, these are patients with previous abdominal operations or septic abdominal complications, intra-abdominal scarring, failed prior infrarenal aortic reconstruction, infected aortic prosthesis, or other retroperitoneal disease. For the appropriate candidates, a thoracofemoral bypass can be superior to the alternative solution of an axillofemoral bypass because of its superior cumulative five-year patency rates of 81–95% versus 54–63%, with axillofemoral bypass usually reserved for higher-risk patients with limb-threatening acute or chronic ischemia [1–4].

Preoperative evaluation includes cardiac stress testing, pulmonary function testing, and optimization of comorbidities. Computed tomographic angiography of the chest, abdomen, and pelvis with bilateral lower extremity runoff is performed to ensure that the thoracic aorta is healthy and there are adequate infrainguinal arterial segments that will serve as good outflow for the distal anastomoses. Major contraindications include aneurysm or occlusive disease of the descending thoracic aorta and the inability to tolerate one-lung ventilation. Relative contraindications include severe obstructive pulmonary disease or prior left thoracotomy with residual dense adhesions [5].

PROCEDURE DESCRIPTION

Positioning

The patient is transferred to the operating table with a vacuum beanbag extending from the shoulders to the proximal thigh. After induction of general anesthesia with the capabilities for one-lung ventilation, the patient's left hemithorax is elevated to an angle of 45–65 degrees, while maintaining the pelvis as flat as possible; this facilitates the thoracotomy while allowing adequate exposure for groin dissections. The left arm is supported in an arm cradle, helping to extend the lower thorax and avoid a brachial plexus injury. A roll is positioned under the right axilla and pillow rests are placed under the knees and between the legs to prevent hyperextension. Legs are secured with a safety strap. Should a full thoracotomy become necessary, a generous operative field should be fully prepared, making sure to include the left scapula and thoracic spine (Figure 42.1).

GROIN INCISIONS AND RETROPERITONEAL ACCESS

The procedure begins in the groins to reduce the length of time that the chest cavity is open, thereby minimizing associated heat and fluid losses. Standard incisions for the exposure of the femoral vessels are used and the femoral vessels are dissected free bilaterally. The left groin skin incision is then extended approximately 10 cm cephalad above the inguinal ligament. At the most cephalad aspect of the left groin incision, the retroperitoneum is accessed to facilitate the creation of the tunnel connecting the left

DOI: 10.1201/9781003452096-42

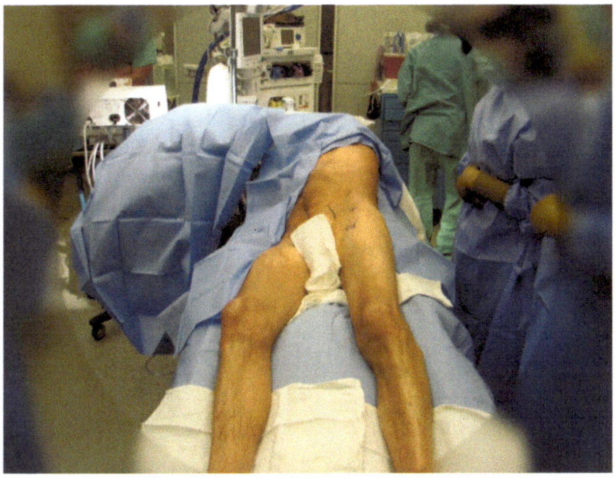

Figure 42.1 The patient is positioned in a right-side down thoracoabdominal position with the left arm in a supportive arm cradle and hips as flat as possible to facilitate exposure of both groins.

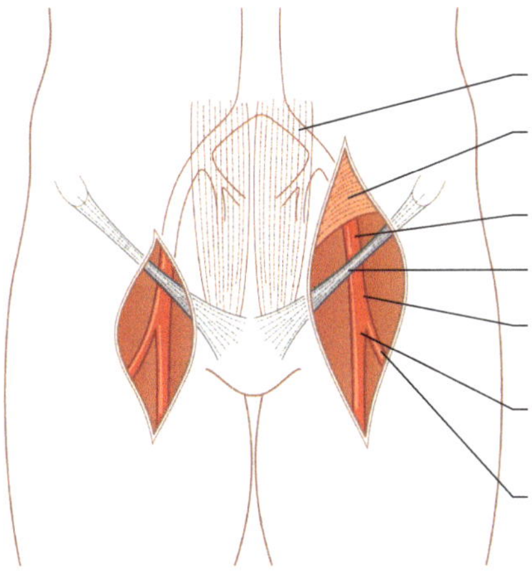

Figure 42.2 Standard groin exposures with left skin incision extending at least 10 cm above the inguinal ligament to allow for retroperitoneal access.

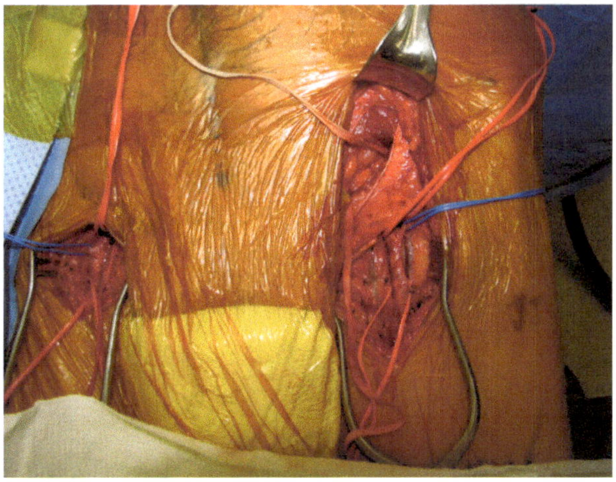

Figure 42.3 Completed groin dissections with controlled femoral vessels and left retroperitoneal incision.

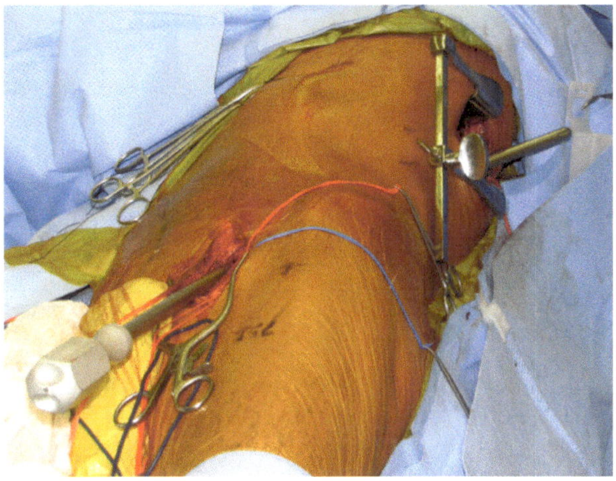

Figure 42.4 A bullet-tipped femoropopliteal tunneler is passed from the left retroperitoneal incision through the previously created retroperitoneal tunnel and into the left chest.

groin to the left thorax (Figures 42.2–42.4). Specifically, a 10 cm incision is made through the aponeurosis of the external and internal oblique muscles and the internal oblique muscles are divided bluntly in the direction of their fibers. The transverse abdominal muscle and transversalis fascia are opened in the lateral aspect of the incision (Figures 42.2–42.3) and the retroperitoneal space is entered medial to the anterior superior iliac crest.

THORACIC AORTA EXPOSURE

Thoracic dissection begins with a limited left posterolateral thoracotomy through the eighth intercostal space to reach the descending thoracic aorta. The specific choice of intercostal space is based on the patient's body habitus and final positioning. The skin incision is extended laterally beyond the margins of the latissimus dorsi muscle, carefully sparing the muscle itself. Superior and inferior skin flaps are then developed to help retract and preserve the muscle. The pleural cavity is entered and a rib spreader is inserted and opened cautiously to prevent rib fractures. If necessary, additional exposure may be obtained by excising the cephalad rib or resecting a short segment under the paraspinous muscles at the posterior margin of the incision. The anesthesia team then deflates the left lung, the inferior pulmonary ligament is taken down to the level of the inferior pulmonary vein, and the lung is retracted into the upper thorax. Two "figure-of-eight" sutures are placed in the center of the left hemidiaphragm using a 0-silk suture. These are brought through the inferior and anterior chest wall and secured to retract the diaphragm caudally and to allow adequate exposure of the distal descending thoracic aorta. The pleura around the distal descending thoracic aorta is incised, and a 6 cm segment of aorta above the diaphragm is exposed. The proximal anastomosis site is chosen by gently palpating

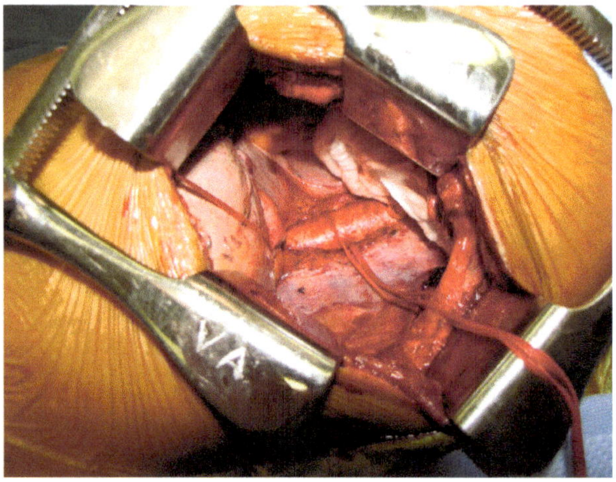

Figure 42.5 A rib spreader in the eighth intercostal space showing exposure of the aorta with umbilical tapes proximal and distal and diaphragm retracted anteriorly and inferiorly with silk suture.

the aorta to find a spot relatively free of atherosclerotic disease. Circumferential dissection is performed both proximally and distally, and umbilical tapes are placed to be used later as "handles" to stabilize the aorta and help position the proximal clamp (Figure 42.5). The authors take special care to preserve all the intercostal arteries because the anterior spinal artery originates from one of the intercostal arteries between the 8th and 12th thoracic vertebrae. The site of the aortotomy is carefully chosen so that it is high enough above the crus of the diaphragm to avoid lateral kinking of the proximal graft after tunneling.

TUNNELING

The authors then create a retroperitoneal tunnel to pass the graft limbs from the thorax to the groins. A 2 cm incision is made in the posteromedial aspect of the left diaphragm under the ribs through the open thoracic incision. The location of the aortotomy and the exit site through the diaphragm must be aligned carefully to avoid lateral kinking of the graft. Additionally, the diaphragmatic opening must be enlarged sufficiently so that the graft is not constricted. The operator's left hand is passed through the left retroperitoneal incision and the right hand through the left thoracic cavity. The left hand then dissects slowly through the left retroperitoneal plane, aiming cephalad and slightly medial, over the external iliac vessels and the psoas major muscle, posterior to the left kidney and posteromedial to the spleen to meet the right hand, which is also following this route starting from the left thorax. A long tunneler is then guided through the tunnel and used to pass an umbilical tape that ultimately facilitates the passage of the graft itself (Figure 42.4). The first option is to use a standard bifurcated prosthetic graft to create a thoracic aorta-bifemoral bypass. In this case, the shaft and two limbs of the graft are tunneled through the retroperitoneal channel and brought through the left retroperitoneal incision. It is imperative to maintain the correct orientation and tension on the limbs to prevent twisting or kinking. Then, a preperitoneal tunnel between the left suprainguinal, retroperitoneal space and the right groin that courses immediately posterior to the rectus muscles and just cephalad to the bladder in the preperitoneal space (retropubic space) is created with blunt finger dissection. If creation of the second tunnel is very difficult, this may be helped by dividing the caudal border of the inguinal ligament on the right. The second option is to use a straight graft to create the thoracic aorta-to-left groin bypass and then use a second cross-femoral bypass graft connecting the left femoral hood of the first graft to the right femoral vessels with a femoral crossover tunneled in a standard subcutaneous plane or a retropubic retroperitoneal tunnel.

ANASTOMOSES AND CHOICE OF GRAFTS

It is the authors' preference to perform the thoracic aortic anastomosis using a partially occluding, side-biting LeMole aortic clamp. This maintains antegrade blood flow through the aorta, potentially limiting the magnitude of the ischemia to the lower torso, visceral vessels, and anterior spinal artery (Figure 42.6). If a partially occluding, side-biting clamp cannot be used, then the aorta may be clamped with an upper vertical and lower-angled clamp; the lower-angled clamp is useful to control intercostal bleeding. After systemic heparinization (100 IU/kg), the jaws of the partially occluding clamp should be directed caudally and secured to prevent accidental dislodgement. The aorta caudal to the clamp should be interrogated with continuous wave Doppler to confirm preserved antegrade flow. An appropriately sized graft is chosen to match the size of the aorta and femoral vessels. When a bifurcated

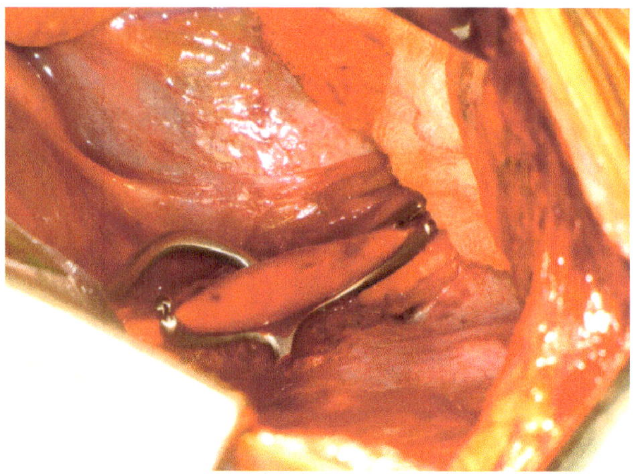

Figure 42.6 A partially occluding LeMole aortic clamp placed on the descending thoracic aorta to allow for continued antegrade blood flow during the proximal anastomosis.

graft is used, a 16 mm × 8 mm or 14 mm × 7 mm graft is appropriate. When a vertical limb from the thoracic aorta to the left groin with a left-to-right femoro-femoral crossover is used, then the authors use 8- or 10-mm grafts for the vertical limb and a 6- or 8-mm graft for the crossover graft. Both Dacron and polytetrafluoroethylene grafts are suitable options. The aortotomy is created and the body of the graft is spatulated appropriately. With the bifurcated graft, the authors leave the body of the graft as long as possible to make sure that there is sufficient length for the right graft limb to reach the right groin without excess stretch or tension. If the graft is not long enough to comfortably reach the right groin, excess graft from the left limb can be used to construct a composite right limb (graft-graft composite). A tension-free aortic anastomosis is created in a continuous fashion with a 2-0 polypropylene monofilament suture. After completing the proximal anastomosis, an atraumatic vascular clamp is positioned on the body of the graft itself to check for leaks.

The distal anastomosis of the left limb is constructed first. The right femoral anastomosis is then completed. If this is a "redo" operation, this may require anastomosis to the previously undissected profunda femoris arteries (PFAs) or anastomoses to the limbs of the older graft. The specific anastomotic configuration is chosen based on the distribution of the occlusive disease. Good flow into the PFAs must be established because the common and superficial femoral arteries are frequently diseased in patients requiring this type of bypass. This may require extending the anastomosis further distally into the PFA and performing a common femoral/PFA endarterectomy. If it is necessary to perform an extensive profundaplasty, the authors usually do a patch angioplasty and then sew the hood of the prosthetic graft onto the patch.

Heparin is usually allowed to wear off or it can be reversed with protamine sulfate after ensuring good distal flow. The thoracic and femoral incisions are closed in layers using standard techniques. A large chest tube (28–32 Fr) is placed through a separate incision and positioned with the tip in the apex of the chest. The lung is reinflated under direct vision. The ribs are approximated using interrupted absorbable suture in a figure-of-eight configuration. Alternatively, to avoid injury to the intercostal neurovascular bundles, a drill might be used to create needle holes through the ribs for placement of interrupted sutures. The chest wall muscles are closed with a running absorbable suture. If skin flaps were created for adequate exposure, closed suction drains are left in the subcutaneous space.

POSSIBLE COMPLICATIONS

Major complications include reoperation for bleeding, respiratory failure, myocardial infarction or cardiac failure, renal failure, and paraplegia.

TRICKS AND TRAPS

- The left groin skin incision is extended approximately 10 cm cephalad above the inguinal ligament to allow access to the retroperitoneum for the creation of the tunnel connecting the left groin to the left thorax.
- The descending thoracic aorta is exposed through a limited left posterolateral thoracotomy using the eighth intercostal space with sparing of the latissimus dorsi muscle.
- Two "figure-of-eight" sutures are placed in the center of the left hemidiaphragm using a 0-silk suture and are passed through the inferior and anterior chest wall and secured to retract the diaphragm caudally and improve exposure of the distal descending thoracic aorta.
- The site of the aortotomy and the exit site of the graft through the diaphragm must be aligned carefully to avoid lateral kinking of the graft.
- Careful slow and smooth creation of the tunnel is crucial to avoid injuring retroperitoneal structures. This tunnel should be created posterior to the left kidney and posteromedially to the spleen.
- Either a bifurcated thoracobifemoral graft or a single vertical thoraco-left femoral graft from the thoracic aorta to the left groin with a left-to-right femoro-femoral crossover can be used. If a bifurcated graft is chosen, leave the body of the graft as long as possible to make sure that there is sufficient length for the right graft limb to reach the right groin without excess stretch or tension.

QUESTIONS

1. Thoracofemoral bypass graft is best indicated for:
   a. Juxtarenal aortic occlusion in a 46-year-old male with hip claudication and erectile dysfunction
   b. Infrarenal aortic and bilateral iliac artery occlusion with rest pain
   c. 6 cm infrarenal AAA with severe iliac artery occlusive disease
   d. Failed aortobifemoral bypass graft in a 46-year-old female (graft occlusion (1) just below the renal arteries) with a history of multiple abdominal operations; (2) presenting with ischemic rest pain

   Answer: d

2. An absolute contraindication for thoracofemoral bypass graft is:
   a. Remote history of MI
   b. Multiple prior laparotomies
   c. Left ventricle ejection fraction of 55%
   d. Circumferential calcification of distal thoracic aorta

   Answer: d

3. Thoracofemoral bypass graft is planned for a 62-year-old male with a prior history of suprapubic cystostomy for bladder pathology.
   a. The right femoral limb of the graft should be brought behind the rectus abdominis in the space of Retzius
   b. The right axillofemoral graft should be considered with a left thoracofemoral bypass graft
   c. The right femoral graft limb is brought from the left groin in the suprapubic subcutaneous tunnel and anastomosed to the right common femoral artery as in a standard crossover femoral-femoral graft
   d. Right femoral limb is brought through the obturator foramen and anastomosed to the proximal right superficial femoral artery

Answer: c

REFERENCES

1. Schneider, J. R. (2010). Extra-anatomic bypass. In J. L. Cronenwett & K. W. Johnston (Eds.), *Rutherford's Vascular Surgery* (7th ed., pp. 1137–1153). Philadelphia, PA: Saunders/Elsevier.
2. Martin, D. & Katz, S. G. (2000). Axillofemoral bypass for aortoiliac occlusive disease. *Am J Surg.*, *180*, 100–103.
3. Passman, M. A., Farber, M. A., Criado, E., et al. (1999). Descending thoracic aorta to iliofemoral artery bypass grafting: a role for primary revascularization for aortoiliac occlusive disease? *J Vasc Surg.*, *29*, 249–258.
4. Igari, K., Kudo, T., Katsui, S., Nishizawa, M. & Uetake, H. (2020, December 20). The comparison of long-term results between aortofemoral and axillofemoral bypass for patients with aortoiliac occlusive disease. *Ann Thorac Cardiovasc Surg.*, *26*(6).
5. Fulton, J. J. & Keagy, B. A. (2006). Redo aortobifemoral and thoracobifemoral bypass for aortoiliac occlusive disease. In G. B. Zelenock (Ed.), *Mastery of Vascular and Endovascular Surgery* (pp. 375–384). Philadelphia, PA: Lippincott Williams & Wilkins.

43

Open surgical management of visceral artery occlusive disease

GRANT B. HUBBARD AND JAE S. CHO

INTRODUCTION

Despite the rise of endovascular therapy in the revascularization of chronic mesenteric ischemia (CMI), there remains a need for open surgery in patients whose anatomy or disease precludes endovascular treatment. Further, open mesenteric revascularization has so far shown superior patency rates when compared with endovascular therapy, as well as lower rates of recurrent symptoms and reintervention. The trade-off for these advantages is higher rates of morbidity and mortality for patients undergoing open revascularization. For these reasons, younger patients with fewer comorbidities may be best served with open surgery rather than endovascular.

Open revascularization for CMI consists of bypass grafting, endarterectomy, or reimplantation. Bypass grafting, the most common method, can be constructed with either an antegrade or a retrograde configuration. Each has its advantages and disadvantages. The salient advantages of an antegrade configuration are that the supraceliac aorta provides the best inflow source because it is usually free of atherosclerosis and it has a higher patency rate compared with a retrograde configuration. The disadvantages are that some vascular surgeons may not be familiar with this anatomic region and there is a higher potential for hemodynamic disturbances with clamping and unclamping of the supraceliac aorta. This latter problem can be reduced by partial aortic occlusion using a side-biting clamp. A retrograde configuration is favored by other vascular surgeons because of their familiarity with this exposure and its inherent lower risk for hemodynamic disturbances. Disadvantages of a retrograde bypass include the following: a potential for graft kinking and occlusion; graft contact with the bowel; and compromised inflow from a diseased infrarenal aortoiliac system. The ultimate choice for bypass configuration is based on surgeon comfort, an adequate inflow source, and minimal disease at the anastomotic inflow site.

Mesenteric endarterectomy with or without patch angioplasty is useful when the disease is focal. Ostial lesions involving the celiac axis (CA) and superior mesenteric artery (SMA) can be treated with transaortic endarterectomy through a trapdoor incision. This can be performed with aortic endarterectomy when the paravisceral aorta is also involved with significant atherosclerotic burden such as a “coral reef” plaque. Isolated reimplantation is most commonly used for the inferior mesenteric artery during abdominal aortic reconstruction.

OPERATIVE TECHNIQUE

Antegrade supraceliac aortomesenteric bypass grafting

A transperitoneal midline incision is made from the xiphoid process to the umbilicus. A bilateral subcostal incision with or without a midline extension to the xiphoid process (transplant incision) may also be used, especially in patients with a large body habitus or in those with a wide costal angle. A self-retaining retractor such as an Integra® Omni-Tract® retractor (Integra LifeSciences Corporation, Plainsboro, NJ, USA) facilitates exposure. The table is placed in a slight reverse Trendelenburg position with superolateral retraction of the costal margins. The left triangular ligament of the liver is divided and the left lateral segment retracted to the patient’s right. The gastrohepatic ligament is incised to enter the lesser sac. Using a nasogastric tube/echocardiography probe, the esophagus is identified and protected by retracting it to the patient’s left. The esophagophrenic ligament is preserved to protect the anterior and posterior vagus nerve fibers. Attention is paid near the lesser curvature

DOI: 10.1201/9781003452096-43

of the stomach to avoid injuries to the vagus nerves and a replaced left hepatic artery, if present.

The median arcuate ligament and interdigitating fibers of the crura are divided longitudinally to expose the aorta, which lies just posteriorly. A sufficient length of the supraceliac aorta is dissected and isolated along the anterior two-thirds of its circumference so that a side-biting clamp can be accommodated. The celiac ganglion that surrounds the CA at its origin is divided. Dissection is continued caudally to the proximal few centimeters of the CA (Figure 43.1). The inferior phrenic artery may be found in about 50% of cases and should be preserved, if possible. The left gastric artery is divided to facilitate end-to-end anastomosis of a graft to the CA.

The SMA can be exposed in its proximal segment or at the root of the mesentery, depending on the extent of disease and the patient's body habitus. When the disease is confined to the orifice of the SMA in a cachectic individual with a short distance between the CA and SMA, the latter vessel can be exposed by continuing dissection of the aorta caudally, aided by caudal retraction of the pancreas. The superior border of the pancreas is mobilized and retracted anteroinferiorly. The origin of the SMA is exposed posterior to the neck of the pancreas and the splenic vein. Care should be taken to avoid injuries

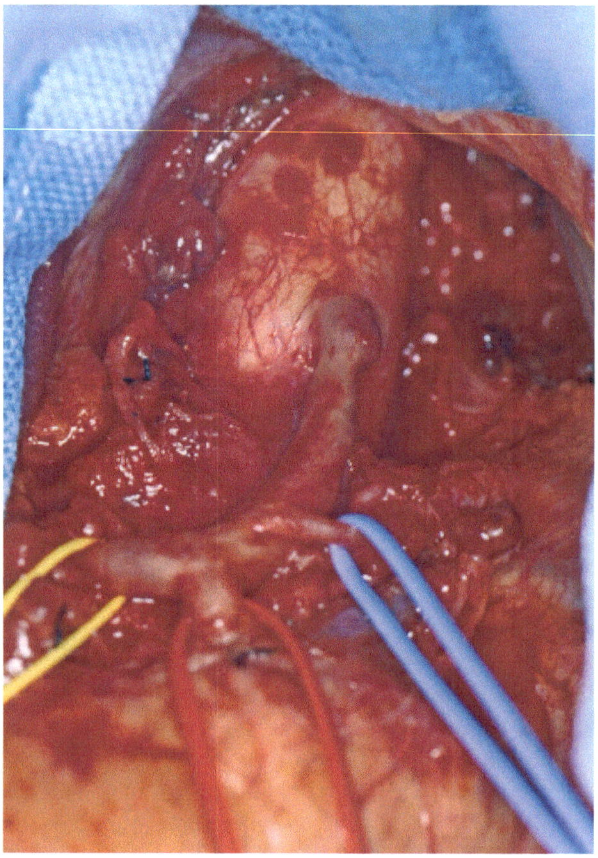

Figure 43.1 The supraceliac aorta, celiac axis, and its branches are dissected free. The blue loop encircles the left gastric artery, the red is for the splenic artery, and the yellow is for the common hepatic artery.

to adjacent vascular structures, such as the inferior pancreaticoduodenal artery. Lymphatics associated with the SMA require careful ligation to avoid a postoperative chyle leak.

The SMA at the base of the mesentery is the most frequently used target because this segment of the artery is more reliably disease-free. The transverse colon is reflected superiorly and the duodenum to the patient's right. The SMA can be easily palpated at the root of the mesentery just to the left of the reflected duodenum. If the artery is not easily localized, the ligament of Treitz is divided to mobilize the fourth portion of the duodenum and the artery can be isolated just cephalad to the duodenum. Alternatively, the middle colic artery can be traced retrograde to the SMA. In patients with CMI who have suffered weight loss, this can be done without much difficulty. About 2.5–3 cm of the vessel should be dissected circumferentially, along with jejunal branches that arise at this level.

A retropancreatic tunnel is prepared using gentle bimanual finger dissection from the supraceliac aorta to the root of the mesentery. It is safest to route this tunnel along the left side of the aorta to avoid injury to adjacent structures. This maneuver should be performed with caution because the tunnel courses are adjacent to the superior mesenteric vein and beneath the splenic vein. Umbilical tape or silastic tubing is placed in the tunnel.

Following systemic heparinization (100 IU/kg), a bifurcated prosthetic graft is selected. The author prefers to use a 12 × 7-mm polyester graft. However, 12 × 6-mm or 14 × 7-mm grafts are good alternatives. Mannitol may be given (0.5 g/kg IV), especially when complete occlusion of the aorta is required. Partial occlusion of the aorta is preferred over complete occlusion because the former prevents back-bleeding through the lumbar arteries, which may be significant. A side-biting clamp, such as a Lemole-Strong aortic clamp (Becton, Dickinson and Company, Franklin Lakes, NJ, USA), is an excellent choice in this location. When partial occlusion is not feasible, complete occlusion is obtained with a standard technique. Following aortic control, a longitudinal aortotomy is made. The graft is configured with the main body as short as possible. Additionally, the heel of the anastomosis should be within 1 cm of the graft bifurcation and the SMA limb should be posterior/posterolateral to the CA limb to avoid kinking of the SMA limb as it enters the retropancreatic tunnel (Figure 43.2).

The main body of the graft is sewn end-to-side to the aorta with a 4-0 polypropylene suture. After anastomotic hemostasis is assured, the CA is divided at its origin and the proximal stump oversewn. The anterior limb of the bifurcated graft is anastomosed end-to-end to the CA with a running 5-0 polypropylene suture. After appropriate back-bleeding and forward-bleeding, the suture line is secured and flow is restored to the CA. Alternatively, the celiac limb can be sewn end-to-side to either the common hepatic or proper hepatic artery.

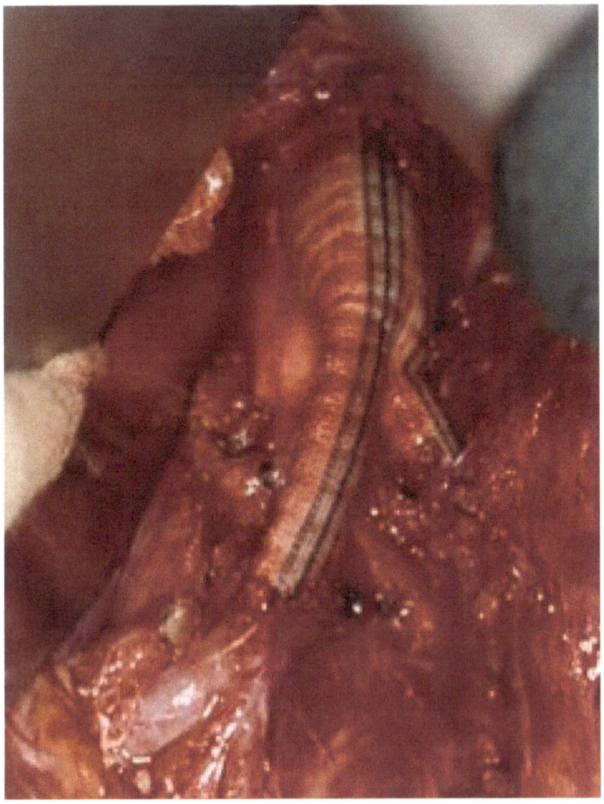

Figure 43.2 Completed antegrade aortoceliac/superior mesenteric artery (SMA) bypass. Note the posterior orientation of the SMA limb to avoid kinking as it enters the retropancreatic tunnel.

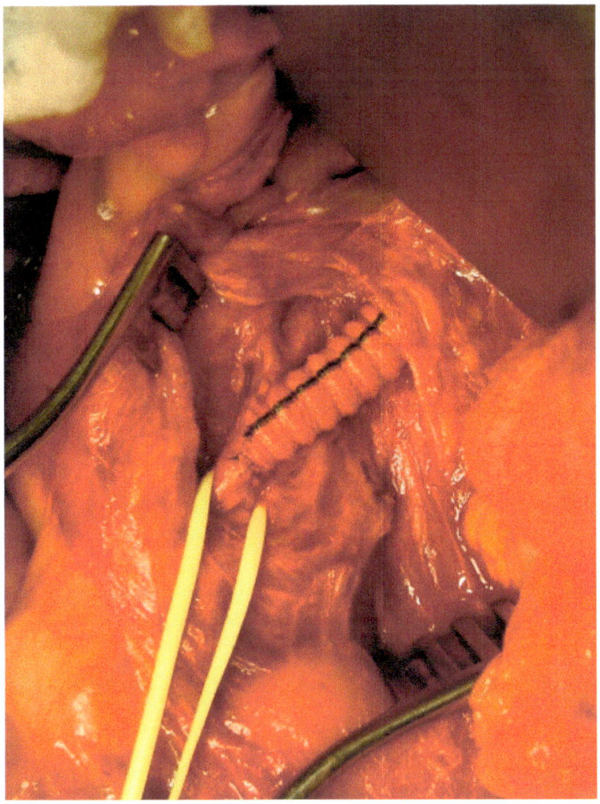

Figure 43.3 The superior mesenteric artery (SMA) limb is sewn end-to-side to the SMA.

The SMA limb is then brought into approximation with the SMA through the retropancreatic tunnel. Control of the SMA and its branches is obtained and a longitudinal arteriotomy is made. The graft is fashioned to fit and sewn end-to-side with a running 6-0 polypropylene suture. After appropriate back-bleeding and forward-bleeding, flow is restored to the SMA (Figure 43.3).

When an isolated bypass to the CA is planned (such as in median arcuate ligament syndrome), a flanged 8-mm limb may be used to bypass to the CA (Figure 43.4). In case of gross contamination with enteric contents, an autogenous (saphenous or femoral vein) conduit or allograft should be used.

Retrograde aortomesenteric bypass grafting

The inflow source for this operation is usually the distal infrarenal aorta, common iliac, or external iliac artery, depending on the quality of the inflow vessel (atherosclerotic burden) and graft configuration. The chosen inflow vessel is isolated and dissected free with standard technique after incising the retroperitoneum. The SMA is dissected and prepared as outlined earlier. The inflow anastomosis is performed first in an end-to-side fashion. The SMA anastomosis is performed in antegrade fashion, end-to-side. It is imperative to allow a gentle curve for the graft as it traverses from the inflow vessel to the target vessel to avoid kinking when the bowel is returned to its normal anatomic position. The graft is covered with the retroperitoneum to protect it from the bowel. Alternatively, the graft may be covered with omentum.

Trapdoor transaortic endarterectomy

The patient is placed in a modified left thoracotomy position. The left hemithorax, shoulder, and arm are positioned at 70 degrees to the table while the left hip is rotated posteriorly as far as possible (usually 30 degrees off the table). Both groins should be accessible, as is the case with any aortic operation. An oblique incision is made from the ninth or tenth intercostal space (ICS) across the abdominal muscles to the umbilicus, with the distal extent to the pubis along the midline as needed. The incision may be extended more proximally as needed along the intercostal space. A self-retaining retractor is invaluable.

Exposure can be provided via the retroperitoneal or transperitoneal route, depending on the need to evaluate the viability of the intestines. The viscera are mobilized medially with the left kidney left in situ; this provides more exposure of the SMA (up to 8–10 cm). When the atherosclerotic burden of the aorta extends beyond the origins of the renal arteries, the left kidney should be mobilized anteriorly along with the viscera. The left crus

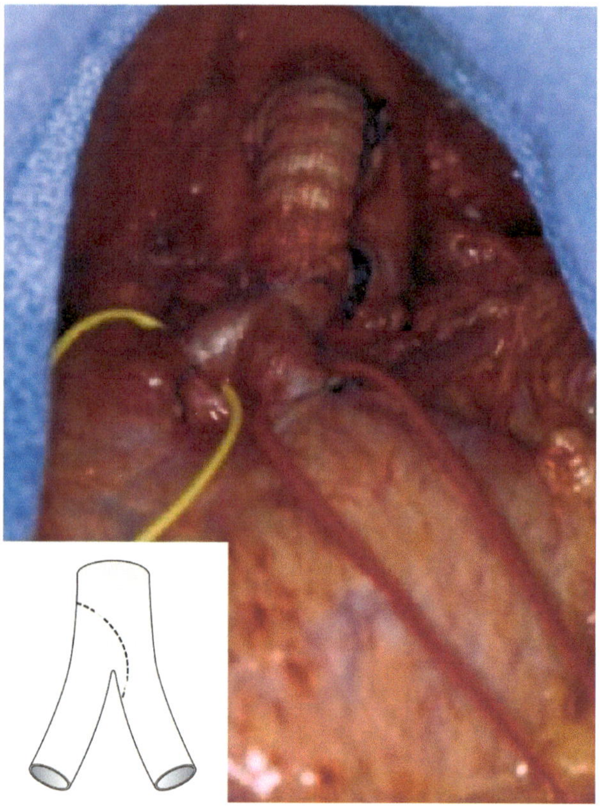

Figure 43.4 Aortoceliac bypass graft using a flanged (inset) polyester graft.

of the diaphragm is divided to expose the paravisceral aorta. Sufficient lengths of the branch vessels are isolated and dissected free. The left renal vein (LRV) is dissected and retracted caudally (Figure 43.5a). When more extensive endarterectomy of the pararenal aorta is needed, or when concomitant aortic reconstruction is planned for occlusive or aneurysmal disease, the left kidney is better reflected anteriorly along with the rest of the viscera.

After control is obtained of the aorta and its branches, a trapdoor aortotomy is made around the orifices of the CA and SMA (Figure 43.5b). The plane of endarterectomy is then developed around the visceral vessel orifices and eversion endarterectomy of these vessels is carried out. The aortotomy is closed primarily with a 4-0 polypropylene suture. On occasion, it may become necessary to extend the endarterectomy of the visceral arteries when plaque extends beyond their orifices. In such a setting, a separate arteriotomy is made in the proximal segment of the visceral artery (usually the SMA), an endarterectomy is performed, and the artery is closed with a patch angioplasty (Figure 43.5c). If renal artery disease is also present, the aortotomy can be extended caudally.

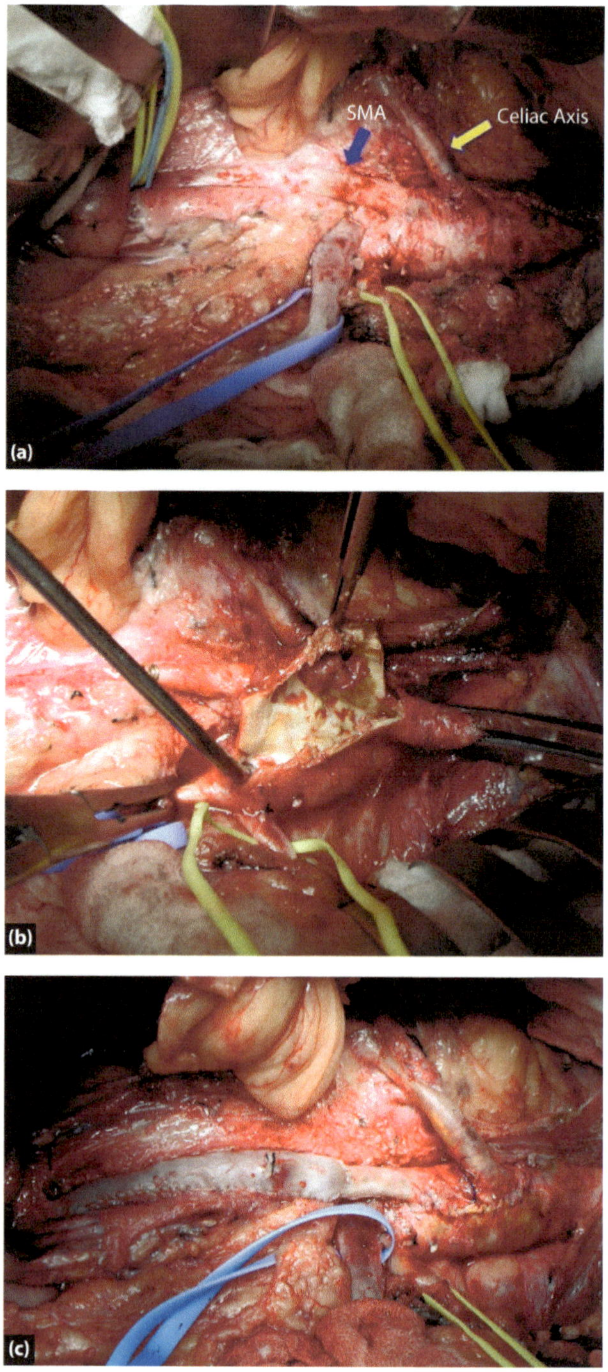

Figure 43.5 Trapdoor transaortic visceral endarterectomy: (a) retroperitoneal exposure of the entire abdominal aorta, celiac axis, superior mesenteric artery (SMA), and left renal artery (yellow loop). The left kidney is left in situ; the left renal vein is encircled with a thick blue loop; (b) a trapdoor aortotomy is made exposing the plaque and acute thrombus at the orifice of the celiac axis; (c) the trapdoor aortotomy is primarily closed. A long SMA endarterectomy with patch angioplasty is also shown.

Thoracovisceral bypass grafting

In the setting of a hostile abdomen, or in the case of inadequate inflow (such as a diseased supraceliac aorta or severe infrarenal aortoiliac occlusive disease that precludes retrograde bypass or warrants concomitant aortic reconstruction), thoracovisceral bypass grafting can be performed. The patient is positioned as described for trapdoor transaortic visceral endarterectomy. An

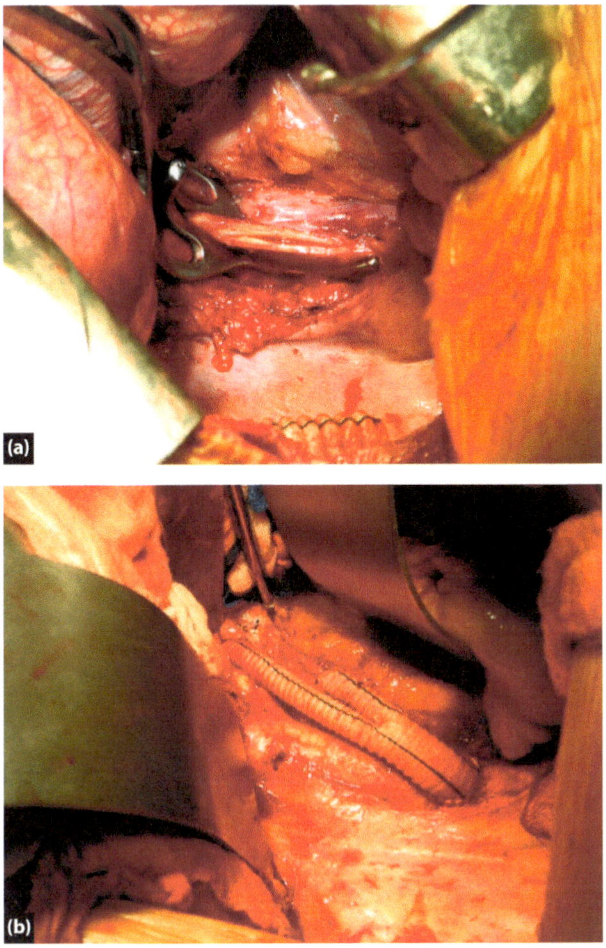

Figure 43.6 Thoracovisceral bypass graft: (a) a Lemole-Strong clamp (Becton, Dickinson and Company, Franklin Lakes, NJ, USA) is applied to the descending thoracic aorta for partial occlusion; (b) descending thoracic aortoceliac/SMA bypass is performed.

oblique incision is made through the seventh ICS across the abdominal muscles to the umbilicus. The diaphragm is divided circumferentially. The viscera are mobilized medially as described earlier. A side-biting clamp is applied to the descending thoracic aorta and a bifurcated graft is then used to reconstruct the visceral vessels with the technique described earlier (Figure 43.6). Once hemostasis of the proximal anastomosis is assured, the patient is systemically heparinized and the distal reconstruction completed.

Transabdominal medial visceral rotation

Access to the paravisceral aorta may also be gained by transabdominal medial visceral rotation through a full-length midline incision. After the small bowel is reflected to the right, the left lateral peritoneal reflection is incised to reflect the left colon medially. Dissection is continued cephalad and the spleen is mobilized. If the left kidney is to be left in situ, a plane of dissection is developed anterior to the left kidney between the pancreas and the Gerota's fascia. Dissection should be kept in the correct plane to avoid bleeding and injury to the pancreas, kidney, and adrenal gland. The stomach, pancreas, spleen, and descending colon are mobilized to the right, leaving the left kidney and associated structures in situ. The left crus of the diaphragm and the triangular ligament are divided. The anterior and posterior trunks of the vagus nerve are preserved. The autonomic ganglia over the SMA and CA are freed to expose the vessels. The LRV crossing the aorta is mobilized to its confluence with the inferior vena cava (IVC). By retracting the LRV caudally, the origins of the renal arteries can be exposed, if needed. The gonadal, adrenal, and lumbar branch veins can be divided as needed to facilitate mobilization of the LRV. The left renal artery can easily be dissected to the hilum. The proximal 2–3 cm of the right renal artery can be exposed with caution by retracting the IVC to the right. The entire abdominal aorta can be mobilized by incising the loose areolar tissue along the left lateral aspect of the aorta and reflecting the entire viscera to the right. The aortic bifurcation and the iliac arteries can be exposed, if necessary (Figure 43.7). Visceral reconstruction, endarterectomy, or bypass grafting can be performed as described earlier.

Closure

Meticulous closure of the abdominal wall is critical to avoid a leak of ascites that frequently develops after mesenteric revascularization because the hyperemic bowel may weep fluid in the early postoperative period.

POSTOPERATIVE COMPLICATIONS

Visceral reperfusion syndrome that can occur after mesenteric revascularization causes both local and remote organ injury, manifested by multisystem organ dysfunction. This multisystem organ dysfunction may not become evident for 48–72 hours postoperatively and may necessitate temporary reintubation. Acute respiratory distress syndrome, elevation of serum hepatic transaminase, thrombocytopenia, coagulopathy resistant to vitamin K supplementation, renal dysfunction, and prolonged postoperative ileus are commonly observed. Prolonged ventilator support and parenteral alimentation may be necessary. Rapid resumption of an oral diet is usually not possible.

Once the patient recovers, vessel patency should be interrogated with radiologic imaging, preferably computed tomography arteriography, to ascertain the adequacy of the reconstruction and to serve as a reference against which future studies may be compared before the patient is discharged.

CONCLUSION

Significant advances have been made over the past 30 years in the management of CMI. The operation must be

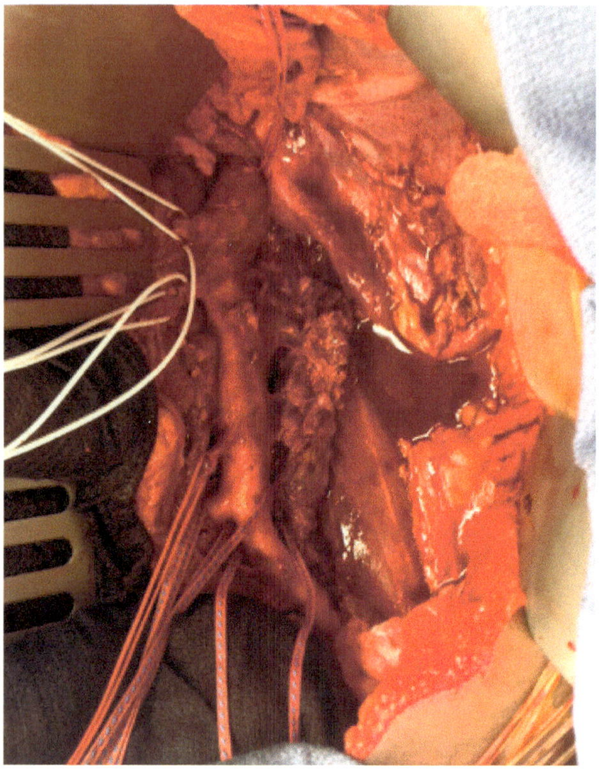

Figure 43.7 Transabdominal left medial visceral rotation, with the left kidney retracted anteriorly to expose the entire abdominal aorta and its branches (except the right renal artery) from hiatus to bifurcation. Upper white vessel loop around celiac; middle white vessel loop (somewhat loose) around superior mesenteric artery (SMA), lower white vessel loop around left renal artery; red vessel loop around inferior mesenteric artery. The three umbilical tapes are around the distal aorta just above bifurcation and both common iliac arteries. Note that the exposure is not much different from that of the retroperitoneal route shown in Figure 43.5 except that only the origin of the SMA can be exposed when the left kidney is reflected anteriorly because of the crossing left renal artery.

individualized to fit the patient's anatomy and risk factors. Not every patient requires complete revascularization, whether it be all mesenteric vessels or concomitant mesenteric and aortic reconstruction, unless it is necessary (i.e., aortic occlusion, symptomatic aortoiliac occlusive disease, or large aortic aneurysm). Unlike in the past, hybrid procedures may obviate the need for aortic reconstruction while minimizing postoperative morbidity.

TRICKS AND TRAPS

- Midline celiotomy and modified thoracoretroperitoneal exposures are frequently utilized, depending on what level of aortic access is required.
- When performing an antegrade bypass from the supraceliac or thoracic aorta, a side-biting clamp is preferred to minimize distal ischemia and to mitigate blood loss from intervening segmental arteries.
- Bypasses are most ideally performed in an antegrade fashion utilizing a bifurcated graft to the SMA and celiac axis.
- When a retrograde SMA bypass is necessary, an adequate length of graft must be used to make a gentle C-loop to avoid kinking. The graft needs to be covered with either retroperitoneum or a piece of omentum.
- In scenarios where occlusive disease is limited to the ostia of the visceral arteries, a transaortic endarterectomy can be performed through a trapdoor aortotomy.
- Additional mesenteric endarterectomy can be performed through a separate visceral branch arteriotomy if needed.
- Close watch must be kept postoperatively for visceral reperfusion syndrome. Prolonged ventilator support and parenteral nutrition may be necessary.

QUESTIONS

1. Which of the following is a disadvantage of antegrade mesenteric bypass grafting compared to retrograde mesenteric bypass?
   a. Potential for grafting kinking and occlusion
   b. Potential graft contact with the bowel
   c. Higher potential for intraoperative hemodynamic disturbances
   d. Lower patency rates

   Answer: c

2. A 56-year-old female is admitted with new onset acute renal failure (serum creatinine 2.5 mg/dL) and an episode of flash pulmonary edema which required temporary mechanical ventilation. A CT angiogram of the chest/ abdomen/ pelvis shows a para-visceral aortic "coral reef" plaque, limited to but involving the ostia of all 4 visceral vessels. Which procedure is best indicated for this patient?
   a. Aortomesenteric bypass, originating from the supraceliac aorta
   b. Iliomesenteric bypass
   c. "Trapdoor" transaortic endarterectomy
   d. Intravascular lithotripsy

   Answer: c

3. During exposure of the supraceliac aorta, division of which structure may lead to injury of the vagus nerve fibers?
   a. Right crus of the diaphragm
   b. Esophagophrenic ligament
   c. Left renal vein
   d. Median arcuate ligament

   Answer: b

4. In an antegrade aortomesenteric bypass, through which tissue plane is the tunnel created for the graft limb to the superior mesenteric artery?
   a. Through the transverse colon mesentery
   b. Anterior to the duodenum
   c. Anterior to the pancreas
   d. Posterior to the pancreas

   Answer: d

5. A 70-year-old male presents to your clinic with a complaint of postprandial abdominal pain, accompanied by a 20 lb weight loss over the last 6 months. Serum albumin is 1.8 g/dL. CT angiogram of the chest/ abdomen/ pelvis shows a 3 cm long, occlusion of the SMA at its origin, an 80 % stenosis of the celiac axis, as well as significant circumferential calcification of the descending thoracic, supraceliac, and infrarenal aortic wall. Which procedure should be performed?
   a. Supraceliac aorta-SMA bypass
   b. Iliomesenteric bypass
   c. Trapdoor transaortic endarterectomy
   d. Median arcuate ligament release

   Answer: b

SUPPLEMENTAL READING

Cho, J. S., Carr, J. A., Jacobsen, G., et al. (2002). Long-term outcome following mesenteric artery reconstruction: a 37-year experience. *J Vasc. Surg., 35*, 453–460.

Foley, M. I., Moneta, G. L., Abou-Zamzam, A. M., Jr, et al. (2000). Revascularization of the superior mesenteric artery alone for treatment of intestinal ischemia. *J Vasc Surg., 32*, 37–47.

Harward, T. R., Brooks, D. L., Flynn, T. C., et al. (1993). Multiple organ dysfunction after mesenteric artery revascularization. *J Vasc Surg., 18*, 459–467.

Jimenez, J. G., Huber, T. S., Ozaki, C. K., et al. (2002). Durability of antegrade synthetic aortomesenteric bypass for chronic mesenteric ischemia. *J Vasc Surg., 35*, 1078–1084.

Reilly, L. M., Ramos, T. K., Murray, S. P., et al. (1994). Optimal exposure of the proximal abdominal aorta: a critical appraisal of transabdominal medial visceral rotation. *J Vasc Surg., 19*, 375–389.

Stoney, R. J., & Effeney, D. J. (1992). *Wylie's Atlas of Vascular Surgery: Thoracoabdominal Aorta and Its Branches*. Philadelphia, PA: J.B. Lippincott Company.

Stoney, R. J., & Wylie, E. J. (1966). Recognition and surgical management of visceral ischemic syndromes. *Ann Surg., 164*, 714–722.

44

Open splanchnic artery aneurysm repair

JOSHUA K. BURK, WOOSUP M. PARK, AND JAE S. CHO

INTRODUCTION

The splanchnic (visceral) vessels are the celiac axis (CA), superior mesenteric artery (SMA), and inferior mesenteric artery (IMA) and their tributaries. Aneurysms of the splanchnic arteries are a rare entity, with an overall incidence in the adult population ranging from 0.1% to 2%. They comprise about 5% of all intra-abdominal aneurysms. The common causes of true aneurysms are degenerative or atherosclerotic in nature. However, fibromuscular dysplasia, collagen vascular diseases, and other rare medical conditions, such as von Recklinghausen disease, periarteritis nodosa, and Behçet's disease have been implicated. Multiparity, portal hypertension, and post-liver transplantation status have been connected to the development of a true splenic artery aneurysm. CA occlusive disease and median arcuate ligament syndrome have been associated with true gastroduodenal artery and pancreaticoduodenal artery aneurysms, presumably due to high compensatory flow through these important collateral pathways. Pseudoaneurysm of the splanchnic beds results from infection or inflammatory etiologies (e.g., pancreatitis), vasculitis, iatrogenic injuries, and trauma.

Of all splanchnic aneurysms, splenic artery aneurysm (SAA) accounts for about 60%; followed by hepatic artery aneurysm (HAA, 20%); SMA aneurysm (SMAA, 6%); celiac axis aneurysm (CAA, 4%); gastric artery aneurysm (4%); jejunal, ileal, and colic artery (4%); pancreaticoduodenal artery aneurysm (PDAA, 2%); and IMA aneurysm (IMAA, <1%) [1]. The indication and exact timing for intervention for true aneurysms hinge on the risk of rupture and thromboembolic complications [2]. The following recommendations have been made for intervention: splenic artery aneurysm, >3 cm (except for women of childbearing age, any size); CA, hepatic artery, jejunal, ileal aneurysm, >2 cm. For aneurysms of the SMA, gastric, gastroepiploic, gastroduodenal, pancreaticoduodenal, and colic arteries, repair is recommended irrespective of size [3]. Pseudoaneurysms, on the other hand, usually grow rather rapidly, thereby they warrant intervention irrespective of size.

Endovascular treatment by means of a covered stent and/or coil embolization is the preferred therapy modality when anatomically feasible and end-organ perfusion can be maintained. However, because of the short lengths of the involved vessels (i.e., CA) and the proximity of major branches that must be preserved (SMA and its branches) or involvement of the branch vessels within the aneurysmal segment, sufficient landing zones are difficult to secure. Furthermore, the flow pattern may be altered or even disrupted after endovascular treatment, thereby necessitating open surgical reconstruction to restore/preserve end-organ perfusion. Thus, open surgical repair is required in many cases.

SURGICAL TREATMENT

Ligation and aneurysmectomy

The simplest surgical repair is ligation without reconstruction. This is the preferred method of repair in the setting of rupture with hemodynamic instability, and even during elective repair if an adequate collateral network is present with preservation of flow to the end organ. Thus, it is critical to have a keen understanding of the splanchnic circulation and its collateral network.

Splenic artery aneurysm (SAA) in the proximal or middle portion of the artery can be treated by proximal and distal ligation and resection of the aneurysm, or more commonly today, with embolotherapy, since the spleen has a rich blood supply from the short gastric arteries and pancreaticoduodenal artery (PDA) network. For those located near the hilum or within the splenic parenchyma, splenectomy is performed. Distal pancreatectomy may be required on occasion.

Celiac axis aneurysm (CAA) can be safely ligated as there is a robust collateral circulation via the PDA and GDA network. However, in patients with mesenteric

DOI: 10.1201/9781003452096-44

ischemia symptoms or in the setting of questionable perfusion to end organs, CA reconstruction should be readily performed.

Hepatic artery aneurysm (HAA) can also be ligated when there is sufficient collateral flow through the SMA, PDA, and gastroduodenal artery (GDA) pathways. When in doubt, temporary occlusion of the hepatic artery during open repair will help decide between reconstruction versus ligation of the HAA. Intrahepatic HAAs usually warrant resection of the involved lobe.

Gastric, pancreaticoduodenal, gastroduodenal, gastroepiploic, jejunal, ileal, and colic artery aneurysms are similarly treated with simple ligation without arterial reconstruction. When intramural aneurysms involve the gastric wall, a wedge resection of the stomach can be performed. When bowel resection is required, special attention needs to be paid to the status of collateral circulation through the marginal artery of Drummond and arc of Riolan in patients with a history of colectomy. Another caveat is that patients with PDAA often have a contributory stenosis or occlusion of the CA, which may warrant surgical revascularization of the CA [4].

Aneurysmorrhaphy may also be performed for saccular visceral artery aneurysms.

Open surgical reconstruction

The necessity for reconstruction depends on the location of the aneurysm and the nature of the collateral mesenteric circulation. As such, open surgical reconstruction is most commonly needed in the setting of CAAs or SMAAs. The standard configuration is supraceliac aorto-celiac/SMA bypass grafting using a prosthetic graft. Other inflow sources may include the iliac, SMA, or renal arteries. When hepatic artery reconstruction is necessary, autologous vein conduit is preferred.

Techniques for reconstruction

ANTEGRADE SUPRACELIAC AORTA-BASED RECONSTRUCTION

A generous midline incision is made from the xiphoid process to just below the umbilicus. A bilateral subcostal incision with midline extension to the xiphoid process may also be used. A nasogastric tube is placed to allow for stomach decompression and facilitate identification of the esophagus during dissection. A self-retaining retractor is placed, and the operating table is positioned in reverse-Trendelenburg positioning to allow gravity to assist with the downward displacement of the viscera. Superolateral retraction of the costal margins facilitates total exposure of the upper abdomen. The left triangular ligament of the liver is divided, and the left lateral segment retracted to the patient's right. The lesser sac is entered with an incision of the gastrohepatic ligament in the avascular plane. With a nasogastric tube in place, the esophagus is identified and protected by retracting it to the patient's left. The esophagophrenic ligament is preserved to protect the anterior and posterior vagus nerves. Increased attention is paid to near the lesser curvature of the stomach to avoid injuries to these nerves and a replaced left hepatic artery, if present.

The median arcuate ligament and left diaphragmatic crus are divided to expose the aorta, which lies posteriorly. A sufficient length of the supraceliac aorta is dissected and isolated free to accommodate a side-biting clamp. Typically, this can be done without entering the left pleura; however, communication with anesthesia when inadvertent pleural entry is encountered is important to avoid ventilation difficulties and postoperative pneumothorax. Dissection is continued caudally on the aorta to the proximal few centimeters of the CA. An inferior phrenic artery originating from the aorta may be found in nearly half of cases and should be controlled [5]. The left gastric artery may be ligated and divided when encountered (Figure 44.1).

If the aneurysm is confined to the CA itself without the involvement of its major branches, the authors prefer aorto-celiac bypass grafting. When the aneurysm involves the splenic artery, the splenic artery is ligated where it is disease-free and aorto-hepatic bypass grafting is performed. Dissection of sufficient hepatic length should be

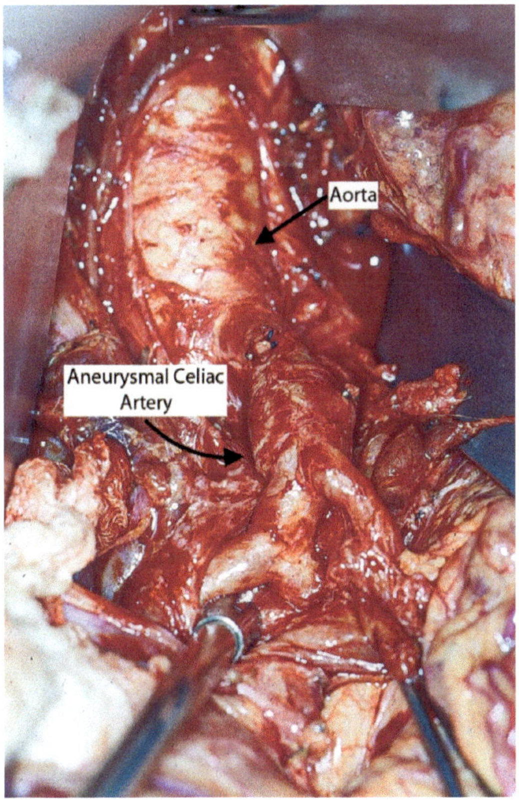

Figure 44.1 Celiac axis aneurysm. A celiac axis aneurysm is dissected out, demonstrating the bifurcation of the artery. A section of the supraceliac aorta is exposed to accommodate a side-biting clamp.

carried out with control of side branches. Mannitol may be given (0.5 g/kg), especially when complete occlusion of the aorta is required.

Following systemic heparinization (100 units/kg), partial control of the aorta is obtained with a side-biting clamp, such as a Lemole-Strong aortic clamp. Partial occlusion of the aorta is preferred over cross-clamping because the former (a) prevents back-bleeding through the segmental arteries, which may be significant; and (b) allows distal perfusion. A longitudinal aortotomy is made and a flanged 8-mm woven polyester graft is fashioned from a 16 × 8 mm bifurcation graft and sewn end-to-side to the aorta with a running 4-0 polypropylene suture. After anastomotic hemostasis is assured, the distal end is anastomosed to the CA in an end-to-end fashion or to the common hepatic artery in an end-to-side fashion, utilizing a running 6-0 polypropylene suture. Before completion of the distal anastomosis, the bypass graft should be thoroughly flushed of debris and air (Figures 44.2 and 44.3).

For SMAA necessitating open reconstruction, the initial exposure proceeds as described to isolate the supraceliac aorta. The SMA at its origin can be accessed from the infrarenal aorta. Dissection along the anterior surface of the aorta at the 12 o'clock position is continued cephalad from the pararenal aorta until the SMA origin is identified. The left renal vein is mobilized by ligating and dividing the left adrenal vein. Division of the renal vein is rarely necessary. The periaortic tissue at this level is rich with lymphatics that should be ligated and divided with

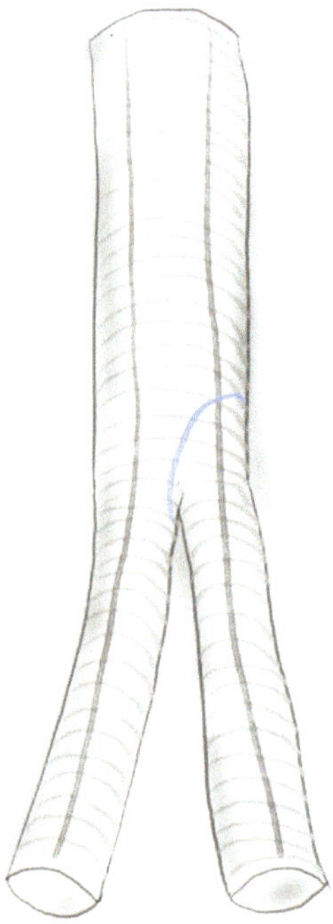

Figure 44.2 Flanged graft. An artist's rendition of a bifurcated polyester graft with a line drawn to demonstrate the appropriate method for fashioning a flanged graft.

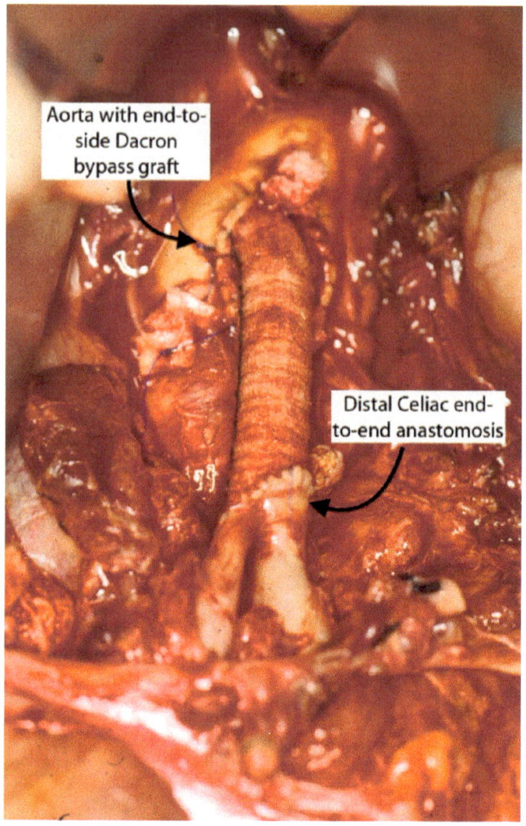

Figure 44.3 Aorto-celiac bypass graft. A celiac axis aneurysm (Figure 44.1) is resected and bypassed with a polyester graft. The proximal anastomosis is fashioned in an end-to-side fashion to the aorta utilizing a side-biting aortic clamp and the distal anastomosis in an end-to-end fashion to the celiac axis bifurcation, distal to the origin of the left gastric artery, which is ligated.

silk ligatures or its equivalent, rather than electrocautery, to avoid postoperative lymphatic leak and possible chylous ascites formation.

Dissection of the mid-SMA is begun by identifying the SMA near the root of the mesentery just superior to the fourth portion of the duodenum. Depending on the location of the aneurysmal segment, significant mobilization may be necessary to ensure side branches feeding the aneurysm are successfully ligated, as demonstrated in Figure 44.4. A retropancreatic tunnel between the supraceliac aorta and the mid-SMA is made with gentle finger dissection to the left side of the aorta so as to avoid any injuries to the mesenteric venous structures or the pancreas itself. An umbilical tape is then passed to secure this tunnel. End-to-end anastomosis can be undertaken if the bypass is being performed to the proximal SMA where (a) size mismatch is not an issue; and (b) bidirectional flow is not necessary to maintain perfusion to critical branches. In many cases, a longer end-to-end configuration is needed to preserve perfusion through major branch vessels (Figure 44.5).

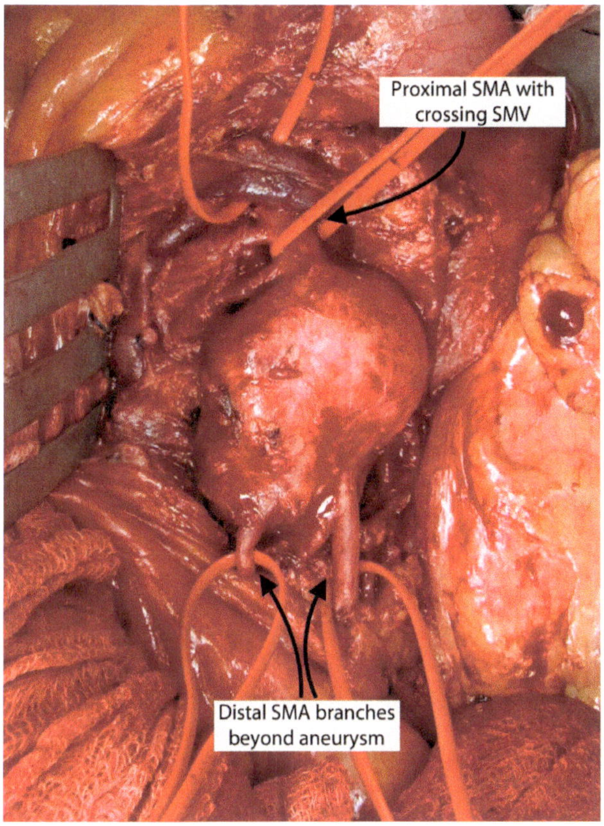

Figure 44.4 SMA aneurysm. A large SMA involving the mid-portion of the artery. Silastic vessel loops are placed around the branches of the artery coming off the aneurysm.

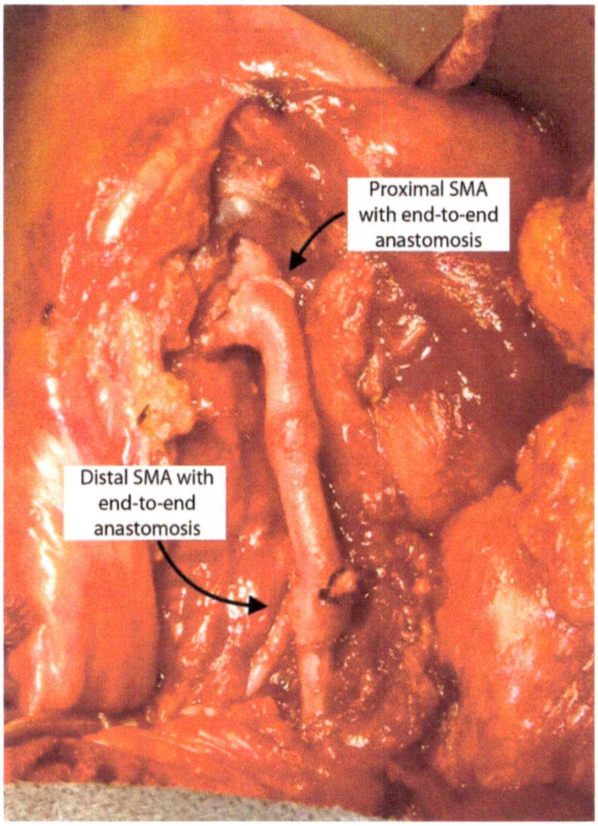

Figure 44.5 SMA aneurysm repair with saphenous vein interposition bypass graft. The SMA aneurysm (Figure 44.4) is resected and bypassed with an interposition saphenous vein graft with both proximal and distal end-to-end anastomoses. Major branch vessels were preserved to maintain perfusion to the bowel.

RETROGRADE INFRARENAL AORTA ILIAC-BASED RECONSTRUCTION

When the supraceliac abdominal aortic wall is calcified and not conducive to clamp placement, inflow can be derived either from the infrarenal aorta or iliac artery. When the infrarenal aorta is chosen, dissection of the aorta is undertaken to the right of the midline to minimize injury to sympathetic nerve fibers to mitigate the risk of sexual dysfunction [6,7]. When the common iliac artery is the inflow source, it is preferred to use the right side for the same reason. The target vessel anastomotic site should be prepared in addition to dissection of the aneurysm. Following systemic heparinization, the inflow anastomosis is completed first using either a 6-mm or 8-mm expanded polytetrafluoroethylene (ePTFE) or polyester graft with a 5-0 polypropylene suture, depending on the size of the target vessel. The aneurysm is then resected and distal anastomosis undertaken either end-to-end or end-to-side, with a 6-0 polypropylene suture. The graft should be covered with the peritoneum, omentum, or a biologic material such as CorMatrix to protect it from the gastrointestinal tract. A gentle curvature of the graft is maintained to avoid kinking when the bowel is returned to its normal anatomic position within the abdomen.

INTERPOSITION BYPASS GRAFTING AND LIGATION

In many cases where there is an aneurysm of the mid-portion of the hepatic or SMA, simple resection with interposition bypass reconstruction is feasible (Figure 44.6). Most commonly, this will be utilized for reconstruction of the SMA. The key to successful reconstruction involves ensuring a healthy, normal proximal artery and a suitable distal target. The proximal and distal artery is dissected out including the intervening branch vessels. Frequently, it may be necessary to sacrifice some of the smaller branches originating off of an aneurysmal segment of the SMA, as demonstrated in Figure 44.7. Test occlusion of these branch vessels is helpful to ascertain the safety of ligation without reconstruction. Interposition grafting is performed using standard vascular surgical techniques. Autogenous saphenous vein conduit is the preferred choice. Upper extremity vein is a good alternative when the former is not available. A prosthetic conduit is the last resort. In cases of infectious etiology, cryopreserved conduit should be used rather than prosthetic material if autologous vein is not available.

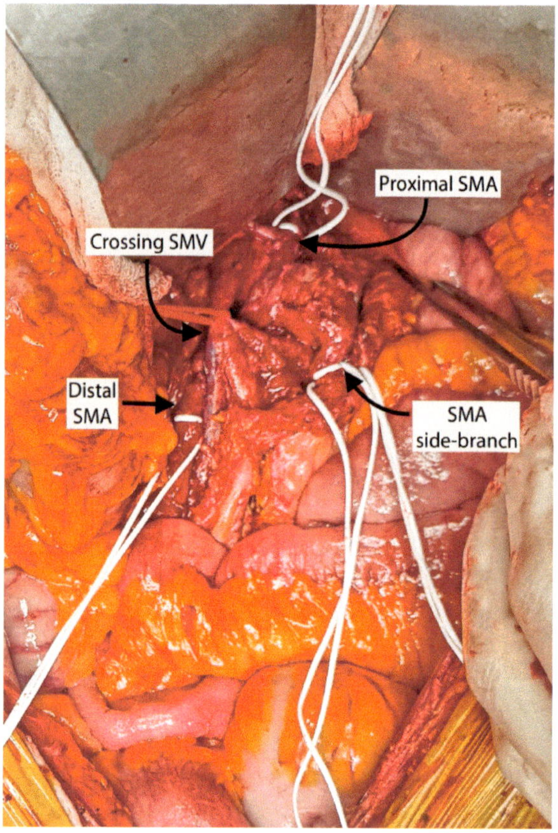

Figure 44.6 Mycotic SMA aneurysm. A mycotic SMA aneurysm involving a proximal branch point of the artery. The superior mesenteric vein (SMV) is retracted to the patient's right to reveal the aneurysm. White silastic vessel loops are placed around the proximal and distal SMA.

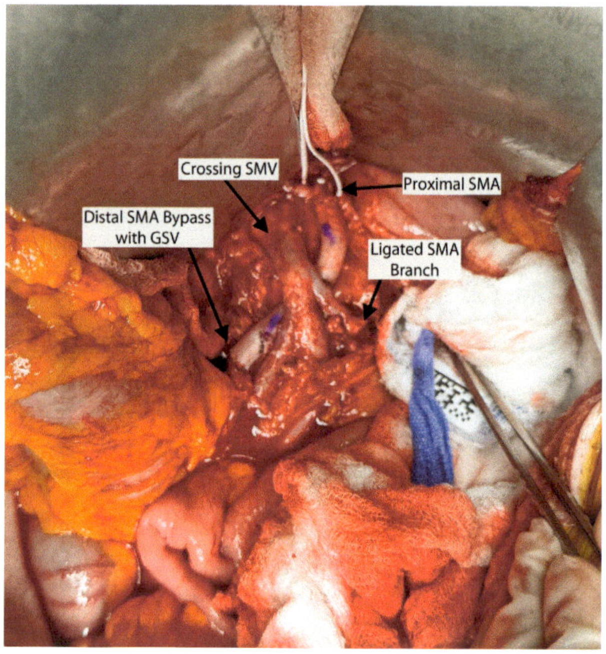

Figure 44.7 Mycotic SMA aneurysm post-repair. The mycotic SMA aneurysm from Figure 44.6 was excised and repair was completed with an interposition bypass graft of the reversed great saphenous vein (GSV). The bypass was tunneled posteriorly to the crossing SMV, which is now in its anatomic position. As demonstrated here, the distal target artery was the main SMA while a smaller side branch was ligated. Prior to ligation of the side branch, test occlusion was performed and the small bowel was grossly inspected and signals along the antimesenteric border verified to ensure bowel viability.

POSTOPERATIVE CARE AND COMPLICATION

Postoperatively, most patients require close monitoring of end-organ perfusion with serial monitoring of liver enzymes and lactate at regular intervals for the first 24 to 48 hours. A benign and self-limited transaminase rise is expected in the immediate postoperative period. While a rise in transaminases is not unexpected, it is paramount to closely monitor the bilirubin and international normalized ratio (INR) as they may be indicative of derangements in hepatic synthetic function. Postoperative lactate level can detect intestinal ischemia.

Nearly all patients should be able to receive aspirin immediately postoperatively. In the authors' experience, most patients with autologous vein reconstruction will do well with 81 mg of aspirin daily and a high-intensity statin. Patients needing ePTFE or polyester reconstruction are typically started on dual antiplatelet therapy with aspirin and clopidogrel 75 mg daily. In the authors' experience, a loading dose is unnecessary. Our follow-up care will typically involve a mesenteric duplex at one, three, and six months, with annual follow-up visits with imaging after the first year. If the patient's body habitus precludes adequate evaluation with duplex, CT angiography can be obtained as an alternative.

CONCLUSION

Open reconstruction of splanchnic aneurysms is frequently required as endovascular solutions may be limited due to the location of the aneurysm and the proximity or involvement of major branch vessels. Vascular surgeons need to be familiar with the indication for repair and be comfortable with a variety of techniques for open reconstructive techniques of the visceral vessels.

TRICKS AND TRAPS

- Understanding the collateral networks of the splanchnic vasculature is critical to determining the necessity of and most appropriate type of reconstruction following splanchnic artery aneurysm resection.
- Upper midline laparotomy or a chevron incision is most frequently employed.
- Utilizing a self-retaining retractor, gastric decompression, and reverse-Trendelenburg positioning can aid in visualizing the upper abdominal structures.

- If an antegrade supraceliac aorta-based bypass grafting is employed, a side-biting aortic clamp should be sufficient in most cases and avoids blood loss from the segmental vessels that may be encountered with cross-clamping.
- In general, an ePTFE or polyester conduit is preferred for aorta or common iliac artery-based reconstruction. For short interposition grafting or in the setting of infection, autogenous vein or a cryopreserved allograft is preferred.
- Care needs to be taken to avoid injury to the superior hypogastric plexus, also known as the preaortic plexus, when dissecting the infrarenal aorta, particularly near the bifurcation and along the iliac arteries. This is accomplished by dissecting to the right of the midline and limiting dissection along the left common iliac artery.
- Always entertain the potential for ligation of aneurysmal segments without reconstruction based on acceptable collateral blood flow.
- Small distal aneurysms of the SMA branches can frequently be treated with short-segment bowel resection.

QUESTIONS

1. Which of the following is the most common splanchnic artery aneurysm?
   a. Hepatic artery aneurysm
   b. Superior mesenteric artery aneurysm
   c. Splenic artery aneurysm
   d. Inferior mesenteric artery aneurysm

   Answer: c

2. What is the recommended size threshold for elective repair of a true splenic artery aneurysm in a woman of a childbearing age?
   a. > 1 cn
   b. > 2 cm
   c. > 3 cm
   d. Any size

   Answer: d

3. A 45-year-old patient presents with symptoms of abdominal pain and is diagnosed with a pancreaticoduodenal artery aneurysm. Which of the following conditions is most frequently associated with this type of aneurysm?
   a. Marfan's syndrome
   b. Celiac axis occlusion
   c. Ehlers-Danlos syndrome
   d. Renal artery stenosis

   Answer: b

4. What of the following factors is not a common cause of splanchnic artery aneurysms?
   a. Atherosclerosis
   b. Fibromuscular dysplasia
   c. Hyperthyroidism
   d. Portal hypertension

   Answer: c

5. Which graft material is generally preferred for an aorto-celiac or SMA bypass grafting in a non-infected setting?
   a. Cryopreserved allograft
   b. Deep femoral vein
   c. Synthetic (Polyester or ePTFE) graft
   d. Bovine pericardial graft

   Answer: c

REFERENCES

1. Deterling RA, Jr. Aneurysm of the visceral arteries. *J Cardiovasc Surg (Torino)*. 1971;12(4):309–22.
2. Corey MR, Ergul EA, Cambria RP, English SJ, Patel VI, Lancaster RT, et al. The natural history of splanchnic artery aneurysms and outcomes after operative intervention. *J Vasc Surg*. 2016;63(4):949–57.
3. Chaer RA, Abularrage CJ, Coleman DM, Eslami MH, Kashyap VS, Rockman C, et al. The Society for Vascular Surgery clinical practice guidelines on the management of visceral aneurysms. *J Vasc Surg*. 2020;72(1S):3S–39S.
4. Sutton D, Lawton G. Coeliac stenosis or occlusion with aneurysm of the collateral supply. *Clin Radiol*. 1973;24(1):49–53.
5. Loukas M, Hullett J, Wagner T. Clinical anatomy of the inferior phrenic artery. *Clin Anat*. 2005;18(5):357–65.
6. DePalma RG, Levine SB, Feldman S. Preservation of erectile function after aortoiliac reconstruction. *Arch Surg*. 1978;113(8):958–62.
7. van Schaik J, van Baalen JM, Visser MJ, DeRuiter MC. Nerve-preserving aortoiliac reconstruction surgery: anatomical study and surgical approach. *J Vasc Surg*. 2001;33(5):983–9.

45

Aortic graft infections

MITCHELL R. WEAVER

INTRODUCTION

The use of prosthetic grafts as conduits for the treatment of aortic aneurysmal or occlusive disease is a cornerstone of vascular surgery. The success of prosthetic grafting is based not only on the technicalities of graft implantation but also on maintaining graft sterility in vivo. Unfortunately, this is not always achieved. Aortic graft infection (AGI) poses a significant morbidity and mortality risk for the patient and is a considerable challenge to the surgeon charged with the patient's care and generates significant socioeconomic costs.

PRESENTATION AND DIAGNOSIS

Diagnosing patients with AGI requires a high index of suspicion in the face of often nonspecific symptomatology. Patient presentations range from generalized malaise and subtle systemic signs all the way to overt sepsis. Laboratory studies are often nonspecific but may include leukocytosis with or without a left-shifted differential count and elevated inflammatory markers, such as erythrocyte sedimentation rate and C-reactive protein. Multiple sets of blood cultures should be obtained, but these may not yield positive results even with obvious infection. Nevertheless, every effort should be undertaken to identify the offending organism. Common pathogens include *Staphylococcus aureus* and *S. epidermidis*, the latter with a penchant for foreign bodies given its biofilm-producing property [1]. Imaging studies usually begin with a high-quality computed tomographic angiogram (CTA), which can confirm the diagnosis, evaluate the extent of the infection, and direct operative planning for definitive treatment. Typical findings include perigraft soft tissue enhancement, adjacent soft tissue stranding, pockets of gas (Figure 45.1), pseudoaneurysm formation, and even frank rupture. In the face of a subtler clinical picture or uncertain findings, a short-term follow-up CTA or a tagged white blood cell scan may further clarify the presence of AGI [2].

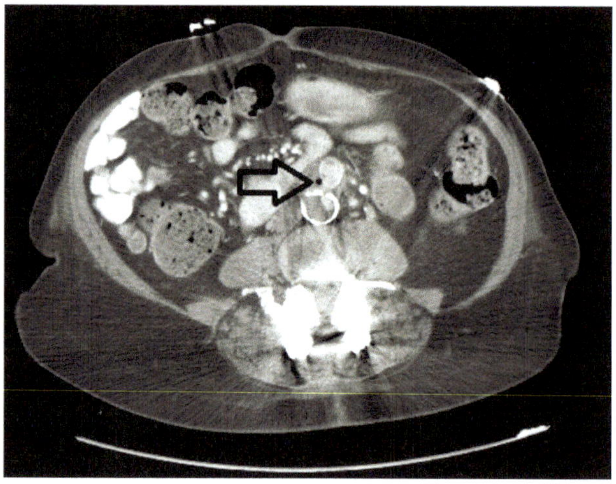

Figure 45.1 Computed tomographic angiogram demonstrating an air pocket (arrow) adjacent to the proximal end of an end-to-side anastomosis of a Dacron aortofemoral bypass graft.

MANAGEMENT PRINCIPLES

Initially, appropriate antibiotic therapy should be administered, and the patient should be physiologically optimized. The goals of treatment include infection eradication, hemorrhage prevention, and maintenance of organ and limb perfusion. Infection eradication typically requires excision of all prosthetic graft material, along with aggressive debridement of surrounding infected and devitalized tissue. In certain cases, graft preservation has been successful when antibiotic therapy has been coupled with multiple washouts and eventual soft tissue coverage. This approach is typically limited to early, nonvirulent,

DOI: 10.1201/9781003452096-45

peripherally located graft infections *not* involving an anastomosis, and is typically not feasible for intracavitary AGI. Percutaneous drainage and antibiotic therapy have been reported to be beneficial in a small number of patients [3]. Options for arterial reconstruction can be divided into either extra-anatomic bypass (e.g., axillobifemoral bypass) with aortic ligation or in situ arterial reconstructions with one of several conduits (femoral vein, cryopreserved allograft, antibiotic-impregnated prosthetic graft, or bovine pericardial grafts). More recent retrospective reviews and meta-analyses suggest the superiority of in situ, in-line arterial reconstruction over extra-anatomic reconstruction [4,5]. As each treatment option has its own benefits and limitations, an individualized approach to AGI with careful surgical judgment is required.

GENERAL OPERATIVE PRINCIPLES

General anesthesia is standard for these operations. Blood products should be available to replace blood loss and correct coagulopathy. Prolonged operative times are the norm; thus, ergonomic patient positioning with appropriate padding is paramount to avoid unintended neurapraxia and pressure-related complications. Warming devices should be used to avoid hypothermia. Both a transperitoneal midline approach and a left flank retroperitoneal approach can be used depending on the operative plan.

A supine position provides the most flexibility when dealing with AGI. The aorta from the diaphragmatic hiatus and as far distally as the external iliac arteries (EIAs) can be exposed through a midline celiotomy incision. While the pararenal aorta can be controlled through a standard inframesocolic approach, more proximal supraceliac control requires partial mobilization of the left lobe of the liver and subsequent division of the gastrohepatic ligament. The supine position also allows for the chest and lower extremities to be prepped into the operative field should an axillobifemoral bypass be planned or to harvest a lower extremity vein. A disadvantage of this approach is the scarring encountered from the initial aortic graft implantation or from previous abdominal surgeries, which makes the identification of tissue planes and subsequent dissection difficult.

A left flank retroperitoneal approach has some significant advantages. First, it avoids a hostile abdomen and provides a direct approach to the aorta without the impediment of the intraperitoneal contents. Second, depending on the interspace chosen for the incision, exposure of the descending thoracic aorta is possible. Disadvantages include the potential difficulty in controlling the distal right iliac artery system and the right femoral artery. This position is not conducive to harvesting lower extremity veins and management of enteric fistulae; exposure and tunneling for the right axillofemoral bypass are impossible from this position.

The first step of the operation involves obtaining exposure for vascular control of the noninfected aorta/artery proximal and distal to the infected graft. One must be cognizant of the risk to adjacent organs during dissection including the ureters, bowel, and major veins. Placement of ureteral stents, to aid in their intraoperative identification, should be considered preoperatively. Should an enteric fistula be present, one must be prepared to repair or resect the bowel. Depending on the level of aortic control, individual visceral branches off the aorta may need to be isolated and controlled. Should the surrounding infection require sufficient debridement to interrupt in-line flow to the renal or visceral branches, cold perfusion techniques should be available.

Aortic cross-clamping requires close and constant communication with the anesthesia team to address hemodynamic fluctuations. Once the patient is anticoagulated and aortic control is established, the goal should be to remove all prosthetic material from the field. Aggressive and thorough debridement of the infected area is *mandatory*. Not only is the graft itself sent for culture, but multiple samples of any obvious purulence encountered, as well as the involved surrounding tissue, should be submitted. The microbiology laboratory should be asked to sonicate graft material and allow for prolonged culture times to identify any slow-growing bacteria within a protective biofilm. In rare circumstances of culture-negative infections, bacterial sequencing may be helpful. Once debridement is completed, attention is focused on in situ revascularization or, less commonly, aortic ligation.

After completing the aortic reconstruction, an attempt is made to provide soft tissue coverage of the graft, typically with a piece of the greater omentum. The greater omentum is carefully freed of its attachments to the transverse colon and lengthened. The omentum can then be divided, creating a tail of omentum to cover the graft. The left side of the omentum with the blood supply based on the left gastroepiploic artery and left omental artery is typically used (Figure 45.2). A fenestration is created at an avascular site within the transverse mesocolon through which the omental flap is passed to cover the graft (Figures 45.3–45.5). Consultation with plastic surgery colleagues is useful when more complex flaps are required for coverage.

ARTERIAL RECONSTRUCTION

Extra-anatomic bypass with aortic ligation

Axillobifemoral bypass with aortic ligation has long been recognized as the standard therapy for AGI involving the infrarenal aorta (Figure 45.6). The benefits of this approach include the ability to stage what are typically long and difficult operations in compromised patients by performing the arterial reconstruction at one setting and graft excision at a second, later (24–72 hours) setting. Another benefit is that the new graft is placed in

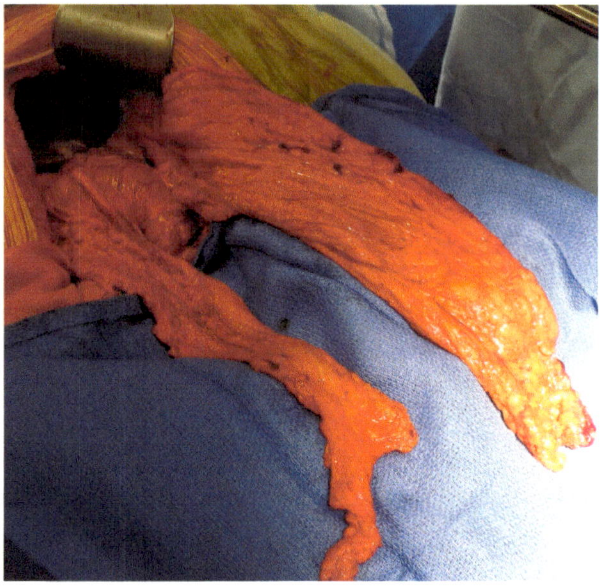

Figure 45.2 Intraoperative image demonstrating the greater omentum after being freed of its attachments to the transverse colon and divided to create a tongue of omentum to cover the graft.

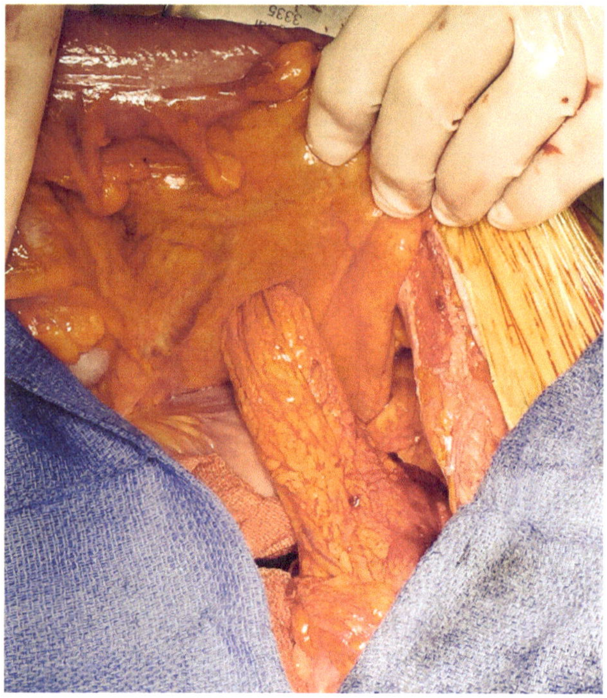

Figure 45.4 Intraoperative image demonstrating a tongue of omentum passed through a mesocolic fenestration.

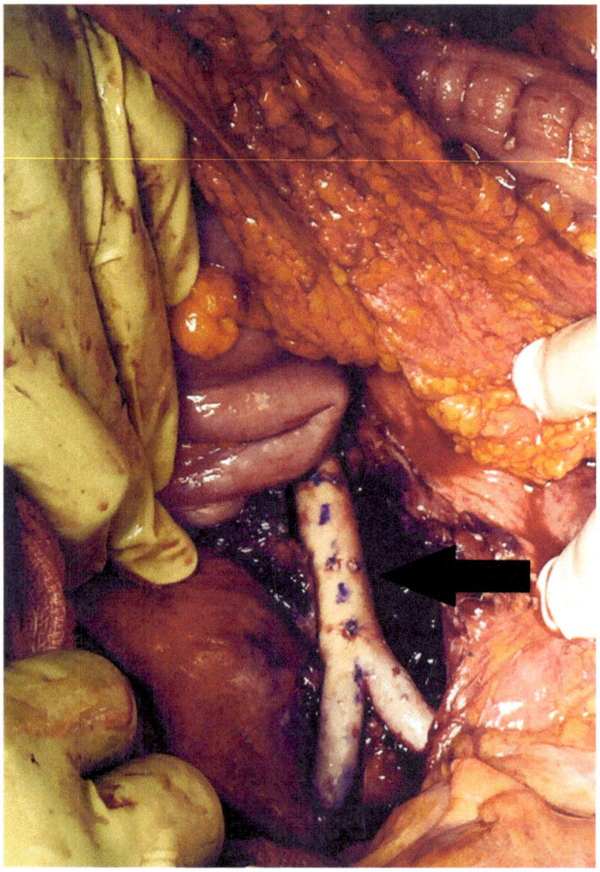

Figure 45.3 Intraoperative image demonstrating a cryopreserved allograft (arrow).

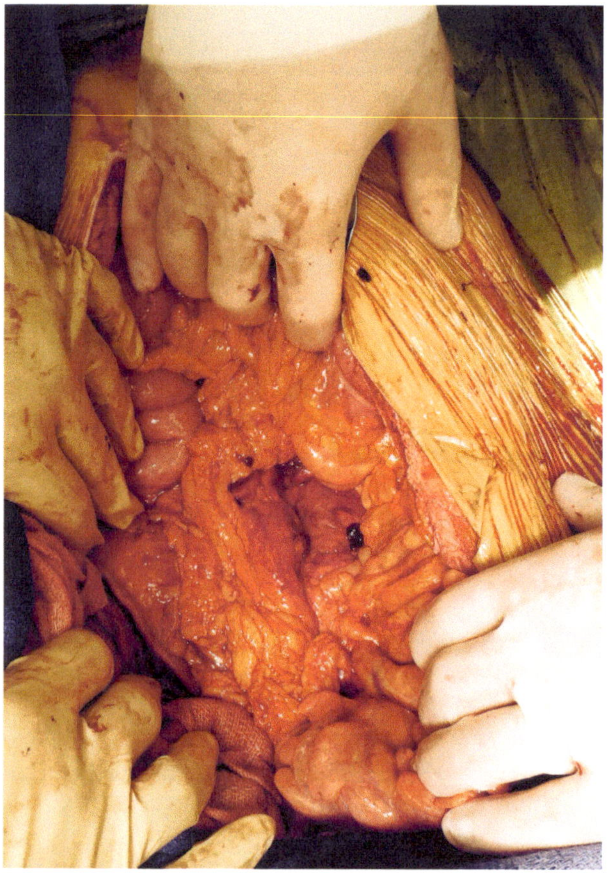

Figure 45.5 Intraoperative image demonstrating complete coverage of a cryopreserved allograft with an omental flap.

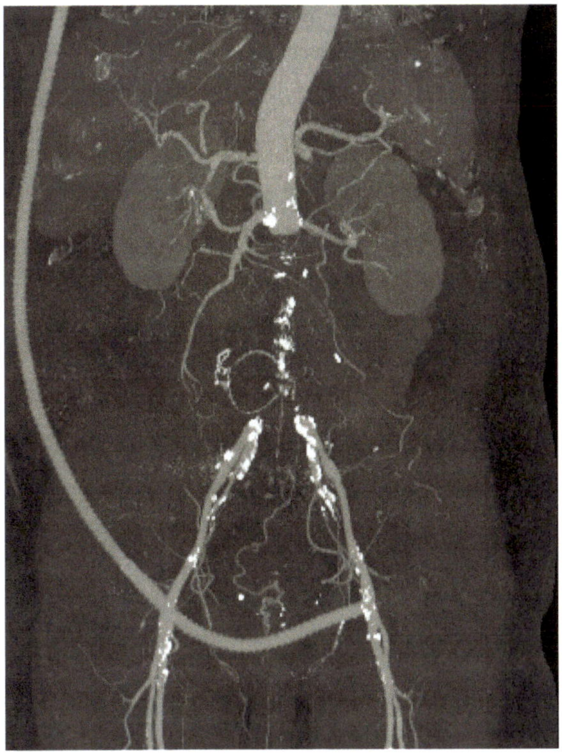

Figure 45.6 Three-dimensional reconstruction of a computed tomographic angiogram obtained two years postoperatively following ligation of the infrarenal aorta and both common iliac arteries with revascularization of the lower extremities via a right axillobifemoral bypass.

clean tissue planes. In cases with severe contamination and virulent organisms, this may be the best option. The major disadvantages of this approach include the poor graft patency of an extra-anatomic reconstruction and the risk of aortic stump blowout [6]. In addition, because emergent cases require addressing the aortic graft before arterial reconstruction, this approach may lead to prolonged and intolerable limb ischemia times. If there is inadequate, healthy infrarenal aorta to allow for oversewing the aortic stump, this method may not be an option.

When the common femoral arteries (CFAs) are not involved with the infection, typically an axillobifemoral bypass may be performed in the usual fashion (see Chapter 41). If the CFAs are involved, bilateral axillary to either superficial femoral artery (SFA) or, more commonly, deep femoral artery (DFA) bypass is required. The distal DFA can be approached along the lateral aspect of the sartorius muscle, thus remaining in clean tissue planes and avoiding a contaminated groin incision. Later, when excising the graft from the CFA, an attempt should be made to preserve flow at the femoral bifurcation.

During the abdominal procedure, care should be taken not to extend the midline incision too far distally and risk exposure/contamination of the cross-femoral limb. Ligation of the aorta is performed with either a stapling device or a 3-0 polypropylene suture in two-layered running fashion. Fascial (*not felt*) pledgets may be helpful to reinforce the closure. If available, the omentum can be sutured in place to bolster the aortic closure.

Historically, operative mortality for this approach was as high as 27% and higher than more recently reported series of in situ reconstructions. A risk of infecting the new extra-anatomic graft exists and approaches 15% in one series. Regarding aortic stump disruption, mortality can exceed 75%. The risk of this occurrence is reported to be as high as 25%. Lastly, limb loss rates have been reported as high as 15%. Overall, patient survival rates of >70% at one year have been achieved with this approach [6–8].

IN SITU AORTIC RECONSTRUCTION

Neoaortoiliac system with femoral vein

Creation of a neoaortoiliac system (NAIS) with the femoral veins is one choice of conduit that may be used for arterial reconstruction in the face of AGI (Figure 45.7). This method involves harvesting the femoral vein from the origin of the deep femoral vein (DFV) to the popliteal vein. Preoperative duplex vein mapping is performed to ensure that the vein is patent and of adequate size, typically >6–7 mm in diameter. Care is taken to preserve the saphenous vein, and especially the DFV, to provide adequate venous drainage for the leg. A longitudinal incision is made along the lateral aspect of the sartorius muscle, which is retracted medially. The vein is mobilized from its confluence with the DFV distally to the above-knee popliteal vein, including dividing the adductor magnus tendon, if necessary, to enter the adductor canal to obtain additional length. During dissection, care is taken to preserve collateral branches of the SFA and popliteal artery. Once exposed, the vein is typically left in place until the required length of vein is determined. When harvested, the vein is divided flush with the DFV, taking care not to leave a stump that may be a nidus for thrombus

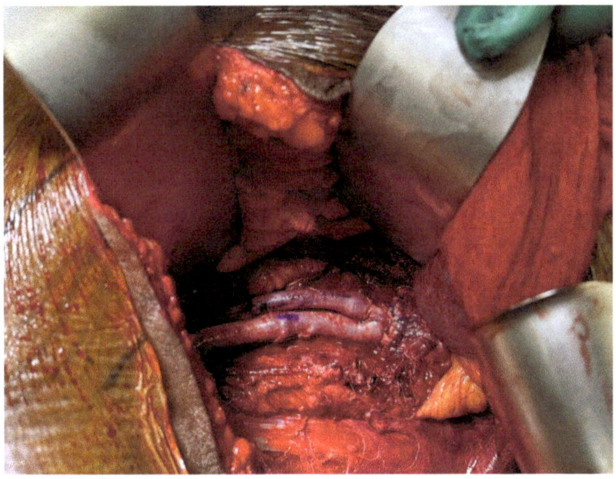

Figure 45.7 Operative photograph demonstrating reconstruction of the infrarenal aorta with a femoral vein (NAIS) graft.

formation. Depending on the size match, the femoral vein can either be reversed or more typically left in its native orientation following valve lysis. Valves are typically lysed by everting the vein and excising them. The vein is then distended and any identified branches are oversewn with fine polypropylene suture. Since a bifurcated reconstruction is typically required, both veins can be harvested and then anastomosed to each other in a side-to-side fashion proximally over a 3 cm distance to create a bifurcated ("pantaloon") graft. Postoperative venous thromboembolic prophylaxis is maintained both mechanically (intermittent pneumatic compression) and pharmacologically (subcutaneous heparin).

NAIS, using autogenous tissue to decrease the risk of reinfection, may allow for a short-duration antibiotic regimen. Overall, recent series reported late mortality to compare favorably with the other methods of reconstruction [8,9]. Disadvantages of NAIS include the added operative time. If available, a second surgical team to harvest the femoral veins can help ameliorate this. Another disadvantage is the size mismatch between the infrarenal aorta, particularly when the initial operation was for aneurysmal disease, and the proximal end of the graft even when a bifurcated vein graft is created. In cases of an unstable patient from hemorrhage or sepsis, an alternative conduit should be considered. NAIS is subject to the same issues affecting lower extremity vein bypasses, namely vein graft stenosis from intimal hyperplasia and aneurysmal degeneration. Finally, postoperative venous complications, including disruption of venous drainage with subsequent leg swelling, deep vein thrombosis, and compartment syndrome with a need for fasciotomy have been reported [9].

CRYOPRESERVED ALLOGRAFTS

Cryopreserved allografts are an alternative conduit for in situ aortic replacement. This approach avoids placement of a prosthetic graft in an infected field, as well as the time and morbidity associated with femoral vein harvest. Current cryopreservation techniques have improved the integrity of these grafts, leading to fewer long-term complications than have been reported in the past. The downside to their use includes cost, and the lead time necessary for their acquisition. Thus, cryopreserved allografts may not be an option in an urgent or emergent situation. Specific handling and storage techniques are also required for the allograft. Once thawed, it is sewn in place in the standard fashion with the one caveat that the lumbar branches are placed facing up to allow for ease of repair if there is any bleeding once the allograft is pressurized.

A recent study detailed the results of a multi-institutional database of 220 patients who underwent the use of cryopreserved aortoiliac allografts for aortic reconstruction in the USA in the setting of infection, including enteric fistula, with a mean follow-up of 30 months. Survival was 75% at one year and 51% at five years. Primary graft patency was 97% at five years. At five years, freedom from graft-related complications was 80%, freedom from graft explant 88%, and freedom from limb loss 97% [10].

ANTIBIOTIC-TREATED GRAFTS

A third option for in-line aortic reconstruction for AGI is the use of an antibiotic-treated prosthetic graft. Currently, available Dacron grafts pretreated with gelatin can be easily impregnated with an antibiotic when soaked in rifampin. Typically, 600 mg of rifampin is reconstituted in 50 mL of solution in which the graft is soaked for 5–30 minutes, after which the excess is allowed to drain off before implantation. Therefore, any chosen graft size may be quickly prepared in the operating room.

The advantages of using antibiotic-treated prosthetic grafts include having a readily available, appropriately sized graft. As with other in-line arterial reconstructions, it avoids aortic stump blowout complications and has superior graft patency compared with an extra-anatomic bypass. Like other in situ reconstructions, limb loss is rare and five-year survival is around 50% [8,11]. Disadvantages of antibiotic-treated grafts are largely related to the risk of reinfection, ranging from 4% to 22% [1,11]. Obviously, antibiotic treatment with rifampin is of no value for nonsusceptible organisms. Reinfection is encountered more frequently with virulent organisms, particularly methicillin-resistant *S. aureus* and may be largely unavoidable. Radical debridement of the aorta and affected retroperitoneal tissue bed and use of an omental wrap are important adjuncts to reduce reinfection rates.

The most recent entrant into the field of AGI grafts is bovine pericardium. Several European groups have achieved good results with grafts constructed on the back table from sheets of bovine pericardium. Such grafts appear to perform at least as well as cryopreserved allografts and are much cheaper. The only disadvantage is the extra time required to construct these grafts [12].

POSTOPERATIVE CARE

The postoperative complications of procedures to treat AGI are like the complications following any infrarenal aortic reconstruction with the additional burden of problems related to infection and sepsis. When femoral artery anastomoses are involved, open groin wounds frequently result and are best managed with negative pressure wound therapy and occasional muscle flaps. The duration of postoperative antibiotic coverage is controversial and depends on several factors, including the offending pathogen, the type of reconstruction, and the patient's immune status. Most patients require a minimum of six weeks of intravenous antibiotics. Some need longer courses; occasionally, lifelong oral suppressive antibiotics are used.

CONCLUSIONS

The diagnosis and treatment of AGI remains a major challenge even for the most experienced vascular surgeon. A variety of reconstructive options are available, but all depend on the administration of culture-specific antibiotics, radical debridement of all infected tissue, and maintenance of vital organ and limb perfusion.

TRICKS AND TRAPS

- When evaluating for AGI, one needs to maintain a high index of suspicion in the face of often nonspecific symptomatology.
- Send multiple cultures to help identify pathogens.
- In most cases in-line arterial reconstruction is preferred.
- Perform radical debridement of all infected and nonviable tissue.
- Use omental wrap for in-line reconstruction.
- Treat with an extended course of antibiotics.

QUESTIONS

1. A 72-year-old man with history of uncomplicated endovascular abdominal aortic aneurysm repair (EVAR) one year ago presents with a four-week history of progressive abdominal and back pain. He has lost his appetite and lacks energy. He is afebrile and hemodynamically stable but has mild upper abdominal tenderness. His sedimentation rate is elevated at 60. CT scan demonstrates air pockets in the aortic sac around his endograft and the duodenum is adherent to the anterior wall of the aneurysm sac. Which of the following statements regarding this clinical scenario is most accurate? Select one:
   a. Aortoenteric erosion is excluded by the history of EVAR
   b. The duodenum can usually be repaired primarily
   c. The endograft can usually be preserved
   d. Broad-spectrum antibiotics are curative

   Answer: b

2. General principles in the treatment of aortic graft infection include:
   a. Excision of entire graft and radical debridement of surrounding involved soft tissues
   b. Targeted antimicrobial therapy
   c. Preserving perfusion to vital organs and extremities
   d. All of the above

   Answer: d

3. Commonly used conduits for in-line reconstruction in the treatment of aortic graft infection include all of the following except:
   a. Rifampin-treated Dacron grafts
   b. Rifampin-treated ePTFE grafts
   c. Cryopreserved allografts
   d. Femoral vein

   Answer: b

4. Mechanisms that can result in prosthetic graft colonization and subsequent infection include:
   a. Intraoperative contamination
   b. Hematogenous spread of bacteria
   c. Contamination of the graft by infection emanating from adjacent infection of soft tissue, gastrointestinal tract, or genitourinary tract
   d. All of the above

   Answer: d

REFERENCES

1. Hodgkiss-Harlow, K. D., & Bandyk, D. F. (2011). Antibiotic therapy of aortic graft infection: treatment and prevention recommendations. *Semin Vasc Surg.*, *24*, 191–198.
2. Lawrence, P. F. (2011). Conservative treatment of aortic graft infection. *Semin Vasc Surg.*, *24*, 199–204.
3. Kennedy, S. A., Kennedy, M. K., Lindsay, T. F., Byrne, J., Jaberi, A., Gold, W. L., et al. (2022, February 18). Selected infected aortic grafts may be successfully managed without graft excision percutaneous drainage for aortic graft infection post-aneurysm repair: a viable option? *Vasc Endovascular Surg.* doi: 10.1177/15385744221075136.
4. Post, I. C. J. H., & Vos, C. G. (2019, August). Systematic review and meta-analysis on the management of open abdominal aortic graft infections. *Eur J Vasc Endovasc Surg.*, *58*(2), 258–281. doi: 10.1016/j.ejvs.2019.03.013. Epub 2019 Jun 7. PMID: 31178356.
5. Janko, M. R., et al. (2022, August). In-situ bypass is associated with superior infection-free survival compared with extra-anatomic bypass for the management of secondary aortic graft infections without enteric involvement. *J Vasc Surg.*, *76*(2), 546–555.e3. doi: 10.1016/j.jvs.2022.03.869. Epub 2022 Apr 23. PMID: 35470015.
6. Berger, P., & Moll, F. L. (2011). Aortic graft infections: is there still a role for axillobifemoral reconstruction? *Semin Vasc Surg*, *24*, 205–210.

7. Charlton-Ouw, K. M., Sandhu, H. K., Huang, G., et al. (2014). Reinfection after resection and revascularization of infected infrarenal abdominal aortic grafts. *J Vasc Surg.*, *59*, 684–692.
8. Kilic, A., Arnaoutakis, D. J., Reifsnyder, T., et al. (2016). Management of infected vascular grafts. *Vasc Med.*, *21*, 53–60.
9. Dorweiler, B., Neufang, A., Chaban, R., et al. (2014). Use and durability of femoral vein for autologous reconstruction with infection of the aortoiliofemoral axis. *J Vasc Surg*, *59*, 675–683.
10. Harlander-Locke, M. P., Harmon, L. K., Lawrence, P. F., et al. (2014). The use of cryopreserved aortoiliac allograft for aortic reconstruction in the United States. *J Vasc Surg.*, *59*, 669674.
11. Lew, W., & Moore, W. (2011). Antibiotic-impregnated grafts for aortic reconstruction. *Semin Vasc Surg.*, *24*, 211–219.
12. Weiss, S., Tobler, E. L., von Tengg-Kobligk, H., et. al. (2017). Self made xeno-pericardial aortic tubes to treat native and aortic graft infections. *Eur J Vasc Endovasc Surg.*, *54*, 646–652.

46

Obturator bypass graft

SEYED S. PAIRAWAN AND ANDI N. PESHKEPIJA

INTRODUCTION

The femoral artery is an important vessel for vascular surgeons. It serves as both a target artery for inflow procedures and as an inflow site itself for infrainguinal bypasses. In patients who have a hostile groin, especially in the setting of an infection, the options for vascular reconstruction are limited. The groin is especially prone to infections because of proximity to the perineum, lymphatic tissue disruption attendant with procedures, and the presence of microbes within the lymphatic channels and/or nodes. Obturator bypass is a viable option in a hostile groin, which serves as a type of extra-anatomical bypass, completely bypassing the femoral triangle. This procedure was first described by Shaw et al. in 1963 [1] and has gained traction over time [2]. Limb-salvage rates have been acceptable, however, patient selection remains key [3]. The aorta or the iliac vessels act as an inflow to the superficial femoral, deep femoral, or popliteal artery target vessels.

INDICATIONS FOR INTERVENTION

This type of extra-anatomical bypass is indicated in patients with the following: (1) infected pseudoaneurysm of the femoral artery; (2) extensive tissue loss in the groin region from radiation necrosis, trauma, or after radical resection of tumors; (3) critical limb-threatening ischemia of the leg with the need for revascularization with concomitant infection in the groin; and (4) metaplastic changes and excessive scarring in the femoral region from previous surgical interventions. Other options include inline reconstruction with native tissue conduits (greater saphenous vein or deep femoral vein) or cryopreserved allograft with healthy tissue flap coverage.

PREOPERATIVE CONSIDERATIONS

There are several steps that need to take place before embarking on an obturator bypass. These include: (1) pretreatment using antibiotics for at least 48 hours; (2) preoperative imaging to evaluate both the extent of the infected groin area and the iliac vessels; and (3) preoperative vein mapping to assess adequacy of possible venous conduits (both superficial and deep veins). Patients may have a history of previous vascular reconstructions including aorto-bi-femoral or even extra-anatomical bypasses. Computed tomography angiography (CTA) imaging allows evaluation of the tissues around these grafts. Other imaging modalities such as tagged white blood cell (WBC) scan or positron emission tomography (PET) CT may be helpful in determining that the inflow artery is not infected. If an anastomosis onto the superficial femoral artery is planned, inline flow to the foot is critical for patency by ensuring adequate outflow. Otherwise, one needs to ensure there is retrograde flow to the profunda or it will need to be revascularized.

OPERATION

Patient positioning

The patient is positioned supine on the operating room table. Depending on the patient body habitus, a self-retracting system may be required. The operation is usually performed under general anesthesia. The entire abdomen, both groins, and the affected lower extremity are prepared and draped circumferentially in a sterile fashion. If there is a presence of an open groin wound, this area would be best prepared with betadine and completely sealed off from the field with an antimicrobial adhesive drape. Appropriate preoperative antibiotics are administered within one hour of skin incision.

DOI: 10.1201/9781003452096-46

Retroperitoneal approach with exposure of the obturator foramen and iliac vessels

A transverse or a curvilinear ("transplant") incision is made in the hypogastric region of the lower abdomen on the side of the revascularization and is deepened to the level of the lateral edge of the rectus muscle; the extraperitoneal space is entered behind the rectus muscle. The external oblique aponeurosis and its muscle fibers are identified and incised in a parallel fashion with electrocautery. This will expose both the internal oblique and its partner, the transversus abdominis muscle, which are both incised in their medial portions, followed by medialization of the peritoneal sac and viscera. A self-retracting system can be positioned at this point, aiming the deeper blades medially and directing the shorter blades laterally toward the anterior superior iliac spine. The iliac vessels should be visualized and the common, external, and internal iliac arteries are dissected out circumferentially and controlled with silastic vessel loops.

The obturator foramen fascia should be visualized or at least identified via palpation at this stage. The obturator foramen is identified by using the obturator artery or superior ramus of the pubic bone as a landmark [4]. The inferior medial portion of the obturator fascia is scored with electrocautery under direct observation, or with a right angle only under guidance by palpation when body habitus does not allow for direct visualization. Once the obturator fascia is incised, the obturator internus muscle is swept away, and the hole in the fascia bluntly enlarged. This hole is created anteromedially in the foramen, away from the obturator artery and nerve that lie more laterally (Figure 46.1). The obturator artery originates from the anterior division of the internal iliac artery in most cases; however, it can also arise from the inferior epigastric artery, allowing a variable course through the membrane.

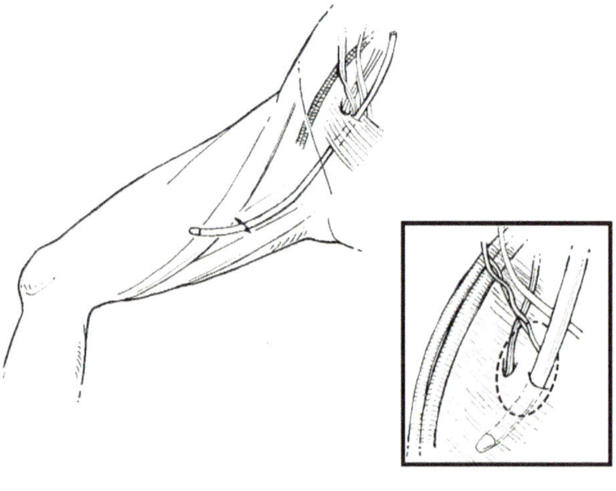

Figure 46.1 Tunneling of graft in the obturator foramen and lower extremity.

Leg dissection and tunnel creation

A vertical incision is made on the medial aspect of the lower or higher part of the thigh, depending on the desired target for distal anastomosis. The superficial femoral artery or proximal popliteal artery is exposed at that level. The goal is to tunnel the bypass graft between the adductor muscles of the thigh. While keeping the leg in a flexed position at the knee, and the hip externally rotated, an intermuscular tunnel toward the distal target artery is created. The authors prefer tunneling the bypass graft starting proximally in the abdomen using a curved tunneler, such as the Atrium AV-2 tunneler (Maquet Cardiovascular, Wayne, NJ, USA) (Figure 46.2), mainly because it allows tunneling through the obturator membrane under direct visualization without risking injury to adjacent viscera (pelvic organs, bladder, colon). The curved nature of the tunneler allows for some guidance control toward the distal exit point. When a more distal anastomosis is desired, like the proximal popliteal artery, other tunneling alternatives include tunneling with a straight Gore vascular tunneler (Gore Medical, Newark, DE, USA) (Figure 46.3). In this case, a plane between the adductor longus and magnus is created (Figure 46.4), with the tunneler advanced proximally from there. The origin of the adductor longus starts just lateral of the pubic symphysis on the anterior surface of the superior pubic ramus, and the origin of the adductor magnus starts just lateral of the pubic symphysis at the inferior pubic ramus, thus the tunneler should arrive on the medial aspect of the obturator foramen. Still, the bimanual technique (with one hand

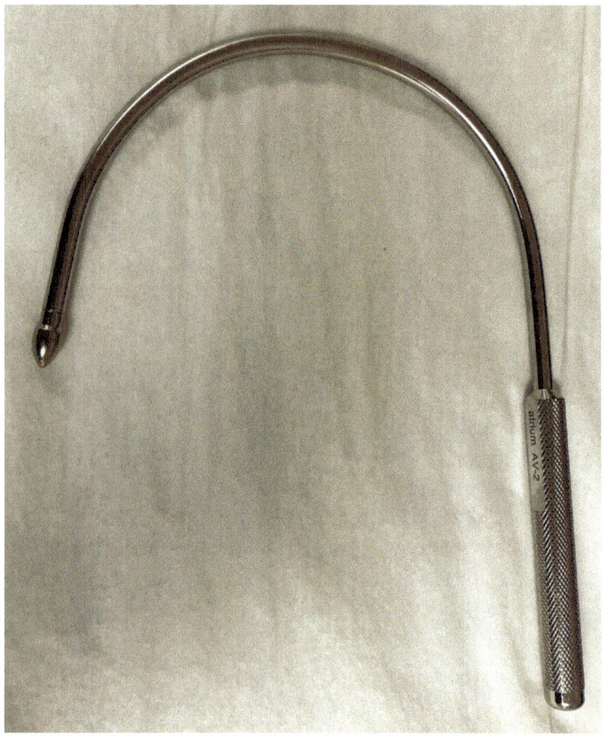

Figure 46.2 Atrium AV-2 vascular tunneler.

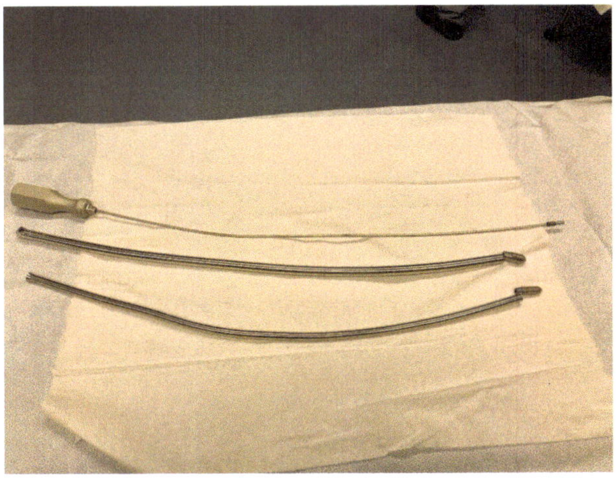

Figure 46.3 Gore tunneler.

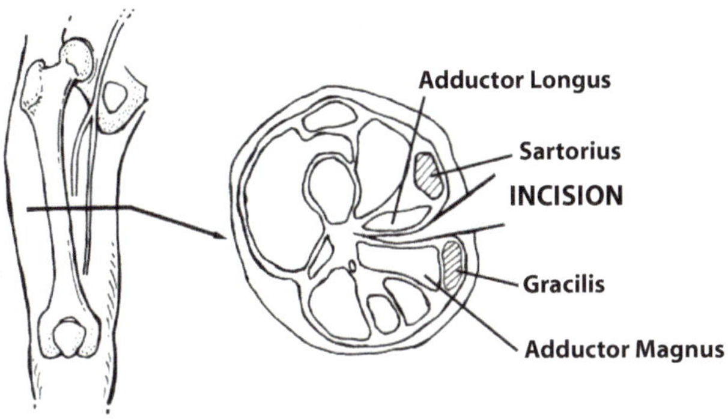

Figure 46.4 Cross-section depicting distal entry point of the tunneler.

behind the obturator membrane) is advised to lessen the risk of injuring the bladder and/or other pelvic organs. It is important to create a tunnel *between* these muscle groups rather than through them.

Graft choices and anastomoses

Many different graft types have been utilized in the literature, including Dacron, saphenous vein (transposed non-reversed versus reversed), and polytetrafluoroethylene (PTFE). The author prefers the ringed PTFE graft because of its resistance to kinking and compression. In an actively infected groin with a graft, using the contralateral transposed non-reversed saphenous vein is an option [5]. Once the patient is fully heparinized (with activated clotting time >250 sec.), the proximal and distal anastomoses are completed in an end-to-side fashion preserving the native inflow and outflow.

Groin wound management

Once the revascularization is completed as described, the incisions are closed and isolated. The infected groin is next addressed. These wounds typically require radical debridement, with excision of all infected tissues and may require muscle flaps, along with vacuum-assisted wound closure therapy. Multiple trips to the operating room for repeated debridements may be required.

COMPLICATIONS

Neuralgia paresthetica. Compression of the lateral femoral cutaneous nerve as it passes medial to the anterior superior iliac spine, which can occur as a result of retraction by laterally placed retractor blades.

Hemorrhage after dissecting the obturator space. The obturator artery has a variable course through the obturator foramen and caution must be exercised when bluntly dissecting this area. It is also important to assess collateral circulation through the obturator foramen preoperatively.

Thigh ischemia. Can occur with ligation of the proximal popliteal artery. End-to-side configuration of this anastomosis is advised to preserve retrograde flow back up the SFA.

Early graft occlusion. As a result of redundancy of the graft or compression of the graft from an inadequate obturator membrane opening.

CASE EXAMPLE

A 59-year-old African American male with a history of aortoiliac occlusive disease, failed iliac stents, and femoral-to-femoral bypass, followed by an aorto-bi-femoral bypass complicated by lymphocutaneous fistulae which were treated by ligation with persistent groin wounds. The patient had a herald bleed from the left groin and was transferred to our hospital for escalation of care. CT scan demonstrated pseudoaneurysms (PSA) at both of the femoral anastomoses (Figure 46.5). The iliac limbs of his aorto-bi-femoral bypass appeared to be uninvolved with infection, with no stranding or fluid collections around them. The left PSA was actively bleeding with hemodynamic instability; he was therefore taken as an emergency to the operating room to address the left side with the technique described previously. A 7 mm ringed PTFE

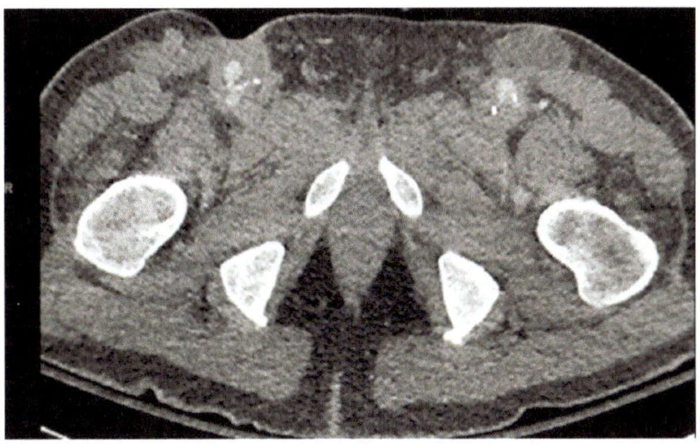

Figure 46.5 Infected pseudoaneurysms at the distal anastomis of aorto-bi-femoral reconstruction (black arrows).

graft was sewn in an end-to-end fashion to the left aorto-iliac graft limb, which was well incorporated in the retroperitoneum without any signs of infection. An Atrium AV-2 tunneler was used to create a tunnel to the superficial femoral artery (SFA), which was the distal target; an anastomosis was created in an end-to-side fashion to this artery. Once the revascularization portion of the procedure was performed, these incisions were closed and isolated and attention was next directed to the left groin where an incision was made over the draining sinus. A hematoma was evacuated, and a lymphocele was encountered. Hemorrhage was identified from the suture line of the graft to the common femoral artery, which had to be ligated, above the origin of the profunda, preserving retrograde flow into it. The graft was excised in its entirety all the way up into the pelvis, avoiding entering the retroperitoneal space of the prior reconstruction. The wound was debrided of all infected and non-viable tissue; hemostasis was achieved and the sartorius muscle was medialized to cover the site of arterial ligation.

A similar operation was performed on the right side during the same hospitalization because of the instability of the right groin PSA. His previous femoral-femoral graft was explanted as well due to concerns about infection. The patient required multiple trips to the operating room for wound debridements but eventually fully healed his incisions. A postoperative CT scan demonstrated open bypass grafts (Figure 46.6).

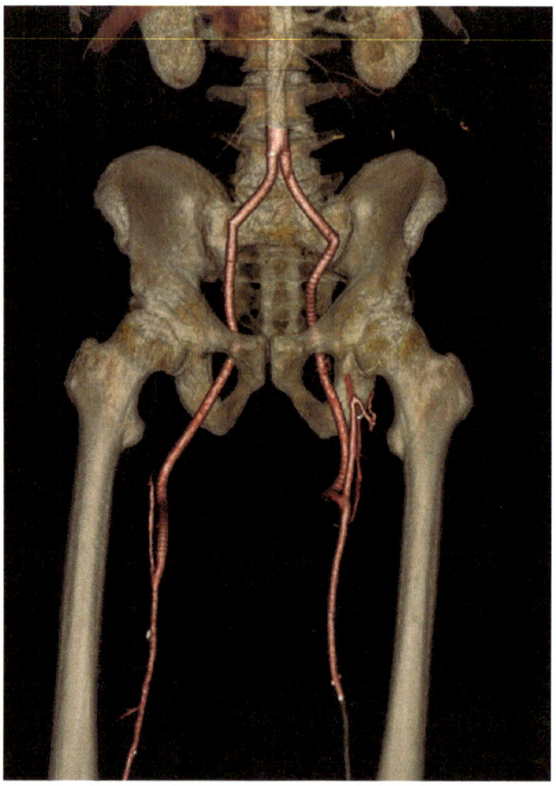

Figure 46.6 Bilateral obturator bypasses passing through the obturator foramen down to the level of the SFA.

TRICKS AND TRAPS

- Lower quadrant retroperitoneal abdominal ("transplant") incision is commonly utilized for proximal exposure/anastomosis. However, a transperitoneal approach can be used as well.
- It is critical to tunnel inferior and medially in the obturator foreman.
- Avoid excessive pressure on lateral retraction blades to prevent compression of the lateral femoral cutaneous nerve.
- Use a curved tunneler (Atrium AV-2) when tunneling from above.
- The tunnel should be created *between* the adductor longus and the adductor magnus rather than through these muscles. Create anastomoses in an end-to-side fashion to preserve retrograde flow to profunda distally if feasible.
- Avoid graft redundancy and create a sizeable opening in the obturator foramen fascia to avoid graft narrowing/compression.
- Use ringed PTFE to minimize kinking or compression of the graft.
- Solate and avoid the infected groin. Complete the bypass, close the wounds, and dress the bypass incisions before opening and debriding the groin.

QUESTIONS

1. A common cause of early obturator bypass graft occlusion is?
   a. Size mismatch of conduit to native artery
   b. Narrow obturator foramen "window"
   c. Graft redundancy
   d. a,b,c
   e. b,c

   Answer: e

2. Retracting the lateral blades against the anterior superior iliac spine with excessive pressure when using a mechanical retraction system can cause compression of which of the following nerves?
   a. Ilioinguinal nerve
   b. Iliohypogastric nerve
   c. Obturator nerve
   d. Lateral femoral cutaneous nerve
   e. None of the above

   Answer: d

3. What is the second-most common location the obturator artery originates from?
   a. Common femoral artery
   b. Internal iliac artery
   c. Inferior epigastric artery
   d. Internal pudendal artery
   e. External iliac artery

   Answer: c

4. In patients with significant SFA/proximal popliteal artery collateral branches, performing an end-to-end popliteal anastomosis increases the risk for which complication?
   a. Acute limb ischemia
   b. Claudication
   c. Intimal hyperplasia
   d. Thigh ischemia
   e. Early graft occlusion

   Answer: d

REFERENCES

1. Shaw, R.S. and A.E. Baue, Management of sepsis complicating arterial reconstructive surgery. *Surgery*, 1963. 53: p. 75–86.
2. Dubouis, A., et al., Obturator bypass remains a useful option. *Ann Vasc Surg*, 2023. 93: p. 1–8. DOI: 10.1016/j.avsg.2022.05.048.
3. Bath, J., et al., Clinical outcomes of obturator canal bypass. *J Vasc Surg*, 2017. 66(1): p. 160–6. DOI: 10.1016/j.jvs.2016.11.049.
4. van Det, R.J. and L.C. Brands, The obturator foramen bypass: an alternative procedure in iliofemoral artery revascularization. *Surgery*, 1981. 89(5): p. 543–7.
5. Panetta, T., V.S. Sottiurai, and R.C. Batson, Obturator bypass with nonreversed translocated saphenous vein. *Ann Vasc Surg*, 1989. 3(1): p. 56–62. DOI: 10.1016/S0890-5096(06)62385-6.

47

Truncal vascular trauma

JAVANEH JABBARI AND SHAHAB A. TOURSAVADKOHI

INTRODUCTION

The management of traumatic injuries to the heart, great vessels, and major abdominal vasculature poses a challenge for surgeons. These are often life-threatening injuries that require emergent intervention; however, the variability of injuries poses a challenge in following algorithms to manage these patients. Although advanced trauma life support (ATLS) is followed while caring for trauma patients, in practice, patients in extremis receive ATLS assessment and treatment concurrently.

DAMAGE CONTROL SURGERY FOR NONCOMPRESSIBLE TORSO HEMORRHAGE

In the setting of life-threatening injuries, damage control surgery is often required as the first stage. Damage control surgery describes a staged or delayed approach to definitive repair of injuries. This allows for immediate control of life-threatening injuries while the patient undergoes resuscitation. In the case of an unknown source of hemorrhage, the best resuscitative maneuver for patients with noncompressible torso hemorrhage and severe shock is thoracic aortic occlusion. Surgically, the thoracic aorta is identified and clamped through a left anterolateral thoracotomy (resuscitative thoracotomy). This allows for a slowing of distal hemorrhage and improvement in cerebral and myocardial perfusion (Figure 47.1).

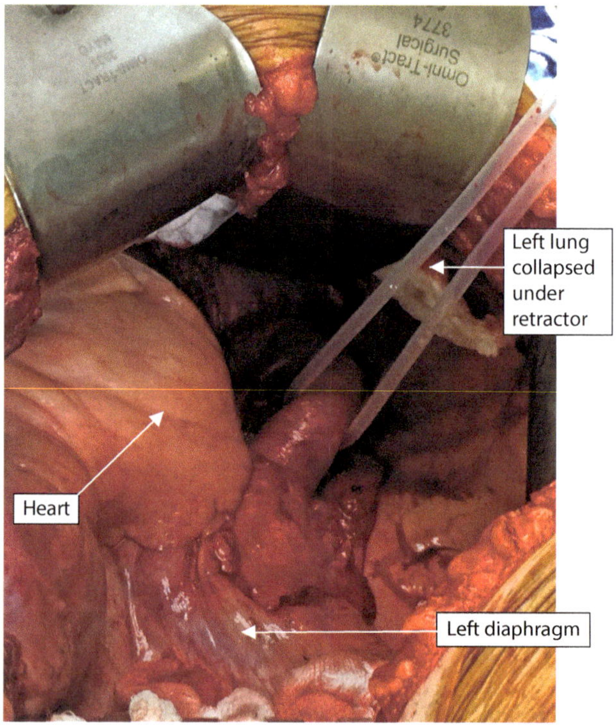

Figure 47.1 Left thoracotomy for control of the descending thoracic aorta.

An alternative to open occlusion is resuscitative balloon occlusion of the aorta (REBOA) using a compliant endovascular balloon (Figure 47.2). Access is gained through the femoral or axillary artery percutaneously under ultrasound guidance or direct cutdown. A 5-Fr sheath is placed. A 150–180-cm, 0.35-inch guidewire is advanced and exchanged for a 180-cm stiff wire (e.g., Amplatz Stiff Wire, Cook Medical Inc., Bloomington, IN, USA). The 5-Fr sheath is then exchanged for a 12-Fr sheath and a 32-mm Coda® Balloon Catheter (Cook Medical Inc.) is inflated in the supraceliac aorta. Occlusion can be achieved at other levels of the aorta as well. It is unclear how long the balloon can be occlusive without causing irreversible organ or neurologic damage.

TEMPORARY FLOW STABILIZATION

If major vascular trauma can be localized, blood flow can be temporarily restored with a vascular shunt. These devices allow for temporary perfusion while the patient undergoes repair of concomitant injuries (e.g., orthopedic fixation), a damage control procedure, or transport to

DOI: 10.1201/9781003452096-47

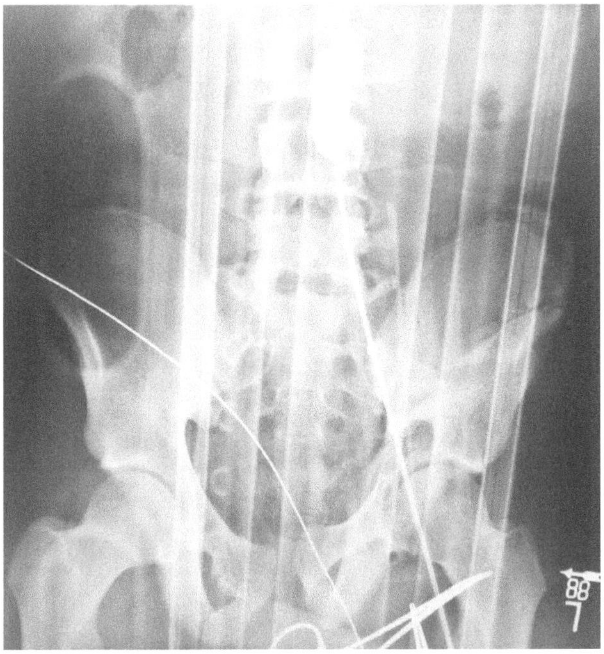

Figure 47.2 Resuscitative endovascular balloon occlusion of aorta (REBOA) for pelvic and abdominal hemorrhage through left femoral access.

a higher-level facility. Inserting a vascular shunt has the potential to cause injury if not done properly. The steps for shunt placement are outlined later in this chapter.

PENETRATING INTRATHORACIC INJURY

Managing patients with severe chest trauma requires an understanding of thoracic surgical approaches. Emergent thoracic exploration is indicated following penetrating thoracic injury in patients with bloody chest tube output >1000–1500 cc immediately after insertion, continued chest tube output or ongoing bleeding >200–300 cc per hour, massive air leak, or evidence of cardiac tamponade [1,2]. A large air leak from a chest tube is concerning for major tracheobronchial injury and can be assessed with bronchoscopy. Up to one-third of patients undergoing thoracic exploration for traumatic hemorrhage require a pulmonary resection because of associated parenchymal injury [3].

The mechanism of injury and the patient's hemodynamics can guide the surgeon on the most appropriate incision to use. Once determined, the next crucial step is identifying the appropriate procedure to perform. Each surgical exposure has its advantages and disadvantages and they are discussed below [4,5].

Anterolateral thoracotomy

A left anterolateral thoracotomy is the most common approach to control bleeding in an unstable patient undergoing emergency resuscitation. It allows rapid access to the thorax with exposure of the heart, aorta, and left lung, and avoids the time-consuming positioning required for a posterolateral thoracotomy. A concomitant exploratory laparotomy can also be performed if needed. Drawbacks include the lack of exposure of the entire lung, posterior mediastinum, and the entire heart. The incision is made in the inframammary crease dividing the pectoralis muscles followed by the intercostal muscles within the desired (usually fourth) intercostal space (ICS). The esophagus needs to be identified and protected. The internal mammary artery and vein are in close proximity medially and should be preserved if possible.

Clamshell thoracotomy

A clamshell thoracotomy is performed by extending an anterolateral thoracotomy across the midline into an anterolateral thoracotomy on the contralateral side. Typically carried from the left to the right when the source of hemorrhage is not identified through a left anterolateral thoracotomy, it provides exposure of the anterior mediastinum, the heart, descending thoracic aorta, both lungs, and pleural cavities. In cutting across the sternum, a Lebsche knife, sternal saw, or Gigli saw may be used followed by ligation of the internal mammary vessels bilaterally.

PENETRATING CARDIAC INJURY

Penetrating injury to the "box" region, defined as the area inferior to the clavicles, superior to the costal margin, and medial to the midclavicular line, should raise the examiner's suspicion for cardiac injury. In a stable patient, a FAST exam can detect pericardial effusion. In patients in extremis who have evidence of a penetrating injury to the box, a left anterolateral thoracotomy is the incision of choice. If necessary, this incision can be extended across the sternum as a clamshell thoracotomy. Atrial injuries can be controlled with a vascular clamp and repaired with 4-0 polypropylene suture, while the right ventricle can be repaired with a horizontal mattress suture. The sutures may be buttressed with pledgets if necessary [6]. If sutures are unavailable, the injuries can be stapled as a damage control approach until the patient is transferred to the operating room.

Injuries to or in close proximity to the coronary arteries can be challenging to repair as the repair can narrow or occlude the native artery. Repair sutures should be placed under the coronary vessels in a horizontal mattress fashion. Distal coronary artery injury and injuries to the diagonal or obtuse marginal branches rarely cause global dysfunction and can be ligated without development of significant cardiac failure.

Mild cardiac dysfunction associated with coronary artery injury can be managed with a mechanical circulatory support device with the goal of avoiding an emergent coronary artery bypass [6,7].

PENETRATING GREAT VESSEL INJURY

Penetrating injuries to the great vessels are found in 5% of thoracic gunshot and 2% of thoracic stab wound victims [8]. On presentation, these patients are frequently in hemorrhagic shock and require emergent surgery. Hemodynamically stable patients can undergo imaging studies prior to intervention. Computed tomography angiography is the imaging modality of choice as it helps identify the injury and allows for operative planning.

In an unstable patient presenting with concern for great vessel injury, a median sternotomy with supraclavicular or neck extension allows rapid control of the proximal great vessels bilaterally. However, many prefer a left anterolateral thoracotomy to control the proximal left subclavian artery (SCA). It is crucial to rule out the internal mammary artery as a potential source of bleeding in a setting of hemorrhagic shock [9].

The role of endovascular repair in treating great vessel injuries is evolving. It is often used as an adjunct to open surgical exploration. Proximal arterial balloon occlusion allows vascular control with minimal dissection while a standard open repair is performed.

BRACHIOCEPHALIC ARTERY INJURY

The standard approach to repair a brachiocephalic artery (BCA) injury is via a median sternotomy. If there is limited injury to the BCA, the injury can be repaired primarily using 4-0 polypropylene suture (Figure 47.3). However, most patients with BCA injury will require a "bypass and exclusion technique." To perform this, a 10-mm Dacron graft is sewn to the ascending aorta using a side-biting aortic clamp for the proximal anastomosis. Distally, the graft is sewn to the BCA beyond the point of injury after the artery has been divided between two clamps. Ideally, the distal clamp should be away from the bifurcation of the carotid and SCA so that collateral perfusion is preserved between the SCA and carotid artery while the proximal inflow is clamped. Once the distal anastomosis is completed, the proximal BCA stump is oversewn. A similar approach is employed for managing proximal left carotid artery injuries that cannot be primarily repaired [10].

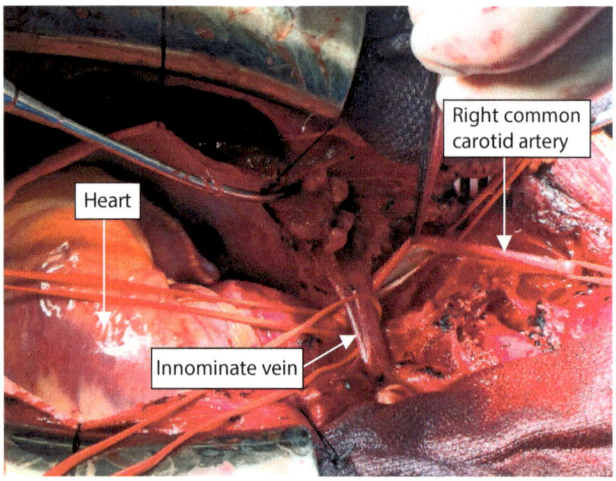

Figure 47.3 Stab wound to posteromedial wall of brachiocephalic artery (BCA) held open by the forceps. The patient's head is to the right. The red vessel loop to the left is cinched down around the proximal BCA for proximal control. On the right, distal control of the right common carotid artery is provided by another red vessel loop, while in the background the right subclavian artery is controlled by a third red vessel loop. In the mid-foreground, there is a loose red vessel loop around the innominate vein.

SUBCLAVIAN ARTERY INJURY

In recent years, most SCA injuries have been repaired endovascularly [11] with stent grafts through femoral and/or brachial access. Due to the challenging location, initial hemorrhage control can be achieved via direct digital compression or insertion of a Foley balloon catheter through the injury tract to tamponade the bleeding. If endovascular options are unavailable, these injuries may require primary repair, patch angioplasty, or interposition grafting. For unstable patients who cannot tolerate immediate definitive surgery, a temporary shunt can be placed.

PULMONARY AND VENOUS INJURY

Injury to the superior vena cava, inferior vena cava (IVC), and pulmonary arteries and veins often cause significant hemorrhage despite their low-pressure systems. Repair can be challenging because of the weaker structural integrity of the vessel walls. Temporary control can be obtained by compressing the vessel distally and proximally. An intestinal Allis or Babcock clamp can be used to partially clamp the site of injury, which can be repaired with a running 4-0 polypropylene suture under the clamps.

INTRA-ABDOMINAL VASCULAR INJURY

Intra-abdominal hemorrhage from vascular injury is often associated with retroperitoneal hematomas. These hematomas are categorized according to their location: zone 1 hematomas are in the midline retroperitoneum (aorta and IVC); zone 2 are located in the upper lateral retroperitoneum (adrenal glands, kidneys, and renal vessels); and zone 3 are confined to the pelvic retroperitoneum (the iliac vessels) (Figure 47.4). Retroperitoneal hematomas following penetrating injury are routinely explored, while only zone 1 injuries or expanding hematomas from blunt trauma are explored (Figure 47.5). Recently, however, this practice has been questioned in light of successful observation of stable, nonexpanding zone 2 penetrating injuries away from the renal hilum and in cases of stable retrohepatic hematomas that may be difficult to access or

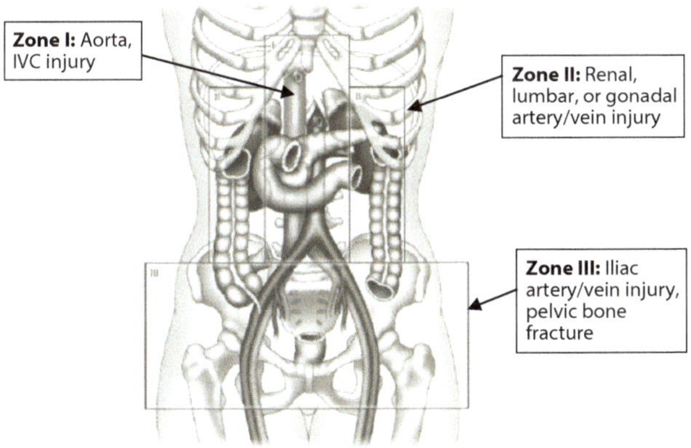

Figure 47.4 Retroperitoneal hematoma zones.

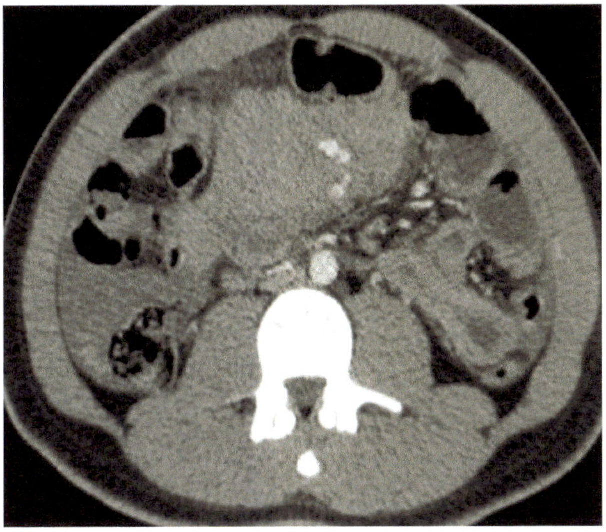

Figure 47.5 Zone 1 hematoma from visceral blunt injury.

control. While early adoption of REBOA may be useful in select cases for initial hemorrhage control, the operative approach to most of these injuries is through a midline laparotomy. REBOA may also be useful in stabilizing select patients with zone 3 blunt injuries, which are difficult to access and control through an open approach and often require endovascular embolization.

Injuries to the superior aspect of zone 1 raise concerns for damage to the aorta or one of its main branches, including the celiac axis, superior mesenteric artery (SMA), or proximal renal arteries. To identify the injury, a left medial visceral rotation (MVR; e.g., Mattox maneuver) is performed to expose the abdominal aorta, the left renal hilum, celiac trunk, and superior and inferior mesenteric arteries. To perform this, the parietal peritoneum is incised along the white line of Told from the sigmoid colon to the splenic flexure. The spleen, tail of pancreas, left kidney, and stomach are mobilized to the right side to expose the aorta and its proximal renal/visceral branches. An aortic compressor or other form of manual compression can provide temporary aortic control of the supraceliac aorta while the surgeon gains exposure.

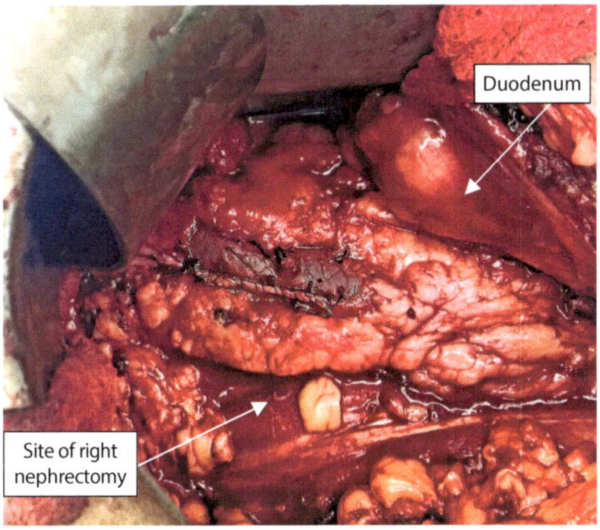

Figure 47.6 Superior mesenteric artery (SMA) interposition graft with great saphenous vein performed to repair an SMA dissection/occlusion after a motor vehicle accident with blunt abdominal trauma. (The patient's head is to the right, feet to the left.)

Injury to the inferior aspect of zone 1 is concerning for injuries to the infrarenal aorta or IVC. In such cases, an inframesocolic approach can be employed retracting the transverse colon cephalad and the small bowel to the right side to expose the retroperitoneum overlying these vessels. Once the left renal vein is identified and retracted cephalad, the underlying infrarenal aorta can be rapidly dissected free and clamped for proximal control.

Injuries to the aorta can be repaired primarily with 3-0 or 4-0 polypropylene sutures. Injuries to the celiac axis or its branches can be repaired primarily, if technically feasible. If not feasible, in an otherwise healthy individual with a patent SMA, such injuries can be ligated if necessary. Proximal SMA injuries are managed with either a shunt for cases requiring rapid damage control or an interposition graft for definitive repair (Figure 47.6).

Zone 2 injuries include renal and renal vascular injuries (Figure 47.7). While small injuries can be repaired primarily or monitored, more complex injuries associated with active bleeding and other intra-abdominal trauma may require a nephrectomy, as long as a contralateral kidney can be identified.

Zone 3 injuries often involve the iliac vasculature. Once proximal and distal control is obtained, direct pressure is applied to the site of injury to control hemorrhage. Exposure to zone 3 is obtained via an MVR, and if uncertain as to which side to mobilize, a right-sided MVR (Cattell-Braasch maneuver) is used as it provides exposure of both proximal iliac vessels, the entire right iliac system, the IVC, and the distal aorta. After obtaining proximal and distal control, iliac artery injuries can be managed with either primary repair for a simple isolated injury, an interposition graft if more significant injury is noted and minimal contamination exists, ligation with

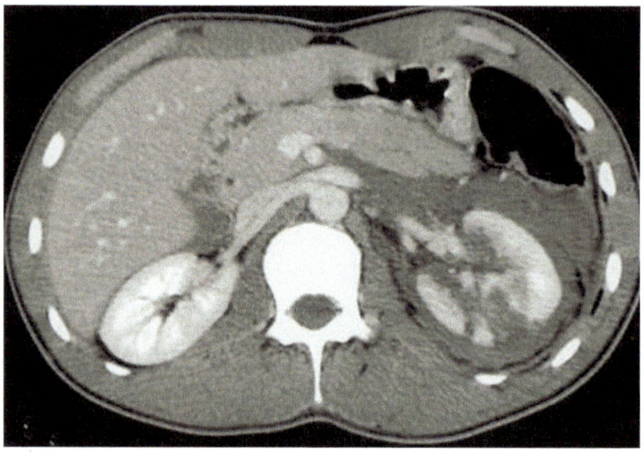

Figure 47.7 Left renal trauma with a zone 2 hematoma.

an extra-anatomic femorofemoral bypass in situations with significant contamination, or a shunt if the patient is hemodynamically unstable and requires a damage control operation.

Operative management of portal vein and retrohepatic IVC (sometimes referred to as zone 4) bleeding is fraught with difficulty. Control of bleeding from the retrohepatic vena cava is especially challenging and is associated with high mortality. Contained hematomas in this area should *not* be explored. Expanding hematomas should be packed first. If exploration is required, complete mobilization of the liver is done by division of the suspensory ligaments, including the right and left triangular, coronary, and falciform ligaments. This provides some mobility to access the retrohepatic portion of the IVC. Attempts to mobilize the liver in this region can result in increased bleeding from a retrohepatic injury, as torquing the liver and IVC may increase the size of the laceration. Hence, hepatic mobilization should only be done in cases of ongoing bleeding not controlled by packing and not amenable to endovascular treatments.

For portal vein injuries, proximal and distal control is obtained with the assistance of direct compression (sponge sticks) while dissecting the vein away from the hepatic artery and bile duct. Once the injury is visualized, it can be gently grasped with Allis clamps and mobilized to allow for suture repair. Small injuries can be primarily repaired. Larger injuries may require formal reconstruction of the vein. Injuries to the proximal portal vein or distal superior mesenteric vein may require mobilization of the pancreas for adequate exposure and control.

POSTOPERATIVE CARE AND COMPLICATIONS

The postoperative care of patients with severe truncal trauma requires a collaborative team effort in the ICU. Early mortality is often due to ongoing hemorrhage from either unrecognized injury or inadequate control of the known injury site. Continuous hemodynamic monitoring is the key to postoperative management and early recognition of complications. Other early complications include access site injury from REBOA and ischemia/reperfusion-induced organ damage. Lower extremity pulses and compartments should be monitored frequently along with serum lactate, creatine phosphokinase levels, and liver function tests. Abdominal compartment syndrome is another complication of torso trauma that needs to be monitored and treated promptly with surgical decompression if present.

Delayed mortality of patients with truncal trauma is usually secondary to uncontrolled sepsis from hollow organ injuries. Source control with definitive surgical repair, surgical drainage, and supportive antibiotics are important post-trauma management steps that can improve overall mortality and morbidity.

TRICKS AND TRAPS

Resuscitative thoracotomy for aortic occlusion:

- Make sure the patient's left arm is extended and stretched above the head.
- Prep the area with betadine.
- Make a generous incision in the inframammary fold (fourth to fifth intercostal space) starting from the sternum to the level of the bed. Follow the curve of the rib if possible.
- Make sure to use your scalpel to cut to the level of the muscle.
- Use heavy curved Mayo scissors to open the pleura.
- Place a Finochietto rib spreader to open the interspace and expose the pleural cavity.
- The pericardium needs to be opened to rule out cardiac tamponade; this also provides access to the heart for repair or cardiac massage.
- Pick up the pericardium with a toothed pickup and make a longitudinal incision to avoid injuring the phrenic nerve.
- Atrial injuries can be controlled with a vascular clamp and repaired with 4-0 polypropylene suture, while the right ventricle can be repaired with a horizontal mattress suture. The sutures may be buttressed with pledgets if necessary.
- If no cardiac injury is noted, you can proceed with cross-clamping of the descending thoracic aorta for proximal aortic occlusion.
- Carefully take down the inferior pulmonary ligament, making sure not to injure the pulmonary vein.
- Once the lung is out of the way, bluntly dissect around the aorta, separating it from the spine and esophagus. Usually, there is a pleural lining that needs to be divided and separated to allow for cross-clamping of the aorta.
- If unable to differentiate the aorta from the esophagus, a nasogastric tube can be placed to help identify the esophagus.
- Once identified, cross-clamp the aorta with an aortic clamp.

QUESTIONS

1. A 32-year-old female presents to the trauma bay for evaluation with a gunshot wound to the left chest. Her vitals are HR 120, BP 90/55, and RR 22. On primary survey, her airway is patent, but she has decreased breath sounds over the left chest and a chest tube is placed in the trauma bay. Which of the following is an indication of emergent thoracic exploration?
   a. bloody output >1500 cc immediately after insertion
   b. An air leak upon entry to the chest
   c. Bloody output of 100 cc per hour for four hours
   d. Ongoing serous output

   Answer: a

2. What imaging modality is recommended for identifying and planning an intervention in hemodynamically stable patients with penetrating injuries to the great vessels?
   a. Magnetic resonance imaging
   b. X-ray angiography
   c. Computed tomography angiography
   d. Ultrasound

   Answer: c

3. A patient with a penetrating injury to zone 1 is best managed by?
   a. Endovascular stenting of the aorta
   b. Midline laparotomy with a left medial visceral rotation
   c. Midline laparotomy with a right medial visceral rotation
   d. Observation if the hematoma is not expanding

   Answer: b

4. What is the standard incision that facilitates obtaining proximal control of the brachiocephalic artery?
   a. Median sternotomy
   b. Neck incisions
   c. Anterolateral thoracotomy
   d. Posterolateral thoracotomy

   Answer: a

REFERENCES

1. Meredith, J. W., & Hoth, J. J. (2007). Thoracic trauma: when and how to intervene. *Surg Clin North Am., 87*, 95–118.
2. Demetriades, D., & Velmahos, G. C. (2002). Penetrating injuries of the chest: indications for operation. *Scand J Surg., 91*, 41–45.
3. Huh, J., Wall, M. W., Jr, Estrera, A. L., et al. (2003). Surgical management of traumatic pulmonary injury. *Am J Surg., 186*, 620–624.
4. DuBose, J. A., O'Connor, J. V., & Scalea, T. M. (2013). Lung, trachea, and esophagus. In E. E. Moore, D. V. Feliciano, & K. L. Mattox (Eds.), *Trauma* (7th ed., pp. 468–484). New York, NY: McGraw Hill.
5. Rabin, J. (2015). The lungs. In T. M. Scalea (Ed.), *The Shock Trauma Manual of Operative Techniques* (pp. 157–172). New York, NY: Springer Science.
6. Kang, N., Hsee, L., Rizoli, S., et al. (2009). Penetrating cardiac injury: overcoming the limits set by nature. *Injury., 40*, 919–927.
7. Wall, M. J., Jr, Mattox, K. L., Chen, C. D., et al. (1997). Acute management of complex cardiac injuries. *J Trauma., 42*, 905–912.
8. Søreide, K. (2009). Epidemiology of major trauma. *Br J Surg., 96*, 697–698.
9. O'Connor, J. V., & Scalea, T. M. (2010). Penetrating thoracic great vessel injury: impact of admission hemodynamics and preoperative imaging. *J Trauma., 68*, 834–837.
10. Mattox, K. L., Wall, M. J. Jr, & Lemaire, S. (2008). Thoracic great vessel injury. In D. V. Feliciano, K. L. Mattox, & E. E. Moore (Eds.), *Trauma* (6th ed., pp. 589–603). New York, NY: McGraw Hill.
11. Carrick, M. M., Morrison, C. A., Pham, H. Q., et al. (2010). Modern management of traumatic subclavian artery injuries: a single institution's experience in the evolution of endovascular repair. *Am J Surg., 199*, 28–34.

48

Extremity vascular trauma

CHINMAYEE POTTI AND MOUNIR J. HAURANI

INTRODUCTION

In civilian trauma, vascular injury is seen in about 2.2% of patients, with 40–75% being peripheral and the majority penetrating [1]. In contrast to occlusive disease, young healthy adults without collateral circulation may have significant ischemia and limb loss following trauma. Management depends on stability and the presence of hard or soft signs of injury. Hard signs include obvious pulsatile bleeding; absent distal pulses; expanding hematoma; and arterial thrill or bruit over or close to the site of suspected arterial injury. Soft signs include the following: a history of significant hemorrhage; diminished distal pulse compared with the contralateral side; distal neurologic abnormalities; and proximity of a vessel to the wound or bone fragments. In the presence of hard signs, it is appropriate to proceed directly to the operating room without further workup. On screening with Doppler-derived ankle-brachial pressure indexes (ABIs), if the ABI is >0.9 and there is no pulse deficit, then the risk of vascular injury is defined as low. If ABI for an extremity is ≤0.9, there is a significant risk for arterial injury and additional imaging is warranted [2]. Anatomic vascular association with orthopedic injuries should aid in diagnosis (Table 48.1).

Table 48.1 Vascular injuries associated with orthopedic injuries

Orthopedic injury	Vascular injury
Supracondylar humerus fracture	Brachial artery
Elbow dislocation	Brachial artery
Distal femoral fracture	Superficial femoral-popliteal artery
Posterior dislocation of the knee	Popliteal artery
Tibial plateau fracture	Popliteal artery, Tibioperoneal trunk

MANAGEMENT PRINCIPLES

Hemorrhage and damage control

Appropriate tourniquet utilization has markedly increased survival rates. Directed digital pressure works extremely well in most extremity vascular injuries. Patients presenting with nonresponsive hemodynamic instability, coagulopathy, acidosis, hypothermia, higher priority life-threatening injuries, unstable orthopedic fractures, and large contaminated wounds without adequate graft coverage options are too unstable for primarily definitive vascular repair. While in the acute resuscitative phase, temporary intravascular shunting allows for rapid restoration of distal limb perfusion. After thrombectomy, regional heparinization, and shunt placement, fixation of associated orthopedic injuries allows a more planned and definitive vascular reconstruction. (Figure 48.1).

The vessel at the site of injury should be dissected proximally and distally to allow for vascular clamp placement and the edges debrided until clean healthy artery. Following proximal and distal Fogarty thrombectomy, good forward and backward bleeding is ensured, and heparinized saline is flushed bidirectionally. Following this, an appropriately sized shunt is inserted distally, allowed to back-bleed, and then inserted proximally, while being careful not to dissect the artery. Shunts are secured using either large caliber ties or Rumel tourniquets. Adequate flow is confirmed using a Doppler flow detector. Shunt placement time should be carefully documented. The shunted arterial segment is covered with soft tissue and/or a negative pressure dressing. Fasciotomy should be considered especially if >6 hours since injury. Definitive repair is recommended <24 hours or as soon as possible.

DOI: 10.1201/9781003452096-48

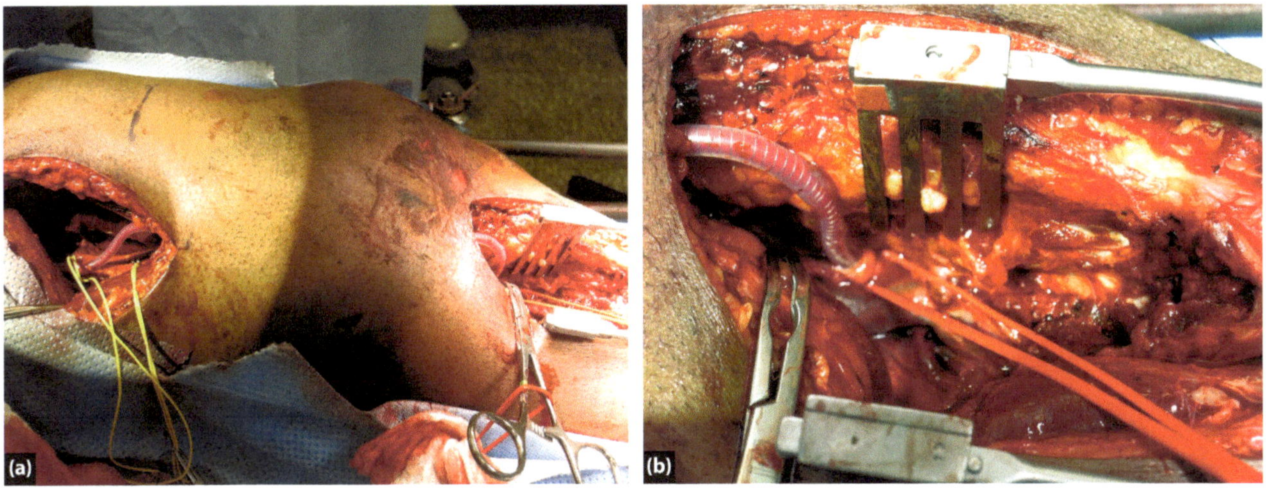

Figure 48.1 An intraluminal (Sundt™, Integra LifeSciences Corporation, Plainsboro, NJ. USA) shunt was placed between the above-knee and below-knee popliteal arteries in a patient with popliteal artery injury: (a) intraluminal shunt in the below-knee popliteal artery; (b) the shunt is held in place with a vessel loop tourniquet.

Imaging modalities in the evaluation of extremity vascular trauma

In patients with long bone fractures, reduction of the fracture and distal pulse reassessment is the first step for evaluating the vasculature, as pulse loss due to arterial entrapment can be resolved with reduction. After a thorough ATLS survey, in the absence of hard signs, with ABI ≤0.9, further imaging can be pursued. CT angiography is routinely used, with sensitivities approaching 100% for vascular injury [1]. Color-flow duplex is an alternative and inexpensive, non-invasive modality that provides rapid and detailed information on extremity blood vessels and surrounding anatomic structures and has a high sensitivity (93%) and specificity (95%) in the evaluation of extremity trauma [3]. A conventional gold standard angiography, although selectively used, can serve as both a diagnostic and therapeutic (endovascular) modality [4]. It is particularly useful in the setting of suspected junctional zone vascular injuries of the subclavian (SCA) and iliac arteries.

Assessment of the mangled extremity and primary amputation

A mangled extremity is defined as an extremity with a complex injury that involves soft tissue, bone, nerve, and vasculature. There are several methods available to calculate the degree of injury and associated outcome after attempted reconstruction. A Mangled Extremity Severity Score (MESS) (Table 48.2) of <4 predicts salvage with 100% accuracy and a score of ≥7 predicts amputation with 100% accuracy. In severe cases, a primary amputation may lead to a superior functional outcome and avoids the misdirection of care when other life-threatening injuries should take priority. The decision to amputate is usually dictated by the degree of soft-tissue injury, Gustilo open fracture classification, the resources available to accomplish and maintain a complex extremity reconstruction (such as an intensive care unit), and the presence of other life-threatening injuries [5].

Treatment planning

Location, severity of injury, hard signs, hemodynamic stability, other injuries, and patient status dictate management. Non-operative management with antiplatelets or anticoagulation is appropriate for vasospasm and for intimal flaps if asymptomatic and not flow-limiting. The "salvageability" of the limb must be considered in the setting of ischemia, hemorrhage, unstable pseudoaneurysm, or arteriovenous fistula necessitating surgery.

DEFINITIVE MANAGEMENT: GENERAL PRINCIPLES

Basic principles of any open vascular repair include obtaining adequate exposure, proximal and distal control, ensuring a prepped potential vein harvest site, thrombectomy and ensuring adequate inflow and backbleeding, debridement of the artery wall back to healthy edges, and definitive tension-free reconstruction (Table 48.3). If exposure is challenging anatomically, endovascular balloon tamponade for control can be considered from a distant site. In the absence of contraindicated injuries, systemic heparinization should be considered. However, flushing regionally with heparinized saline after thrombectomy is essential. Doppler confirmation of flow following shunting and completion angiogram after reconstruction is recommended.

Longer ischemia times prelude significantly worse outcomes, necessitating expeditious repair within three hours of injury. Fasciotomies should be considered especially if greater than six hours of ischemia. Great saphenous vein (GSV) is the most commonly used conduit/patch. To

Table 48.2 Mangled Extremity Scoring System (MESS)

Injury type	Characteristics	MESS score
Skeletal/soft-tissue injury	Low energy (stab wound, simple fracture, pistol gunshot wound)	1
	Medium energy (open or multiple fractures, dislocation)	2
	High energy (high-speed motor vehicle accident or rifle gunshot wound)	3
	Very high energy (high-speed trauma + gross contamination)	4
Limb ischemia	A pulsatile limb without signs of ischemia	0
	Pulse reduced or absent but perfusion normal	1[a]
	Pulseless, paresthesia, diminished capillary refill	2[a]
	Cool, paralyzed, insensate, numb	3[a]
Shock	Systolic blood pressure always >90 mmHg	0
	Transient hypotension	1
	Persistent hypotension	2
Age, years	<30	0
	>30–50	1
	>50	2

[a]Multiply by two if the injury >6 hours.

Table 48.3 General principles and adjuncts of open vascular repair

Type of repair	Indication	Examples
Vessel ligation	Damage control situations	Subclavian, brachial, radial, ulnar, and isolated tibial arteries
Lateral repair	<50% loss in vessel diameter	Repair of common femoral artery with a patch
Direct anastomosis	No tension after debridement of nonviable vessel wall	Repair of brachial artery after sharp transection
Bypass	Inability to perform a direct repair or a primary anastomosis without undue tension	Not suitable in hemodynamically unstable patients. Conduit considerations

ensure access to such, both lower limbs should be prepped into the operative field. Contralateral GSV harvest is recommended to preserve sufficient venous drainage on the injured limb as venous injuries are commonly associated with arterial trauma. Many prosthetic conduits are available with polytetrafluoroethylene (PTFE) being the most used. All prosthetic grafts perform with similar patency rates, which are inferior to autogenous grafts for arterial or venous reconstructions, especially in infrapopliteal vessels. They also have a higher rate of graft infections in contaminated wounds (Table 48.3).

It is vital to stabilize long bone fractures, with temporary or definitive methods prior to vascular repair. In stable patients without other life-threatening injuries, repair of venous injuries is recommended to improve limb outcomes, especially for axillary, subclavian, popliteal, femoral, common femoral, and iliac injuries.

SPECIFIC INJURIES: LOWER EXTREMITIES

Open management of iliofemoral injuries

Standard femoral exposure is obtained in most situations. Identifying and lateralizing the inguinal ligament and transecting it will aid in more proximal control. Further proximal control can be obtained with retroperitoneal iliac exposure or intraluminal balloon control from the contralateral groin. In an unstable limb salvage situation, re-establishing in-line flow takes precedence over reconstructing the femoral bifurcation. Either the femoral vein or the profunda femoris vein, but not both, can be ligated, but the common femoral vein should be reconstructed if possible to avoid postoperative limb morbidity (e.g., swelling, compartment syndrome, post-thrombotic state).

Open management of the popliteal artery

Popliteal artery exposure is gained through standard medial distal thigh and proximal calf incisions. In severe popliteal fossa injuries, above- and below-knee incisions can be connected by cutting through all medial tendon attachments to the knee (Figure 48.2). Due to documented improvement in limb salvage, it is strongly recommended that concomitant popliteal venous injuries be repaired prior to definitive arterial repair while using a temporary arterial shunt. As previously referenced, it is recommended that unstable orthopedic injuries be fixed prior to definitive arterial repair. These injuries have a

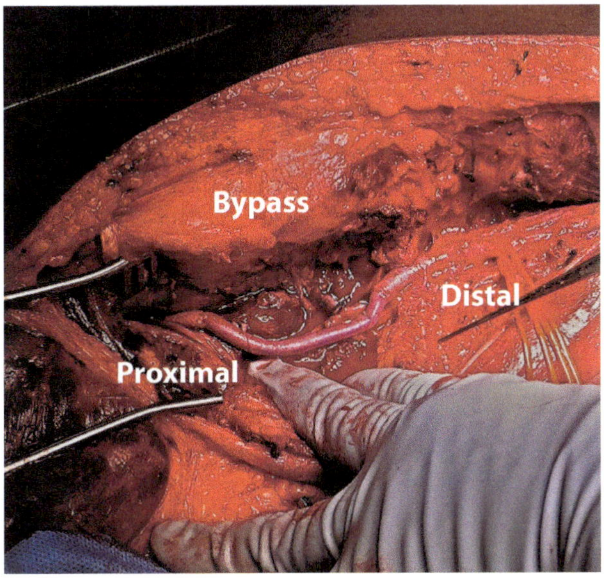

Figure 48.2 Gunshot wound to the popliteal artery was repaired with an interposition (contralateral saphenous vein) bypass graft.

high risk of compartment syndrome and there should be a low threshold for fasciotomies.

Open management of tibial arteries

When managing tibial vascular injuries, one must control bleeding, reduce any fractures, warm and resuscitate the patient, and examine the foot with continuous-wave Doppler. In most cases, after these maneuvers, an arterial signal will be present in the foot indicating viability and obviating the need for additional maneuvers. If there is no Doppler signal after these steps, one must consider that there may be injury to more than one tibial vessel or to the tibial peroneal trunk. The options in this scenario are: (1) attempt to restore flow with a small-caliber, temporary vascular shunt; (2) perform vascular reconstruction with a below-knee popliteal-to-tibial bypass or interposition graft using the saphenous vein; or (3) accept ligation and continue expectant management. One should be mindful that in some cases, primary amputation should be performed when ischemic damage has been present for more than six hours, there is severe orthopedic injury to the foot or ankle with associated injuries, or when the severity of the mangled extremity is such that a safe attempt at limb salvage is precluded. In general, patency of at least two tibial vessels is considered optimal.

SPECIFIC INJURIES: UPPER EXTREMITIES

Management of SCA and axillary arteries

The proximal right SCA can be exposed through a median sternotomy. The left SCA originates and follows a posterior course from the aortic arch. A high left anterolateral thoracotomy, typically performed at the third or fourth intercostal space, provides optimal exposure. Further exposure requires a separate clavicular incision, with or without resection of the clavicular head. When more distal exposure is required, a supraclavicular incision is made parallel to the clavicle, and a horizontal, infraclavicular incision is made at the middle third of the clavicle and extended laterally. Prosthetic grafts are used for reconstruction with excellent patency and low infection risk. If the medial clavicle is resected, it should not be replaced to prevent callus formation.

Reconstruction of venous injuries is preferred over ligation to mitigate the risk of long-term disability [6].

Management of the brachial artery

Brachial artery injuries should be reconstructed primarily or with autogenous veins (GSV or ipsilateral basilic vein, assuming there is no concomitant ipsilateral deep venous injury). Prosthetic conduits should be avoided because of poor patency. Care must be exercised to avoid injury to the brachial vein and median nerve during exposure and reconstruction (Figures 48.3–48.7) [7].

Management of radial and ulnar arteries

An S-shaped incision over the antecubital fossa allows access to the distal brachial artery and the proximal radial and ulnar arteries. Identifying the brachial artery and tracing it distally may aid in identifying these forearm arteries. The radial artery follows the medial border of the brachioradialis muscle, and the medial groove of this muscle can be used as a landmark to make an incision in the mid-forearm. The ulnar artery dives deep to the pronator teres muscle slightly beyond the bifurcation and remains deep to the flexor muscles of the proximal forearm before emerging into a more superficial course at the midpoint of the forearm. Injury to only one artery (radial or ulnar) can be managed with simple ligation if the palmar arch is complete. Otherwise, these injuries should be repaired with an autogenous vein graft.

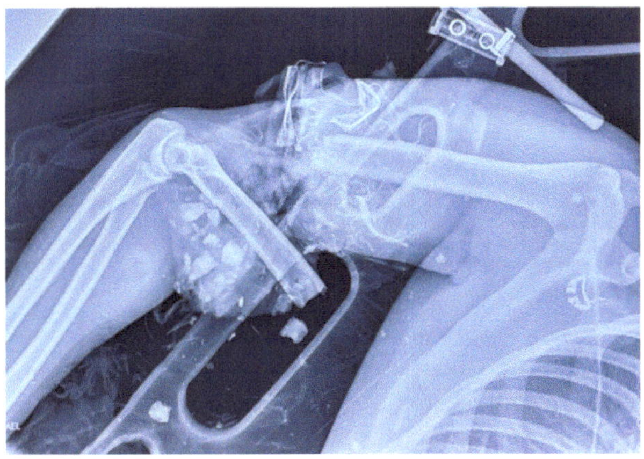

Figure 48.3 Traumatic upper arm injury: X-ray.

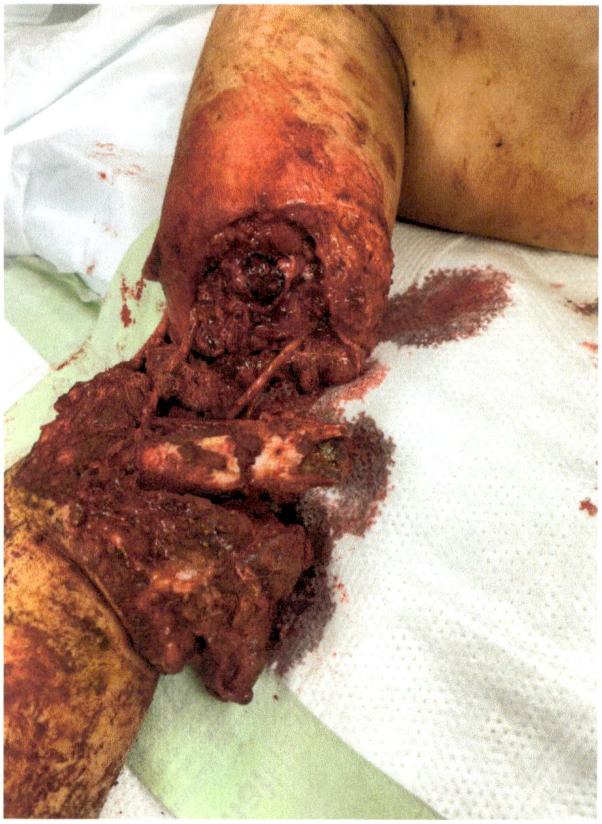

Figure 48.4 Almost complete transection of the arm except for the ulnar and radial nerves.

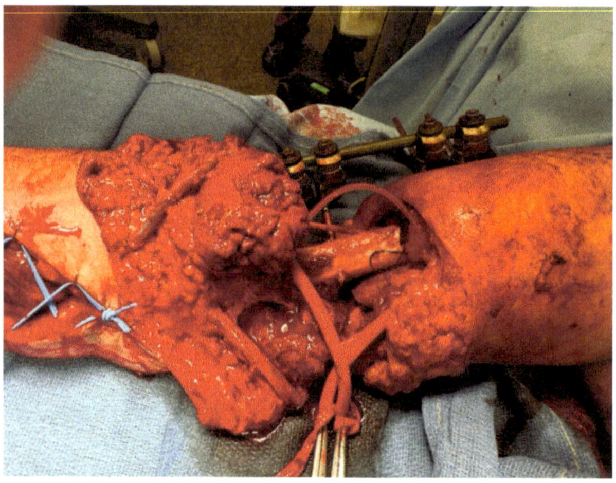

Figure 48.5 Argyl shunt with Rumel tourniquets and external fixator stabilizing the bone. Note very dilated veins due to severe venous hypertension with no intact vein/venous return.

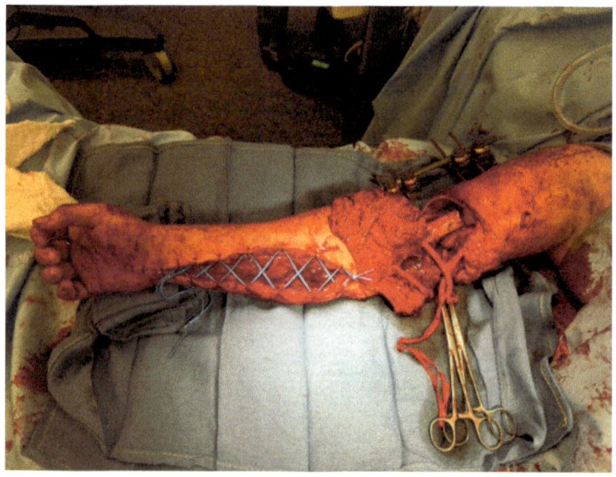

Figure 48.6 Fasciotomies completed prior to definitive arterial repair.

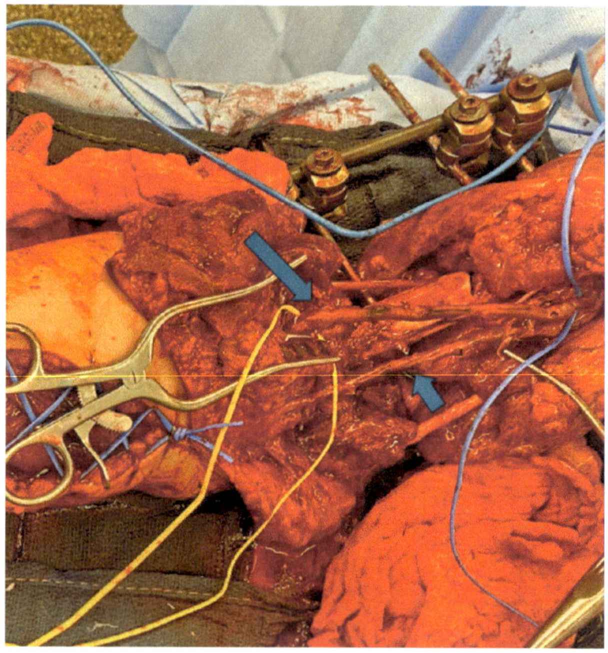

Figure 48.7 Arterial and venous bypass (blue arrows) using reversed saphenous vein for artery and saphenous vein without reversal for vein bypass.

ENDOVASCULAR MANAGEMENT

Endovascular treatment is emerging to be a suitable alternative for both penetrating and blunt trauma in feasible situations, especially in central junction zones. When available, CTA is a valuable resource for preoperative planning. For lower extremity injuries, based on location, patient stability, and presence of other injuries, one can consider antegrade or retrograde femoral access from the contralateral limb. For upper extremity access, axillary, radial, or brachial arteries can be used. Once wire access is obtained through and beyond the injury, covered stents (e.g., iCast™ Balloon Expandable Covered Stent, Atrium Medical Corporation, Hudson, NH, USA; Fluency, BARD Peripheral Vascular, Inc., Tempe, AZ, USA; GORE® VIABAHN® Endoprosthesis, W. L. Gore & Associates, Flagstaff, AZ, USA) can be placed across the site of injury. More aggressive oversizing (>20%) is recommended for upper extremities due to very compliant vessels with a higher risk of endoleak compared with lower extremities (<20%) (Table 48.4).

Table 48.4 Open versus endovascular techniques

Objective	Open techniques	Endovascular techniques
Temporary control of flow	Arterial clamping, sponge stick control of venous bleeding	Balloon control (REBOA) for lower extremities; occlusive sheath control
Permanent occlusion of flow	Surgical ligation	Amplatz vascular plug, coil occlusion, stent graft plugs
Mass control of bleeding	Open surgical packing	Mass embolization with coils or sterile compressed sponge/thrombin
Control of bleeding and restoration of flow	Open bypass, patch repair, primary repair, shunts	Stent graft repair, covered stent coverage, or closed cell stenting/coiling

POSTOPERATIVE CARE

Reperfusion injury is constituted by a myriad of electrolyte abnormalities, myoglobinuria, and systemic inflammatory reactions from free radical washout into the systemic circulation. In addition to trauma and injury-related goal-directed resuscitation, aggressive resuscitation should be pursued to prevent acute kidney injury from myoglobinuria. It is especially important to perform frequent neurovascular checks and monitor for compartment syndrome if fasciotomies were not already performed [8]. All patients without contraindications should receive aspirin and prophylactic doses of subcutaneous low-molecular-weight heparin. Consider a therapeutic dose of anticoagulation in cases of venous reconstruction.

Other complications include bleeding, infection, complications from other injuries, trauma-related coagulopathy, and graft thrombosis, which should be addressed immediately if the patient is stable.

TRICKS AND TRAPS

1. Planning: knowing other injuries and coordinating with the teams involved are key to good patient outcomes, e.g., is it safe to heparinize?
2. Equipment: ensure the availability of shunts, sutures, bypass conduit, ACT machine, options for fluoroscopy, and duplex ultrasound.
3. Prepping: prep widely and adequately for proximal control, as well as possible contralateral vein harvest.
4. Discuss with your orthopedic colleagues the sequence of procedures: shunt, temporary fixation, then bypass *or* arterial repair first.
5. When proximal control is challenging, consider possible endovascular balloon control sites and prepare for backup.
6. Ensure the injury site is adequately irrigated, and devitalized tissue completely debrided to minimize infection risk.
7. If able to, consider harvesting vein conduit while awaiting another team's procedure in polytrauma. Do not transect the vein until you adequately debride proximal and distal vessel ends. Always harvest more vein than you consider necessary. If there is a valve at the anastomosis site, even if reversed, perform a valvulotomy.
8. Attempt to tunnel your bypass away from the injury site if possible. If not, ensure adequate coverage of the arterial repair or bypass.
9. Always perform a Fogarty thrombectomy proximally and distally prior to performing arterial repair.
10. The authors strongly recommend doing fasciotomies. If you think about it, do it.
11. Most patients are hemoconcentrated with falsely elevated hemoglobin values. If hypotensive intraoperatively, have a low threshold to transfuse.

QUESTIONS

1. A 33-year-old man presents to the trauma bay after kicking a glass door and lacerating his left thigh. His vital signs are stable and primary survey identifies no other injuries. He is noted to have a small hematoma over the left thigh that is soft and non-expanding. What is the next step in the management of this patient?
   a. Ankle-brachial index
   b. Duplex ultrasound of the leg
   c. CT angiography of the leg
   d. Surgical exploration of the leg
   e. Non-contrasted CT of the leg

   Answer: a

2. A 29-year-old female presents as a trauma activation after a stab wound to the left upper extremity. Which of the following is an indication for immediate operative exploration?
   a. Diminished pulse compared with the other side
   b. Bruit on auscultation
   c. Small hematoma at the injury site
   d. Distal neurological abnormalities

   Answer: b

3. A 35-year-old male presents after multiple gunshot wounds to the chest, abdomen, and extremities. You have been paged that there is a noticeable deformity with exposed bone in the right upper extremity. Which of the following is an appropriate orthopedic and vascular injury association?
    a. Fracture of surgical neck of the humerus: posterior circumflex artery
    b. Midshaft of humeral fracture: ulnar collateral artery
    c. Fracture of the medial epicondyle: brachial artery
    d. Supracondylar fracture: profunda brachii artery

    Answer: a

4. A 40-year-old male presents after a gunshot wound to the left thigh, hypotensive to systolic blood pressure of 70, and has pulsatile bleeding from the site. He is taken emergently for exploration. An injury is noted in the mid-thigh SFA. After extensive debridement of devitalized overlying skin and tissue, it is a 2 cm long tear, <50% circumferential. What is the best option for repair?
    a. Patch angioplasty with a vein patch
    b. Stent across the tear after appropriate heparinization
    c. Polytetrafluoroethylene bypass
    d. Primary repair since this is a dirty wound without good coverage options

    Answer: a

REFERENCES

1. Alam, H. B., & DiMusto, P. D. (2015). Management of lower extremity vascular trauma. *Curr Trauma Rep.*, *1*, 61–68. https://doi.org/10.1007/s40719-014-0007-2
2. Conrad, M. F., Patton, J. H., Jr, & Parikshak, M., et al. (2002). Evaluation of vascular injury in penetrating trauma: angiographers stay home. *Am Surg.*, *68*, 269–274.
3. Busquéts, A. R., Acosta, J. A., Colón, E., et al. (2004). Helical computed tomography angiography for the diagnosis of traumatic arterial injuries of the extremities. *J Trauma.*, *56*, 625–628.
4. de Mestral, C., Sharma, S., Haas, B., et al. (2013). A contemporary analysis of the management of the mangled lower extremity. *J Trauma Acute Care Surg.*, *74*, 597–603.
5. Dua, A., Desai, S. S., Shah, J. O., et al. (2014). Outcome predictors of limb salvage in traumatic popliteal artery injury. *Ann Vasc Surg.*, *28*, 108–114.
6. Franz, R. W., Skytta, C. K., Shah, K. J., et al. (2012). A five-year review of management of upper-extremity arterial injuries at an urban level I trauma center. *Ann Vasc Surg.*, *26*, 655–664.
7. Ergunes, K., Yilik, L., Ozsoyler, I., et al. (2006). Traumatic brachial artery injuries. *Tex Heart Inst J.*, *33*, 31–34.
8. Donaldson, J., Haddad, B., & Kahn, W. S. (2014). The pathophysiology, diagnosis, and current management of acute compartment syndrome. *Open Orthop J.*, *8*, 185–193.

49

Penetrating extracranial carotid and vertebral artery trauma

CHINMAYEE POTTI AND MOUNIR J. HAURANI

INTRODUCTION

Penetrating neck trauma constitutes 10% of all injuries, with a mortality rate of up to 20% when the carotid artery is affected [1]. Imaging and endovascular advancements are replacing traditional surgery, reshaping the management of these injuries. Nevertheless, surgical exploration and open vascular repair skills remain crucial due to the substantial morbidity and mortality linked to major vascular injuries in the neck.

EXTRACRANIAL PENETRATING CAROTID INJURY

Management hinges on patient stability, anatomic zone, and the presence of hard or soft signs of vascular injury (Table 49.1). Traditional neck zones provide a framework for anatomic and technical considerations, but a recent shift toward a patient-focused "no-zone" technique has emerged with advanced imaging [2]. Surgically exploring unstable patients with "hard signs" of vascular injury is imperative, irrespective of the zone. Additional indications include damage to aerodigestive structures leading to crepitus, respiratory distress, or air bubbling from the wound, as well as neurologic deficits suggesting cerebral ischemia. All stable patients without hard signs should undergo advanced imaging (Figure 49.1).

Table 49.1 Signs of cervical penetrating vascular injury

Signs/indications	Description
Hard signs (surgical exploration warranted)	1. Pulsatile bleeding 2. Palpable thrill 3. Audible bruit 4. Expanding hematoma
Soft signs (further diagnostic imaging warranted)	1. History indicative of moderate hemorrhage 2. Diminished pulse 3. Small, stable hematoma
Additional indications (surgical exploration warranted)	1. Evidence of cerebral ischemia a. Hemiparesis/neurologic deficit b. Altered mental status 2. Evidence of tracheobronchial/ esophageal disruption a. Crepitus b. Air bubbling from wound c. Respiratory distress

Zone I injuries pose challenges due to restricted access to the proximal common carotid artery (CCA) by the clavicle and sternum. Zone III injuries are difficult to control because the internal carotid artery (ICA) enters into the skull base. Zone II injuries are easily accessible through a cervical incision for proximal and distal control.

Traditionally, angiography has been the gold standard for zone I or zone III injuries. It provides a comprehensive assessment of the extracranial arteries from intrathoracic origin to intracranial termination but demands significant expertise. For zone II injuries with platysma muscle violation, diagnostic neck exploration was mandatory, resulting in historically high rates (ranging from 30% to 89%) of negative explorations [3]. CT angiography or duplex ultrasonography is becoming the initial modality of choice in lieu of arteriography to rule out an arterial injury [4] in all stable patients because of speed, widespread availability, technical ease, and non-invasive nature. The sensitivity of computed tomography angiography (CTA) for vascular injury approaches 100%, with

DOI: 10.1201/9781003452096-49

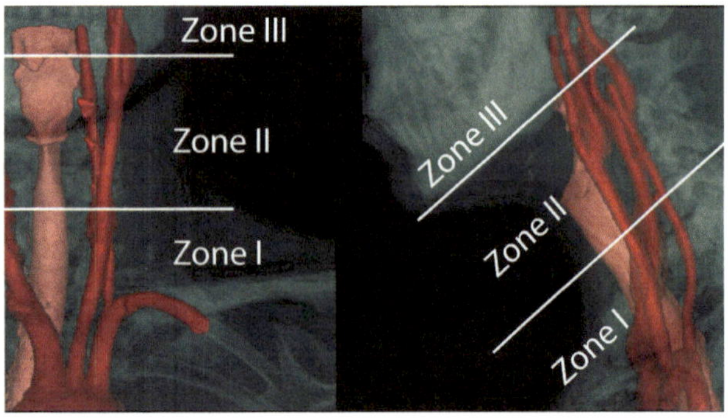

Figure 49.1 Zones of injury. Zone I: below the cricoid cartilage and above the clavicles at the thoracic inlet. Zone II: between the cricoid cartilage and the angle of the mandible. Zone III: above the angle of the mandible.

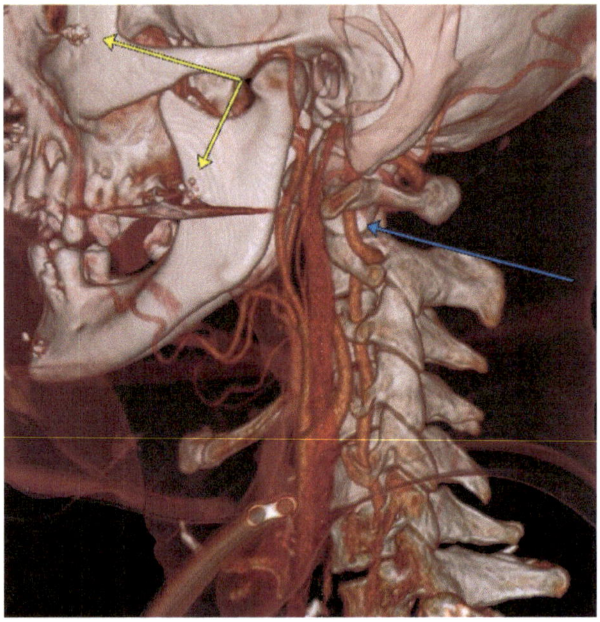

Figure 49.2 Computed tomography angiography (CTA) reconstruction of a patient shot in the neck. The blue arrow marks the bullet entry site. The yellow arrows mark bullet fragments. In this case, CTA effectively ruled out vascular injury.

the additional benefit of identifying aerodigestive tract injuries [5] (Figure 49.2).

SPECIAL OPERATIVE CONSIDERATIONS IN OPEN NECK EXPLORATION AND VASCULAR REPAIR

The authors recommend prepping both lower extremities for access to the great saphenous veins, facilitating vein patching or interposition grafting as needed. Wide prepping, extending from the angle of the mandible to the chest below the xiphoid, is beneficial in case further exposure becomes necessary.

Controlling carotid bleeding often involves direct manual pressure. When manual pressure is insufficient, temporary control can be achieved by using balloon catheter tamponade—inserting a balloon catheter or Foley catheter into the wound tract.

An oblique incision is made along the anterior border of the sternocleidomastoid muscle (SCM). The platysma is divided along the medial border (Figure 49.3). Retracting the SCM laterally exposes the internal jugular vein, followed along its anterior border to the facial vein. Division of the facial vein provides complete access to the carotid sheath and bifurcation. This incision can be extended proximally along the SCM to the sternal notch or distally to the angle of the mandible. Once the injury is identified, proximal and distal control is obtained. Digastric muscle division allows further distal access. Carefully inflating a No.2- or 3-Fr Fogarty balloon catheter provides temporary distal control until the internal carotid artery (ICA) is better exposed for repair (or ligation). Mandibular or zygomatic arch osteotomy can enhance distal exposure but this is a time-consuming and disfiguring step. In hemodynamically unstable patients, placing a temporary shunt allows resuscitation and rewarming before complex repairs.

Obtaining proximal control of zone I carotid injuries proves challenging due to their posterior course below the sternoclavicular joint. To control the proximal arch vessels, a partial or full median sternotomy can be performed (Figure 49.4). For left-sided injuries, accessing the proximal subclavian artery (SCA) is achievable with an anterolateral thoracotomy through the fourth intercostal space (ICS). If additional proximal control is necessary on the right, splitting and "T-ing off" the manubrium into the second ICS provides access to the origin of the brachiocephalic artery and aortic arch (Figure 49.4). A side-biting clamp can be placed on a noncalcified aortic arch to provide effective control of the brachiocephalic origin.

Once control is achieved, the decision to repair or ligate the carotid artery depends on the injury severity and patient status. Despite the associated mortality and morbidity, every effort should be made to revascularize the carotid artery [6–8]. In cases of hemodynamic instability or challenging injuries, carotid ligation may be considered. Revascularization is contraindicated if there is no back-bleeding from the distal carotid in patients with profound neurologic deficits due to the risk of distal embolization [9] after revascularization. Carotids with distal stump pressure >70 mmHg can safely be ligated [10].

Devitalized arterial wall is debrided to healthy edges. Smaller defects are primarily repaired, while patch angioplasty is used for larger ones (<50% wall circumference). Injuries >50% of the circumference or those repairs associated with significant tension require interposition bypass preferably with saphenous vein. If vein is unavailable, prosthetic grafts have been successfully used with patency equivalent to autogenous repair [8]. However, prosthetic grafts in a contaminated surgical field pose a higher risk for postoperative infection.

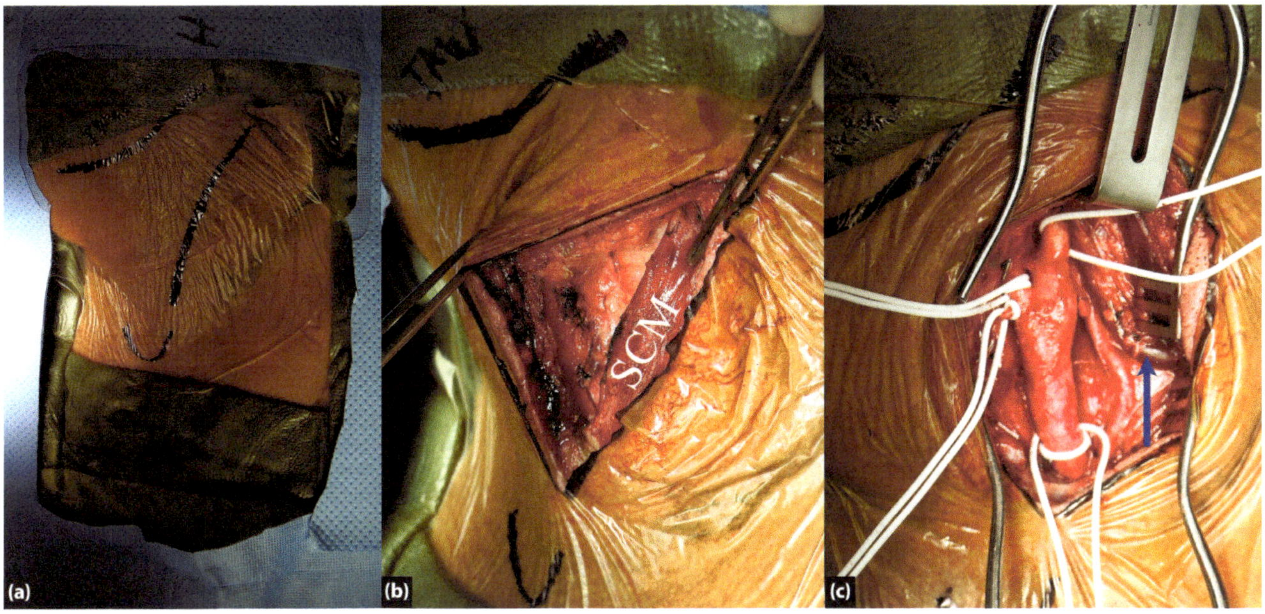

Figure 49.3 Incision should be made along the anterior border of the SCM: (a) the sternal notch and the angle of the jaw are marked; (b) the SCM is dissected along the anterior border and retracted laterally along with the IJV; (c) the common, external, and internal carotid arteries can be quickly explored and controlled. The blue arrow shows ligated facial vein to fully mobilize the IJV.

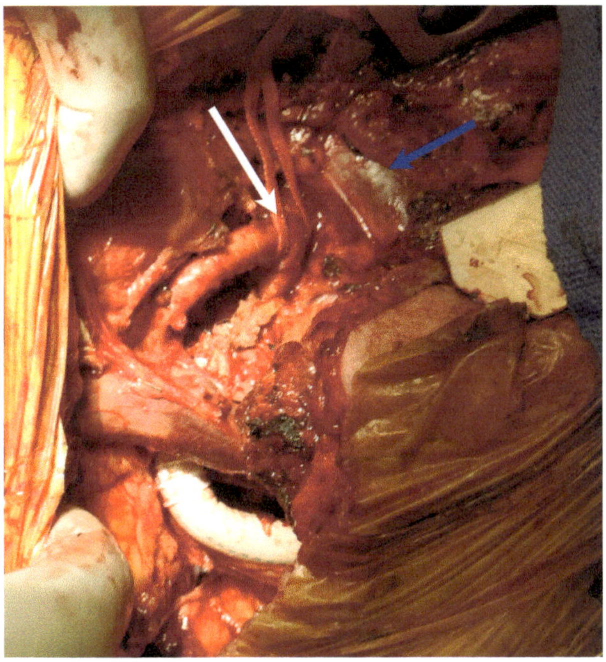

Figure 49.4 Proximal control of the arch vessels for zone I injuries. The patient's head is to the left, with a Finochietto rib spreader to the right holding the edges of the divided manubrium apart, which is further mobilized by division into the second ICS. The umbilical tapes and white arrow show the brachiocephalic artery, with the brachiocephalic (blue arrow) vein crossing over the artery. Distally, the subclavian artery needed to be reconstructed with a short interposition prosthetic graft.

ENDOVASCULAR APPROACH TO CAROTID ARTERY INJURIES

Regardless of the imaging modality, common vascular injury features include an intimal flap, long tapered narrowing or occlusion, vessel dilation with a dissecting aneurysm pattern, or the presence of crescentic intramural hematoma [11]. For hemodynamically stable patients with zone I and zone III injuries, endovascular repair is preferred due to anatomic challenges. A four-vessel cervical and cerebral angiogram assesses the injury's location, extent, and collateral circulation.

Endovascular repair depends on the type of injury. For small intimal irregularities and dissections with <25% luminal stenosis, short-term imaging and conservative management on antiplatelet medications are prudent, as up to 70% heal within weeks to months [11]. Symptomatic patients or disease progression may warrant endovascular management [11]. Treatment aims to prevent false lumen expansion, thrombolysis/thrombectomy for acute stroke, and stenting for larger dissections. Self-expanding stents, preferred for their tolerance to flexion and external compression, are more commonly used than balloon-expandable stents. Complete or nearly complete transection, usually with a large pseudoaneurysm, may not be amenable to stenting. In such cases, balloon occlusion of the internal carotid artery (ICA) can quickly control hemorrhage, although with an increased risk of neurologic morbidity. This allows for adequate resuscitation and improved cerebral perfusion pressure through collateral blood flow. Pseudoaneurysms can be managed with covered

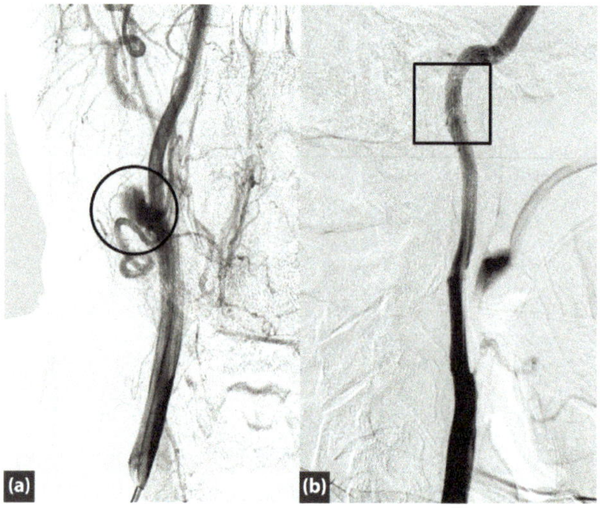

Figure 49.5 Stent repair of carotid artery pseudoaneurysm: (a) patient with unstable neck fractures and carotid artery pseudoaneurysm (circled). Given his concurrent neck injury, the injury was treated with a stent graft; (b) notice the embolic protection device in place (squared).

endovascular stent grafting or pseudoaneurysm coiling and exclusion (Figure 49.5).

COMPLICATIONS

Carotid ligation carries significant morbidity, with a stroke rate of 30% [12] and a mortality rate of 45% [7]; it is primarily utilized on comatose patients with generally poor prognoses. Open repair in patients without neurologic deficit poses a 1% risk of permanent deficit [6]. Patients with neurologic deficits have a 50% chance of improvement with revascularization [6]. Additionally, complications such as cranial nerve injury, wound/graft infection, and postoperative bleeding can occur.

Carotid stent grafting demonstrates an overall primary patency of 80% at two years, with procedural mortality below 1% and a stroke risk of 3.5% [13]. Long-term outcomes data is limited. Other complications associated with endovascular therapy include a less than 1% incidence of femoral artery pseudoaneurysm [11] and a 6.6% rate of contrast-induced nephropathy in trauma patients [14].

FOLLOW-UP

Standard follow-up with surveillance carotid duplex imaging post-repair is recommended. The authors advocate antiplatelet therapy following any open repair. While data is limited, lifelong antiplatelet therapy is advised for patients with carotid or SCA stents [15].

EXTRACRANIAL PENETRATING VERTEBRAL ARTERY INJURY

Penetrating vertebral artery injuries (VAIs) are rare and usually discovered incidentally [16]. The vertebral artery comprises four segments: V1, V2, V3, and V4, with V2 most frequently injured [16] (Figure 49.6). Due to the difficulty in exposing these areas for open repair, all injuries should be addressed endovascularly if possible. The robust collateral circulation of the vertebrobasilar system makes vertebral artery ligation significantly less likely to result in an ischemic insult compared with carotid ligation. Vertebral artery intervention is aimed at hemorrhage control and the prevention of posterior circulation embolic stroke through ligation or embolization, rather than revascularization (Figure 49.6).

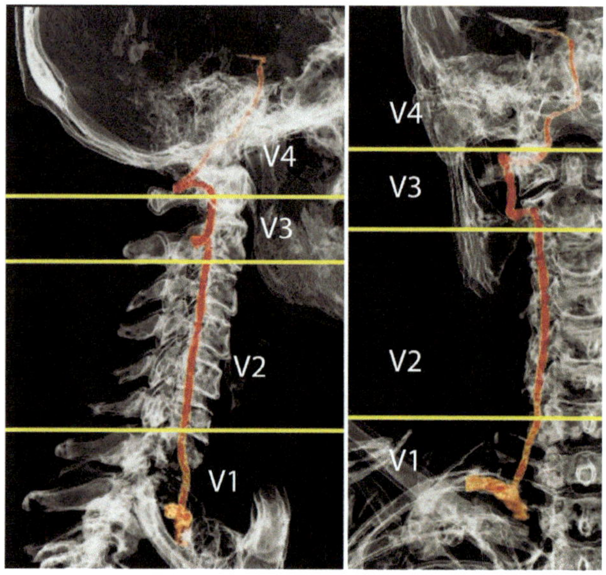

Figure 49.6 The segments of the vertebral artery (V1–V4). The V1 segment is accessible via the cervical incision just superior to the clavicle or through an extended incision parallel to the anterior border of the sternocleidomastoid muscle. The V1 segment extends from its origin off the subclavian artery to the C6 transverse process. The V2 segment runs from the C2 to the C6 transverse process. Once the artery enters the C6 transverse process and until it exits again at C2, it is relatively protected but challenging to access surgically. The V3 segment is the extracranial segment between the C2 transverse process and the vertebral canal of the skull base. The V4, or intracranial segment, continues until it joins with the contralateral vertebral artery to form the basilar artery at the lower border of the pons.

OPERATIVE CONSIDERATION IN OPEN NECK EXPLORATION INVOLVING THE VERTEBRAL ARTERY

When endovascular therapy is unavailable, an open surgical approach is determined by injury location. Standard neck exploration—oblique incision along the anterior SCM from below the mastoid to the sternoclavicular junction provides access. For more proximal control needed for vertebral artery ligation at its origin on the subclavian artery (SCA), the incision can be extended laterally, parallel to, and approximately 1–2 cm above the clavicle.

For V1 injuries, transection of the clavicular head of the SCM and anterior scalene muscle (ASM) may be necessary. Care is taken to avoid injury to the phrenic nerve on the ASM. Branches of the thyrocervical trunk are divided to access the vertebral artery and the subclavian vertebral junction. Proximal control may require median sternotomy to expose the SCA. A small Fogarty catheter is useful for obtaining temporary control, and the vertebral artery is then ligated above and below the injury.

V2 injuries can be challenging to ligate due to their interosseous canal location. An incision along the anterior border of the SCM is made, and the carotid sheath is retracted laterally. Division of the middle thyroid vein allows access to the prevertebral space. Bone wax is applied firmly into the bleeding interspace between the transverse processes for control. Direct exposure of the interosseous vertebral artery is not necessary, as the space between the transverse processes can be palpated. Metal clip appliers are guided along a probing index finger to the vertebral artery segments above and below the injured vessel under the longus colli muscle. Metal clips are placed above and below the site of injury within the same interspace, or one interspace above and below if necessary. To avoid inadvertent nerve root injury during clipping, the clips should be applied from an anterior approach, just below the transverse process [17].

ENDOVASCULAR APPROACH TO VAIS

Endovascular intervention is preferred as there are no anatomic constraints. Pseudoaneurysms or arteriovenous fistula formation necessitate intervention with coil embolization due to the high risk of posterior circulation embolic stroke. Proximal balloon control of the subclavian artery and distal balloon control of the vertebral artery are useful adjuncts when anticipating complex open vascular repair. Patients with vertebral dissection without other sequelae can be managed with antiplatelet or anticoagulation therapy, with many of these lesions resolving over time [18].

COMPLICATIONS

Post-traumatic pseudoaneurysms can occur in 15–26% of patients [16]. Vertebrobasilar insufficiency after ligation is reported in 1.8–3.1% of patients, characterized by neurologic symptoms such as altered mental status, dysphagia, dysarthria, diplopia, and nystagmus [19]. The literature on blunt trauma VAIs indicates a risk of posterior circulation stroke ranging from 5% to 24%, with neurologic symptoms typically emerging four to five days after the initial trauma [20]. Access-related complications and contrast-induced nephropathy can occur [14].

FOLLOW-UP

Patients with VAIs should remain on either anticoagulation or antiplatelet therapy. Heparin therapy reduced neurologic events from 20–35% to 0–14%, and subsequent studies found no significant difference in patients receiving antiplatelet therapy (either clopidogrel or aspirin) compared with anticoagulation [8,20,21]. The degree of injury, from partial dissection to complete transection, does not predict posterior circulation stroke [19,20]. Current recommendations advocate treating all asymptomatic patients, regardless of severity, with antiplatelet therapy or anticoagulation. Symptomatic patients without contraindications should receive anticoagulation therapy. All VAIs should be treated with antithrombotic therapy for three to six months or until resolution on radiographic imaging.

TRICKS AND TRAPS

Penetrating carotid injury:

- Prep both extremities into the field for access to the great saphenous veins.
- Apply direct manual pressure and consider balloon catheter tamponade using a Foley or compliant balloon catheter.
- For distal ICA control, consider dividing digastric muscle, mandibular osteotomy, and balloon tamponade control.
- Incision along the anterior border of SCM.
- Identify injury and proximal and distal control.
- Debride artery ends to clean healthy edges.
- Primary repair/patch closure/interposition grafting/ligation based on the extent of the injury.
- Thrombosed carotid arteries should be ligated.
- Vertebral artery injuries are best managed with endovascular techniques given the difficulties associated with exposure.

QUESTIONS

1. The best method of repair for a carotid artery injury involving >50% of the wall circumference is:
   a. Ligation
   b. Primary repair
   c. Patch closure
   d. Interposition grafting with saphenous vein
   e. Interposition grafting with internal jugular vein

   Answer: d

2. A 60-year-old woman presents following a motor vehicle collision. She is hemodynamically stable. On primary survey, she is noted to have multiple facial fractures. A laceration was noted over the right neck below the angle of the mandible with a visibly expanding hematoma. What is the next step in the evaluation for carotid vascular injury?
   a. Carotid duplex
   b. Surgical exploration
   c. CT angiography of the neck
   d. Non-contrast CT neck
   e. MR angiography of the neck

   Answer: b

3. A 30-year-old man presents with a stab wound to the neck following a robbery attempt. After completion of primary and secondary surveys, a 2 cm wound is noted in the neck above the angle of the mandible without active bleeding or hematoma. A CTA of the head and neck demonstrates an irregularity along the mid V2 vertebral artery consistent with a pseudoaneurysm. What is the next step in the management of this patient?
   a. MR angiography of the neck
   b. Open operative intervention and ligation of pseudoaneurysm
   c. Endovascular intervention for coil embolization of the pseudoaneurysm
   d. Non-contrast CT neck
   e. Carotid duplex

   Answer: c

4. A 74-year-old man is brought to the trauma bay after falling from a ladder onto a tree branch below. He was hemodynamically stable on presentation. His primary survey reveals a 4 cm neck laceration above the clavicle and below the cricoid cartilage. Upon further exploration, the wound is noted to be superficial to the platysma. What is the next step in the management of this patient?
   a. Esophagram
   b. Bronchoscopy
   c. Operative neck exploration
   d. CT angiogram of the neck
   e. Wound closure and observation alone

   Answer: e

REFERENCES

1. Blitzer, D. N., et al. (2020). Penetrating injury to the carotid artery: characterizing presentation and outcomes from the National Trauma Data Bank, *J Vasc Surg.*, 67, 192–199.
2. Ibraheem, K., et al. (2018). "No zone" approach in penetrating neck trauma reduces unnecessary computed tomography angiography and negative explorations. *J Surg Res.*, 221, 113–120.
3. Múnera, F., et al. (2002). Penetrating neck injuries: helical CT angiography for initial evaluation. *Radiology.*, 224, 366–372.
4. Tisherman, S. A., et al. (2008). Penetrating neck injuries, management of citation. *J Trauma.*, 64(5), 1392–1405.
5. Demetriades, D., et al. (1996). Complex problems in penetrating neck trauma. *Surg Clin North Am.*, 76, 661–683.
6. Liekweg, W., et al. (1978). Management of penetrating carotid arterial injury. *Ann Surg.*, 188, 587–592.
7. du Toit, D. F., et al. (2003). Neurologic outcome after penetrating extracranial artery trauma. *J Vasc Surg.*, 38, 257–262.
8. O'Brien, P. J., et al. (2011). A modern approach to cervical vascular trauma. *Perspect Vasc Surg Endovasc Ther.*, 23, 90–97.
9. Thal, E. R., et al. (1974). Management of carotid artery injuries. *Surgery.*, 76, 955–962.
10. Ehrnefeld, W. K., et al. (1983). Relation of carotid stump pressure to safety of carotid artery ligation. *Surgery*, 93, 299–305.
11. Vellimana, A. K., et al. (2021, March). Endovascular considerations in traumatic injury of the carotid and vertebral arteries. *Semin Intervent Radiol.*, 38(1), 53–63.
12. Lawrence, K. B., et al. (1948). Wounds of common carotid arteries: report of 17 cases from World War II. *Am J Surg.*, 76, 29–37.
13. DuBose, J., et al. (2008). Endovascular stenting for the treatment of traumatic internal carotid injuries: expanding experience. *J Trauma.*, 65, 1561–1566.
14. Matsushima, K., et al. (2011). Posttraumatic contrast-induced acute kidney injury: minimal consequences or significant threat? *J Trauma.*,70, 415–419.
15. Bhatt, D. L., et al. (2001). Dual antiplatelet therapy with clopidogrel and aspirin after carotid artery stenting. *J Invasive Cardiol.*, 13, 767–771.
16. Asensio, J. A., et al. (2020, June). A systematic review of penetrating extracranial vertebral artery injuries. *J Vasc Surg.*, 71(6), 2161–2169.
17. Hatzitheofilou, C., et al. (1988). Surgical approaches to vertebral artery injuries. *Br J Surg.*, 75, 234–237.
18. Franz, R. W., et al. (2010). Postdischarge outcomes of blunt cerebrovascular injuries. *Vasc Endovascular Surg.*, 44, 198–211.

19. Thomas, G. I., et al. (1959). The significance of anomalous vertebral-basilar artery communications in operations on the heart and great vessels: an illustrative case with review of the literature. *Surgery.*, 46, 747–757.
20. Biffl, W. L., et al. (2000). The devastating potential of blunt vertebral arterial injuries. *Ann Surg.*, 231, 672–681.
21. Alterman, D. M., et al. (2013). Contemporary outcomes in vertebral artery injury. *J Vasc Surg.*, 57, 741–774.

50

Blunt thoracic aortic injury

ALISON O. FLENTJE AND SHAHAB A. TOURSAVADKOHI

INTRODUCTION

Blunt thoracic aortic injury (BTAI) is rare and is a potentially lethal injury most commonly seen as a result of high-speed motor vehicle accidents with an overall incidence of <1%. It includes a spectrum of lesions in the aortic wall ranging from an abnormality seen only on modern imaging to injury resulting in sudden death. BTAI is the second leading cause of death among blunt trauma patients after head injury. It is estimated that only 13–15% of BTAI patients make it to the hospital alive. Risk factors correlated with BTAI from a motor vehicle crash are age >60, front-seat occupancy, non-use of seatbelt, velocity changes >25 mph, front or side impact, and intrusion into the vehicle. The etiology of BTAI is a deceleration injury from a point of anatomic tethering (aortopulmonary ligament) [1]. The standard diagnostic imaging modality is a computed tomography angiogram (CTA); an example of a BTAI requiring treatment is shown in Figure 50.1 [2].

BTAI is graded as: grade I, an intimal tear (minimal aortic injury); grade II, an intramural hematoma; grade III, a pseudoaneurysm; and grade IV, a rupture or transection (Figure 50.2). The natural history depends on the severity, or grade, of injury [3].

BACKGROUND

BTAI was historically treated in the 1960s–1980s with immediate open repair. The 1990s brought the delayed management concept: medically controlling blood pressure (BP) and heart rate (beta-blockade) while addressing other life-threatening injuries first. Thoracic endovascular aortic repair (TEVAR) was first reported as a treatment for BTAI in 1997. A covered stent graft uses radial force to remain in position, along with proximal barbs, hooks, or struts. Specific concerns in the younger trauma population are more acute angles of curvature, smaller aortic diameters, smaller access vessels, and longer life

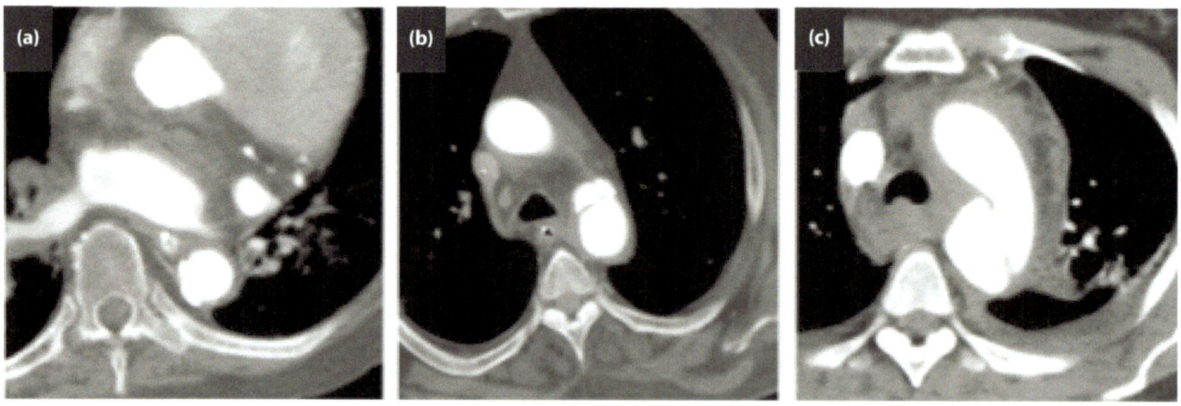

Figure 50.1 Computed tomography of blunt thoracic aortic injury: low; moderate; and high-risk traumatic aortic pseudoaneurysms: (a) small pseudoaneurysm with trace periaortic hematoma managed with surveillance imaging; (b) moderately sized pseudoaneurysm with minimal periaortic hematoma, managed with delayed endovascular repair during the patient's index admission; (c) large lesion with extensive mediastinal hematoma and left hemothorax managed with emergency endovascular repair. (Courtesy of Harris DG, Rabin J, Bhardwaj A, et al. Nonoperative management of traumatic aortic pseudoaneurysms. *Ann Vasc Surg.* 2016, 35, 75–81.)

DOI: 10.1201/9781003452096-50

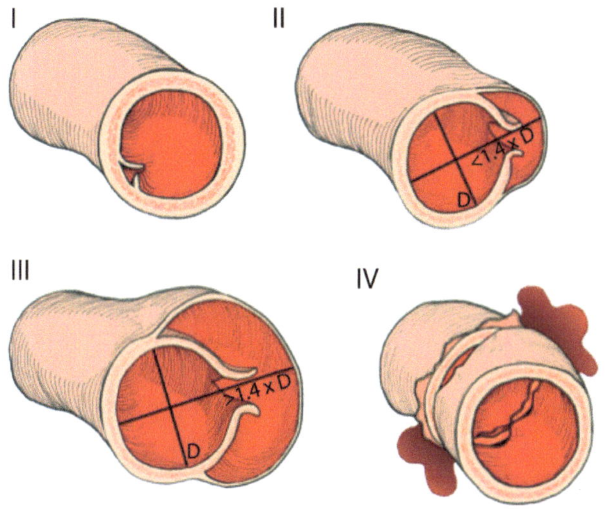

Figure 50.2 Proposed grades of blunt traumatic aortic injury: I: intimal; II: small pseudoaneurysm <50% circumference and injury diameter <1.4 × normal diameter; III: large pseudoaneurysm >50% circumference or injury diameter >1.4 × normal diameter; IV: frank rupture. (Courtesy of Rabin J, Harris DG, Drucker C, et al. The evolution of management strategies for blunt aortic injury. *Curr Surg Rep.* 2016, 4, 3.)

expectancy (possible aortic diameter growth) potentially causing "bird beaking," endoleaks, or graft migration, fracture, and collapse. Challenges to stent grafting the thoracic aorta as compared with the abdominal aorta include the following: increased hemodynamic forces and variability over the cardiac cycle; greater elasticity and movement of the aortic wall; and a curvature. Because our understanding of the natural history of BTAI has changed, management has evolved from immediate "clamp and sew" open repair of all operative candidates to a selective approach with often delayed repair (largely endovascular). The updated Western Trauma Association management algorithm is outlined in Figure 50.3 [4].

SCREENING

In high-speed MVCs, screening has traditionally been done with CXR. Some of the concerning findings include a widened/abdominal mediastinum (present in 93% of patients with TBAI), left hemothorax, loss of aortic nob, first/second rib fractures, tracheal deviation, depressed left bronchus, and left apical cap. The sensitivity of CXR is as low as 41%, so additional imaging is needed for diagnosis in high-risk patients [4].

DIAGNOSIS

CTA of the chest, abdomen, and pelvis through the midthighs is the imaging modality of choice for diagnostic and operative planning with a sensitivity of 95–100% and a negative predictive value of 99–100%. Previously, conventional aortography was considered the standard diagnostic modality but is an invasive procedure that involves additional resource utilization and an additional risk of a lower sensitivity to identifying lower-grade injuries. CTA also offers enhanced preoperative planning abilities to measure and size grafts. Aortic diameters at the proximal and distal landing zones are measured, as is the length of required coverage. Aortic arch angulation, location of the left subclavian artery (SCA), vertebral artery, and left common carotid origins, and the presence of anatomic variations are also evaluated. Access vessels are assessed for diameter extent and disease. This helps make the decision regarding cut-down versus percutaneous access and whether a conduit is needed. The iliac vessels need to be a minimum of 6 mm to accommodate a 16–25-Fr delivery sheath.

MEDICAL MANAGEMENT

Medical management with anti-impulse control should be initiated immediately upon identification of a BTAI. Although there are no optimal hemodynamic parameters established, in general, target a goal systolic blood pressure <100 mmHg and a heart rate <100 beats per minute. This attempts to prevent the progression of a contained lesion by reducing aortic wall stress and has been shown to reduce the risk of rupture from 12% to 1.5% in one study [5]. The first line of therapy is a short-acting β-blocker infusion like esmolol. If goals are not achieved, there is the addition of a calcium channel blocker like diltiazem or a vasodilator like nitroprusside. There should be a multidisciplinary discussion to determine optimal goals in patients with concomitant traumatic brain injuries where hypotension should be avoided [4].

INDICATIONS FOR SURGERY

The majority of low-grade (grade I or II) injuries can be managed with medical therapy alone, with repeat CTA 48–72 hours later to evaluate for progression of injury. Early evidence showed most type I injuries heal spontaneously, usually by eight weeks, so these patients should continue to be followed with repeat CT. Definitive indications for surgery include grade IV injuries and all grade III injuries with active extravasation and other high-risk features. Patients without secondary signs of injury (pseudocoarctation, mediastinal hematoma, or large left hemothorax) are generally safe to wait for delayed repair, especially if they have other significant associated injuries. A novel BTAI score was developed to predict early rupture in high-grade injuries more accurately than with clinical assessment. This score is based on the size of the pseudoaneurysm-to-aortic diameter ratio (>1.4), the presence of a descending thoracic aortic hematoma (>10 mm), and lactate (>4 mmol/L). There is a high risk for rupture when two or more of these three risk factors are present, suggesting the need for immediate repair in these cases (Figure 50.4) [6].

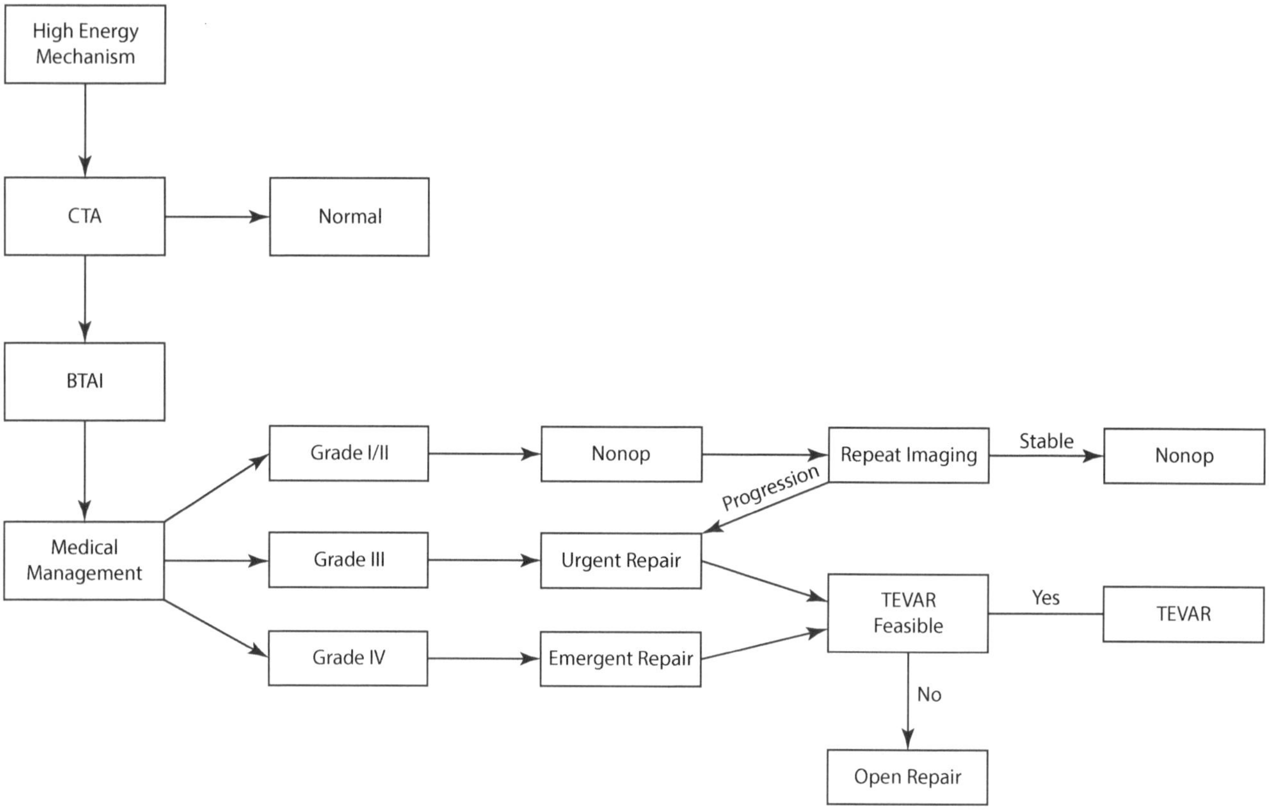

Figure 50.3 Western Trauma Association algorithm of management of blunt thoracic injury. (Adapted from Brown C, Moya D, Martin M, et al. Blunt thoracic aortic injury: A Western Trauma Association critical decisions algorithm. *J Trauma Acute Care Surg.* 2022, 94, 113–116.)

Risk Score Criteria:

Lactate >4 mM
Mediastinal hematoma >10 mm
Lesion/normal aortic ratio >1.4

High risk for aortic rupture when any 2 factors are present.

Figure 50.4 Risk score criteria for predicting aortic injury rupture. (Courtesy of Harris DG, Rabin J, Kufera JA, et al. A new aortic injury score predicts early rupture more accurately than clinical assessment. *J Vasc Surg.*, 61, 332–338.)

GENERAL PROCEDURAL GUIDELINES

TEVAR for high-grade injuries is currently recommended over open or non-operative management. The goal of TEVAR is injury coverage, usually with the shortest-length device suitable for the lesion. The advantages of TEVAR for the older thoracic aneurysm patients with multiple comorbidities have been well documented. But what about TEVAR for BTAI in the young trauma patient, with a longer life expectancy and no comorbidities? Recent meta-analyses have demonstrated decreased short-term mortality, spinal cord ischemia (SCI), and stroke with TEVAR compared with open repair. The first prospective trial of TEVAR versus open repair for BTAI was carried out by the American Association for the Surgery of Trauma. It demonstrated superior results for TEVAR, with decreased in-hospital mortality (23.5% versus 7.2%) and decreased blood transfusion requirements [6]. Looking only at patients without critical extrathoracic injuries, TEVAR resulted in a 13-fold mortality reduction. The benefits of TEVAR include decreased anticoagulation intensity and avoidance of thoracotomy, single-lung ventilation, and left heart bypass [7]. The Society for Vascular Surgery (SVS) clinical practice guidelines recommend TEVAR over open repair for grade II–IV injuries [2] and this has been the authors' practice for nearly a decade [8]. The devices used primarily in the USA are listed in Table 50.1.

Other injuries are assessed to ensure the feasibility of heparinization and patient positioning. The need for general anesthesia and spinal drainage is assessed based on the patient's clinical status and anatomic considerations. Routine performance of the procedure without heparinization has been described and can be performed with minimal additional morbidity.

Predeployment aortography should be performed with the device and stiff wire in place. Techniques for

Table 50.1 Thoracic endovascular aortic repair stent grafts currently on the market in the USA

Product	Diameter (mm)	Delivery profile (F)	Proximal end	Material
GORE®TAG® Conformable Thoracic Endoprosthesis with Active Control System[a]	21–45	18–24 ID	Partially uncovered stent	Expanded PTFE, nitinol stent
GORE®TAG® Thoracic Brach Endoprosthesis[a]	21–45	20–26 ID	Partially uncovered stent	Expanded PTFE, nitinol stent
Valiant NavionThoracic Stent Graft[b]	20–46	18–22 OD	Covered or uncovered stent	Woven polyester graft, nitinol stent
Cook Zenith Alpha™ Thoracic Endovascular Graft[c]	24–46	16–20 ID	Uncovered stent	Woven polyester graft, nitinol stent
Terumo Aortic Relay Device Plus[d]	22–46	22–26 OD	Covered or uncovered stent	Woven polyester graft, nitinol stent

[a]W. L. Gore & Associates, Flagstaff, AZ, USA.
[b]Medtronic, Minneapolis, MN, USA.
[c]*Cook Medical Inc., Bloomington, IN, USA. PTFE:* polytetrafluoroethylene.
[d]Bolton Medical, Sunrise, FL, USA.

deployment are specific to each device. In general, familiarity with a device is key to technical success. Postdeployment angiography should be performed to evaluate great vessel and iliac artery patency, stent graft patency, injury coverage, seal, and possible endoleaks. Ballooning is almost never required and should be avoided.

Guidelines from the SVS recommend against routine cerebrospinal drainage for TEVAR in the setting of BTAI (2). The risk of SCI is lower with TEVAR for BTAI compared with TEVAR for other pathologies. Specific risk factors for SCI with TEVAR are as follows: aortic coverage length; intraoperative hypotension; renal insufficiency; atherosclerosis or prior coverage of the left SCA; patency of internal iliac or vertebral arteries; and history of prior abdominal aortic aneurysm repair. Because most of these factors are not present with BTAI and because most lesions are covered with one 10 cm stent graft, the authors do not recommend routine spinal drainage. High-risk individuals can be monitored with motor and sensory evoked potentials and drained selectively.

SVS guidelines recommend routine revascularization of the left SCA after coverage with elective TEVAR (2); there is no supportive level I evidence. Revascularization is important with patent left internal mammary grafts, left-sided arteriovenous dialysis fistulas, left-hand dominance, LVA off the aortic arch, and supra-aortic pathology (carotid or vertebral artery stenoses) [8]. Most trauma patient coverage of the left SCA can be performed safely, especially if a small amount of thoracic aorta is covered. However, we recommend interval revascularization, especially if the patient develops left arm symptoms with a carotid-SCA bypass or SCA-to-carotid transposition.

FOLLOW-UP

Follow-up is with CT scans at one, six, and 12 months. Without concerning findings, annual surveillance is resumed.

GENERAL PROCEDURAL GUIDELINES FOR OPEN REPAIR

Although TEVAR is the procedure of choice for BTAI, open repair has a role depending on the availability of urgent TEVAR at some facilities. If pursuing open repair, single-lung ventilation is usually required, and the most appropriate exposure is obtained through a fourth intercostal space posterolateral thoracotomy incision. The site of injury is left undisturbed and the aorta is preferentially clamped distal to the left SCA, although control between the left carotid and left SCA is sometimes necessary. Following distal control in the mid-descending thoracic aorta, an interposition Dacron graft is sewn in place with a 3-0 or 4-0 polypropylene suture. Techniques to maintain distal perfusion via left heart bypass or total cardiopulmonary bypass are associated with better outcomes and lower rates of SCI.

COMPLICATIONS

Complications of TEVAR for BTAI include a 1% risk of stroke compared with 3–5% for all TEVARs [9]. There is an approximate risk of 1% for SCI, but this increases with certain risk factors (Table 50.2). Endoleaks, bird beaking, and accidental excessive aortic coverage are also low but not insignificant risks. Mortality at 30 days is 6% after

Table 50.2 Complications of thoracic endovascular aortic repair for blunt thoracic aortic injury

Complication	Description
Stroke	Increases with left subclavian artery (SCA) coverage
Spinal cord ischemia	Increases with risk factors: prior infrarenal aortic surgery; renal failure; hypotension; occluded hypogastric or lumbar arteries
Endoleak	Types I–IV
"Bird beaking"	Graft encroaches into the aortic arch, leading to endograft collapse or migration
Excessive aortic coverage	Left SCA, left common carotid, or celiac artery coverage
Retrograde type A aortic dissection	Rare; risk increased with proximal ballooning
Access	Iliac artery rupture, femoral artery dissection, distal embolization

TEVAR for BTAI compared with 14% for open repair of BTAI; mortality is largely influenced by associated injuries (9).

CONCLUSIONS

Management of BTAI has undergone a transformation over the last several decades from universally early, open repair to selective, expectant, non-operative medical treatment for grade I and II injuries, urgent versus delayed repair for grade III injuries, and immediate treatment for grade IV injuries. TEVAR for BTAI is recommended over open repair whenever anatomically feasible.

TRICKS AND TRAPS

- Obtain high-quality preoperative CTA for planning.
- If a contained rupture, avoid unnecessary stimulation that increases blood pressure and avoid induction until access is obtained and you are approaching graft deployment.
- Once deployed, do not push the aortic graft forward, as this can create retrograde dissection.
- Avoid ballooning the aorta if ruptured unless required to seal the endoleak.
- Attempt left subclavian revascularization if possible.

QUESTIONS

1. Which grade is correctly paired with its description?
   a. Grade I: intramural hematoma
   b. Grade II: pseudoaneurysm
   c. Grade III: intimal tear
   d. Grade IV: rupture or transection

   The correct answer is d. This is the most lethal of all the grades of injury. Grade I is an intimal tear (minimal aortic injury), grade II is an intramural hematoma, and grade III is a pseudoaneurysm.

2. Which is NOT a risk factor that correlates with BTAI from a motor vehicle crash?
   a. Age >60
   b. Front-seat occupancy
   c. Non-use of seatbelt
   d. Velocity changes >10 mph
   e. Intrusion >15 into the vehicle

   The correct answer is d. A velocity change of >25 mph is a risk factor for BTAL.

3. What are the definitive indications for surgery for BTAI?
   a. Grade IV injuries and all grade III injuries with active extravasation and other high-risk features
   b. All injuries should receive surgical therapy given the risk of rupture
   c. Pregnant and pediatric patients
   d. These injuries should be managed medically and not with surgical intervention

   The correct answer is b. Grade IV injuries and all grade III injuries with active extravasation and other high-risk features.

4. Why is medical management with anti-impulse control used in BTAI?
   a. To reduce the risk of stroke
   b. To reduce chest pain and symptom management
   c. Prevent the progression of a contained lesion by reducing aortic wall stress and reducing the risk of rupture
   d. To minimize bleeding during surgical intervention

   The correct answer is c. To prevent the progression of a contained lesion by reducing aortic wall stress and reducing the risk of rupture.

REFERENCES

1. Parmley, L. F., Mattingly, T. W., Manion, W. C., et al. (1958). Nonpenetrating traumatic injury of the aorta. *Circulation.*, *17*, 1086–1101.
2. Harris, D. G., Rabin, J., Bhardwaj, A., et al. (2016). Nonoperative management of traumatic aortic pseudoaneurysms. *Ann Vasc Surg.*, *35*, 75–81.
3. Rabin, J., Harris, D. G., Drucker, C., et al. (2016). The evolution of management strategies for blunt aortic injury. *Curr Surg Rep.*, *4*, 3.
4. Brown, C., Moya, D., Martin, M., et al. (2022). Blunt thoracic aortic injury: a Western Trauma Association critical decisions algorithm. *J Trauma Acute Care Surg.*, 94, 113–116.
5. Hemmila, M. R., Arbabi, S., Rowe, S. A., et al. (2004). Delayed repair for blunt thoracic aortic injury: is it really equivalent to early repair? *J Trauma*, 56, 13–23.
6. Harris, D. G., Rabin, J., Kufera, J. A., et al. (2015). A new aortic injury score predicts early rupture more accurately than clinical assessment. *J Vasc Surg.*, *61*, 332–338.
7. Cheng, D., Martin, J., Shennib, H., et al. (2010). Endovascular aortic repair versus open surgical repair for descending thoracic aortic disease: a systematic review and meta-analysis of comparative studies. *J Am Coll Cardiol.*, *55*, 986–1001.
8. Lee, W. A., Matsumura, J. S., Mitchell, R. S., et al. (2011). Endovascular repair of traumatic thoracic aortic injury: clinical practice guidelines of the Society for Vascular Surgery. *J Vasc Surg.*, *53*, 187–192.
9. Fortuna, G. R., Jr, Perlick, A., DuBose, J. J., et al. (2016). Injury grade is a predictor of aortic-related death among patients with blunt thoracic aortic injury. *J Vasc Surg.*, *63*, 1225–1231.

51

Dialysis access

ALICE LEE

INTRODUCTION

Patients with chronic kidney disease (CKD) and end-stage renal disease (ESRD) are 25% and 1% of the Medicare population, respectively. Costs related to the care of ESRD account for 9% of all Medicare payments. Management and recommendations are based on the Kidney Disease Outcomes Quality Initiative (KDOQI) Clinical Practice Guideline for Vascular Access (2019). Prior editions were focused on the premise of "Fistula First"; however, the latest guideline advocates for an individualized End Stage Kidney Disease (ESKD) Life-Plan. Consideration for access is not based on vein availability and sizes but takes into account a patient's needs and preferences. Guidelines also include the likely complications of current access and plans for next access.

Options for upper extremity access are radiocephalic, brachiocephalic, and brachial-basilic fistulas and graft configurations are straight and loop. Arterial requirements include the absence of a pressure differential of 20 mmHg between arms and in the distal forearm, and a patent palmar arch and arterial luminal diameter of at least 2.0 mm. Venous requirements include the following: a diameter >2.5 mm; absence of obstruction; straight segment for cannulation; and continuity with proximal central vein. For consideration of a graft, vein diameter should be >4 mm. Any abnormalities should be further evaluated with arteriography/venography.

RADIOCEPHALIC FISTULA

For a radiocephalic fistula (Figure 51.1), a longitudinal incision is made at the wrist and subcutaneous tissues are divided. Identify the cephalic vein and isolate it from the surrounding structures. Next, isolate the radial artery and encircle with vessel loops. Anticoagulate with 3000–5000 units of heparin is given. Divide the distal end of the cephalic vein after confirmation that enough length has been dissected. Some prefer to also mark the vein prior to ligation to minimize the chance of twisting the vein. The vein is then dilated gently with heparinized saline solution with an olive tip. Clamp the radial artery and create an arteriotomy with an 11 blade. Arteriotomy is then lengthened with Potts scissors. Stay sutures using 7-0 Prolene can be placed on the radial artery to improve exposure for the anastomosis. The vein can be slightly beveled to match the arteriotomy. Cephalic vein end to radial artery side anastomosis is done using 6-0 or 7-0 Prolene. Prior to tying the suture, back and forward bleed the artery. Assess the fistula by palpating a thrill. If there are visible branches, recommend ligating them to facilitate maturation of the fistula. In addition, a pulse exam should be completed. The incision can be closed alone with a 4-0 absorbable suture or 3-0 for the subcutaneous tissues followed by 4-0 for the skin.

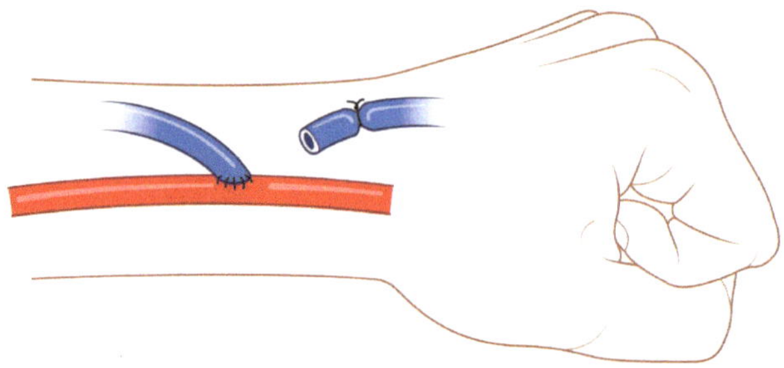

Figure 51.1 Radiocephalic arteriovenous fistula.

BRACHIOCEPHALIC FISTULA

A transverse incision can be placed above or below the antecubital fossa. This will be determined by the location of the radial/ulnar bifurcation. Subcutaneous tissues are divided, and the cephalic vein is identified. If the median cubital vein is large enough, this branch is useful to use for fistula creation because it is in the direction of the brachial artery. Isolate the cephalic vein from its surrounding structures with enough length to reach the brachial

DOI: 10.1201/9781003452096-51

artery without tension. Next, identify the brachial artery by opening the fascia and dividing the bicipital aponeurosis. Isolate the brachial artery and encircle it with vessel loops. The patient is anticoagulated with heparin (3000–5000 units). The distal end of the cephalic vein is divided, ensuring there is enough length to create the anastomosis without tension. Once divided, the vein is gently dilated with heparinized saline administered via an olive tip syringe. The brachial artery is controlled with vascular clamps and an arteriotomy is created; 7-0 Prolene can be used for stay sutures for better visibility of the arterial lumen. The end of the cephalic vein may be beveled to match the arteriotomy. Then using fine Prolene suture (6-0 or 7-0), an end cephalic vein to side brachial artery anastomosis is created. Prior to tying the stitch, allow the brachial artery to back and forward bleed. Check for thrill and complete a pulse exam of the radial and ulnar arteries. Subcutaneous tissues are closed with a 3-0 absorbable suture and skin incision is closed with a 4-0 absorbable suture.

BASILIC VEIN TRANSPOSITION

In one-stage procedures, the basilic vein is mobilized through a single-arm incision or skip incisions along the course of the basilic vein (Figure 51.2); if necessary, the incision is extended transversely to the antecubital fossa. The medial antebrachial cutaneous nerve is carefully protected. The basilic vein is disconnected and dilated with heparinized solution and then transposed inside an anterolateral subcutaneous tunnel; following patient heparinization (3000–5000 units), the basilic vein is anastomosed to the brachial artery using 6-0 Prolene.

In a two-stage procedure, a transverse incision is made either above or below the antecubital fossa. The benefit of an incision distal to the antecubital fossa is that the working length of the basilic vein for the second stage is longer. The steps are similar to a brachiocephalic fistula: isolate the basilic vein and brachial artery and create an

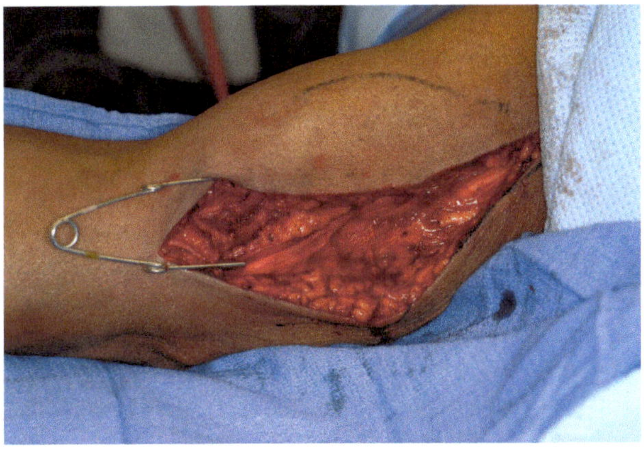

Figure 51.2 Basilic vein mobilized through a single incision along the medial aspect of the arm in preparation for a one-stage transposition procedure.

anastomosis using 6-0 Prolene. After the anastomosis, a period of four to six weeks is allowed for vein maturation.

The second stage is mobilization or transposition of the basilic vein. The basilic vein is isolated generally through skip incisions but can also be done through a single long incision (Figure 51.3). Branches are ligated as the vein is dissected out. The brachial artery can be isolated through the distal incision but be sure that the portion of the brachial artery that is being isolated matches the length of basilic vein that is available. A superficial anterolateral tunnel is created being mindful not to create a tight angle of the basilic vein by the axilla; 3000–5000 units of heparin is given. To minimize twisting of the vein, mark the basilic vein prior to dividing it. Pass the basilic vein through the tunneler without twisting. Location of the anastomosis will depend on how the divided ends of the basilic vein lay in relation to each other. If the ends of the vein are parallel, anastomose the ends using 6-0 Prolene. If the ends of the vein are not parallel, clamp the brachial artery, make an arteriotomy, and create an anastomosis of the basilic vein end to the brachial artery side using 6-0 Prolene. Prior to tying the suture, be sure to back and forward bleed the artery as well as back bleed the basilic vein.

ARTERIOVENOUS GRAFT

A longitudinal skin incision is made above the antecubital fossa and is deepened through the subcutaneous tissue. The fascia is entered and the brachial artery is identified, isolated, and surrounded with vessel loops. A second longitudinal incision is made in the proximal upper arm near the axilla. The distal brachial vein/axillary vein is then identified and isolated with vessel loops. A tunnel is created in an anterior lateral fashion between the two incisions and the graft is introduced through the tunnel; 3000–5000 units of heparin are given for anticoagulation. After clamping the brachial artery, an arteriotomy is created. The graft is beveled to match the arteriotomy and anastomosis is made using 6-0 Prolene. Prior to tying the stitch, the artery is back and forward bled. The graft is irrigated with heparinized saline and a clamp is placed on the arterial side of the graft. Clamps are placed on the vein and a venotomy is made. The graft is beveled to match the venotomy and anastomosis is made using 6-0 Prolene. Prior to tying the stitch, the vein and graft are allowed to back bleed. Inspect for thrill and conduct a pulse exam of the radial/ulnar arteries.

For a loop graft, a single longitudinal incision is made in the axilla and deepened through to the subcutaneous tissue and the fascia is entered. The distal brachial/axillary vein and axillary artery are identified and dissected out. A tunnel is created with a counter-incision in the lower upper arm. Arterial and venous anastomoses are created in a standard fashion as a straight graft.

For loop grafts, avoid angling the graft as it has a propensity to kink. This author prefers to have the graft lay parallel on the artery/vein rather than at an angle.

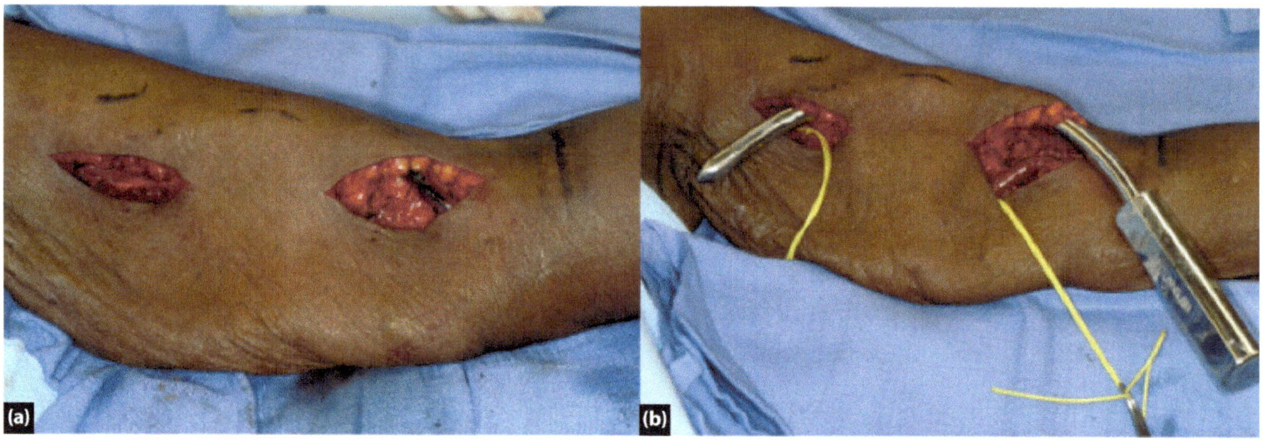

Figure 51.3 Basilic vein transposition: (a) second stage of a two-stage procedure with mobilization of the basilic vein through two longitudinal small "skip" incisions along the course of the basilic vein, one over the distal part of the basilic vein near its anastomosis and one at the level of the proximal part; (b) the basilic vein is divided and tunneled with a tunneler over the anterolateral aspect of the arm.

TRICKS AND TRAPS

- Rule of "6s": diameter of at least 6 mm, depth from skin <6 mm, and flow volume of 600 ml/min or greater.
- Fistula vessel requirements are 2 mm for the artery and 2.5 mm for the vein. For a graft, vein >4 mm.
- Pre-incision examination of vessels with ultrasound to confirm optimal fistula type/location. This may reveal a site that was not suitable on the initial vein mapping.
- For fistula creation, take small "bites" on the vein to prevent narrowing of the hood.
- If duplex shows heterogenous calcification of the artery, access creation is still possible but the artery must be able to be clamped. Arteriotomy location should be determined if there is a soft spot of the artery.

QUESTIONS

1. An 80-year-old female was recently diagnosed with CKD. Medical history includes hypertension, atrial fibrillation, and diabetes mellitus. She is right-hand dominant with a left-sided pacemaker. Bilateral brachial and cephalic veins are suitable for access creation. Which access would you recommend?
   a. Left arm brachiocephalic fistula
   b. Right arm brachiocephalic fistula
   c. Peritoneal dialysis catheter
   d. Left arm arteriovenous graft

   Answer: b

2. A 65-year-old male underwent a left radiocephalic fistula creation and is seen in clinic for evaluation for usage. Duplex shows flows of 300 ml/min, diameter of cephalic is 4 mm, and there are several large branches. What is the next step in management?
   a. Abandon access and vein map for next access creation
   b. Balloon-assisted maturation
   c. Ligate branches as they are diverting flow away from the main cephalic vein
   d. Have the patient return in four weeks

   Answer: c

3. A 35-year-old male with CKD is looking for recommendations on access. His medical history includes hypertension and diabetes mellitus. He has no prior surgical history. Bilateral brachial and cephalic wins are suitable for access creation. Right-arm dominant. Which access would you recommend?
   a. Tunneled dialysis catheter
   b. Left arm brachiocephalic fistula
   c. Left arm arteriovenous graft
   d. Peritoneal dialysis catheter

   Answer: d

4. A 90-year-old female with CKD presents for access creation discussion. Medical history includes severe chronic obstructive pulmonary disease on 3 L oxygen, congestive heart failure with an ejection fraction of 10%, hypertension, and diabetes mellitus. Bilateral radial and cephalic veins are suitable for access creation. Left-arm dominant. Which access would you recommend?
   a. Tunneled dialysis catheter
   b. Left arm radiocephalic fistula creation
   c. Peritoneal dialysis catheter
   d. Right arm radiocephalic fistula creation

   Answer: a

REFERENCES

Arroyo, Michael R., et al. "Primary and staged transposition arteriovenous fistulas." *Journal of Vascular Surgery* 47.6 (2008): 1279–1283.

Cull, David L., et al. "The fistula elevation procedure: a valuable technique for maximizing arteriovenous fistula utilization." *Annals of Vascular Surgery* 16.1 (2002): 84–88.

Lok, C. E., Huber, T. S., Lee, T., et al; KDOQI Vascular Access Guideline Work Group. "KDOQI clinical practice guideline for vascular access: 2019 update." *American Journal of Kidney Diseases*. 75.4(suppl 2) (2020): S1–S164.

Schinstock, Carrie A., et al. "Outcomes of arteriovenous fistula creation after the Fistula First Initiative." *Clinical Journal of the American Society of Nephrology* 6.8 (2011): 1996–2002.

52

Complications of dialysis access

CHRYSANTHI P. PAPAGEORGOPOULOU AND STAVROS K. KAKKOS

INTRODUCTION

Complications related to vascular access for dialysis continue to be a major problem for hemodialysis patients, as they have a negative impact on morbidity and mortality. Dysfunction of vascular access is one of the most important factors that affects blood flow and has detrimental effects on the quality of dialysis. Three main types of vascular accesses are used in daily clinical practice to provide renal replacement therapy in hemodialysis patients. These basic options include the native arteriovenous fistula (AVF), the prosthetic arteriovenous graft (AVG), and tunneled hemodialysis catheters (central venous catheter [1]. The arteriovenous fistula is a creation, surgically, of an anastomosis between an artery and a vein. The vein for about four to six weeks, or more, undergoes maturation and can be used for dialysis. On the contrary, the arteriovenous graft is created by anastomosing a mostly polytetrafluoroethylene tube (PTFE) to the side of an artery and the end or side of a vein. The PTFE tube, after a period of time for common graft types, will be punctured for dialysis. Finally, the tunneled hemodialysis catheters are inserted in a central vein and can be used immediately for dialysis therapy. Although these options can all provide successful hemodialysis, they are associated with multiple early and late complications that can affect the quality of dialysis therapy and the lifetime of the vascular access or jeopardize the limb or life. The most common complications continue to plague vascular access. These include true and false access aneurysms, infection, vascular access stenosis and restenosis, vascular access thrombosis, central venous occlusive disease, vascular access-induced limb ischemia, and ischemic monomelic neuropathy.[2] Major progress has been made in understanding these complications and changes in therapeutic management, due to the advances of endovascular surgery. A regular surveillance program with clinical assessment of vascular access, venous dialysis pressures, recirculation studies, and color Doppler ultrasonography is essential for a successful dialysis program. In this chapter, we discuss the most common complications associated with dialysis and provide algorithms for therapeutic options.

TRUE AND FALSE ACCESS ANEURYSMS

True vascular access aneurysms are localized dilatations involving all layers of the vessel wall affecting an AVF or even the brachial artery, whereas false aneurysms (pseudoaneurysms) can affect both AVFs and AVGs and have a wall defect [2]. True aneurysms are reported in up to 17% of AVFs and false aneurysms in 7% of AVGs [1]. Aneurysms are usually caused or accompanied by pre-aneurysm or post-aneurysm, downstream, stenosis [2]. Repeated needling in the same area may cause segmental aneurysms. Rapidly growing aneurysms can lead to necrosis of the overlying skin, with the risk of rupture and profuse hemorrhage. AVGs do not dilate, but destruction of the wall due to repeated punctures or at the anastomosis can lead to false aneurysms (Figures 52.1 and 52.2).

When a vascular access aneurysm is complicated with stenosis, partial resection of the wall of the aneurysm, known as aneurysmorrhaphy, and patch angioplasty along the stenosis is a common procedure [2]. The resected material can be used as a patch. Ligation of the aneurysm and bypass grafting, or graft interposition, is an alternative. AVG false aneurysms are treated by resection and bypass grafting, or graft interposition. When the aneurysmal segment is complicated with infection, complete resection of the graft is usually therapeutic. Endovascular treatment using different types of stent grafts for exclusion of the aneurysm should be the second choice when the surgical option can preserve the cannulation sites [2].

INFECTION

Vascular access infection remains the second most frequent cause of death in hemodialysis patients with the first cause being cardiovascular events [3]. Diabetes,

DOI: 10.1201/9781003452096-52

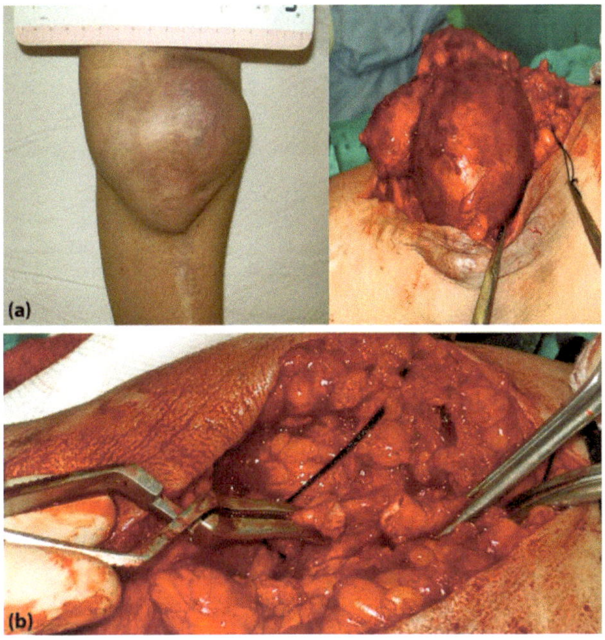

Figure 52.1 (a) True anastomotic aneurysm of the brachial artery after a brachiocephalic AVF. Operative exposure of the aneurysm; (b) Successful resection, just before primary, end-to-end anastomosis of the brachial artery.

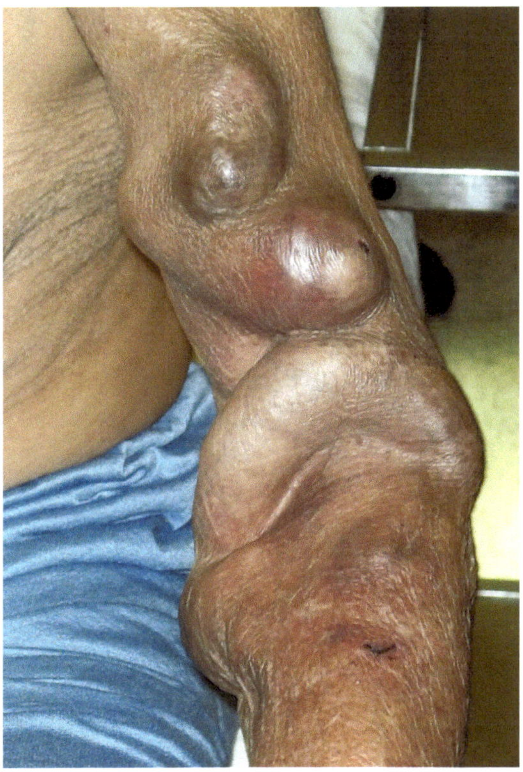

Figure 52.2 Giant, serpentine-like aneurysms of a native AVF.

multiple comorbidities, uremia, central venous catheters, and repeated cannulation of the AVF or AVG have been identified as major risk factors for infection of the access. Central venous catheters are more prone to infection, followed by AVGs and rarely AVFs [2]. The typical clinical presentation of the VA infection includes local signs such as redness, tenderness, warmth, swelling, and purulent discharge or ulceration. However, fever can be present as the only symptom. Gram-positive cocci (*Staphylococcus aureus* 50–90%) are the major cause of the infection, but also Gram-negative microorganisms are isolated in about one-third of the infections. All VA late infections should be treated with broad-spectrum antibiotics for both Gram-positive and Gram-negative organisms. AVG infection can be complicated with sepsis and profound life-threatening hemorrhage. In AVG infection, total resection of the graft is suggested in patients with clinical signs of infection, peri-graft fluid, and sepsis [2]. For infection with *S. aureus,* total excision should be planned, while in *S. epidermidis* infection and localized infection to a segment, with no peri-graft fluid along the rest of the graft, partial excision can be performed. Subtotal excision, with resection of the whole graft but a small stump on the arterial side, can be used in selected cases to avoid extensive dissection of the artery and nerve damage (Figure 52.3).

In AVFs, infection at the anastomosis is rare, but in such cases, immediate treatment with antibiotics and resection of the infected tissue is necessary. Infection in cannulation sites, especially when the buttonhole technique is used, can be more frequent; antibiotic treatment and change of cannulation site are required [4].

VASCULAR ACCESS STENOSIS AND RECURRENT STENOSIS

Stenosis of the VA can occur at any level, but only stenoses that cause a hemodynamic effect ($\geq 70\%$ of the lumen)

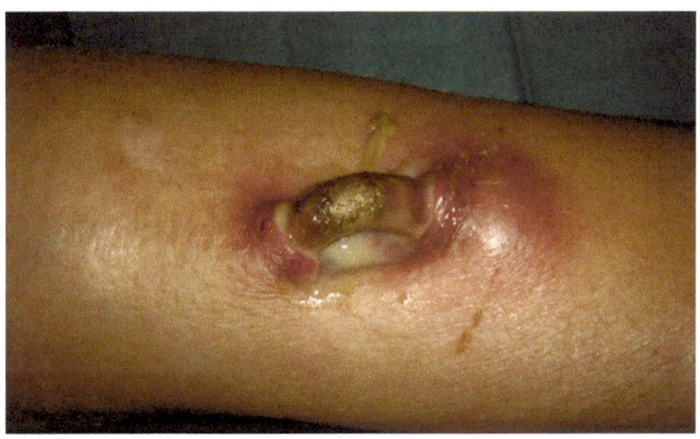

Figure 52.3 AVG infection complicated with sepsis and erosion of the outer wall of the graft.

and are associated with abnormal physical examination (reduced thrill or pulsatile AVF), decreased flow, and elevated venous pressures should be treated [4].

Inflow arterial stenosis (subclavian, brachial, radial or ulnar artery) is more frequent in the elderly, diabetics, and hypertensive patients. The arteriovenous anastomosis of the AVF and the arterial anastomosis of the AVG are the most common sites for stenosis [4]. Percutaneous transluminal angioplasty (PTA) has been proven safe and effective, with a low rate of re-intervention treatment. Stenting has specific indications including elastic recoil, rapidly recurrent stenosis, and residual stenosis after PTA [4]. Bypass grafting and endarterectomy, as open surgical treatments, are rarely performed [4].

For venous outflow stenosis, balloon angioplasty is recommended as a first-line treatment, especially when the lesion is short (less than 2 cm). For long lesions, balloon angioplasty remains ambivalent, and bypass grafting should be considered as an alternative. Stenoses of the venous outflow are usually resistant to balloon angioplasty, requiring high-pressure balloons or cutting balloons. Stents, stent grafts, and, mentioned earlier, surgical options should be considered in complicated cases when PTA fails. Stent-graft placement should be considered for the treatment of cephalic arch stenosis. Vein transposition or bypass grafting should be considered as alternatives or bailout techniques (Figure 52.4).

VASCULAR ACCESS THROMBOSIS

Thrombosis is usually the final complication after VA dysfunction due to stenosis of the access or the venous outflow.

For AVFs, early thrombus removal is urgent and should be started as soon as possible. Although the treatment was originally open thrombectomy, since the 1980s, great advances have been made, and pharmacological thrombolysis, pharmaco-mechanical thrombectomy, mechanical thrombectomy, or a combination of these can be used as first-line treatment. However, thrombus removal alone is not sufficient to maintain long-term patency, because a flow-limiting stenosis is present in more than 85% of the cases and re-occlusion is frequent [2]. PTA of the underlining stenosis or open surgical intervention is required.

For AVGs, early de-clotting is not urgent, but should be managed without risking VA function for the next hemodialysis. Thrombus remaining more than five days is often fixed to the vessel wall, making surgical extraction more difficult than interventional treatment. Surgical thrombectomy is performed with a thrombectomy catheter designed for grafts. Intra-operative angiography is essential to check for remaining thrombus and to identify and treat the underlying cause of the thrombosis, including central venous stenosis. Meta-analysis has proven that endovascular therapy and surgical thrombectomy have similar results in terms of primary and primary assisted patency at one year [5].

CENTRAL VENOUS OCCLUSIVE DISEASE

Central venous occlusive disease (CVOD) is a common cause of VA dysfunction with an incidence of up to 40% [2,6]. Only 12–13% of patients have symptomatic CVOD that requires treatment. The vast majority of patients have asymptomatic CVOD causing minor swelling of the upper extremity, increased venous outflow resistance, post-cannulation bleeding, and AVF aneurysms leading eventually to VA loss. Clinical suspicion should be followed by access angiography and computed tomography angiography (CTA) of the extremity. For symptomatic CVOD, PTA is an acceptable treatment with good short-term patency, but due to elastic recoil and recurrent neointimal hyperplasia, repeated interventions are often required [6]. According to most studies, bare metal stents do not have superior results in long-term patency over PTA and are not recommended in mobile axillary vein or subclavian vein segments (Figure 52.5) [6].

VASCULAR ACCESS-INDUCED LIMB ISCHEMIA

Vascular access-induced limb ischemia, also known as "steal syndrome," occurs in 5–10% of AVFs using brachial artery as inflow, but in less than 1% of radiocephalic AVFs.

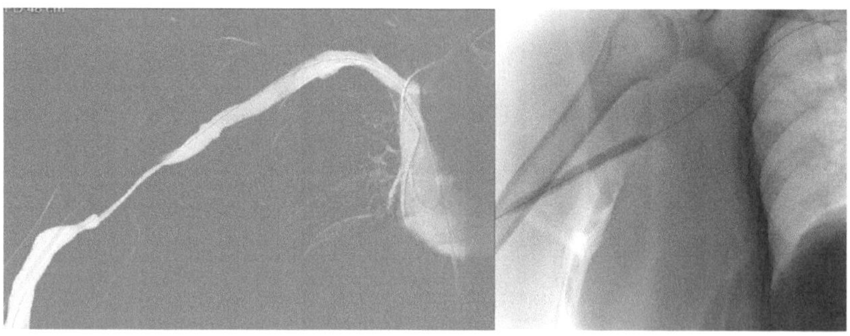

Figure 52.4 PTA of the basilic vein was performed on a patient with reduced AVF flow due to venous outflow stenosis.

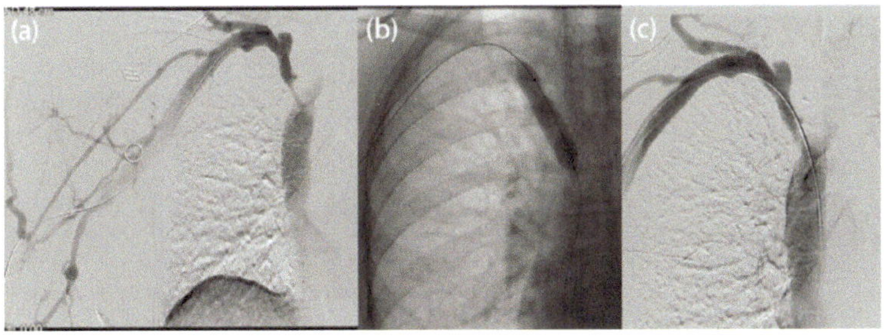

Figure 52.5 (a) Pre-dilatation venography; (b) PTA; (c) and post-dilatation venography of a central venous stenosis causing reduced VA flow and prolonged bleeding times.

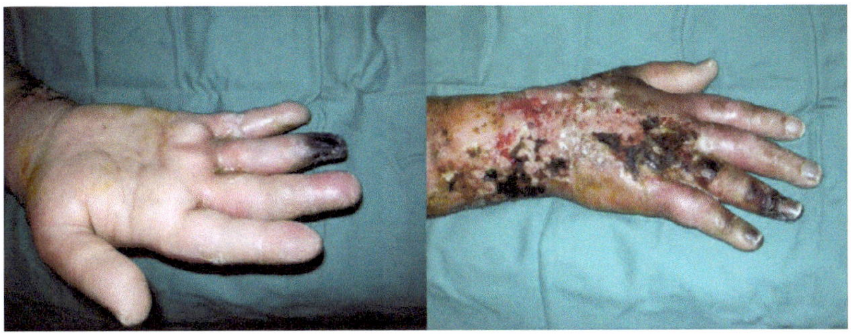

Figure 52.6 Non-healing ulcers of the forearm and digital necrosis in a patient with steal syndrome. Due to the delay in vascular consultation and the advanced necrotic lesions, VA ligation was inevitable.

Diabetes and older age in hemodialysis patients increase the incidence of symptomatic VA-induced limb ischemia [7]. When non-healing ulcers and digital necrosis are present, VA ligation is the only therapeutic option (Figure 52.6). In cases of rest pain or symptoms during exercise, preservation of the VA and treatment of the distal ischemia should be planned. Arterial stenosis proximal to the anastomosis should be treated with PTA. Steal syndrome due to high flow of the VA can be treated with either external banding of the AVF or a revision using distal inflow (RUDI) procedure. Improvement of distal perfusion, with a normal VA flow, can be obtained by either a distal revascularization interval ligation (DRIL) or a proximalization of the arteriovenous anastomosis (PAVA) procedure [2].

ISCHEMIC MONOMELIC NEUROPATHY

The nerve function of the distal upper extremity can be affected by the VA creation when the brachial artery is used as the arterial inflow. Ischemic monomelic neuropathy (IMN) is a rare but serious complication caused by axonal ischemia of the peripheral nerves, especially the radial nerve, leading to irreversible limb dysfunction [8]. Suspicion of this clinical entity will lead to diagnosis, especially in patients with diabetes, pre-existing neuropathy, and distal arterial disease. The clinical presentation of IMN is present immediately after the creation of the VA and includes motor dysfunction (wrist drop), sensory dysfunction (paresthesia and numbness), and/or striking pain [8]. Immediate ligation of the VA is the only option to prevent further neurological deficit.

TRICKS AND TRAPS

- Regular surveillance programs with clinical assessment of vascular access and color Doppler ultrasonography are essential for a successful dialysis program.
- True anastomotic aneurysms of the brachial artery after a brachiocephalic AVF can be treated with complete excision of the aneurysm and primary repair, usually end-to-end anastomosis, of the brachial artery.
- When AVG infection or pseudoaneurysm is complicated with an acute life-threatening hemorrhage, control of the bleeding using a fistula clamp or even a sphygmomanometer on the brachial artery can be life-saving.
- In order to avoid steal syndrome in brachiocephalic fistulas in elderly patients, the arteriotomy on the brachial artery should not exceed 5 mm in length.
- A thrill is associated with a blood flow >450 ml/min: in case the patient notices that the thrill is reduced or it cannot be felt, immediate consultation by a vascular access surgeon or interventionalist is required.

QUESTIONS

1. True vascular access aneurysms are localized dilatations affecting:
   a. An arteriovenous fistula
   b. The brachial artery
   c. a + b
   d. None of the above

   Answer: c

2. Vascular access infection is a rare complication and can easily be treated with broad-spectrum antibiotics.
   a. True
   b. False

   Answer: b

3. Central venous occlusive disease is a common cause of VA dysfunction treated with primary stenting.
   a. True
   b. False

   Answer: b

4. Steal syndrome due to high flow of the VA can be treated with:
   a. External banding of the AVF
   b. RUDI procedure
   c. DRIL of the brachial artery
   d. All of the above
   e. None of the above

   Answer: d

REFERENCES

1. Masud A, Costanzo EJ, Zuckerman R, Asif A. The complications of vascular access in hemodialysis. *Semin Thromb Hemost.* 2018;44(1):57–59. doi: 10.1055/s-0037-1606180. PMID: 28898900.
2. Clinical practice guidelines for haemodialysis adequancy, update 2006. *Am J Kidney Dis.* 2006;48:S2–90.
3. Li PK, Chow KM. Infectious complications in dialysis: epidemiology and outcomes. *Nat Rev Nephrol.* 2011;8(2):77–88. doi: 10.1038/nrneph.2011.194. PMID: 22183504.
4. Schmidli J, Widmer MK, Basile C, de Donato G, Gallieni M, Gibbons CP, Haage P, Hamilton G, Hedin U, Kamper L, Lazarides MK, Lindsey B, Mestres G, Pegoraro M, Roy J, Setacci C, Shemesh D, Tordoir JHM, van Loon M, Esvs Guidelines Committee, Kolh P, de Borst GJ, Chakfe N, Debus S, Hinchliffe R, Kakkos S, Koncar I, Lindholt J, Naylor R, Vega de Ceniga M, Vermassen F, Verzini F, Esvs Guidelines Reviewers, Mohaupt M, Ricco JB, Roca-Tey R. Editor's Choice – vascular access: 2018 Clinical practice guidelines of the European Society for Vascular Surgery (ESVS). *Eur J Vasc Endovasc Surg.* 2018 Jun;55(6):757–818. doi: 10.1016/j.ejvs.2018.02.001. PMID: 29730128.
5. Kuhan G, Antoniou GA, Nikam M, Mitra S, Farquharson F, Brittenden J, Chalmers N. A meta-analysis of randomized trials comparing surgery versus endovascular therapy for thrombosed arteriovenous fistulas and grafts in hemodialysis. *Cardiovasc Intervent Radiol.* 2013;36(3):699–705. doi: 10.1007/s00270-013-0564-8. PMID: 23381773.
6. Ronald J, Davis B, Guevara CJ, Pabon-Ramos WM, Smith TP, Kim CY. Treatment of central venous in-stent restenosis with repeat stent deployment in hemodialysis patients. *J Vasc Access.* 2017;18(3):214–219. doi: 10.5301/jva.5000705. PMID: 28430317.
7. Al Shakarchi J, Stolba J, Houston JG, Inston N. Surgical techniques for haemodialysis access-induced distal ischaemia. *J Vasc Access.* 2016;17(1):40–46. doi: 10.5301/jva.5000467. PMID: 26349875.
8. Thermann F, Kornhuber M. Ischemic monomelic neuropathy: a rare but important complication after hemodialysis access placement—a review. *J Vasc Access.* 2011;12(2):113–119. doi: 10.5301/jva.2011.6365. PMID: 21360465.

53

Thoracic outlet syndrome

JOE KARAM

INTRODUCTION

The thoracic outlet region is comprised of three anatomic spaces: the scalene triangle, the costoclavicular space, and the pectoralis minor space. The neurovascular bundle, which consists of the subclavian artery (SCA), subclavian vein (SCV), and brachial plexus, courses through the scalene triangle to the costoclavicular space and then through the pectoralis minor space. Compression of the various structures within the neurovascular bundle anywhere along this trajectory can result in the symptomatology of thoracic outlet syndrome. Compression can be caused by variations in anatomy, injuries, and repetitive physical activities. Neurogenic thoracic outlet syndrome (NTOS) results from brachial plexus compression, which leads to a constellation of neurologic symptoms of the upper extremity. It is the most common form of thoracic outlet syndrome, accounting for more than 90% of cases. Venous thoracic outlet syndrome (VTOS) occurs from compression and repetitive injury to the subclavian vein between the first rib and clavicle, accounting for 7–9% of all thoracic outlet cases. Arterial thoracic outlet syndrome (ATOS) is the least frequent form of TOS. It represents 1–3% of all TOS. We reserve the definition of ATOS for patients who have fixed arterial lesions (stenosis, occlusion, or aneurysmal dilation) of the subclavian artery as it passes over the first rib. This is usually due to compression by an osseous abnormality (cervical rib or another bony anomaly).

NEUROGENIC THORACIC OUTLET SYNDROME

Epidemiology

There are approximately 2000–2500 first rib resection procedures performed annually in the USA; of these, NTOS accounts for >90% of all cases [1]. However, the lack of objective diagnostic criteria and inconsistent reporting standards for NTOS make it difficult to estimate the true incidence and prevalence. Also, the condition is likely underdiagnosed clinically in patients who seek medical attention and in symptomatic patients who fail to seek medical care [2].

DIFFERENTIAL DIAGNOSIS

Because of the nonspecific and diffuse nature of symptoms, the differential diagnosis for NTOS can be broad and includes a variety of upper extremity neurologic and musculoskeletal conditions. Various cervical spine disorders can produce similar neurologic symptoms, including arthritis, degenerative disc disease, post-traumatic strain, and spinal stenosis. Several impingement syndromes, such as acromioclavicular impingement, ulnar nerve (cubital tunnel) entrapment, and median nerve (carpal tunnel) compression syndrome, are also frequently on the differential diagnosis. Shoulder tendinitis, epicondylitis, and fibromyalgia should also be considered.

PHYSICAL EXAMINATION

Symptoms of NTOS include pain, dysesthesia, numbness, and weakness that do not localize to a specific neuroanatomic distribution. These neurologic symptoms are typically exacerbated by maneuvers that compromise the thoracic outlet, such as raising the arms overhead or stretching the brachial plexus, such as dangling the arms. Various clinical tests are designed to elicit positional or effort-related sensory disturbances. With the Elevated Arm Stress Test (EAST; Roos Stress Test), patients are asked to adduct the shoulder to 90 degrees, flex the elbow to 90 degrees, and face the palms forward. With the arms in this position, the patient is asked to open and close the hands repeatedly for up to three minutes, or until the maneuver becomes intolerable. In addition, Adson's maneuver is conducted by having the patient turn their head toward the affected side while extending the

DOI: 10.1201/9781003452096-53

symptomatic arm and inhaling. Pulse changes and symptom exacerbation are then assessed. Although this test often does not specifically demonstrate nerve root compression, a positive Adson's sign suggests thoracic outlet compromise and can be associated with NTOS. Various other maneuvers, such as the Upper Limb Tension Test, also attempt to compromise the thoracic outlet and reproduce or exacerbate distal symptoms.

Tenderness to palpation over certain areas is also an important physical examination finding in the patient with NTOS. Palpation over the scalene triangle typically results in severe local discomfort, elicits pain that radiates down the axilla, or leads to the reproduction of distal sensory symptoms. Similarly, palpation over the pectoralis minor insertion can also lead to pain and symptom reproduction. Positive results on these physical examination tests and maneuvers serve to strongly support the diagnosis of NTOS in combination with a consistent clinical history [3].

DIAGNOSTIC WORKUP

The diagnosis of NTOS is made clinically, with the assistance of specific clinical tests. Often, specific diagnostic testing for NTOS yields negative or equivocal results, thus diagnostic studies are frequently most useful for the exclusion of other conditions. Plain radiographs can aid in the diagnosis of NTOS if an osseous cervical rib is identified, but other imaging tests are typically uninformative.

Computed tomography or magnetic resonance imaging (MRI) studies are usually negative because the factors causing brachial plexus compression are presumably beyond the resolution of such tests. Even if thoracic outlet anomalies are identified, correlation with the patient's symptoms cannot be definitively proven. However, exclusion of other conditions, such as degenerative disc disease or rotator cuff pathology, with these imaging modalities is important. Additionally, electromyography (EMG) and nerve conduction studies (NCS) are often performed when evaluating a patient with suspected NTOS and are also frequently negative in this condition. NTOS is not typically associated with permanent neurologic dysfunction; however, if EMG or NCS testing is positive in a patient with NTOS, the prognosis is poor even with adequate surgical decompression [4].

PHYSICAL THERAPY

Before invasive intervention, trying physical therapy that is specifically directed toward the relief of NTOS symptoms is warranted. The approach to NTOS physical therapy is unique from therapy for other related conditions; thus, it should be conducted by a therapist with expertise in NTOS care. The Edgelow Neurovascular Entrapment Syndrome Treatment protocol has been tested extensively in patients with pain originating from the thoracic outlet. This approach focuses on correcting breathing and core motor control dysfunction and calming brachial plexus hyperesthesia. Adjunctive treatments, such as anti-inflammatory medications or muscle relaxants, can also provide benefit [5].

DIAGNOSTIC BLOCKS

Test muscle blocks are frequently performed to help provide diagnostic information and guide NTOS therapy [6]. Anterior scalene muscle (ASM) and pectoralis minor blocks are performed under ultrasound guidance by injecting local anesthetic (lidocaine).

The response to the anesthetic injection is then assessed. Within a few minutes, the patient should start to have reduced symptoms at rest and improved tolerance during repeat physical examination. A positive response with muscle block correlates with good outcomes for NTOS decompression surgery.

OPERATIVE TECHNIQUE

We focus our discussion on the supraclavicular approach for thoracic outlet decompression because it provides excellent exposure to the first rib, a cervical rib (if present), scalene muscles, and the brachial plexus. We also describe the adjunctive pectoralis minor tenotomy procedure via the deltopectoral approach.

Positioning

After the initiation of general anesthesia, the patient is positioned supine with the head of the bed elevated to 30 degrees. The neck is then extended and turned toward the opposite side from the surgical site.

Exposure

The procedure begins with a transverse incision made one to two fingerbreadths above the clavicle within the supraclavicular fossa. On the medial side, the incision starts at the lateral border of the sternocleidomastoid muscle; laterally, the incision extends 6–8 cm, approaching the anterior edge of the trapezius muscle. The platysma muscle layer is then transected, exposing the supraclavicular scalene fat pad and the diagonally traversing omohyoid muscle, which is divided routinely. The scalene fat pad is then mobilized, starting at the lateral edge of the internal jugular vein, and is progressively dissected away from the surface of the ASM. As the fat pad is reflected, the ASM should be exposed, with the phrenic nerve crossing its surface. The surgeon should proceed with caution until the phrenic nerve is positively identified. Typically, the phrenic nerve can be easily distinguished because it is the only peripheral nerve to run from lateral to medial as it courses distally. After the phrenic nerve is identified, the fat pad can be mobilized far enough laterally to expose the underlying brachial plexus roots; subsequently, it can be reflected on its pedicle and secured out of position with silk suture or a retractor (Figure 53.1).

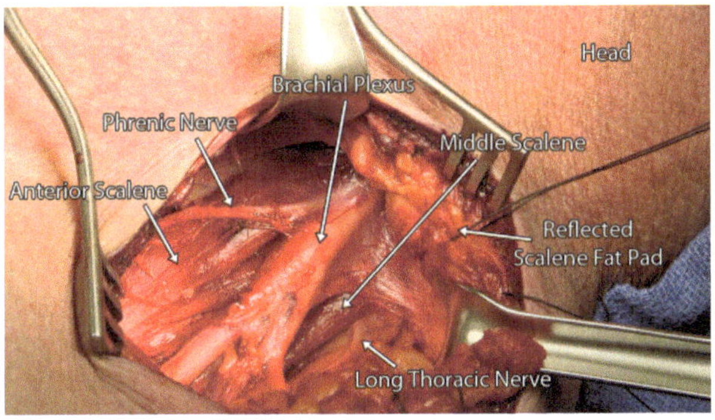

Figure 53.1 Operative image of the critical view of the essential structures in a standard supraclavicular thoracic outlet decompression.

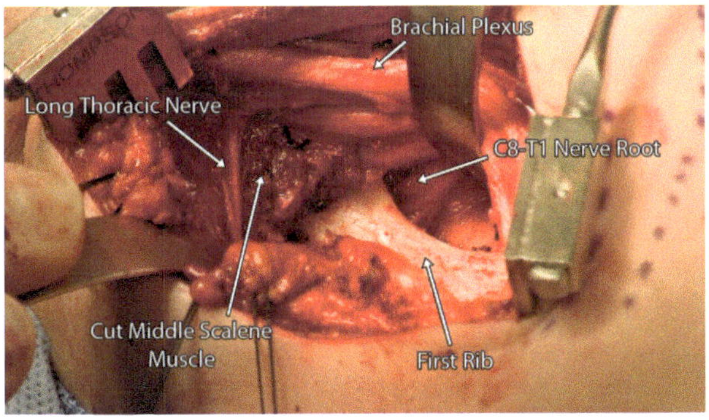

Figure 53.2 Operative image of the posterior aspect of the first rib with exposure of the C8– T1 nerve roots.

Scalenectomy

During dissection of the ASM, it is important to note the locations of the phrenic nerve, C5-C6 nerve roots, and the SCA to avoid injury to these structures. In preparation for excision, the ASM should be mobilized circumferentially, down to the level of the attachment to the first rib. When the surgeon can pass a right-angle clamp under the ASM at its osseous attachment, the muscle can be divided at this location using curved Mayo scissors. It is preferable to perform this step with scissors because cautery may induce thermal injury to adjacent structures. The muscle can then be lifted superiorly and detached from the underlying structures, typically using gentle finger dissection, to its origin at the C6 transverse process. Frequently, muscle fibers can interdigitate with roots of the brachial plexus; thus, care must be taken to avoid causing injury to these structures throughout the dissection. At its origin, the muscle can then be sharply divided while protecting adjacent nerve roots. Additionally, the scalenus minimus muscle, characterized by fibers that originate posteriorly to the C5-C6 nerve roots in the plane of the middle scalene muscle (MSM), may be apparent at this point. Because the scalenus minimus fibers pass between the brachial plexus nerve roots, it may be an additional source of neural compression and should also be excised.

With the ASM removed, the brachial plexus will be very apparent. It should be brought forward with gentle retraction to expose the MSM. Before dividing the MSM, the long thoracic nerve must be identified. This nerve exits the anterolateral border of the MSM and courses inferolateral. The MSM insertion on the first rib is identified and dissected off the rib surface with electrocautery. Proximally, the MSM is sharply transected just distal to the course of the long thoracic nerve.

First rib resection

The posterior neck of the first rib is exposed with a periosteal elevator. The lateral musculofascial attachments to the first rib are then released anteriorly from its posterior neck to the scalene tubercle. The pleural apex is bluntly dissected away from the inferior surface of the rib along its entire course. With the brachial plexus roots well protected, the neck of the first rib is sharply divided with a Stille bone cutter (Stille AB, Torshälla, Sweden). The cut edge of the posterior first rib is remodeled to a smooth surface with a Kerrison bone rongeur, protecting the C8 and T1 nerve roots from injury to a level parallel with the transverse process; its edge is then sealed with bone wax (Figure 53.2).

The anterior portion of the first rib is then exposed underneath the clavicle and similarly divided just medial to the level of the scalene tubercle, with protection of the SCV, SCA, and brachial plexus nerve roots. The anterior edge of the rib is remodeled to a smooth surface and sealed with bone wax. After dividing additional intercostal muscle attachments, the first rib is removed from the operative field.

Cervical rib removal

When a cervical rib is present, we typically resect it after the middle scalenectomy is completed. It is exposed at its posterior origin and the neck of the rib is divided, protecting the nerve roots origin (C8 and T1) from injury. The proximal end of the cervical rib is detached from its attachment of the first rib and removed as a specimen.

Brachial plexus neurolysis

Inspection of the brachial plexus nerve roots typically shows an extensive amount of dense post-inflammatory scar tissue. This fibrous tissue is removed by performing a complete brachial neurolysis. During this step of the procedure, the nerve roots contributing to the brachial plexus are thoroughly identified and carefully protected from injury, including the C5-C8 spinal segments and T1.

To prevent or limit the development of perineural scar tissue that might contribute to recurrent NTOS, we use an absorbable adhesion barrier wrapped around the brachial plexus as a temporary physical barrier between the nerves and adjacent tissues.

Pectoralis minor tenotomy

A small, vertical infraclavicular incision is made in the deltopectoral groove and carried through to the subcutaneous tissues. The pectoralis fascia is entered, and the lateral edge of the pectoralis major is lifted and retracted medially. The space between the pectoralis muscles is developed bluntly; the pectoralis minor tendon is identified, encircled, and then divided under direct vision close to the coracoid process with electrocautery for hemostasis. The clavipectoral fascia is also divided sharply just beneath the clavicle. This gives a palpable improvement in the subpectoral space, allowing relief if any neurovascular compression is found at this site.

Wound closure

We irrigate the wound with saline, obtain hemostasis, and pay careful attention to any detectable lymphatic leak. The authors also check for any air leaks from the lung parenchyma. If there is an opening in the pleural space, we suction the pleural cavity. A closed-suction 10F round Blake drain is brought through a lateral stab wound and placed extending into the pleural space. The scalene fat pad is approximated over the brachial plexus and the wound is closed in layers.

POSTOPERATIVE CARE

We do not restrict arm movement postoperatively; physical therapy is initiated on the first postoperative day. The drain is typically removed on the second postoperative day after 24 hours of a low-fat diet if no chyle leak is apparent. Daily chest x-rays are performed to monitor for pleural effusion with the last x-ray being done after the drain is pulled.

Pain control can be challenging in this patient population; care is taken to titrate narcotic medication. A strict bowel regimen is set in place.

Patients often complain of mild paresthesia in the C8–T1 distribution. An elevated hemidiaphragm can result from traction injury to the phrenic nerve.

It is imperative to establish a long-term follow-up plan for patients with NTOS. They require frequent medication alteration, evaluation for persistent or recurrent symptoms, and most importantly, continued physical therapy.

VENOUS THORACIC OUTLET

Effort-induced axillary-subclavian vein thrombosis, also known as Paget-Schroetter syndrome, is an underrecognized cause of upper extremity DVT. This condition is considered the venous manifestation of thoracic outlet syndrome (TOS), where the underlying cause is the compression of and repetitive injury to the subclavian vein (SCV), between the first rib and clavicle [7].

Patients with VTOS typically present with spontaneous, sudden-onset swelling in the entire affected limb, with symptoms of pain, heaviness, and cyanosis. They are typically young (15–45 years) and otherwise healthy, physically active individuals. They typically report a history of frequent intense exercise, repetitive overhead activity, or heavy lifting [8,9].

On physical examination, patients with VTOS usually exhibit a markedly swollen upper extremity. Multiple subcutaneous collateral veins may be visible in the affected arm, shoulder, and anterior chest.

Although attractive from a theoretical standpoint, Duplex imaging of the SCV is limited by the clavicle.

The thrombosis might be apparent on Duplex if the clot extends into the axillary vein or the distal SCV below the clavicle. Venous obstruction and collateral flow can also affect hemodynamic parameters and waveform analyses.

Contrast-enhanced upper extremity computed tomography or magnetic resonance venography are often used as a first step in imaging evaluation. This allows the presence, location, and extent of the thrombosis to be accurately assessed. In acute presentations (<6 weeks from the onset of symptoms), we prefer catheter-based contrast venography as the first step in imaging evaluation, as it can provide accurate diagnostic information and immediate therapeutic intervention in cases where thrombolysis and possible balloon angioplasty are options.

In patients with acute-to-subacute presentation of VTOS, we focus our initial approach on restoring a patent SCV. This is critical for evaluating residual stenosis and positional venous compression and is most rapidly achieved by pharmacomechanical thrombolysis. Balloon angioplasty to diameters of 10–12 mm can give good radiographic results; however, the benefit is usually incomplete and short-lived unless the source of extrinsic compression has been addressed. Placement of stents in the SCV should not be performed as part of the initial treatment because mechanical deformation and stent fractures are predictable outcomes that can cause more harm than benefit.

After thrombolysis, patients are maintained on systemic anticoagulation to prevent early recurrent thrombosis. In general, we do not believe that long-term anticoagulation as a stand-alone treatment for VTOS is sufficient, whereas surgical treatment offers optimal outcomes. The goal of surgical intervention is complete thoracic outlet decompression and definitive treatment of residual subclavian stenosis or occlusion. Surgical treatment is typically conducted within four to six weeks of thrombolysis.

Surgical techniques

Surgical management of VTOS can be performed with several different strategies and approaches. The transaxillary approach to VTOS was promoted in the early

1990s, as exemplified by Freischlag [10], who provided detailed descriptions and outcomes of this technique.

The infraclavicular approach to VTOS was developed and described by Molina and colleagues [11]. In this protocol, all patients suspected to have VTOS undergo venography and initial thrombolysis. Patients with long-segment occlusions of the axillary vein and SCV are excluded from surgical management and receive lifelong anticoagulation. All other patients undergo surgery through an infraclavicular approach, with the first rib resected along with portions of the anterior scalene and subclavius muscles. The SCV is exposed along its length underneath the clavicle and vein patch angioplasty with saphenous vein is performed in all patients. The incision is extended medially to a partial median sternotomy, if needed, for completion of a long-patch angioplasty or a SCV bypass graft. In this protocol, a venogram is performed the day after the operation and a stent is placed in the treated SCV.

We favor the paraclavicular approach for VTOS, which allows for complete decompression of the thoracic outlet and possible reconstruction of the SCV, if needed, in the same operation. Compared with the trans-axillary and infraclavicular approaches, the paraclavicular approach provides the following advantages: (1) direct surgical treatment for all patients with VTOS by complete thoracic outlet decompression; (2) the potential to treat the SCV by thorough external venolysis, when appropriate; and (3) the potential to reconstruct the SCV, when necessary, with either vein patch angioplasty or bypass grafting, with no need for a sternotomy or postoperative stent placement.

Paraclavicular thoracic outlet decompression for VTOS involves several additional considerations to the standard, previously described supraclavicular exploration for NTOS. Positioning is like NTOS (semi-Fowler's) on a fluoroscopic table. A 4-Fr micropuncture sheath is placed in the basilic vein for the initial venogram to confirm the level of disease and to serve as a baseline for comparison at the end of the procedure.

Following the standard supraclavicular decompression, the authors focus on two critical aspects of surgery for VTOS: complete medial resection of the first rib and external venolysis of the SCV.

To completely resect the anteromedial portion of the first rib, a second transverse skin incision is made 1 cm below the head of the clavicle and immediately over the medial first rib. Flaps are created at the level of the pectoralis major fascia. The tissue plane between the lower and middle portions of the pectoralis major muscle is spread in a muscle-sparing manner until the cartilaginous portion of the first rib is encountered. The rib is exposed and dissected free of surrounding tissue attachments with electrocautery. The clavicle is elevated with protection of the SCV, and all intercostal muscle attachments to the rib are divided along with the tendon of the subclavius muscle on its upper surface. The anteromedial aspect of the first rib is transected at the level of the sternum with a bone rongeur and the whole first rib is removed as a single specimen. The cut edge of the bone is remodeled to a smooth surface and sealed with bone wax. The remaining subclavius muscle and its tendon are resected to provide additional exposure to the SCV.

External venolysis of the SCV

The axillary vein is then identified and exposed from the infraclavicular incision where it emerges from underneath the clavicle. When necessary, the pectoralis minor muscle may be divided at its insertion on the coracoid process to allow more distal exposure of the axillary vein. The authors then turn their attention to the proximal SCV by tracing it up to the supraclavicular space. From the supraclavicular exposure, the SCV, the lower aspect of the internal jugular vein, and the upper aspect of the brachiocephalic vein are all exposed. Circumferential external venolysis is performed by excising the thick fibrous tissue that typically encases the SCV. Once venolysis is complete, a venogram is performed to assess the lumen of the SCV and determine the need for further reconstruction (Figure 53.3).

SCV reconstruction

If SCV reconstruction is required, the patient is systemically anticoagulated with intravenous heparin. The decision on patch angioplasty or bypass grafting is made using the venogram, visualization of the vein, and digital palpation. We use cryopreserved femoral vein grafts for patch bypasses and bovine pericardium for patch angioplasty (Figures 53.4 and 53.5).

POSTOPERATIVE CARE

The patient is started on 500 units of heparin an hour six hours postoperatively, then using a low-intensity protocol, a heparin infusion is taken to therapeutic with a goal PTT between 60 and 90 sec. Once PTT levels are therapeutic with no evidence of bleeding, they are transitioned to oral anticoagulation with the drain typically pulled out

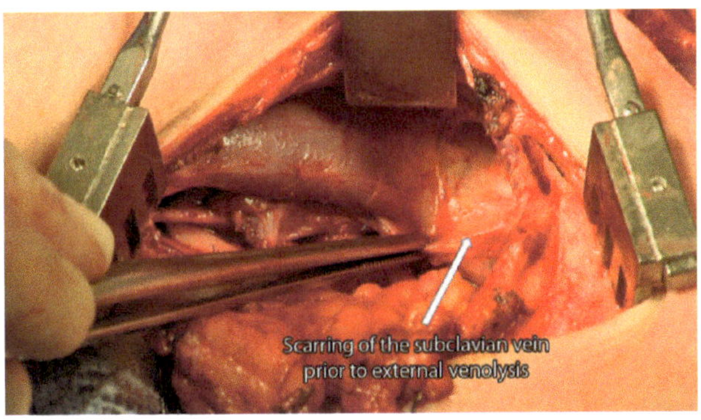

Figure 53.3 Typical appearance of the scarred subclavian vein before external venolysis.

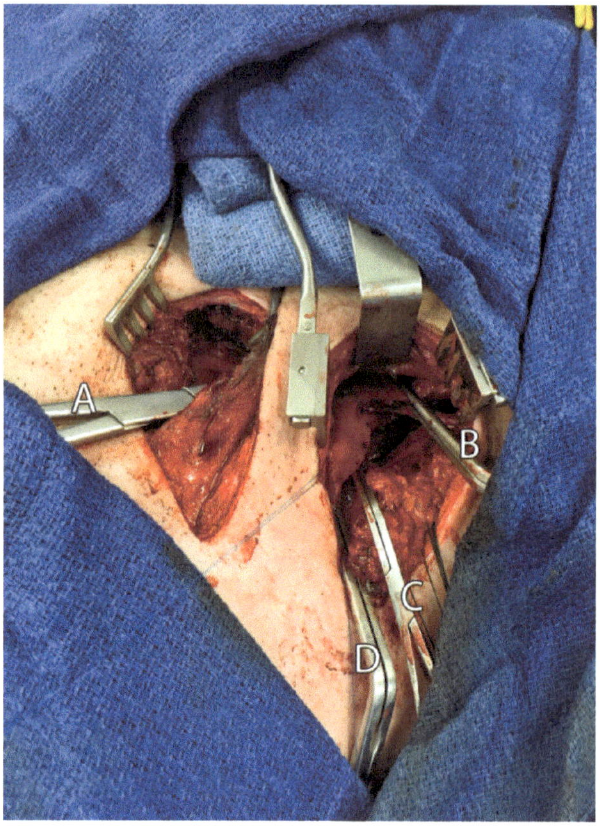

Figure 53.4 Clamp placement for venous reconstruction in the paraclavicular approach: (a) brachiocephalic vein clamp; (b) internal jugular vein clamp; (c) clamp on large collateral veins; (d) distal subclavian vein clamp.

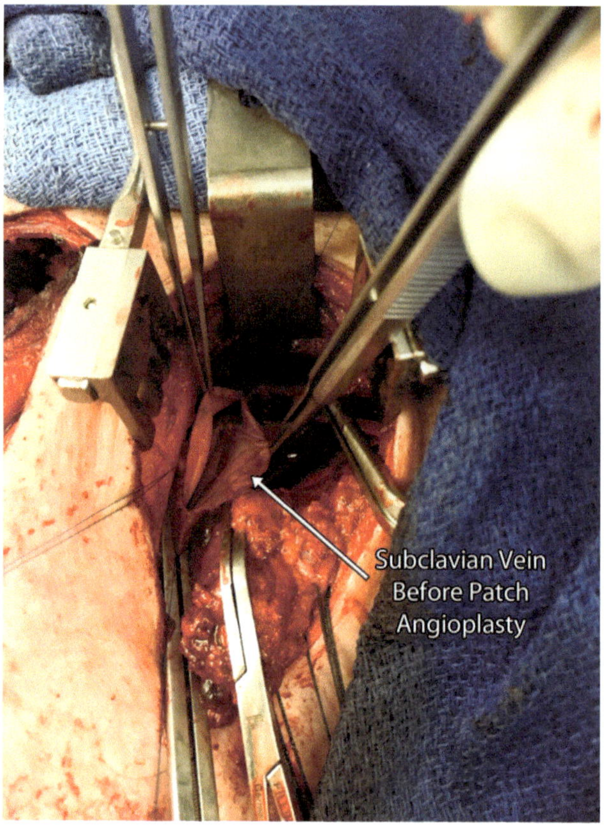

Figure 53.5 Preparation of the subclavian vein before patch angioplasty (arrow).

on postop day three. We continue anticoagulation for up to three months postoperatively.

ARTERIAL THORACIC OUTLET SYNDROME

ATOS is the least frequent form of TOS. It represents 1–3% of all TOS. The majority of ATOS patients (up to 75%) had cervical ribs, whereas anomalous first ribs and tight fascial bands accounted for the rest of the structural anomalies causing compression of the SCA [12].

There are two clinical manifestations of ATOS: one related to the injury to the SCA; the second related to distal manifestations of arterial ischemia caused by embolic or thrombotic occlusions. The treatment for ATOS focuses on relieving arterial compression and removing the source of the emboli to restore normal circulation to the arm.

Patients presenting with acute arm ischemia from ATOS are treated first with thrombectomy. After distal circulation is restored, the patients are prepared for ATOS repair within a few days of the initial procedure.

The approach is like that used for NTOS, in that the focus is on complete decompression of the thoracic outlet with anterior and middle scalenectomy and removal of the first rib and cervical rib, if present (Figures 53.6–53.9).

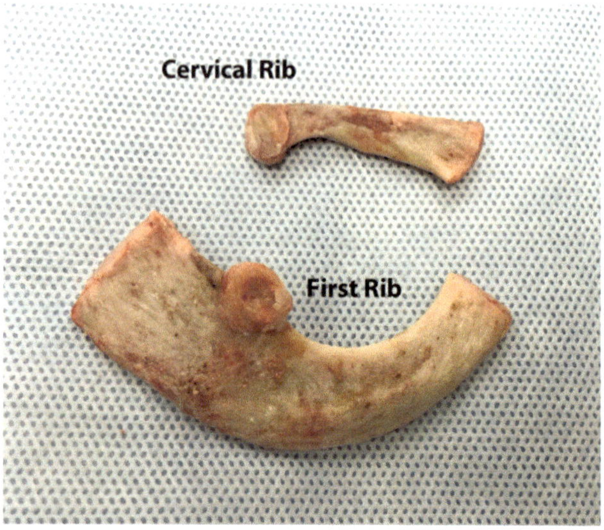

Figure 53.6 First rib with cervical rib, typically connected by a joint.

The decision to repair the SCA with a bypass graft versus patch angioplasty depends on the extent of the aneurysm or embolizing lesion along its course. A paraclavicular approach is sometimes needed to perform SCA-axillary artery bypasses. Those are typically performed using cryopreserved femoral vein graft.

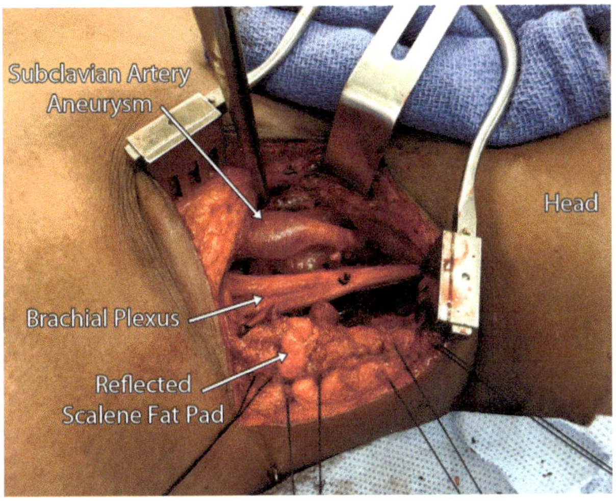

Figure 53.7 Subclavian artery aneurysm after scalenectomy and first rib removal.

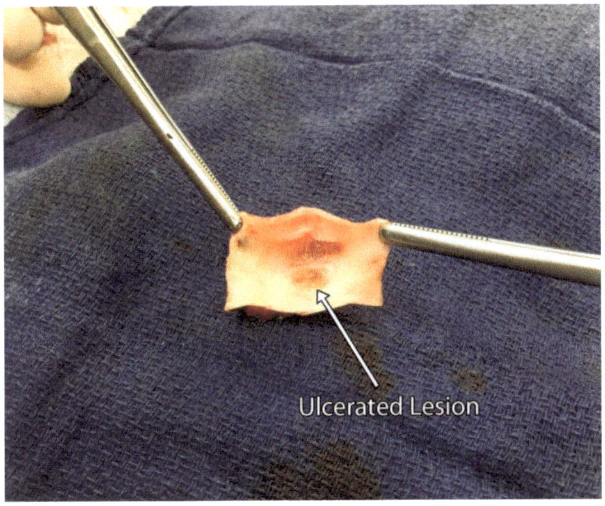

Figure 53.8 Ulcerated lesion inside a subclavian aneurysm (arrow). This is typically the cause of distal embolization.

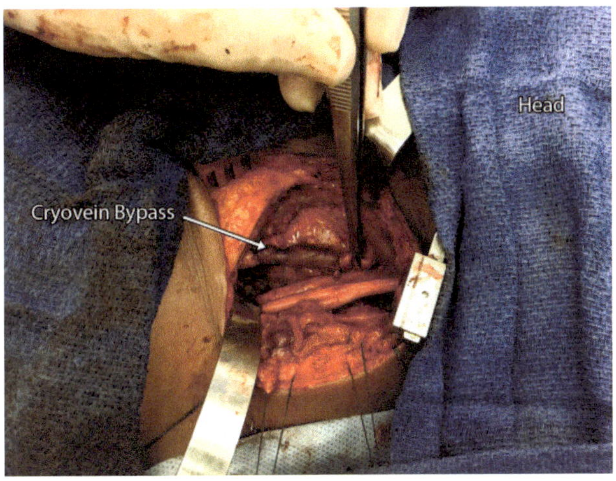

Figure 53.9 Arterial reconstruction with cryopreserved femoral vein graft.

TRICKS AND TRAPS

Neurogenic thoracic outlet syndrome:

- Remember to look for pectoralis minor syndrome during the initial evaluation of the patient with NTOS.
- Supraclavicular thoracic outlet decompression is the preferred approach for treating neurogenic thoracic outlet syndrome.
- The critical view of safety includes visualizing the phrenic nerve, long thoracic nerve, and brachial plexus.

Venous thoracic outlet syndrome:

- Venogram with thrombectomy/lysis should be performed on all patients with suspected venous thoracic outlet syndrome.
- Full exposure of the subclavian vein is done through a paraclavicular approach.
- Meticulous dissection around the IJ confluence with the subclavian vein decreases the risk of lymph leak and thoracic duct injury.
- Venography at completion of decompression guides the decision for venous reconstruction.

Arterial thoracic outlet syndrome:

- Cross-sectional imaging of all patients presenting with acute upper extremity ischemia helps rule out subclavian artery injury from ATOS.
- Treat the ischemia first, then proceed with ATOS decompression, ideally 24–48 hours after index procedure.

QUESTIONS

1. What is the course of the phrenic nerve and its relationship to the anterior scalene muscle?
    a. Crossing over the muscle medial to lateral
    b. Crossing over the muscle lateral to medial
    c. Crossing under the muscle medial to lateral
    d. Crossing under the muscle lateral to medial

    Answer: b

2. Which of the following is true about the long thoracic nerve?
    a. Pierces through the anterior scalene muscle
    b. Courses medial to the middle scalene muscle
    c. Innervates the trapezius muscle
    d. Fans out from the middle scalene muscle and courses lateral to it

    Answer: d

3. Which of the following is true about the scalene minimus muscle?
   a. It is always present within the scalene triangle
   b. It is attached to the middle scalene muscle and the medial first rib and courses through the brachial plexus
   c. Should not be divided during thoracic outlet decompression
   d. It is an essential muscle for neck flexion

   Answer: b

4. When a young healthy patient is diagnosed with a subclavian vein DVT, which of the following steps in management are appropriate?
   a. Start on anticoagulation
   b. Catheter-based venogram with lysis versus thrombectomy at the time of diagnosis
   c. Referral to vascular surgery
   d. All of the above

   Answer: d

5. The majority of patients diagnosed with arterial thoracic outlet syndrome have cervical ribs:
   a. True
   b. False

   Answer: a

REFERENCES

1. Hempel, G. K., Shutze, W. P., Anderson, J. F., et al. (1996). 770 consecutive supraclavicular first rib resections for thoracic outlet syndrome. *Ann Vasc Surg., 10*, 456–463.
2. Juvonen, T., Satta, J., Laitala, P., et al. (1995). Anomalies at the thoracic outlet are frequent in the general population. *Am J Surg., 170*, 33–37.
3. Thompson, R. W., Petrinec, D., & Toursarkissian, B. (1997). Surgical treatment of thoracic outlet compression syndromes. II. Supraclavicular exploration and vascular reconstruction. *Ann Vasc Surg., 11*, 442–451.
4. Freischlag, J., & Orion, K. (2014). Understanding thoracic outlet syndrome. *Scientifica (Cairo)., 2014*, 248163.
5. Watson, L. A., Pizzari, T., & Balster, S. (2010). Thoracic outlet syndrome part 2: Conservative management of thoracic outlet. *Man Ther., 15*, 305–314.
6. Sanders, R. J., Hammond, S. L., & Rao, N. M. (2007). Diagnosis of thoracic outlet syndrome. *J Vasc Surg., 46*, 601–604.
7. Flinterman, L. E., Van Der Meer, F. J., Rosendaal, F. R., et al. (2008). Current perspective of venous thrombosis in the upper extremity. *J Thromb Haemost., 6*, 1262–1266.
8. Azakie, A., McElhinney, D. B., Thompson, R. W., et al. (1998). Surgical management of subclavian-vein effort thrombosis as a result of thoracic outlet compression. *J Vasc Surg., 28*, 777–786.
9. Sanders, R. J., Hammond, S. L., & Rao, N. M. (2007). Diagnosis of thoracic outlet syndrome. *J Vasc Surg., 46*, 601–604.
10. Freischlag, J. (2008). Venous thoracic outlet syndrome: transaxillary approach. *Oper Tech Gen Surg., 10*, 122–130.
11. Molina, J. E., Hunter, D. W., & Dietz, C. A. (2007). Paget-Schroetter syndrome treated with thrombolytics and immediate surgery. *J Vasc Surg., 45*, 328–334.
12. Criado, E., Berguer, R., & Greenfield, L. (2010). The spectrum of arterial compression at the thoracic outlet. *J Vasc Surg., 52*, 406–411.

54

Open and endovascular venous reconstruction

MILES JACKSON, JACOB W. GUERRANT, AND ERIN PANG

INTRODUCTION

Venous reconstruction is commonly used to treat chronic sequela of deep vein thrombosis (DVT) and chronic venous insufficiency (CVI) and is less frequently employed in oncologic or traumatic reconstructions. Endovascular intervention is accepted as the first-line interventional approach for most of these cases, though open surgery is still performed for patients with unsuccessful endovascular intervention or whose anatomy or pathology favors open surgical reconstruction.

PATHOLOGY

Acute DVT is initially managed with systemic anticoagulation, including heparin infusion for inpatient settings and frequent transition to oral or parenteral regimens at discharge. Anticoagulation alone can provide adequate management and risk reduction for DVT progression or PE occurrence; however, it relies heavily on intrinsic thrombolytic mechanisms that do not reliably produce venous recanalization. Extensive iliofemoral DVT may take months to recanalize and 30–50% of patients will develop symptoms consistent with post-thrombotic syndrome (PTS) and/or CVI [1]. Current catheter-based interventions, including thrombolysis or thrombectomy, can yield expeditious removal or reduction of thrombus burden and produce significant benefits in the reduction of PTS symptoms, especially in patients presenting with iliofemoral DVT [2].

Chronic venous disease and venous insufficiency are frequent sequelae of DVT secondary to venous valvular destruction related to venous inflammation. Patients with PTS have a similar symptomatic presentation to CVI patients albeit with slightly different etiology. These patients frequently present with extremity edema, aching, heaviness, skin changes including hemosiderin deposition, fibrosis, and ulceration. The American Venous Forum and Society of Vascular Surgeons classify venous disease using the Clinical, Etiological, Anatomical, Pathophysiological (CEAP) system. Originally developed in 1994 and most recently revised in 2020, the system was created to standardize discussion of venous pathology and develop management guidance. The CEAP classification system is summarized in Table 54.1.

First-line management for venous disease is generally non-operative. The cornerstone is compression, especially graduated compression with elastic wraps or garments, elevation at rest, and regular low-impact exercise with weight loss to normal BMI [4]. Chronic venous disease primarily affects quality of life. Patients with persistent symptoms despite non-operative interventions should be considered for endovascular or open interventions to restore patency or vein function to the affected extremity with the goal of improving quality of life. Indications additionally include recurrent DVT, severe PTS, and significant lifestyle impairment or inability to complete activities of daily living. Current endovascular techniques include thrombolysis and thrombectomy, recanalization, venoplasty, and venous stenting. Open surgical intervention is reserved for patients with long-segment and/or chronic occlusions that have been unsuccessfully treated using endovascular management. The underlying etiology of the venous occlusion will dictate the operative approach necessary. There are many open surgical venous reconstructions previously described; however, many of them are infrequently employed given the recent establishment and widespread use of endovascular approaches. Several procedures still employed include saphenopopliteal bypass (SPB) for unilateral femoral vein occlusion, the Palma procedure or cross-pubic femorofemoral venous bypass for unilateral external or common iliac vein occlusion, and popliteal vein aneurysm plication.

DOI: 10.1201/9781003452096-54

Table 54.1 CEAP Classification System

Clinical	
C0	No visible or clinical signs of venous disease
C1	Telangiectasias or reticular veins
C2	Varicose veins
C2r	Recurrent varicose veins
C3	Edema
C4	Changes in skin and subcutaneous tissue secondary to chronic venous disease
C4a	Pigmentation, eczema
C4b	Lipodermatosclerosis, atrophie blanche
C4c	Corona phlebectatica
C5	Healed ulcer
C6	Active venous ulcer
C6r	Recurrent active venous ulcer
Etiological	
P	Primary
S	Secondary
Si	Secondary, intravenous
Se	Secondary, extravenous
C	Congenital
N	No cause identified
Anatomical	
S	Superficial
D	Deep
P	Perforator
N	No venous anatomic location identified
Pathophysiological	
R	Reflux
O	Obstruction
R,O	Reflux and obstruction
N	No pathophysiology identified

Adapted from the 2020 update of the CEAP classification system and reporting standards [3].

ENDOVASCULAR TECHNIQUES

As mentioned, endovascular techniques are the first-line approach for most patients. General principles include wire access across the lesion or occlusion, venoplasty, and stenting of all recanalized segments. Isolated venoplasty without stenting is usually not a durable option given the propensity for perivenous fibrotic scarring to produce recurrent stenosis or occlusion. Ideal timing for intervention in acute DVT is generally within the first four weeks; otherwise, most interventionalists will wait until the latter part of the sub-acute period, around three to four months, when thrombus has become more organized and partially contracted to permit full balloon and stent expansion during recanalization.

Notably, peripheral venous interventions are rarely employed to treat femoral venous occlusions as low flow and extensive collateralization significantly compromise stent longevity. The vast majority of interventions are focused on proximal venous outflow.

Iliocaval chronic venous disease

Access for proximal venous intervention is ideally performed in the mid-thigh GSV or femoral vein, allowing for the placement of long, large bore sheaths, ideally 11Fr. There should be appropriate attention paid to peri-operative anticoagulation with weight-based heparin to prevent iatrogenic thrombus formation. Venous recanalization should begin with the use of a 0.035" hydrophilic angled tip wire such as a standard or stiff GLIDEWIRE (Terumo Medical Corporation, Somerset, NJ, USA) in addition to an angled tip crossing catheter such as a NAVICROSS (Terumo Medical Corporation). If there is repeated buckling despite advancement of the crossing catheter, the sheath should be advanced in stepwise fashion with the wire and catheter to provide proximal support and aid in the establishment of a flow channel through the occluded iliocaval venous segment.

Recanalization is typically performed in distal to proximal fashion. Antegrade venography is used to establish collateral pathways and any trace contrast filling through the target vein to roadmap wire trajectory. Retrograde imaging from above is significantly less useful for this purpose and IVUS catheters (Volcano Corporation, San Diego, CA, USA) have no utility until the lesion is traversed. Progress is often slow and multiple attempts and pathways may be required to traverse an occlusion. Ideally, the wire will bypass the occlusion or sheaths advanced from the femoral and internal jugular veins are able to be advanced into adjacent positions, allowing for venoplasty or wire and snare capture to establish "body-floss."

Bilateral iliac venous or caval reconstructions require bilateral access in addition to right internal jugular venous access. This can allow for the "body-floss" technique to provide strength and pushability of balloons and stents. In patients with dense chronic thrombotic occlusive disease that is resistant to standard techniques, serial venoplasty using small caliber, high-pressure balloons can help to establish a flow lumen through stepwise advancement. Sharp recanalization techniques are well documented and frequently employ the stiff end of a GLIDEWIRE (Terumo Medical Corporation), BRK-1 Transeptal needle (St. Jude Medical, Inc., St. Paul, MN, USA), Chiba biopsy needle (Cook Medical Inc., Bloomington, IN, USA), or a variety of interventional radiology needles, which can be used to traverse dense or difficult lesions. Once a lesion is traversed, the needle should be captured by a snare placed on the proximal side of the occlusion from internal jugular access. The inner stylet is exchanged for a wire, which is then externalized through the internal jugular sheath. Once through-and-through wire access is established, standard techniques including venoplasty and stenting are employed with the use of venography and IVUS to

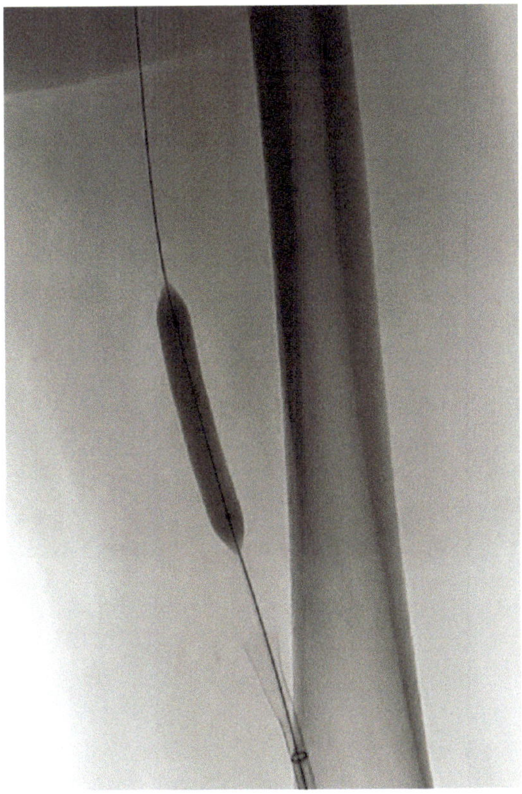

Figure 54.1 Stepwise venoplasty can significantly improve outflow in chronic venous thrombosis.

determine flow patterns, adequate stent sizing, and complete expansion of all deployed stents (Figure 54.1).

Once the occlusion is traversed, confirmatory venography or IVUS is necessary to ensure appropriate intraluminal position of wires and catheters. IVUS provides the additional benefits of reduced contrast use, determines anatomic relationships with nearby structures, and provides planimetry, which is essential prior to venoplasty and stent placement. If not previously given, it is recommended to give peri-operative anticoagulation at this time. Sequential venoplasty with increasing balloon diameters is performed; flow channels are frequently established using long 6–8 mm balloons that can treat the entire iliocaval segment. Following this first venoplasty, venography should be performed to evaluate for contrast extravasation. If negative, then proceeding with venoplasty to standard diameters is performed with IVC dilated to 18–20 mm, common iliac vein to 16 mm, and external vein and common femoral vein to 14 mm. The IVC is typically treated using an 18–20 mm self-expanding stent. Ideally, IVUS is used to select iliac vein stent size to allow for complete stent-wall apposition. Alternative methods for selecting stent size include the "rule of squares." Patients with chronically thrombosed IVC filters either require filter removal or filter exclusion with a large self-expanding stent with re-establishment of a patent IVC lumen.

OPEN TECHNIQUES

Operative planning for femoral venous insufficiency requires identification of incompetent valves with imaging. The purpose of open venous surgery is to reconstruct and re-establish valvular function. Tibial venous valves number three to 12 and are generally evenly distributed. Popliteal veins have one to three valves, femoral veins have one to five valves, and profunda femoris veins have one to four valves. Most surgeons will selectively repair the profunda femoris vein or the femoral and profunda femoris veins if both are incompetent. This decision depends upon the location of disease, accessibility, and suitability for valve repair. Proximal veins have larger valves and are technically easier to repair. Open surgery techniques for valve repair are often described and infrequently performed techniques include internal valvuloplasty, external valvuloplasty, external banding, and vein transplant or transposition. Any open surgery technique requires a healthy and otherwise usable segment of vein for treatment to re-establish venous competence. Outcomes are generally highly variable and published data are limited to individual institutions or small series with no clearly superior modality.

Autogenous grafts have the best chance for long-term patency. Ideally, the GSV can be used because of availability, length, and low thrombogenic rates. Remember to preserve the GSV conduit in patients with known coronary and peripheral arterial disease. Larger caliber replacements include ePTFE, which is widely available, customizable, and externally supported. The use of arteriovenous fistulae has also been demonstrated to improve the patency of grafts placed in the venous system [5]. These will increase flow through grafts and decrease platelet and fibrin deposition in prosthetic grafts. Autogenous fistulas require less flow than prosthetic grafts to prevent thrombosis. Generally, a large GSV side branch is employed and anastomosed to the superficial femoral artery. The creation of arteriovenous fistula is recommended in all prosthetic femoral vein grafts and iliocaval grafts >10 cm in length and left in place for six weeks.

Saphenopopliteal bypass with arteriovenous fistula

Initially described in the 1970s, saphenopopliteal bypass (SPB) is used to treat femoral vein occlusion and is especially useful if the profunda femoris vein is unable to adequately drain the affected extremity. Planning includes venous Duplex with specific evaluation of the femoral vein, profunda femoris vein, and GSV. Pre-operative venography should also be performed to determine flow patterns. Suitable patients should demonstrate patent inflow from the popliteal vein, patent GSV and saphenofemoral junction, and patent outflow through the ipsilateral iliocaval segments. Alternatively, this procedure can also be performed in conjunction with a cross-pubic femorofemoral venous bypass to preserve outflow if ipsilateral iliac venous occlusion is present. The addition of arteriovenous fistula can be performed to promote patency based on an assessment of bypass flow.

Venous bypass is performed in a similar fashion to an arterial bypass. Patients should be mapped preoperatively in PACU with the GSV delineated as well as large venous branches identified. General anesthesia is employed. The patient should be placed in a supine position with the operative leg gently bent and externally rotated for circumferential prep. Standard pre-operative antibiotics and VTE prophylaxis should be performed.

Exposure includes above-knee longitudinal cutdown with exposure and dissection of the GSV and ligation of all branches with 3-0 or 4-0 silk ties. Next, dissection into the popliteal fossa in the standard fashion with exposure and isolation of the popliteal vein is performed, and proximal and distal control is obtained using silastic vessel loops. Adequate GSV length can be determined using a silk tie for measurement to ensure it is able to reach the popliteal vein without significant tension while the knee is in full extension. Once satisfied, the surgeon should provide full intraoperative anticoagulation with weight-based heparin for an ACT >250 seconds. The popliteal vein is then occluded using the vessel loops and a longitudinal venotomy is created. The GSV is marked along its exposed surface to prevent twisting and then transected and the distal aspect is ligated using 2-0 or 3-0 silk ties. A distal end-to-side GSV to popliteal vein anastomosis is created using interrupted 6-0 Prolene. As always, immediately prior to completion of the suture line, forward and back bleeding should be performed on all vessels to prevent embolization of residual air or debris. Flow is then evaluated using a GSV side branch with any arteriovenous fistulae created using a distal venous branch or interposition graft and the popliteal artery can be performed distal to the venous bypass anastomosis. This can be easily performed using a segment of distal GSV stump as an interposition conduit. The popliteal artery is controlled using vessel loops or clamps and occluded and an aortic punch can be used to create an end-to-side vein to artery bypass, which is then anastomosed to the SPB in an identical fashion using 6-0 Prolene. As with all fistulas, palpation should demonstrate a thrill indicative of adequate flow (Figure 54.2).

After closure, patients should be placed on intravenous heparin infusion, LMWH, or oral anticoagulation. Below-knee compression garments and ambulation are encouraged to promote flow through the bypass. Arteriovenous fistulae should be ligated or embolized six to 12 weeks post-operatively to prevent neointimal hyperplasia of the venous portion of the fistula.

Cross-pubic femorofemoral venous bypass (Palma procedure) with arteriovenous fistula

Initially described over 60 years ago by Palma and Esperon [6], the Palma procedure has remained clinically

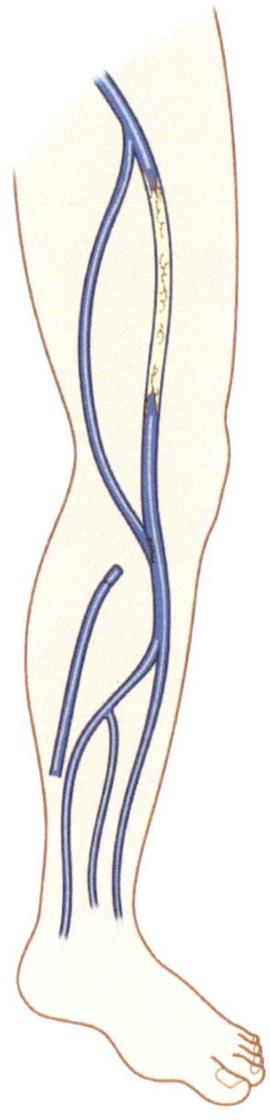

Figure 54.2 Saphenopopliteal bypass (illustration showing surgical incision, occluded vein segment, route of bypass). Note the distal GSV disconnected from the GSV used for the bypass.

relevant for the management of unilateral iliofemoral venous occlusions. The operation requires a normal patent contralateral iliofemoral venous system and GSV and involves transposition of the contralateral GSV to the ipsilateral CFV. Notably, this is an excellent option for young women with residual chronic iliac venous occlusive disease following acute iliofemoral DVT from May–Thurner syndrome and is also indicated in patients unsuitable for iliac vein stenting or with failed prior endovascular interventions. Suitability should be determined by venous Duplex and venography to determine patency and adequacy of the contralateral GSV and flow patterns consistent with usable drainage.

Patients should be mapped pre-operatively in PACU with the GSV delineated as well as large venous branches identified. General anesthesia is employed. The patient should be placed in a supine position with the legs gently bent and externally rotated for circumferential prep to also include the abdomen. Standard pre-operative antibiotics and VTE prophylaxis should be performed (Figure 54.3).

A standard vertical incision is made over the femoral vein in the patent groin with dissection and exposure of the SFJ. Distal medial thigh exposure of the GSV can be performed using a single long incision or multiple skip incisions; either method is acceptable for mobilization

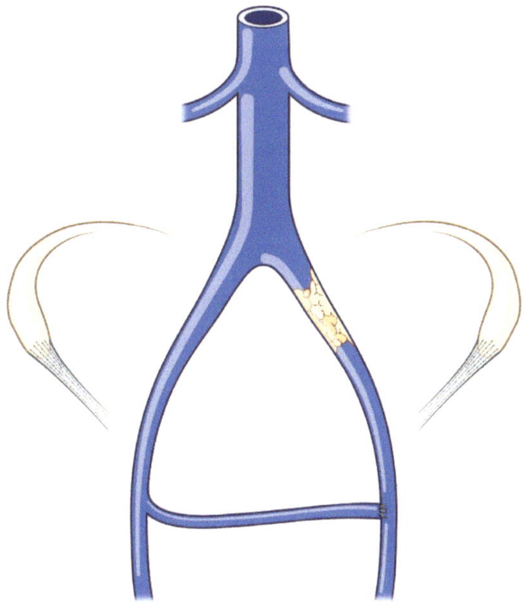

Figure 54.3 Palma procedure (illustration showing occluded left iliac vein segment and route of bypass).

of the GSV to the level of the knee. All GSV branches should be ligated using 3-0 or 4-0 silk as encountered. Next, an identical vertical groin incision is made in the affected extremity, and dissection and exposure of the CFV, femoral vein, and PFV are performed. These vessels are typically engorged and delicate secondary to venous hypertension from proximal occlusion. Existing venous collaterals should be preserved if possible. A curved tunneler is then introduced from the affected side to the GSV donor groin. Care should be taken in creating this tunnel as many cross-pelvic collaterals may be present and can contribute to significant bleeding. Once satisfied, the surgeon should provide full intra-operative anticoagulation with weight-based heparin for an ACT >250 seconds. The contralateral distal GSV is then marked along its length and distal ligation is performed using 2-0 silk. The GSV is transected and passed through the suprapubic tunnel with care taken to prevent kinking or twisting. The CFV is then controlled using a side-biting clamp and a longitudinal venotomy is created. An end-to-side GSV to CFV anastomosis is created using interrupted 6-0 Prolene in standard fashion. Flow is assessed using a GSV branch and an arteriovenous fistula can be created to augment flow (Figures 54.4 and 54.5).

After closure, patients should be placed on intravenous heparin infusion, LMWH, or oral anticoagulation. Below-knee compression garments and ambulation are encouraged to promote flow through the bypass. Arteriovenous fistulae should be ligated or embolized six to 12 weeks post-operatively to prevent neointimal hyperplasia of the venous portion of the fistula.

ANTICOAGULATION AND ANTIPLATELET THERAPY

Peri-operative use of weight-based heparin is standard during venous interventions and endothelial injury should be treated with anticoagulation for a minimum of six weeks. There is broad variation in accepted anticoagulation protocols, but we recommend Plavix 75 mg daily at a minimum following bypass or stent placement for a minimum of six weeks. Long-term anticoagulation can be employed in patients with thrombophilia and/or recurrent thrombosis, ISR, or extensive stenting.

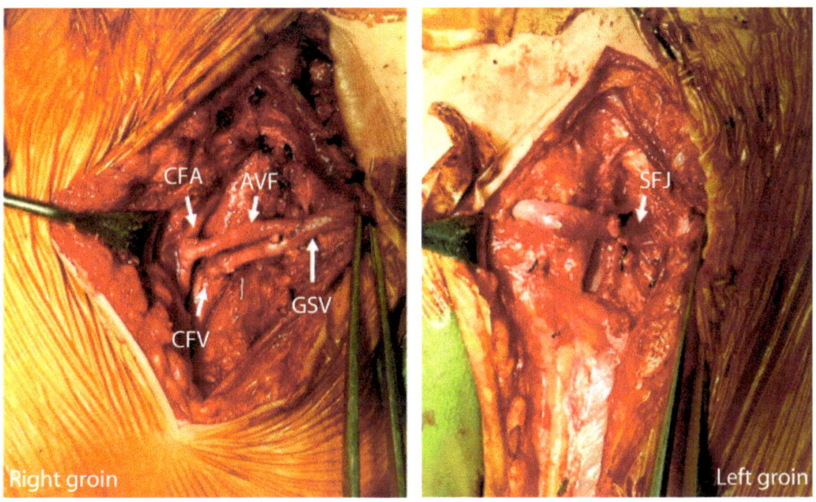

Figure 54.4 Completion of Palma procedure with arteriovenous fistula in a 28-year-old woman (case example 3). AVF, arteriovenous fistula; CFA, common femoral artery; CFV, common femoral vein; GSV, greater saphenous vein; SFJ, saphenofemoral junction.

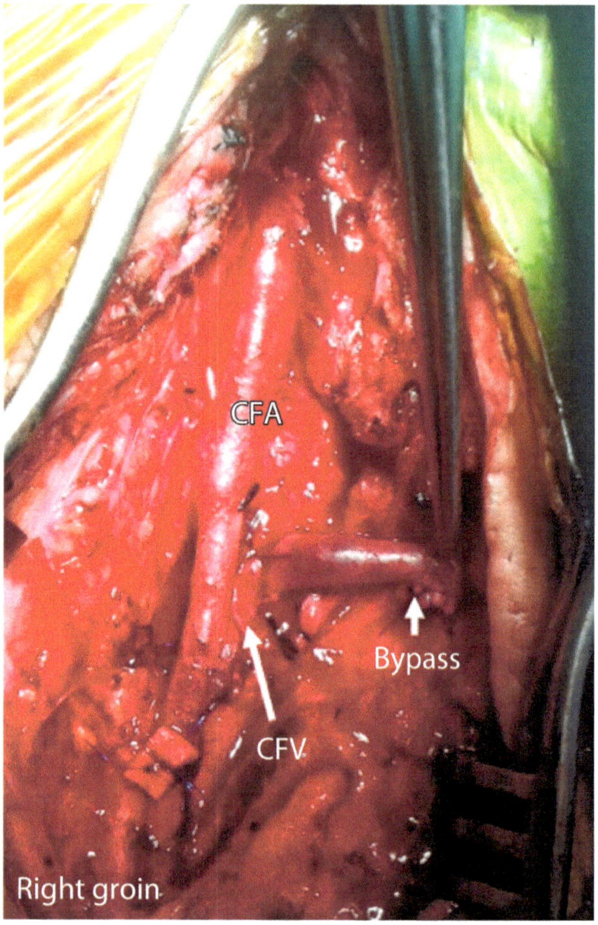

Figure 54.5 Revision of the Palma procedure with take-down of arteriovenous fistula (AVF) and use of the AVF vein segment as an interposition between the common femoral vein and the patent portion of the bypass (case example 3). Note the interval removal of the AVF. CFA, common femoral artery; CFV, common femoral vein.

ONGOING MANAGEMENT AND FOLLOW-UP

All patients should continue with compression therapy and leg elevation at rest as previously established. Surveillance should be established early and regularly; patients should undergo venous Duplex imaging at one week, four to six weeks, and then every six months for stent malfunction. May–Thurner stents have lower rates of occlusion whereas post-thrombotic veins should be monitored every three months to detect early in-stent restenosis prior to occlusion. Symptomatic change should prompt earlier evaluation.

TRICKS AND TRAPS

- All attempts should be made to proceed with endovascular intervention prior to open surgery, if possible, to maximize opportunities for intervention should minimally invasive approaches fail.
- Mid-thigh femoral vein access and large sheaths allow for good pushability and working length.
- A 0.035" GLIDEWIRE is often a great wire for identifying a lumen through trabeculated vein; the majority of lesions can be traversed using this wire and a low-profile crossing catheter in stepwise fashion with a sheath being progressively advanced into the occluded segment.
- Several attempts may be required to traverse a difficult lesion, which may end in perforation or impassable portions of the occlusion; you may have to pull back and start again multiple times to find a true path.
- The use of IVUS is imperative in all iliac vein cases and is superior to isolated venography for the determination of appropriate stent size and length for adequate lesion coverage.
- Always post-dilate iliac vein stents to at least their nominal diameter or higher and confirm adequate expansion using post-dilation IVUS and venography.
- Difficult lesions may require antegrade access from the ipsilateral CFV and retrograde access using the right internal jugular vein with a looped snare to establish the "body-floss" technique.
- Some venous lesions may not be traversable and these patients should be considered for open venous bypass if necessary; this is especially true in patients with recurrent in-stent restenosis and occlusion.
- Open venous bypass techniques require adequate inflow and outflow to maintain patency; the judicious use of short-term arteriovenous fistulae should be considered for most cases.
- As with arterial cases, autogenous conduit selection is ideal and minimizes thrombogenicity and infection risk.
- Use of prosthetic conduits in large venous reconstructions should always be performed with an arteriovenous fistula as adjunct to prevent early thrombosis.
- Anticoagulation in the peri-operative period is not standardized but widely used to promote patency.

QUESTIONS

1. Recommended initial venous access for iliac stenting includes:
   a. Mid-femoral vein with long 11Fr sheath
   b. Prone patient with popliteal access and 7Fr sheath
   c. Right internal jugular vein with 5Fr sheath
   d. Contralateral common femoral vein with 11Fr sheath

Answer: a

2. Extensive iliocaval venous reconstructions can require multiple points of venous access with the addition of which technique to increase pushability?
   a. Rule of squares
   b. Body-floss technique
   c. CEAP
   d. Sheath telescoping

   Answer: b

3. Palma procedure uses the _______ GSV to treat _______ proximal iliac occlusion.
   a. Ipsilateral, ipsilateral
   b. Contralateral, ipsilateral
   c. Ipsilateral, contralateral
   d. Contralateral, contralateral

   Answer: b

4. The use of arteriovenous fistulae can promote flow through venous bypasses. These should be ligated or embolized by which time?
   a. One to two weeks
   b. Six weeks
   c. Six months
   d. One year

   Answer: b

REFERENCES

1. Kahn S, Comerota A, Cushman M, et al. The post-thrombotic syndrome: evidence-based prevention, diagnosis, and treatment strategies: a scientific statement from the American Heart Association. *Circulation*. 2014;130:1636–1661.
2. Vedantham S, Goldhaber SZ, Julian JA, et al. Pharmacomechanical catheter-directed thrombolysis for deep-vein thrombosis. *N Engl J Med*. 2017;377:2240–2252.
3. Lurie F, Passman M, Meisner M, et al. The 2020 update of the CEAP classification system and reporting standards. *J Vasc Surg Venous Lymphat Disord*. 2020; 8(3): 342–352.
4. Raju S, Hollis K, Neglen P. Use of compression stockings in chronic venous disease: patient compliance and efficacy. *Ann Vasc Surg*. 2007;21(6):790–795. PMID: 17980798.
5. Menawat SS, Gloviczki P, Mozes G, et al. Effect of a femoral arteriovenous fistula on lower extremity venous hemodynamics after femorocaval reconstruction. *J Vasc Surg*. 1996;24:793. PMID: 8918326.
6. Palma EC, Riss F, Del Campo F, Tobler H. Tratamiento de los trastornos postflebiticos mediante anastomosis venosa safeno-femoral cotrolateral. *Bull Soc Surg Uruguay*. 1958;29:135.

Index

B

C

P

Q

R

S

V

W

Z